Chest Disease (Fourth Series)
Test and Syllabus

AMERICAN COLLEGE OF RADIOLOGY
PROFESSIONAL SELF-EVALUATION AND CONTINUING EDUCATION
PROGRAM

BARRY A. SIEGEL, M.D., *Co-Editor in Chief*
> Professor of Radiology and Medicine and Director, Division of Nuclear Medicine, Edward Mallinckrodt Institute of Radiology, Washington University School of Medicine, St. Louis, Missouri

ELIAS G. THEROS, M.D., *Co-Editor in Chief*
> Isadore Meschan Distinguished Professor of Radiology, Bowman Gray School of Medicine of Wake Forest University, Winston-Salem, North Carolina

SET 27:
CHEST DISEASE (FOURTH SERIES) TEST AND SYLLABUS

Editor

ANTHONY V. PROTO, M.D., Professor of Radiology and Interim Chairman, Department of Radiology, Medical College of Virginia, Virginia Commonwealth University, Richmond, Virginia

Co-Authors

LARRY R. BROWN, M.D., Consultant, Mayo Clinic, and Associate Professor, Mayo Medical School, Mayo Clinic, Rochester, Minnesota

ROBERT H. CHOPLIN, M.D., Associate Professor of Radiology, Bowman Gray School of Medicine of Wake Forest University, Winston-Salem, North Carolina

LAWRENCE R. GOODMAN, M.D., Professor of Radiology and Director, Chest Radiology Section, Medical College of Wisconsin, Milwaukee, Wisconsin

CARL E. RAVIN, M.D., Professor and Chairman, Department of Radiology, Duke University Medical Center, Durham, North Carolina

PAUL STARK, M.D., Professor of Radiology, Loma Linda University School of Medicine, and Director, Division of Thoracic Radiology, Loma Linda University Medical Center, Loma Linda, California

WILLIAM D. WEHUNT, M.D., Radiologist, Community Radiology Associates, Montgomery General Hospital, Olney, Maryland

Publishing Coordinators: G. Rebecca Haines and Thomas M. Rogers
Publishing Consultant: Earle V. Hart

AMERICAN COLLEGE OF RADIOLOGY
Reston, Virginia 1989

Copyright © 1989
The American College of Radiology
1891 Preston White Drive
Reston, Virginia 22091

Made in the United States of America

Sets Published
Chest Disease
Bone Disease
Genitourinary Tract Disease
Gastrointestinal Disease
Head and Neck Disorders
Pediatric Disease
Nuclear Radiology
Radiation Pathology and Radiation
 Biology
Chest Disease II
Bone Disease II
Genitourinary Tract Disease II
Gastrointestinal Disease II
Head and Neck Disorders II
Nuclear Radiology II
Cardiovascular Disease
Emergency Radiology
Bone Disease III
Gastrointestinal Disease III
Chest Disease III
Pediatric Disease II
Nuclear Radiology III
Head and Neck Disorders III
Genitourinary Tract Disease III
Diagnostic Ultrasound
Breast Disease
Bone Disease IV
Pediatric Disease III
Chest Disease IV

Sets in Preparation
Neuroradiology
Gastrointestinal Disease IV
Nuclear Radiology IV
Magnetic Resonance
Biological Effects of Diagnostic and
 Other Low-Level Radiation
Cardiovascular Disease II
Emergency Radiology II
Interventional Radiology
Genitourinary Tract Disease IV
Head and Neck Disorders IV

Library of Congress Cataloging-in-Publication Data

Chest disease (fourth series) test and syllabus / editor, Anthony V. Proto; co-authors, Larry
R. Brown . . . [et al.].
  p. cm. — (Professional self-evaluation and continuing education program ; set 27)
  On cover: Committee on Professional Self-Evaluation and Continuing Education,
Commission on Education, American College of Radiology.
  Includes bibliographical references.
  ISBN 1-55903-027-5 (set 27) : $125.00. — ISBN 1-55903-000-3 (set)
  1. Chest—Radiography—Examinations, questions, etc. 2. Chest— Radiography—
Outlines, syllabi, etc. I. Proto, Anthony V. II. Brown, Larry R. (Larry Randolph), 1938–
III. American College of Radiology. Commission on Education. Committee on Professional
Self Evaluation and Continuing Education. IV. Series.
  [DNLM: 1. Thoracic Radiography—examination questions. W1 PR606 set 27 /
WF 18 C525]
RC941.C535 1989]
617.5′4—dc20
DNLM/DLC   89-18173
for Library of Congress   CIP

Committee Chairman's Preface

As Chairman of the Committee for Chest Disease Syllabus IV, I was afforded the opportunity to fashion the contents of this volume. It was clear from a review of the prior three chest volumes that the numerous cases presented discussed a variety of topics. Moreover, Syllabus III emphasized the basic approaches to interpretation of images in chest disease (radiographic correlations with anatomy, pathology, airway physiology, and vascular physiology), providing "primers" for airway and vascular physiology as well. To duplicate prior efforts would be repetitive, and to provide a volume that would be inclusive of all topics in radiology of the chest would be impossible. Accordingly, the best approach seemed to be to select as both committee members and authors radiologists with a special interest in chest disease whose different experiences would be reflected in their case material and points of focus. Their charge was to submit cases that would promote discussion of differential diagnoses and update the reader's knowledge.

It has truly been a pleasure to work with the members of the Committee—Drs. Larry R. Brown, Robert H. Choplin, Lawrence R. Goodman, Carl E. Ravin, Paul Stark, and William D. Wehunt. They have all given freely and extensively of their time to prepare a series of cases that are replete with information and reflect their detailed knowledge of and experience with the topics discussed. As Committee Chairman I have taken the liberty to edit the manuscripts freely, not to change the individual author's information or point of view but to impart an overall consistency in presentation of the cases and discussions of the options for each question.

Thanks are due to many people, too numerous to mention, whose time and effort have resulted in this Syllabus. I would, however, like to single out some to whom special thanks are due: the members of the Committee listed above, without whose contributions this volume would not have been possible; Dr. John H. Harris, Jr., whose support has been appreciated; Dr. Barry A. Siegel, whose outstanding editorial expertise and attention to detail have provided valued and insightful contributions; Earle V. Hart, Jr., and Thomas M. Rogers, editorial consultant and production editor, respectively, who have both made numerous important suggestions; and G. Rebecca Haines, whose enthusiasm and expertise have been responsible in a major way for developing an improved mechanism for more timely production of the ACR syllabi.

Last, but certainly not least, very special thanks are due to Dr. Elias G. Theros. Watching him in action during the various committee meetings, as cases were chosen and questions scrutinized, emphasized to me his untiring commitment to developing challenging material, material that "...will provoke the reader into thinking closely about alternatives...," as stated by Dr. Theros in his Introduction to Chest Disease Syllabus I. As we publish the fourth syllabus dealing with chest disease, it is appropriate to dedicate this volume to Dr. Theros, a most admired colleague, whose devotion and unique talents have made the Self-Evaluation Program the success that it is.

Anthony V. Proto, M.D.
Editor and Committee Chairman

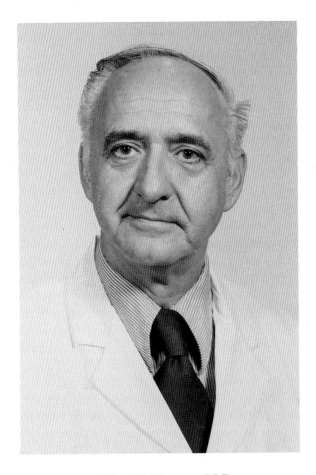

Elias G. Theros, M.D.

Editor's Preface

The Professional Self-Evaluation and Continuing Education Program of the American College of Radiology was formally inaugurated in 1972 with the publication of the first Chest Disease Syllabus. The eminent success of this program is well known to all radiologists and reflects the dedication of the many physicians who have donated their expertise and tireless efforts to this series. Dr. Anthony V. Proto and the members of his committee have more than maintained this tradition by producing another outstanding self-evaluation test and syllabus, the 27th in the series and the fourth devoted to the radiologic aspects of diseases of the chest.

In the preface, Dr. Proto addresses a concern of many of the authors developing packages for the fourth cycle of the Self-Evaluation Program, namely that the selection of material seems increasingly difficult because of the profound depth of coverage in prior syllabi. A perusal of this volume will quickly demonstrate that this issue was not a problem for this committee. This test and syllabus deal with important clinical problems that diagnostic radiologists are quite likely to encounter in their practices. Moreover, it is clear that the accelerating pace of advances in medicine and, particularly, in radiology will continue to create new knowledge that will present appropriate content for future tests and syllabi. The chest radiographic features of the acquired immunodeficiency syndrome and of amiodarone toxicity, which are considered in this volume, are cogent examples of clinical problems not even recognized at the time of publication of the third Chest Disease Syllabus.

My sincere appreciation and that of my co-editor, Elias G. Theros, M.D., are due to Dr. Proto and his colleagues—Drs. Larry Brown, Robert Choplin, Lawrence Goodman, Carl Ravin, Paul Stark, and William Wehunt—for their extraordinary efforts consummating in this outstanding volume. All members of the radiologic community will be the benefactors of their important contribution to continuing education. Working with these individuals has been both highly rewarding and pleasurable. Dr. Proto, as principal editor of this work, has brought exceptional skill to this task; it is with great satisfaction that Dr. Theros and I welcome Dr. Proto as an Associate Editor of the Self-Evaluation Program, commencing with the next volume in the series. Dr. Theros and I hope that in our roles as series editors we have helped to hone the material in this volume so that the test is logical, clear, and relevant to practicing diagnostic radiologists and so that the syllabus fully guides the readers through the reasoning leading to the correct diagnosis or answer of each question. Throughout, we have strived to maintain the individual flavor of each author's prose as well as the authors' expert opinions regarding the clinical problems discussed herein.

The publications staff of the American College of Radiology deserve special thanks. This dedicated and highly professional group of individuals, and especially Rebecca Haines and Tom Rogers, have structured the arduous task of syllabus production into a very efficient process without accepting any compromises in the quality of the final product. Mr. Earle V. Hart, Jr., whose many years of service to this program and to the College are well known, continues to keep his watchful eye on details of style and production as a consultant to the ACR.

Dr. Proto has chosen to dedicate this volume to Dr. Elias G. Theros. This is an entirely appropriate tribute—one of many made to Dr. Theros by the radiologic community—to the man who developed the concept for this Self-Evaluation Program over 20 years ago, was the principal editor of the first Chest Disease Syllabus, chaired the Committee on Professional Self-Evaluation and Continuing Education from its inception until 1985, and has given his untiring effort and exceptional wisdom to this program while serving continuously as its Editor in Chief for nearly two decades. All radiologists owe Lee Theros a great debt of gratitude for the Self-Evaluation Program, an exceptional teacher's labor of love that has proven to be such an important contribution to our specialty. Beginning with the next volume in this series, Dr. Theros will become Editor Emeritus of the Self-Evaluation Program, and I will assume the role of Editor in Chief. To Dr. Proto's thanks and to those of the American College of Radiology, I add my personal gratitude to Lee for all he has taught me about radiology and the art of self-evaluation.

Barry A. Siegel, M.D.
Co-Editor in Chief

viii

Chest Disease (Fourth Series) Test

For you to derive the maximum benefit from this program, you should complete the following test, and send your answer sheet to the ACR for scoring, before you proceed to the syllabus.

If for any reason you refer to the syllabus material, or any other references, in answering the questions, please be sure to answer "yes" to Question 158, the first demographic data question. Your score will then *not* be used in developing the norm tables.

NOTE: You must return your answer sheet for scoring, whether or not you use reference materials, in order to claim the 15 hours of Category I credit.

CASE 1: Questions 1 through 3

Routine posteroanterior (Figure 1-1) and lateral (Figure 1-2) chest radiographs taken on this 72-year-old man showed a mass that was later evaluated by contrast-enhanced computed tomography (CT) (Figures 1-3 and 1-4). The CT numbers of the mass were higher than those of water but lower than those of adjacent muscle.

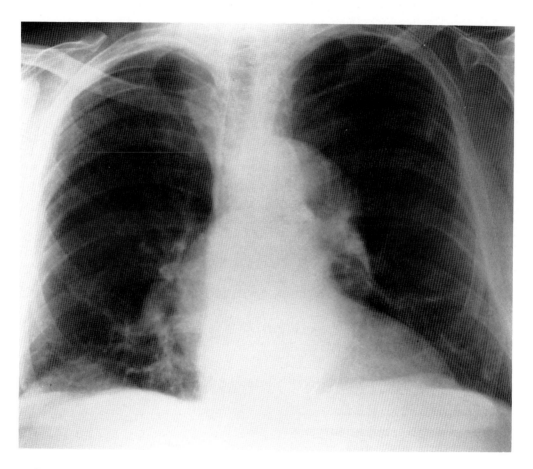

Figure 1-1

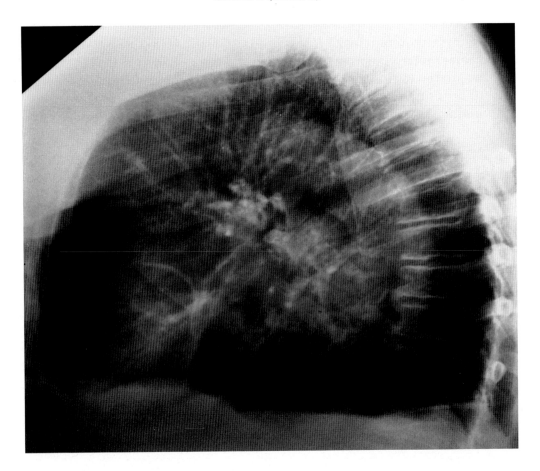

Figure 1-2

1. Which *one* of the following is the MOST likely diagnosis?

    (A) Teratoma
    (B) Aortic aneurysm
    (C) Bronchogenic cyst
    (D) Achalasia
    (E) Adenopathy

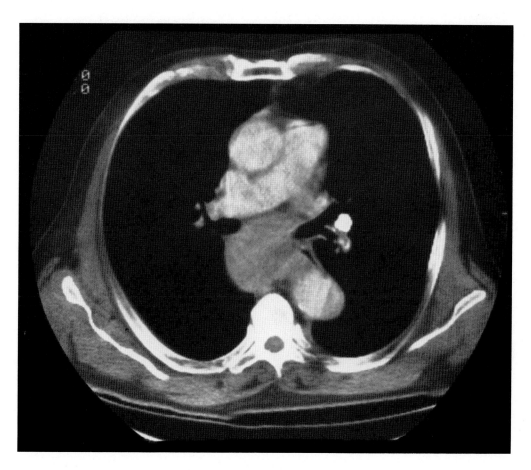

Figure 1-3

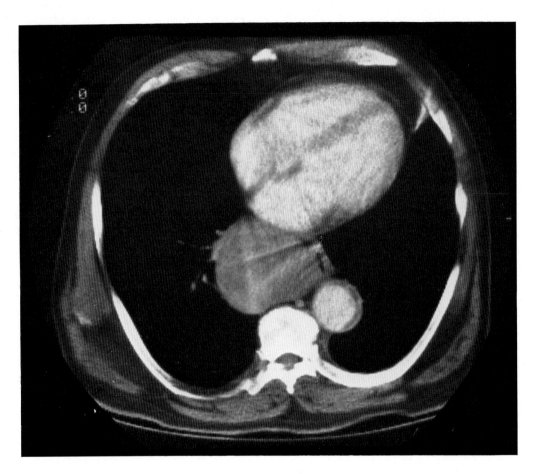

Figure 1-4

CASE 1 (Cont'd)

QUESTIONS 2 AND 3: MARK YOUR ANSWER SHEET TRUE (T) OR FALSE (F) FOR EACH OF THE RESPONSE CHOICES.

2. Regarding CT numbers in the evaluation of mediastinal masses,

    (A) they reliably separate schwannomas from meningoceles
    (B) they reliably separate mediastinal cysts from solid lesions
    (C) they characterize fatty lesions more reliably than do conventional radiographic techniques
    (D) they detect lymph node calcification more reliably than does conventional tomography
    (E) a rise after administration of contrast medium as an intravenous drip indicates a vascular structure

3. Concerning middle mediastinal masses in adults,

    (A) they are most commonly benign
    (B) they are more likely to be a cause of respiratory distress in adults than in children
    (C) partial calcification favors a neoplastic etiology
    (D) they are more easily delineated by CT than by conventional radiography
    (E) following detection by chest radiography, biopsy is the diagnostic procedure of choice

CASE 2: Questions 4 through 7

This 29-year-old woman presented with a history of recurrent respiratory infections since childhood. She had previously undergone a lobectomy for bronchiectasis. You are shown an anteroposterior bronchogram (Figure 2-1).

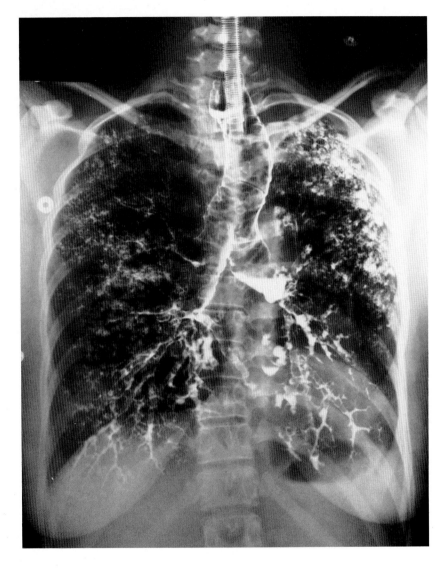

Figure 2-1

4. Which *one* of the following is the MOST likely diagnosis?

    (A) Tracheopathia osteochondroplastica
    (B) Chronic relapsing polychondritis
    (C) The Mounier-Kuhn syndrome
    (D) Hypogammaglobulinemia
    (E) The Kartagener syndrome

QUESTIONS 5 THROUGH 7: MARK YOUR ANSWER SHEET TRUE (T) OR FALSE (F) FOR EACH OF THE RESPONSE CHOICES.

5. Concerning tracheopathia osteochondroplastica,

    (A) it is frequently associated with tracheal diverticulosis
    (B) it is a premalignant condition
    (C) it is associated with mucosal ulcerations in the tracheobronchial tree
    (D) it is characterized by osteocartilaginous masses along the inner anterolateral surfaces of the trachea
    (E) it typically involves a short segment of the trachea or main bronchi

6. Concerning the Mounier-Kuhn syndrome,

    (A) it is frequently associated with bronchiectasis
    (B) it is characterized by congenital diverticula of the trachea and bronchi
    (C) it radiographically resembles tracheobronchial amyloidosis
    (D) it usually occurs secondary to chronic recurrent infections

7. Concerning diverticula of the trachea and bronchi,

    (A) rudimentary bronchus is a type
    (B) the congenital type arises from the distal bronchi
    (C) the acquired type results from chronic irritation or infection
    (D) tracheocele is a type that develops from high levels of intratracheal pressure
    (E) redundant nonmuscular membranous tissue is a cause

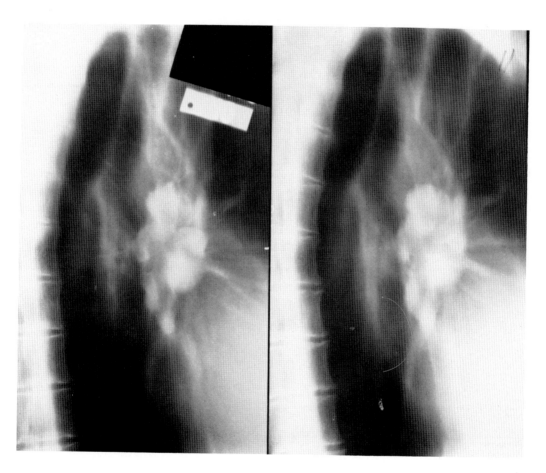

Figure 3-1

For each of the numbered 55° oblique hilar tomograms shown (Figures 3-1 through 3-5), select the *one* lettered structure or diagnosis (Option A, B, C, D, or E) MOST closely associated with it. Each lettered structure or diagnosis may be selected once, more than once, or not at all.

 8. Figure 3-1. Left hilar tomogram
 9. Figure 3-2. Left hilar tomogram
10. Figure 3-3. Left hilar tomogram
11. Figure 3-4. Right hilar tomogram
12. Figure 3-5. Left hilar tomogram

 (A) Hilar adenopathy
 (B) Superior pulmonary vein
 (C) Bronchogenic carcinoma with metastases
 (D) Endobronchial obstructive lesion
 (E) Prominent venous confluence

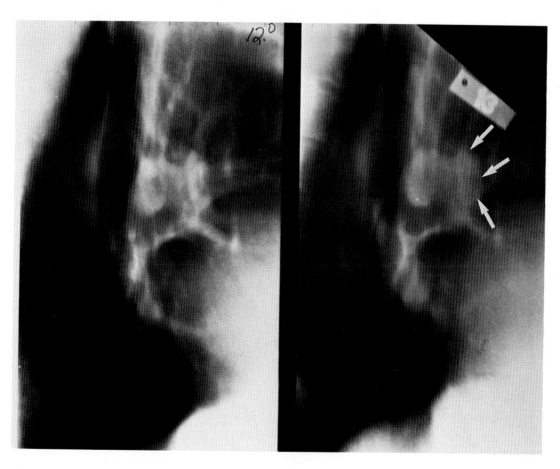

Figure 3-2

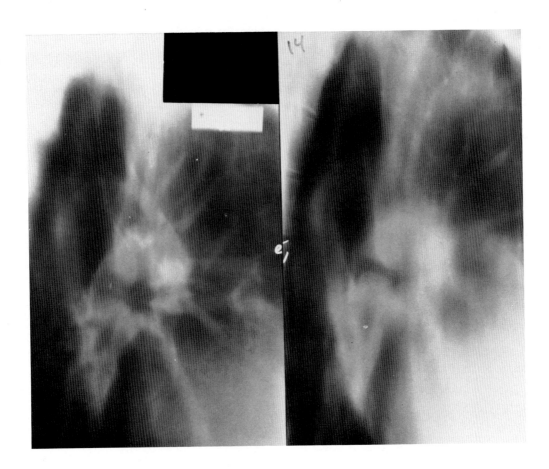

Figure 3-3

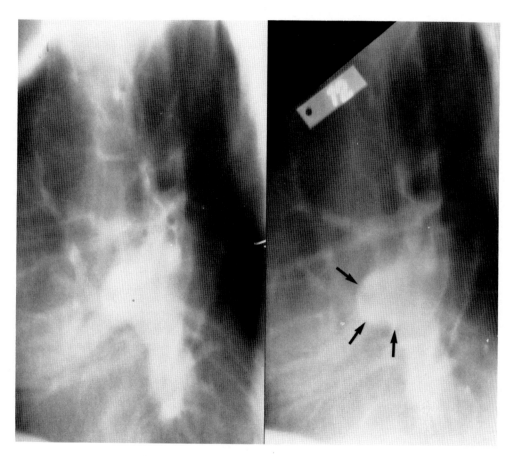

Figure 3-4

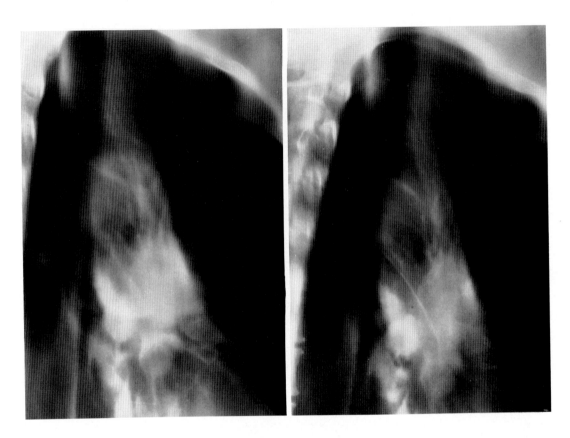

Figure 3-5

CASE 3 (Cont'd)

QUESTIONS 13 AND 14: MARK YOUR ANSWER SHEET TRUE (T) OR FALSE (F) FOR EACH OF THE RESPONSE CHOICES.

13. Concerning 55° oblique hilar tomography,

    (A) to study the left hilum, the patient's left side is closest to the tabletop

    (B) the x-ray tube is angled 55° posteriorly

    (C) the paramediastinal areas are well evaluated

    (D) a wedge filter is usually helpful in obtaining good-quality studies

    (E) the presence of a few flecks of calcium within a hilar mass excludes malignancy

    (F) nonvisualization of a bronchus indicates obstruction

14. Concerning normal anatomy in 55° oblique hilar tomography,

    (A) the left pulmonary artery is located above the left upper lobe bronchus

    (B) the right inferior pulmonary vein is located anterior to the right hilum

    (C) the left superior pulmonary vein is located anterior to the left upper lobe bronchus

    (D) multiple large rounded structures in the bronchial angles represent arteries and veins

    (E) the middle lobe bronchus is usually too small to be visualized

    (F) major fissures are usually visualized

    (G) the azygos vein is less visible than on anteroposterior tomography

CASE 4: Questions 15 through 18

This 60-year-old man has a history of recurrent pneumonias. You are shown posteroanterior (Figure 4-1) and lateral (Figure 4-2) chest radiographs.

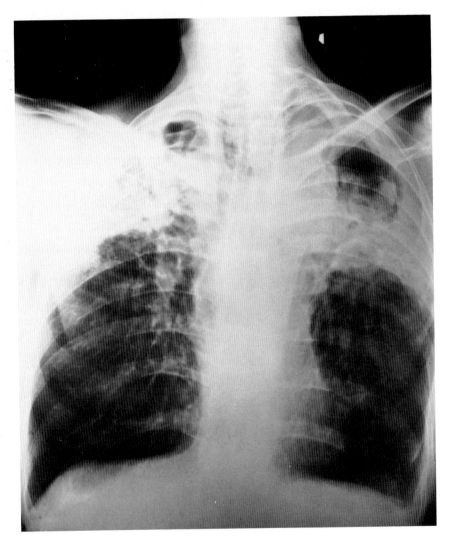

Figure 4-1

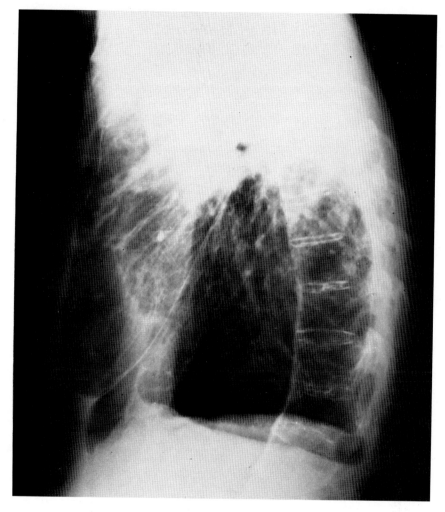

Figure 4-2

15. The constellation of radiographic findings seen in Figures 4-1
    and 4-2 is BEST explained by which *one* of the following?

    (A) Sarcoidosis
    (B) Atypical mycobacterial infection
    (C) Silicosis
    (D) Collagen vascular disease
    (E) Semi-invasive aspergillus infection

CASE 4 (Cont'd)

QUESTIONS 16 THROUGH 18: MARK YOUR ANSWER SHEET TRUE (T) OR FALSE (F) FOR EACH OF THE RESPONSE CHOICES.

16. Regarding cystic and fibrobullous changes in the upper lobes,

   (A) progressive adjacent pleural thickening usually indicates complicating malignancy
   (B) hemoptysis is common in uncomplicated cases
   (C) allergic bronchopulmonary aspergillosis is a common complication
   (D) tomography is frequently helpful in the diagnosis of mycetomas

17. Concerning silicosis,

   (A) most small opacities are found in the mid- and lower lung zones
   (B) radiographically, it is classified as "complicated" only if an opacity larger than 3 cm is detected
   (C) cavitation due to infection of a conglomerate mass is most often caused by fungal disease
   (D) a diffuse bilateral alveolar pattern on the chest radiograph indicates the advanced chronic form
   (E) conglomerate masses begin centrally and migrate peripherally

18. Concerning semi-invasive aspergillosis,

   (A) it usually is preceded by cavities
   (B) mycetomas are a feature
   (C) it is associated with mild immunosuppression
   (D) mucoid impaction is a common feature

This 20-year-old man had a 6-month history of mild dyspnea on exertion. No specific treatment was given. You are shown a series of posteroanterior chest radiographs (Figures 5-1 through 5-3).

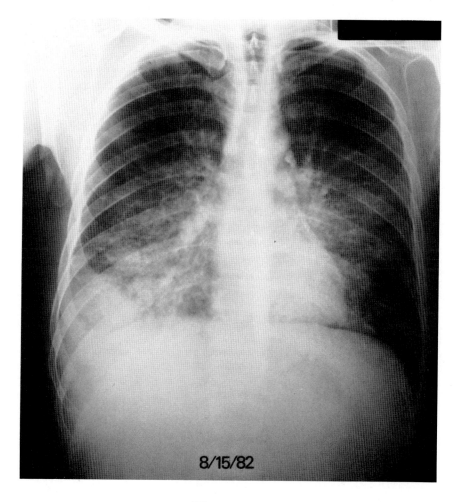

8/15/82

Figure 5-1

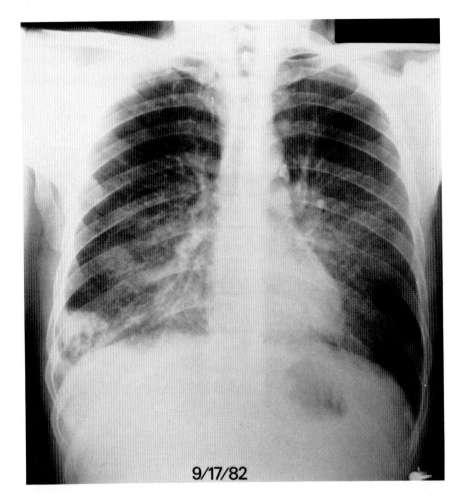

9/17/82

Figure 5-2

19. Which *one* of the following is the MOST likely diagnosis?

   (A) Bronchioloalveolar cell carcinoma
   (B) Hydrostatic pulmonary edema
   (C) Lymphoma
   (D) Alveolar proteinosis
   (E) Pulmonary hemorrhage

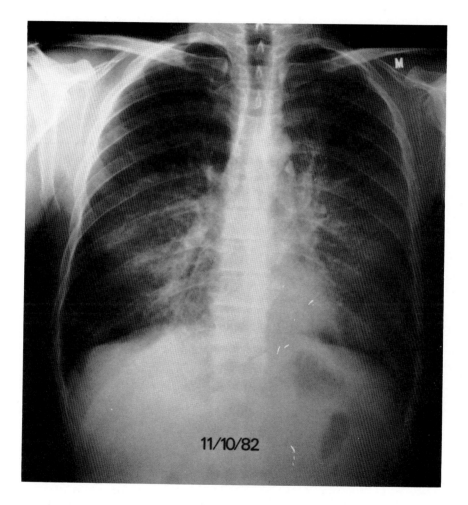

11/10/82

Figure 5-3

QUESTIONS 20 THROUGH 23: MARK YOUR ANSWER SHEET TRUE (T) OR FALSE (F) FOR EACH OF THE RESPONSE CHOICES.

20. Conditions that can appear alveolar but primarily involve the interstitium include:

   (A) microlithiasis
   (B) lobar pneumonia
   (C) sarcoidosis
   (D) primary pulmonary lymphoma

21. Hallmarks of an alveolar pattern on the chest radiograph include:

   (A) ill-defined vessels
   (B) air bronchograms
   (C) fluffy margins
   (D) segmental or lobar distribution
   (E) small irregular shadows

22. Concerning alveolar proteinosis,

   (A) the infiltrate consists primarily of intra-alveolar red blood cells and a variable number of chronic inflammatory cells
   (B) the infiltrate is caused by an antigen-antibody reaction in the pulmonary capillary
   (C) the severity of the radiographic appearance correlates closely with the clinical condition of the patient
   (D) the radiographic appearance is identical in adults and children
   (E) the radiographic appearance changes rapidly

23. Concerning pulmonary hemorrhage,

    (A) when it occurs in the idiopathic form, it frequently results in marked, radiographically visible chronic interstitial changes
    (B) when it occurs in the Goodpasture syndrome, hemoptysis is a frequent feature
    (C) it occurs infrequently in patients given anticoagulants
    (D) it is found as a manifestation of lupus erythematosus

CASE 6: Questions 24 through 30

This 46-year-old patient had a routine chest radiograph (Figure 6-1) and a subsequent computed tomographic (CT) examination (Figure 6-2).

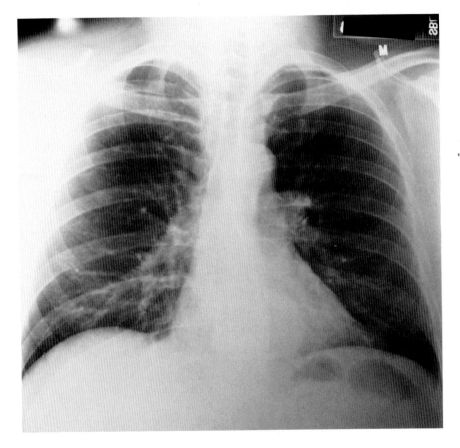

Figure 6-1

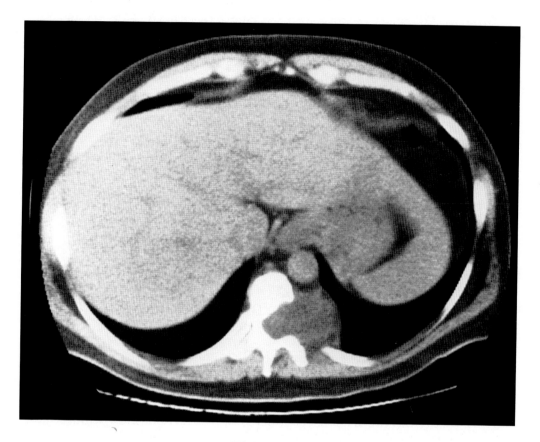

Figure 6-2

QUESTION 24: MARK YOUR ANSWER SHEET TRUE (T) OR FALSE (F) FOR EACH OF THE RESPONSE CHOICES.

24. Diseases that should be considered in the differential diagnosis include:

    (A) lateral meningocele
    (B) neurofibroma
    (C) extramedullary hematopoiesis
    (D) neurenteric cyst
    (E) pheochromocytoma

For each of the numbered masses listed below (Questions 25 through 28), select the *one* lettered characteristic (A, B, C, D, or E) MOST closely associated with it. Each lettered characteristic may be selected once, more than once, or not at all.

25. Neuroblastoma
26. Ganglioneuroma
27. Schwannoma
28. Neurofibroma

(A) occurs most commonly in the third and fourth decades
(B) is a round cell tumor arising from sympathetic ganglia
(C) occurs most commonly early in the third decade
(D) is associated with localized congenital vertebral abnormalities
(E) age of peak occurrence is over 65

QUESTIONS 29 AND 30: MARK YOUR ANSWER SHEET TRUE (T) OR FALSE (F) FOR EACH OF THE RESPONSE CHOICES.

29. Concerning schwannomas (neurilemmomas),

(A) they are tumors arising from both sheath and nerve cells
(B) they are the most common posterior mediastinal tumors
(C) most are elongated and oriented vertically
(D) they are the most common tumors in neurofibromatosis
(E) on CT, they are frequently denser than adjacent skeletal muscle

30. Concerning neurofibromatosis,

(A) when the lung is involved, cystic air collections are often present
(B) scoliosis spanning the upper 7 to 10 thoracic vertebral bodies is characteristic of thoracic spine involvement
(C) associated middle mediastinal masses represent mediastinal adenopathy
(D) patients with the central, rather than peripheral, form seldom have mediastinal neurofibromas

CASE 7: Questions 31 through 36

This 66-year-old man with known poorly differentiated granulocytic leukemia presented with pleuritic left chest pain. You are shown the posteroanterior chest radiograph taken on the day of admission (Figure 7-1).

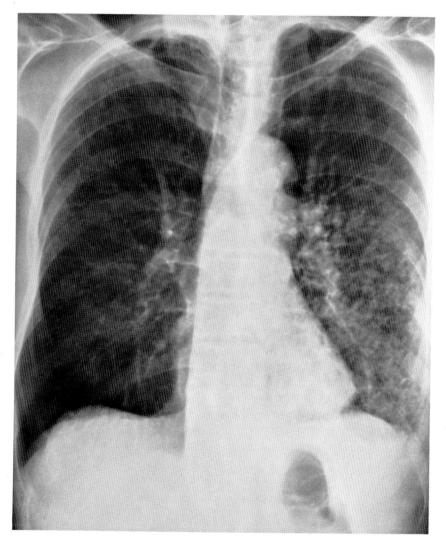

Figure 7-1

31. Which *one* of the following is the MOST likely diagnosis?

    (A) Infectious pneumonia
    (B) Leukemic infiltration of the lung
    (C) Amyloidosis
    (D) Hemorrhage
    (E) Drug reaction

32. Which *one* of the following is the MOST likely etiologic agent to be isolated in leukemic patients with infectious pneumonia?

    (A) A gram-negative bacillus
    (B) A fungus
    (C) A gram-positive coccus
    (D) *Pneumocystis carinii*
    (E) A virus

QUESTION 33: MARK YOUR ANSWER SHEET TRUE (T) OR FALSE (F) FOR EACH OF THE RESPONSE CHOICES.

33. Leukemic involvement of the thorax produces:

    (A) mediastinal and hilar lymph node enlargement
    (B) pneumothorax
    (C) ill-defined lung infiltrates
    (D) pleural effusion
    (E) lung nodules

34. Which *one* of the following is the LEAST likely radiographic pattern to be associated with thoracic amyloidosis?

   (A) Cardiomegaly
   (B) Pulmonary nodules
   (C) Hilar and mediastinal lymph node enlargement
   (D) Pleural plaques
   (E) Reticular lung infiltrate

QUESTION 35: MARK YOUR ANSWER SHEET TRUE (T) OR FALSE (F) FOR EACH OF THE RESPONSE CHOICES.

35. Which of the following drugs used in the treatment of leukemia may result in pulmonary toxicity?

   (A) Busulfan
   (B) Prednisone
   (C) Methotrexate
   (D) Daunorubicin
   (E) Vincristine

36. Which *one* of the following is the LEAST likely radiographic pattern to result from cytotoxic drug-induced pulmonary injury?

   (A) Ill-defined peripheral infiltrates
   (B) Central "butterfly" infiltrates
   (C) Localized parenchymal infiltrates
   (D) Bilateral basilar reticular infiltrates
   (E) Bilateral apical reticular infiltrates

This woman had a pneumonectomy for metastatic breast carcinoma at age 45 years. Five years later, she developed dyspnea and orthopnea. You are shown chest radiographs taken at ages 47 and 50 years (Figures 8-1 and 8-2).

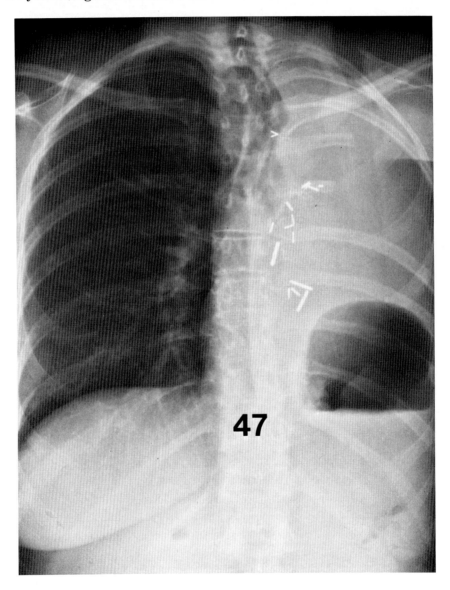

Figure 8-1

QUESTION 37: MARK YOUR ANSWER SHEET TRUE (T) OR FALSE (F) FOR EACH OF THE RESPONSE CHOICES.

37. Diagnoses that should be considered at age 50 years (Figure 8-2) include:

   (A) normal postpneumonectomy appearance
   (B) bronchopleural fistula
   (C) empyema
   (D) recurrent carcinoma
   (E) bronchoesophageal fistula

38. Which *one* of the following would be the next MOST effective imaging study?

   (A) Conventional tomography
   (B) Computed tomography
   (C) Ga-67 scintigraphy
   (D) Barium esophagram
   (E) Tc-99m methylene diphosphonate (MDP) scintigraphy

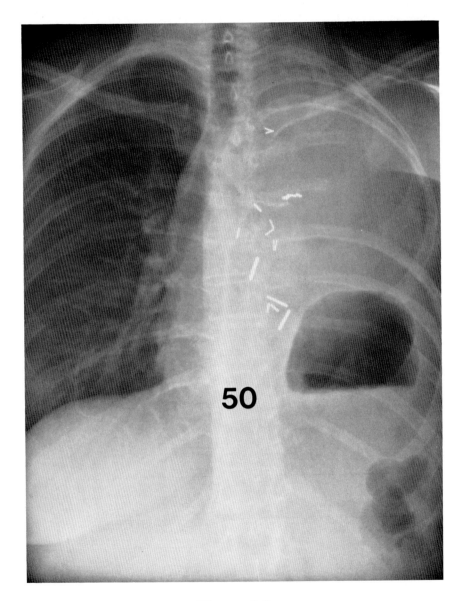

Figure 8-2

QUESTION 39: MARK YOUR ANSWER SHEET TRUE (T) OR
FALSE (F) FOR EACH OF THE RESPONSE CHOICES.

39. Concerning the postpneumonectomy patient,

   (A) the aortic arch undergoes rotation to a more sagittal
   orientation after a right pneumonectomy
   (B) fluid is completely resorbed from the pleural space
   within 1 year
   (C) compensatory lung growth by formation of new alveoli
   takes place in a patient who undergoes a pneumonectomy at age 12 years
   (D) chronic overdistention of the remaining lung results
   in emphysema with destruction of alveolar walls
   (E) the risk of respiratory failure is high when the
   predicted postoperative forced expiratory volume in 1
   second (FEV_1) is less than 1.0 L

40. Which *one* of the following is the LEAST likely cause of
acquired bronchoesophageal fistula?

   (A) Mediastinal neoplasm
   (B) Mediastinal granuloma
   (C) Tuberculosis
   (D) Trauma
   (E) Wegener's granulomatosis

41. Which *one* of the following is LEAST likely to cause an
empyema?

   (A) *Mycobacterium tuberculosis*
   (B) Anaerobic bacilli
   (C) Fungi
   (D) *Streptococcus pneumoniae* (pneumococci)
   (E) *Pneumocystis carinii*

CASE 9: Questions 42 through 48

This 48-year-old man had progressively increasing dyspnea and wheezing for 1 year. A posteroanterior chest radiograph was taken at the time of a hand injury (Figure 9-1). Note that the opacity at the level of the left third anterior rib is an artifact.

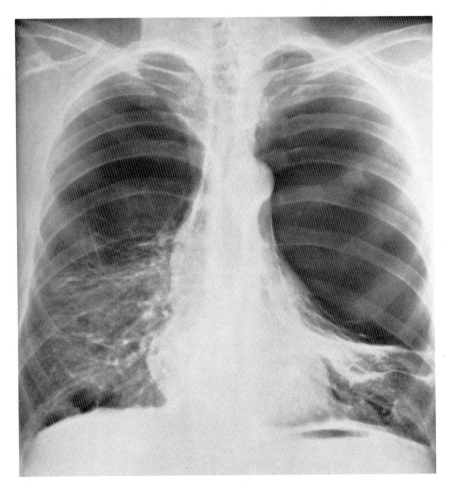

Figure 9-1

42. Which *one* of the following is the MOST likely diagnosis?

   (A) Bilateral pneumothorax
   (B) Bilateral lower lobe atelectasis
   (C) The Swyer-James syndrome
   (D) Giant bullous cysts
   (E) Alpha-1-antitrypsin deficiency

For each of the conditions listed below (Questions 43 through 46), select the *one* histopathologic designation (A, B, C, D, or E) MOST closely associated with it. Each histopathologic designation may be used once, more than once, or not at all.

43. The Swyer-James syndrome
44. Giant bullous cysts
45. Alpha-1-antitrypsin deficiency
46. "Smoker's lung"

   (A) Paraseptal emphysema
   (B) Centrilobular emphysema
   (C) Panacinar emphysema
   (D) Alveolar overdistention without alveolar wall disruption
   (E) Subpleural fibrosis with focal emphysema

47. Which *one* of the following is the LEAST likely to be associated with lower lobe atelectasis?

   (A) Depression of the ipsilateral interlobar pulmonary artery
   (B) Development of an ipsilateral juxtaphrenic peak
   (C) Obscuration of the ipsilateral posterior hemidiaphragm on the lateral view
   (D) Vertical orientation of the ipsilateral lower lobe bronchus
   (E) Mediastinal shift toward the atelectatic side

QUESTION 48: MARK YOUR ANSWER SHEET TRUE (T) OR FALSE (F) FOR EACH OF THE RESPONSE CHOICES.

48. Concerning alpha-1-antitrypsin deficiency,

   (A) adult heterozygous patients are at high risk of developing emphysema even in the absence of smoking
   (B) severe emphysema will develop in almost all homozygous patients, even in the absence of smoking
   (C) cirrhosis of the liver is present in the majority of adult patients
   (D) hilar enlargement results from the associated lymphadenopathy

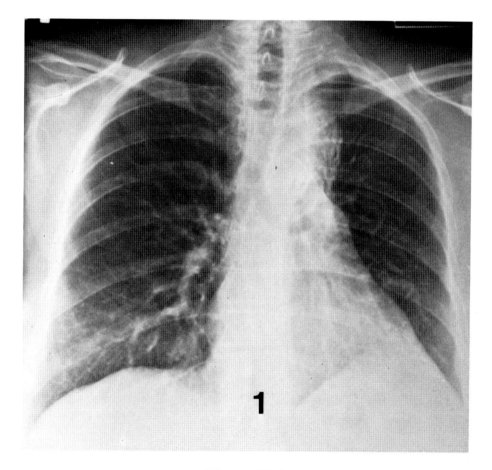

Figure 10-1

For each of the numbered posteroanterior chest radiographs (Figures 10-1 through 10-5), select the *one* lettered description (A, B, C, D, or E) MOST closely associated with it. Each statement may be used once, more than once, or not at all.

49. Figure 10-1
50. Figure 10-2
51. Figure 10-3
52. Figure 10-4
53. Figure 10-5

    (A) Acute-phase radiation effect; port for treatment of lung carcinoma

    (B) Acute-phase radiation effect; mantle port for treatment of lymphoma

    (C) Acute-phase radiation effect; port for treatment of breast carcinoma

    (D) Fibrotic-phase radiation effect; port for treatment of lung carcinoma

    (E) Fibrotic-phase radiation effect; mantle port for treatment of lymphoma

54. Which *one* of the following is the LEAST likely effect of radiation therapy?

    (A) Pleural effusion
    (B) Pericardial effusion
    (C) Pulmonary opacities
    (D) Superior vena cava obstruction
    (E) Regional volume loss

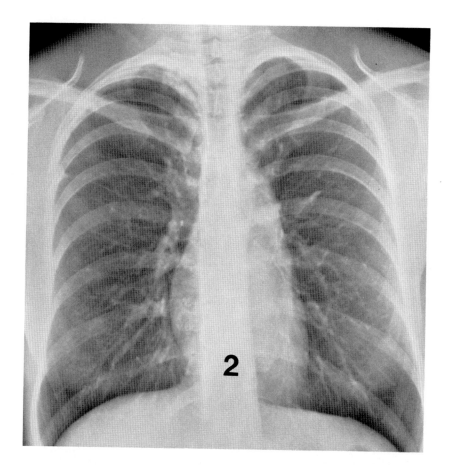

Figure 10-2

55. After the completion of radiation therapy, patients who develop symptomatic radiation pneumonitis most commonly present within:

    (A) 1 to 5 weeks
    (B) 3 to 6 months
    (C) 6 to 12 months
    (D) 12 to 18 months
    (E) 18 to 24 months

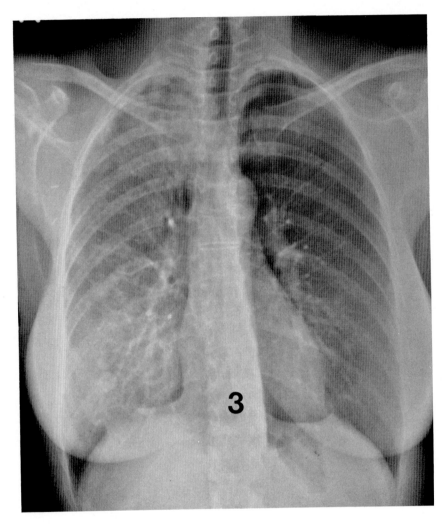

Figure 10-3

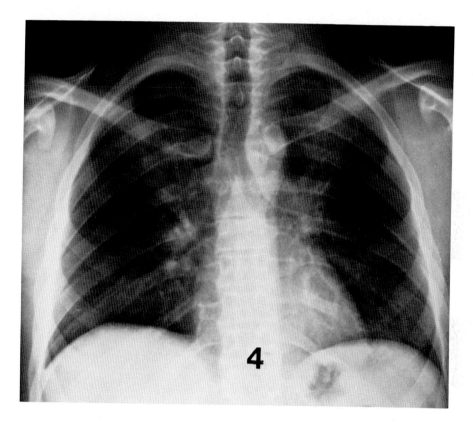

Figure 10-4

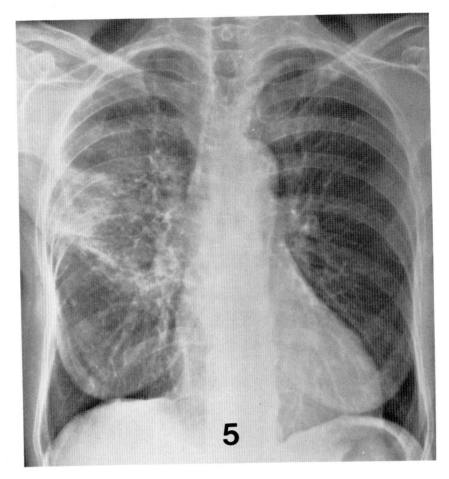

Figure 10-5

56. Which *one* of the following is NOT a risk factor for developing radiation pneumonitis?

    (A) Large lung volume irradiated
    (B) Short radiation delivery time
    (C) Concomitant chemotherapy
    (D) Concomitant pneumonia
    (E) Previous radiation therapy

This 60-year-old woman developed swelling of the chest wall. You are shown scans from her computed tomographic (CT) examination (Figures 11-1 and 11-2).

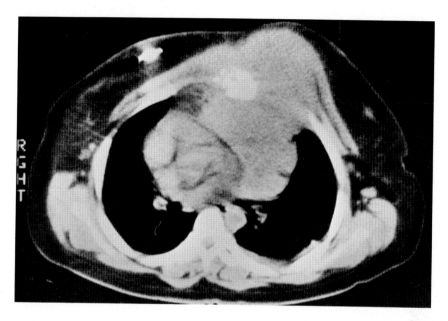

Figure 11-1

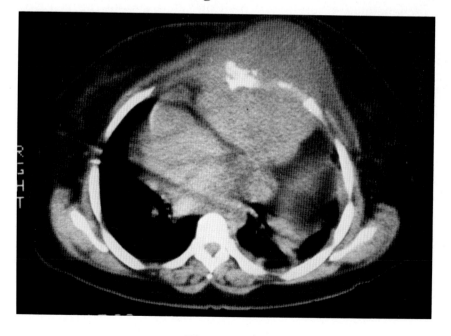

Figure 11-2

57. Which *one* of the following is the MOST likely diagnosis?

    (A) Actinomycosis
    (B) Malignant mesothelioma
    (C) Lymphoma
    (D) Candidiasis
    (E) Invasive thymoma

58. When a disease process arises in the thorax, abdominal CT is LEAST likely to provide additional information for which *one* of the following?

    (A) Blastomycosis
    (B) Malignant mesothelioma
    (C) Lymphoma
    (D) Candidiasis
    (E) Invasive thymoma

59. On imaging studies, which *one* of the following is LEAST likely to result from malignant mesothelioma?

    (A) Pleural mass
    (B) Hilar mass
    (C) Opaque hemithorax
    (D) Pericardial thickening
    (E) Chest wall invasion

QUESTION 60: MARK YOUR ANSWER SHEET TRUE (T) OR FALSE (F) FOR EACH OF THE RESPONSE CHOICES.

60. Concerning actinomycosis,

    (A) the most commonly involved site is the thorax
    (B) when extension occurs across normal anatomic boundaries, it is due to elaboration of proteolytic enzymes
    (C) the left lung is more frequently involved than the right one
    (D) sulfur granules contain the responsible organism

This 56-year-old man had a long history of ventricular arrhythmia and moderate rheumatoid arthritis. He had a 48-hour history of progressive dyspnea on exertion, mucoid sputum production, and mild chills. There was no hemoptysis, paroxysmal nocturnal dyspnea, or orthopnea. Medications included digitalis, amiodarone, and nonsteroidal anti-inflammatory drugs. The pulmonary capillary wedge pressure was 8 cm of water. A radiograph obtained 1 month earlier (not shown) demonstrated clear lungs and moderate cardiomegaly. You are shown the admission frontal radiograph (Figure 12-1).

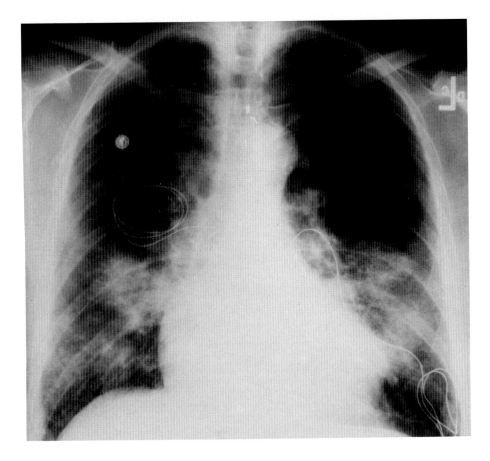

Figure 12-1

61. Considering the history and radiographic findings, which *one* of the following is the MOST likely diagnosis?

    (A) Congestive heart failure
    (B) Rheumatoid lung
    (C) Digitalis toxicity
    (D) Amiodarone toxicity
    (E) Aspiration pneumonia

QUESTION 62: MARK YOUR ANSWER SHEET TRUE (T) OR FALSE (F) FOR EACH OF THE RESPONSE CHOICES.

62. Concerning collagen vascular diseases that affect the lung,

    (A) the most frequent intrathoracic manifestation of rheumatoid arthritis is rheumatoid nodules
    (B) pulmonary opacities in systemic lupus erythematosus are most often due to diseases other than lupus pneumonitis
    (C) drug toxicity is responsible for approximately 10% of cases of systemic lupus erythematosus
    (D) radiographically, pulmonary fibrosis in scleroderma is characteristically perihilar
    (E) patients with polymyositis/dermatomyositis commonly develop diaphragmatic weakness

For each of the drugs listed below (Questions 63 through 67), select the *one* lettered side effect (A, B, C, D, or E) MOST closely associated with it. Each side effect may be used once, more than once, or not at all.

63. Nitrofurantoin (Furadantin)
64. Methysergide
65. Sulfonamides
66. Methadone
67. Adriamycin

    (A) Acute pneumonitis or chronic fibrosis
    (B) Pleural fibrosis
    (C) Cardiac toxicity
    (D) Noncardiac edema
    (E) Loeffler-type pneumonitis

CASE 13: Questions 68 through 71

This otherwise healthy 38-year-old woman presented with a 10-day history of productive cough (watery sputum) and a 3-day history of chills, fever, nausea, vomiting, and diarrhea. Her temperature was 40.4°C, her respiratory rate was 20/minute, and her leukocyte count was 5,200/μL (84% segmented neutrophils, 2% bands, and 14% lymphocytes). There was no growth on routine sputum cultures or blood cultures. You are shown posteroanterior and lateral chest radiographs (Figures 13-1 and 13-2).

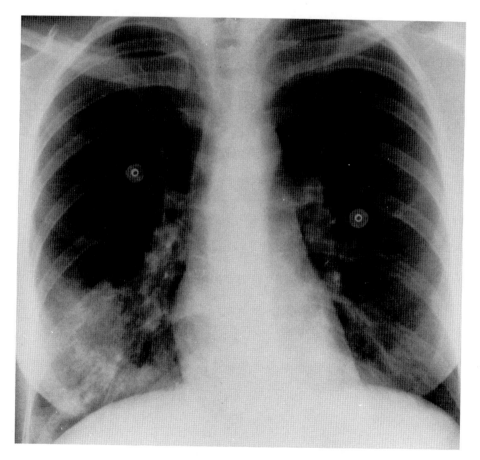

Figure 13-1

68. Considering the history and radiographic findings, which *one* of the following is the MOST likely diagnosis?

    (A) Legionnaires' disease
    (B) *Pneumocystis carinii* pneumonia
    (C) Blastomycosis
    (D) Pneumococcal pneumonia
    (E) Primary tuberculosis

QUESTIONS 69 THROUGH 71: MARK YOUR ANSWER SHEET TRUE (T) OR FALSE (F) FOR EACH OF THE RESPONSE CHOICES.

69. Concerning the radiographic appearance of Legionnaires' disease,

    (A) at presentation, patchy or confluent lower lobe air-space disease is most frequent
    (B) with time, the disease progresses to multilobar involvement in most patients
    (C) progression to lobar consolidation occurs in under 10% of patients
    (D) cavitation occurs in under 10% of nonimmunocompromised patients
    (E) pleural effusion is present in one-third to one-half of the cases
    (F) hilar or mediastinal adenopathy is present in about one-half of the cases

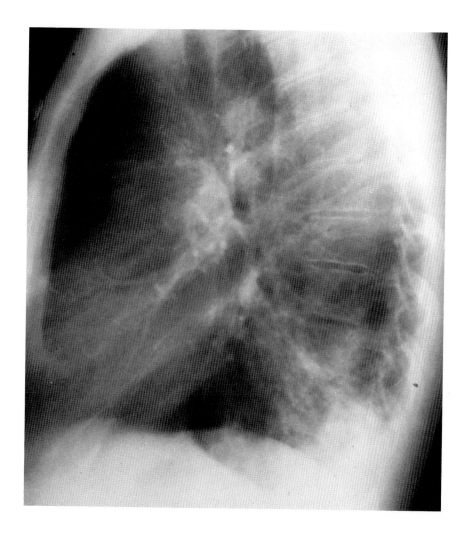

Figure 13-2

70. Concerning primary tuberculosis,

    (A) adenopathy is more frequent than in postprimary tuberculosis
    (B) the predominant location is in the apical or apical posterior segments of the upper lobes
    (C) the majority of effusions are empyemas
    (D) the Ghon focus is a residuum
    (E) it is rarely seen after 15 years of age

71. Concerning acute bacterial pneumonias,

    (A) adenopathy is more frequent in children than in adults
    (B) pneumatoceles secondary to staphylococcal pneumonia are more frequent in children than in adults
    (C) empyemas are more frequent with staphylococcal than with pneumococcal pneumonia
    (D) airborne pseudomonas pneumonia tends to be lobar

This erect portable radiograph (Figure 14-1) was taken immediately after right internal jugular catheterization. An arrowhead indicates the tip of the internal jugular catheter.

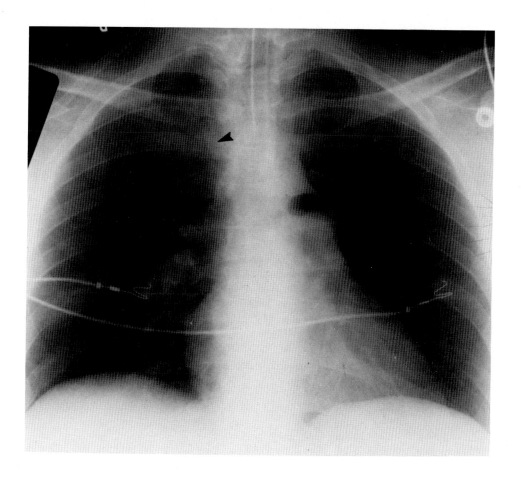

Figure 14-1

72. Which *one* of the following is the MOST likely diagnosis?

   (A) Mediastinal air
   (B) Paramediastinal bulla
   (C) Pulmonary ligament air
   (D) Pericardial air
   (E) Pulmonary artery air

QUESTIONS 73 THROUGH 75: MARK YOUR ANSWER SHEET TRUE (T) OR FALSE (F) FOR EACH OF THE RESPONSE CHOICES.

73. Concerning ventilator-induced barotrauma,

   (A) pneumothorax is usually due to rupture of a peripheral bulla or bleb through the pleura
   (B) interstitial air, although usually present, is seldom visible radiographically in adults
   (C) when pneumoperitoneum or pneumoretroperitoneum is a complication, pneumomediastinum is visible in only one-half of patients

74. Concerning the various substances that may embolize to the lung,

    (A) death occurs with venous air embolization only if the air crosses a patent foramen ovale to enter the systemic circulation

    (B) coagulopathy is a major cause of morbidity and mortality following amniotic fluid embolization

    (C) the fat embolism syndrome more closely resembles the adult respiratory distress syndrome than it does venous thromboembolism

    (D) intravenous metallic mercury injections usually cause minimal symptoms and dramatic radiographs

    (E) oil embolism complicating lymphangiography causes a mild to moderate decrease in diffusing capacity in the majority of patients

75. Concerning support and monitoring devices,

    (A) to ensure accurate central venous pressure readings, a central venous pressure catheter is ideally positioned in the right atrium

    (B) on the radiograph, a Swan-Ganz catheter is ideally positioned in a segmental pulmonary artery

    (C) pulmonary capillary wedge pressures are affected by positive pressure ventilation

    (D) aortic counter-pulsation catheters are ideally positioned with the tip in the aortic knob

    (E) flexion of the neck advances an endotracheal tube toward the carina

CASE 15: Questions 76 through 79

This elderly man presented with a 1-week history of shortness of breath. You are shown a posteroanterior chest radiograph (Figure 15-1) taken at the time of admission.

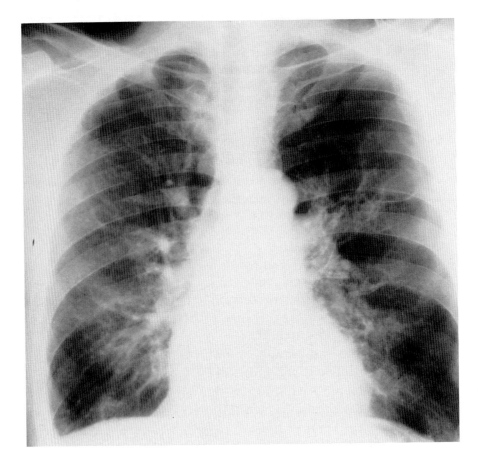

Figure 15-1

76. Which *one* of the following is the MOST likely diagnosis?

    (A) Emphysema with pulmonary edema
    (B) Adult respiratory distress syndrome
    (C) Emphysema with pneumonia
    (D) Swyer-James syndrome
    (E) Alpha-1-antitrypsin deficiency

QUESTIONS 77 THROUGH 79: MARK YOUR ANSWER SHEET TRUE (T) OR FALSE (F) FOR EACH OF THE RESPONSE CHOICES.

77. Concerning the adult respiratory distress syndrome,

    (A) shock is a prerequisite for its development
    (B) the radiographic opacities usually lag behind the patient's symptoms for the first 24 to 36 hours
    (C) pulmonary opacities usually start peripherally and progress centrally
    (D) increased pulmonary capillary permeability is a prominent feature
    (E) its diagnosis requires lung biopsy

78. Conditions associated with unilateral or asymmetrical pulmonary edema include:

    (A) rapid re-expansion of the lung after a pneumothorax or hydrothorax
    (B) pulmonary embolism
    (C) left atrial myxoma
    (D) gravitational shift in a patient with congestive heart failure

79. Regarding obstructive pulmonary disease,

   (A) the chest radiograph is a sensitive indicator of mild emphysema

   (B) redistribution of blood flow to the upper lobes in a patient with emphysema indicates concomitant left heart failure

   (C) hyperinflation is a more prominent feature of centrilobular than of panacinar emphysema

   (D) a unilateral hyperinflated lung with a large hemithorax strongly suggests the Swyer-James syndrome

CASE 16: Questions 80 through 86

This 56-year-old woman presented with insidious onset of shortness of breath over the last 6 to 12 months. You are shown anteroposterior (Figure 16-1) and oblique (Figure 16-2) radiographs of the upper thorax.

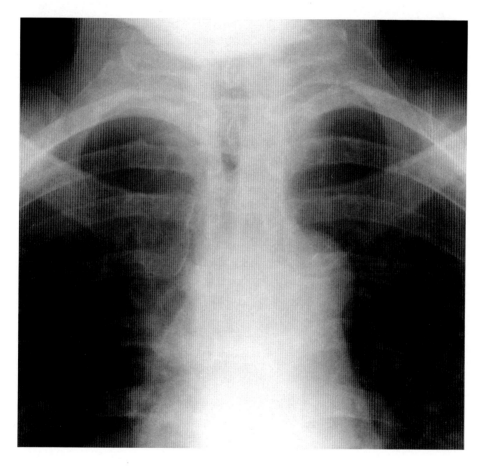

Figure 16-1

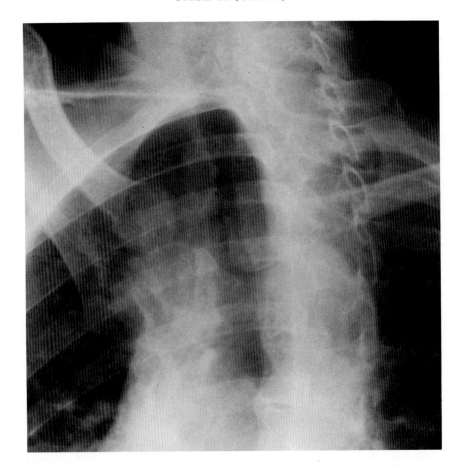

Figure 16-2

80. Which *one* of the following is the MOST likely diagnosis?

(A) Saber-sheath trachea
(B) Laryngotracheal papillomatosis
(C) Mounier-Kuhn syndrome
(D) Postintubation tracheal stenosis
(E) Tracheoesophageal fistula

QUESTION 81: MARK YOUR ANSWER SHEET TRUE (T) OR FALSE (F) FOR EACH OF THE RESPONSE CHOICES.

81. Concerning tracheal narrowing,

    (A) computed tomography is the most definitive imaging study for tracheal stenosis secondary to trauma or intubation

    (B) when viewed fluoroscopically, areas of tracheomalacia in the thorax collapse upon inspiration

    (C) dyspnea seldom occurs until the tracheal diameter is narrowed at least 50%

    (D) on spirometry, the forced expiratory volume in 1 second (FEV_1) is sufficient to evaluate tracheal function

For each of the tracheal abnormalities listed below (Questions 82 through 85), select the *one* lettered statement (A, B, C, D, or E) MOST closely associated with it. Each statement may be used once, more than once, or not at all.

82. Mounier-Kuhn syndrome
83. Laryngotracheal papillomatosis
84. Saber-sheath trachea
85. Rhinoscleroma

    (A) is believed to be viral in origin

    (B) is characterized by tracheobronchial diverticula

    (C) is associated with pneumothorax

    (D) may involve nasal sinuses, nose, and pharynx

    (E) is strongly correlated with chronic obstructive pulmonary disease

QUESTION 86: MARK YOUR ANSWER SHEET TRUE (T) OR FALSE (F) FOR EACH OF THE RESPONSE CHOICES.

86. Concerning an acquired tracheoesophageal fistula,

   (A) respiratory symptoms usually exceed esophageal symptoms
   (B) when due to prolonged intubation, it usually presents with mediastinal emphysema
   (C) the most frequent etiology is infection
   (D) it frequently follows intubation with a Sengstaken-Blakemore tube

This elderly man, examined 10 days after esophageal repair for the Boerhaave syndrome, had recurring low-grade fever and an increasingly abnormal chest radiograph. You are shown an anteroposterior erect portable radiograph (Figure 17-1), with arrowheads indicating the course of a chest tube, and three computed tomographic scans (Figures 17-2, 17-3, and 17-4) done on the same day. The abnormal opaque areas seen on the computed tomographic scans were of fluid density.

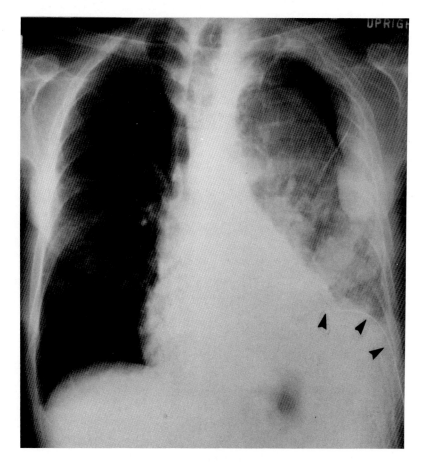

Figure 17-1

QUESTIONS 87 THROUGH 90: MARK YOUR ANSWER SHEET TRUE (T) OR FALSE (F) FOR EACH OF THE RESPONSE CHOICES.

87. Concerning this patient's images,

   (A) there is fluid in the anterior mediastinum
   (B) there is fluid in the major fissure
   (C) there is dense consolidation of the left upper lobe
   (D) the chest tube does not communicate with the pleural collections

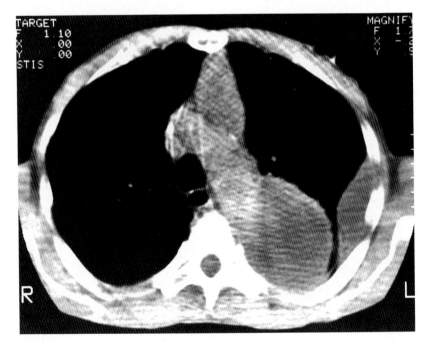

Figure 17-2

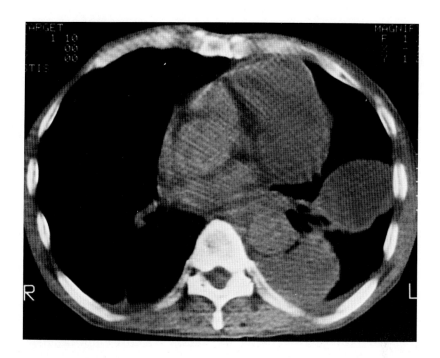

Figure 17-3

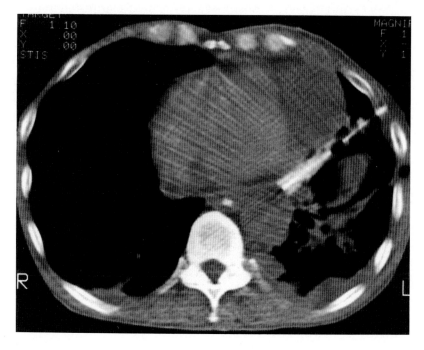

Figure 17-4

88. Concerning the computed tomographic differentiation between lung abscesses and empyemas,

   (A) a lung abscess characteristically has a thin wall
   (B) a lung abscess characteristically displaces adjacent lung markings (vessels, bronchi)
   (C) a lung abscess has a distinct interface with normal lung
   (D) an empyema is usually elliptical rather than round

89. Concerning potential complications following median sternotomy,

   (A) a 20% increase in mediastinal width in the first 48 hours after coronary bypass surgery implies the need for reoperation
   (B) pulmonary edema secondary to cardiopulmonary bypass is present radiographically in the majority of patients
   (C) after the first postoperative week, computed tomography is of little value in separating postoperative changes from pathologic processes
   (D) a thin midline lucency in the sternum is a reliable radiographic predictor of impending sternal dehiscence
   (E) left lower lobe atelectasis after coronary artery surgery is partially attributable to temporary paralysis of the left hemidiaphragm

90. Concerning postoperative fluid collections,

   (A) after laparotomy, pleural effusions are present in approximately 50% of patients

   (B) the initial radiographic signs of subphrenic abscess, such as pleural effusion, atelectasis, or diaphragmatic elevation, are usually present by the fifth postoperative day

   (C) immediately following hemorrhage, a hemothorax is usually isodense with respect to unopacified soft tissue (muscle) on computed tomographic scans

   (D) a pleural effusion developing 2 to 6 weeks after cardiac surgery is more likely due to the postpericardiotomy syndrome than to infection

CASE 18: Questions 91 through 94

This 26-year-old woman presented with complaints of dyspnea and hemoptysis. You are shown posteroanterior and lateral chest radiographs (Figures 18-1 and 18-2).

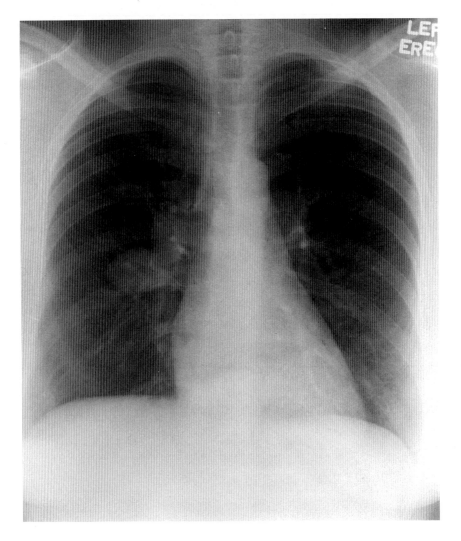

Figure 18-1

CASE 18 (Cont'd)

91. Which *one* of the following is the MOST likely diagnosis?

(A) Carcinoid tumor
(B) Metastatic carcinoma
(C) Primary tuberculosis
(D) Hodgkin's lymphoma
(E) Arteriovenous malformation

QUESTIONS 92 THROUGH 94: MARK YOUR ANSWER SHEET TRUE (T) OR FALSE (F) FOR EACH OF THE RESPONSE CHOICES.

92. Concerning carcinoid tumors,

(A) they are benign bronchial adenomas
(B) they are most common in the sixth decade of life
(C) hemoptysis is a common feature
(D) the majority are located in the peripheral airways
(E) calcification is commonly recognized on conventional chest radiographs

93. Concerning Hodgkin's lymphoma,

(A) at the time of presentation, it involves the lung parenchyma in approximately 30% of cases
(B) when pulmonary parenchymal involvement is present, associated mediastinal or hilar lymph node enlargement is seen in less than 60% of cases
(C) at the time of presentation, it involves the thorax more commonly than does non-Hodgkin's lymphoma
(D) involvement of the anterior mediastinal lymph nodes is infrequent
(E) at the time of presentation, pleural effusion is seen in approximately 50% of patients

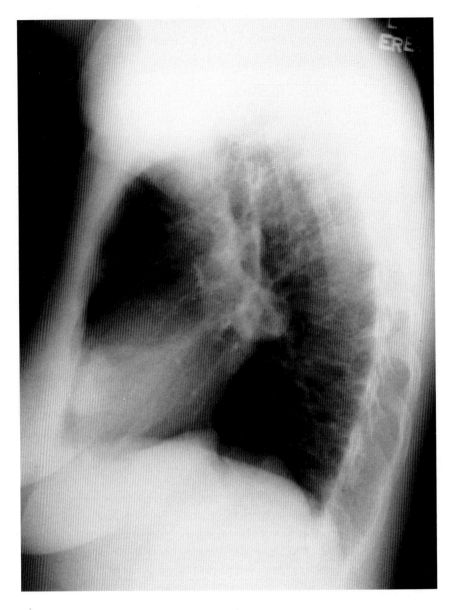

Figure 18-2

94. Concerning pulmonary arteriovenous malformations,

   (A) they occur most often in the upper lobes
   (B) they are associated with hypertrophic osteoarthropathy
   (C) most are found in patients with hereditary hemorrhagic telangiectasia
   (D) bronchial artery embolotherapy is an accepted method of treatment
   (E) an associated complication is brain abscess

This 60-year-old alcoholic patient presented with shortness of breath. You are shown a posteroanterior chest radiograph (Figure 19-1).

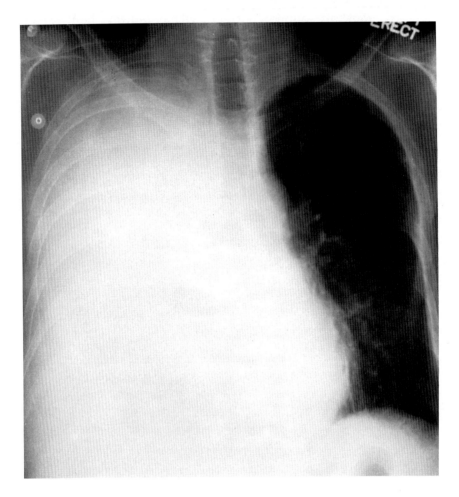

Figure 19-1

95. Which *one* of the following is the LEAST likely diagnosis?

   (A) Malignant mesothelioma
   (B) Atelectasis of the right lung
   (C) Meigs' syndrome
   (D) Hepatic hydrothorax
   (E) *Klebsiella* pneumonia

QUESTIONS 96 THROUGH 98: MARK YOUR ANSWER SHEET TRUE (T) OR FALSE (F) FOR EACH OF THE RESPONSE CHOICES.

96. Concerning mesothelioma,

   (A) the benign form is associated with previous exposure to asbestos
   (B) the association of hypertrophic osteoarthropathy and a localized pleural mass suggests the benign form
   (C) pleural effusions are commonly seen in association with the benign form
   (D) when there is pleural effusion with the malignant form, the mediastinum is usually shifted contralaterally
   (E) the malignant form frequently has metastasized to distant sites at the time of initial detection

97. Concerning Meigs' syndrome,

   (A) the original description included both benign and malignant ovarian tumors
   (B) pleural effusion indicates metastatic spread
   (C) ascitic fluid is generally absent
   (D) right-sided pleural effusions are more common than left-sided ones

98. Concerning hepatic hydrothorax,

   (A) the associated liver disease is cirrhosis
   (B) right-sided pleural effusions are more common than left-sided ones
   (C) ascites is uncommon
   (D) it is most likely secondary to pulmonary infection

This 32-year-old woman has cardiac disease secondary to the carcinoid syndrome. You are shown a posteroanterior chest radiograph (Figure 20-1).

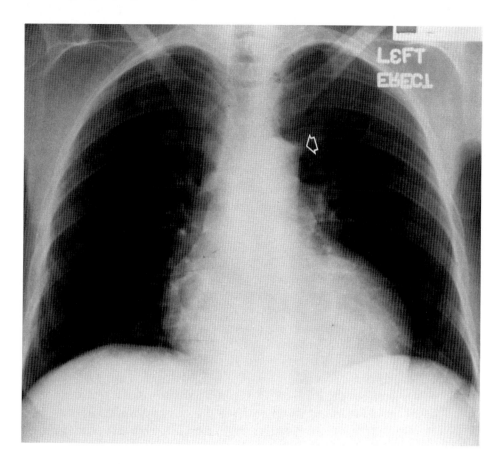

Figure 20-1

99. Which *one* of the following is indicated by the arrow in Figure 20-1?

    (A) Aortic diverticulum
    (B) Lymph node
    (C) Ductus arteriosus
    (D) Left superior intercostal vein
    (E) Persistent left superior vena cava

QUESTIONS 100 AND 101: MARK YOUR ANSWER SHEET TRUE (T) OR FALSE (F) FOR EACH OF THE RESPONSE CHOICES.

100. Concerning "carcinoid heart disease" secondary to an intra-abdominal primary carcinoid tumor,

(A) metastatic spread of tumor to the liver is implied

(B) it is generally secondary to metastatic involvement of the myocardium

(C) the tricuspid and pulmonic valves are most commonly involved

(D) echocardiography reveals metastasis to the valves

101. Concerning an aortic diverticulum,

(A) when visible, that found in adults at the aortoductal junction is generally seen better on the lateral than on the posteroanterior chest radiograph

(B) that seen with an aberrant right subclavian artery and a left aortic arch is thought to represent incomplete regression of the primitive distal right aortic arch

(C) that associated with a right aortic arch and an aberrant left subclavian artery is seen on the posteroanterior chest radiograph as a soft tissue opacity in the left paratracheal region

(D) that associated with a left aortic arch and an aberrant right subclavian artery is termed the "diverticulum of Kommerell "

History withheld. You are shown posteroanterior (Figure 21-1) and lateral (Figure 21-2) chest radiographs of a 32-year-old woman.

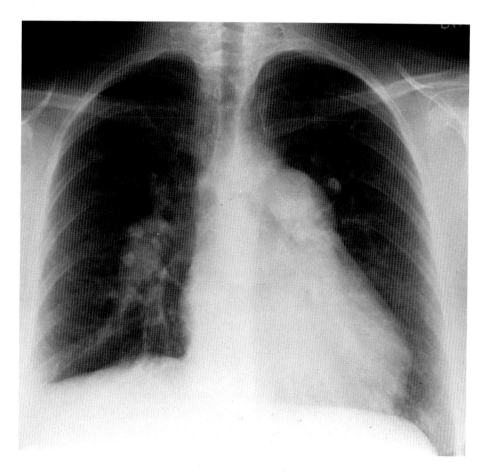

Figure 21-1

102. Which *one* of the following is the MOST likely diagnosis?

    (A) Lymphoma
    (B) The Hughes-Stovin syndrome
    (C) Pulmonic valvular stenosis
    (D) Pulmonary arterial hypertension
    (E) Sarcoidosis

QUESTIONS 103 THROUGH 106: MARK YOUR ANSWER SHEET TRUE (T) OR FALSE (F) FOR EACH OF THE RESPONSE CHOICES.

103. Concerning the Hughes-Stovin syndrome,

    (A) findings include aneurysms of large and small pulmonary arteries
    (B) most cases are associated with congenital cardiovascular defects
    (C) it occurs more commonly in women than in men
    (D) peripheral venous thrombosis is a feature
    (E) hemoptysis is uncommon

104. Concerning pulmonic valvular stenosis,

    (A) radiographically, dilatation more commonly involves the main and left pulmonary arteries than the right pulmonary artery
    (B) the associated dilatation of the main pulmonary artery is readily distinguished on chest radiographs from idiopathic dilatation of that artery
    (C) there is poor correlation between the prominence of the pulmonary artery and the severity of valvular stenosis
    (D) when complicated by both right ventricular hypertrophy and a right-to-left shunt at the atrial level, it is termed the "trilogy of Fallot"

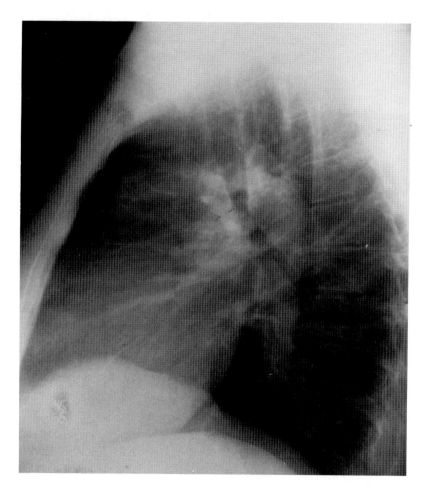

Figure 21-2

105. Concerning primary pulmonary arterial hypertension,

    (A) the diagnosis is essentially one of exclusion
    (B) the disease most commonly affects young women
    (C) dyspnea on exertion is a common presenting complaint

106. Concerning sarcoidosis,

    (A) pleural effusion is rarely, if ever, associated with it
    (B) "eggshell" calcifications are an uncommon residuum
    (C) enlargement of anterior mediastinal nodes occurs in approximately 15% of patients
    (D) enlargement of subcarinal nodes is rare

This 43-year-old woman suffered from progressive exertional dyspnea. You are shown a posteroanterior chest radiograph (Figure 22-1).

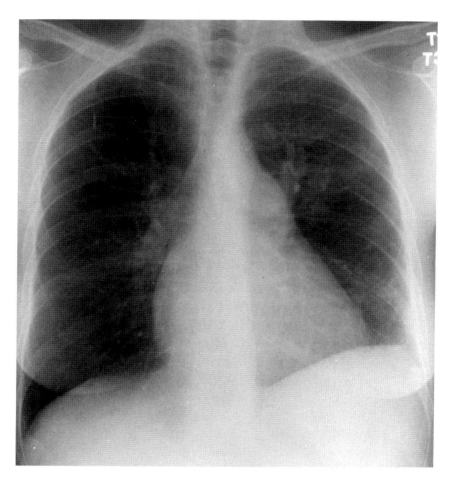

Figure 22-1

107. Which *one* of the following is the MOST likely diagnosis?

   (A) Atrial septal defect
   (B) Ventricular septal defect
   (C) Pulmonary thromboembolism
   (D) Acute myocardial infarction
   (E) Chronic congestive heart failure

QUESTIONS 108 THROUGH 110: MARK YOUR ANSWER SHEET TRUE (T) OR FALSE (F) FOR EACH OF THE RESPONSE CHOICES.

108. Concerning atrial septal defect,

   (A) the ostium primum type is often part of a complex malformation known as an endocardial cushion defect
   (B) the left atrium is generally enlarged
   (C) fixed splitting of the second heart sound is noted on physical examination
   (D) it is more common in male patients
   (E) it is a common cause of heart failure in infancy
   (F) it is the only left-to-right shunt in which the pulmonary flow can be massive and the murmur not apparent

109. Concerning ventricular septal defect

   (A) in newborns, a murmur is immediately apparent
   (B) it is the most common left-to-right shunt present in adults
   (C) spontaneous closure occurs in 15 to 30% of patients
   (D) left atrial enlargement is the rule in adult patients

110. Concerning pulmonary thromboembolism,

    (A) pulmonary angiography is unsafe in patients suspected of having the chronic form

    (B) the presence of stenoses or webs in pulmonary arteries suggests the acute form

    (C) surgery has no role in the management of the chronic form

    (D) pulmonary arterial hypertension is an absolute contra-indication to pulmonary angiography

    (E) when right ventricular end-diastolic pressures exceed 20 mm Hg there is increased risk of death during pulmonary angiography

CASE 23: Questions 111 through 114

This 35-year-old woman with myasthenia gravis is being evaluated for thymoma. You are shown posteroanterior and lateral chest radiographs (Figures 23-1 and 23-2) and computed tomographic scans (Figures 23-3 through 23-5).

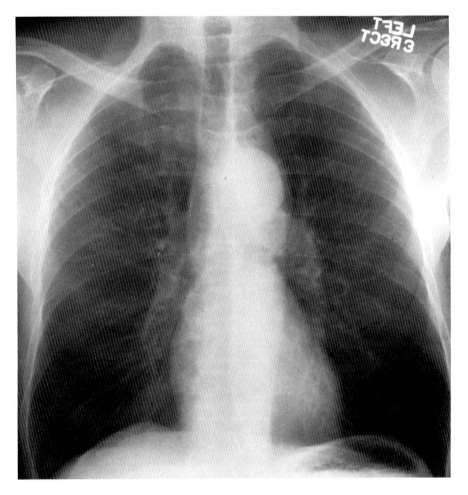

Figure 23-1

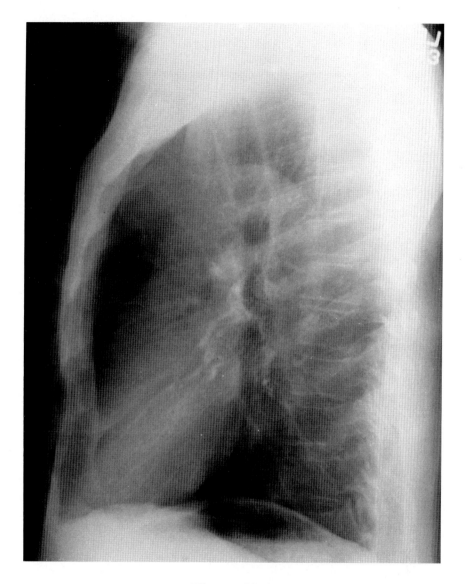

Figure 23-2

111. Which *one* of the following is the MOST likely diagnosis?

    (A) Thymic hyperplasia
    (B) Thymolipoma
    (C) Substernal thyroid
    (D) Thymoma
    (E) Normal thymus

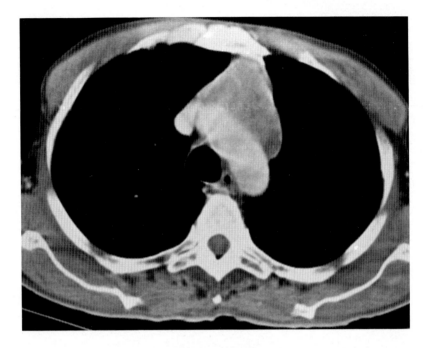

Figure 23-3

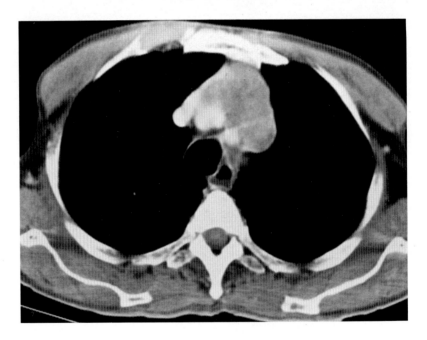

Figure 23-4

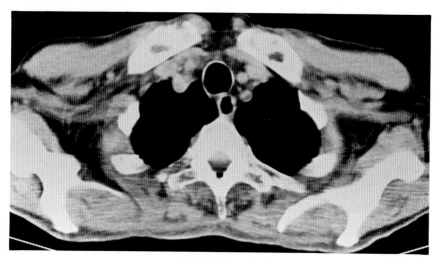

Figure 23-5

QUESTIONS 112 THROUGH 114: MARK YOUR ANSWER SHEET TRUE (T) OR FALSE (F) FOR EACH OF THE RESPONSE CHOICES.

112. Concerning patients with myasthenia gravis,

(A) posteroanterior and lateral chest radiographs will demonstrate fewer than 10% of associated thymomas
(B) approximately 10 to 15% have thymomas
(C) 25 to 50% of patients with thymomas have the disease
(D) distant metastases from malignant thymomas are common

113. Concerning thymolipomas,

(A) they contain both fat and epithelial elements of the thymus gland
(B) they characteristically cause symptoms early in their course
(C) when large they mold to the cardiac and diaphragmatic contours
(D) they constitute approximately 50% of thymic tumors

114. Concerning thymomas,

    (A) they are common in children

    (B) benign and malignant lesions are distinguished readily by histologic examination

    (C) approximately 50% are predominantly cystic

    (D) they are present in 50% of patients with aregenerative erythrocytic anemia

    (E) on computed tomography, fat plane obliteration indicates mediastinal invasion

This 30-year-old man presented with a cough. You are shown a portable chest radiograph (Figure 24-1).

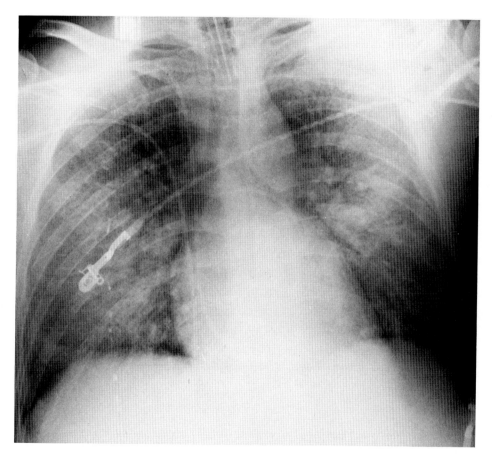

Figure 24-1

CASE 24 (Cont'd)

QUESTIONS 115 THROUGH 118: MARK YOUR ANSWER SHEET TRUE (T) OR FALSE (F) FOR EACH OF THE RESPONSE CHOICES.

115. Conditions that should be considered in the differential diagnosis include:

    (A) *Pneumocystis carinii* pneumonia in a patient with acquired immunodeficiency syndrome (AIDS)

    (B) chronic eosinophilic pneumonia

    (C) atypical mycobacterial infection

    (D) pulmonary edema due to heroin abuse

    (E) pulmonary alveolar proteinosis

116. Concerning *Pneumocystis carinii* pneumonia,

    (A) it is diagnosable by transbronchial biopsy

    (B) the organism is rarely obtained with bronchial washings

    (C) the typical radiograph shows multifocal patchy pneumonia

    (D) a normal chest radiograph virtually excludes it in a patient with AIDS

117. Concerning atypical mycobacterial infections,

    (A) they are rare in patients with AIDS

    (B) they are difficult to differentiate radiographically from tuberculosis

    (C) they do not destroy lung parenchyma

    (D) treatment regimens are similar to those used for typical tuberculosis

    (E) they are transmitted by person-to-person contact

118. Concerning pulmonary alveolar proteinosis,

    (A) initially it involves the interstitial compartment of the lung
    (B) it classically produces the "photographic-negative" image of pulmonary edema
    (C) it is associated with *Nocardia asteroides* infections
    (D) asbestos workers develop a similar radiographic appearance when massively exposed to asbestos fibers
    (E) the alveoli are filled with a surfactant-like material

This 27-year-old woman presented with progressive wheezing. You are shown a posteroanterior view (Figure 25-1), a cone-down view (Figure 25-2), and a lateral view with barium in the esophagus (Figure 25-3).

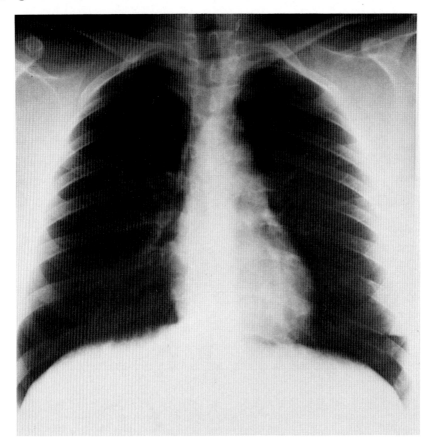

Figure 25-1

119. Which *one* of the following is the MOST likely diagnosis?

    (A) Pulmonary sling
    (B) Leiomyoma of the esophagus
    (C) Tracheal neoplasm
    (D) Bronchogenic cyst
    (E) Double aortic arch

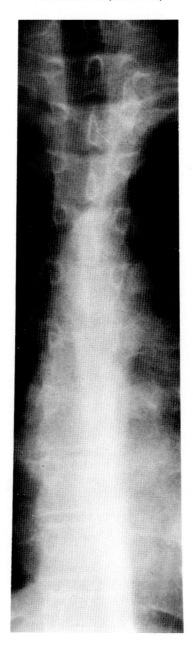

Figure 25-2

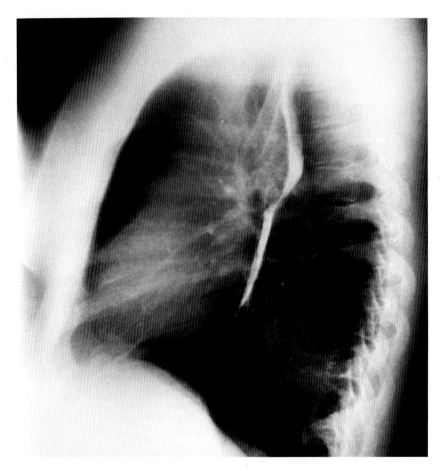

Figure 25-3

CASE 25 (Cont'd)

QUESTIONS 120 THROUGH 122: MARK YOUR ANSWER SHEET TRUE (T) OR FALSE (F) FOR EACH OF THE RESPONSE CHOICES.

120. Concerning a pulmonary sling,

    (A) it is usually detected in adulthood
    (B) the left pulmonary artery originates from the right pulmonary artery
    (C) the anomalous vessel produces an anterior imprint on the trachea
    (D) the right main bronchus is not affected
    (E) the left hilus is larger and higher than the right one

121. Concerning tracheal neoplasms in adults,

    (A) they are usually benign
    (B) adenoid cystic carcinomas (cylindromas) are more common than squamous cell carcinomas
    (C) adenoid cystic carcinomas are more common in the sixth than in the third decade of life
    (D) adenoid cystic carcinomas usually arise from the posterolateral tracheal wall
    (E) carcinoid tumors are among the most common

122. Concerning double aortic arch,

    (A) typically, the left arch is larger than the right
    (B) usually, the right arch is lower than the left
    (C) it is usually associated with a bicuspid aortic valve
    (D) it is the most common vascular ring in adults

This 38-year-old man was examined because of mild fever and cough. You are shown posteroanterior (Figure 26-1) and lateral (Figure 26-2) chest radiographs.

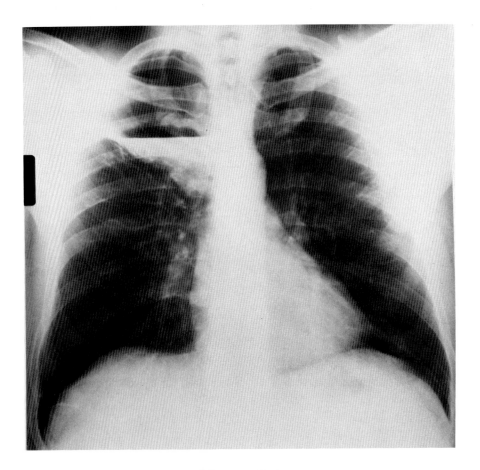

Figure 26-1

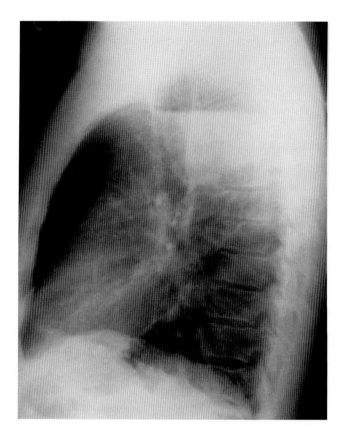

Figure 26-2

123. Which *one* of the following is the MOST likely diagnosis?

    (A) Anaerobic lung abscess
    (B) Empyema
    (C) Tuberculosis
    (D) Wegener's granulomatosis
    (E) Infected bulla

CASE 26 (Cont'd)

QUESTIONS 124 THROUGH 126: MARK YOUR ANSWER SHEET TRUE (T) OR FALSE (F) FOR EACH OF THE RESPONSE CHOICES.

124. Concerning lung abscesses,

    (A) they usually result from aspiration

    (B) fewer than 1% occur as a result of hematogenous dissemination

    (C) CT is required to distinguish them from empyemas in most cases

    (D) the middle lobe is a common location

    (E) the treatments of abscesses and empyemas are similar

125. Concerning Wegener's granulomatosis,

    (A) it typically produces a solitary cavity in the lung

    (B) it usually involves the upper airways and the kidneys

    (C) the limited form involves the kidneys

    (D) approximately 20% of patients develop lymphoma

126. Concerning bullae,

    (A) they are more common in emphysematous than in otherwise normal lungs

    (B) their walls usually are less than 3 mm thick

    (C) when infected, surgical intervention is the treatment of choice

    (D) they are usually found in the lower lobes

    (E) they are more likely to be infected by fungal than by bacterial pathogens

You are shown routine posteroanterior (Figure 27-1) and lateral (Figure 27-2) chest radiographs of a 53-year-old man. A computed tomographic (CT) scan was obtained subsequently (Figure 27-3).

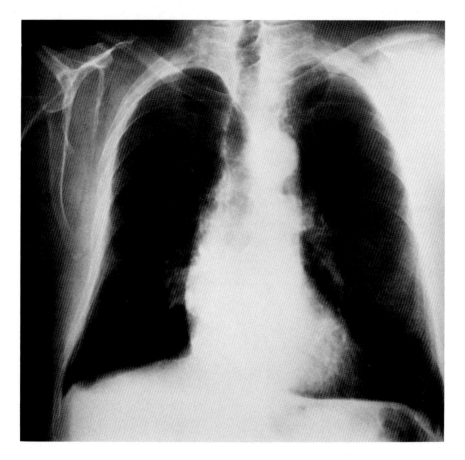

Figure 27-1

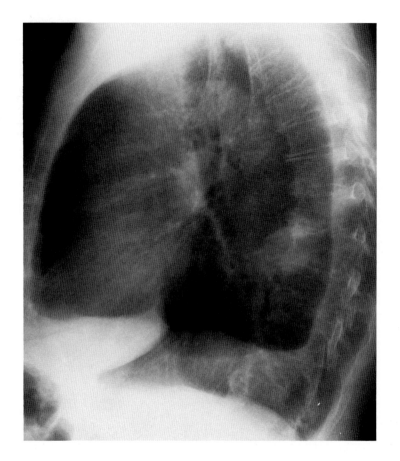

Figure 27-2

127. Which *one* of the following is the MOST likely diagnosis?

    (A) Bronchogenic carcinoma
    (B) Organized pulmonary infarct
    (C) Cryptococcal granuloma
    (D) Rounded atelectasis
    (E) Plasma cell granuloma

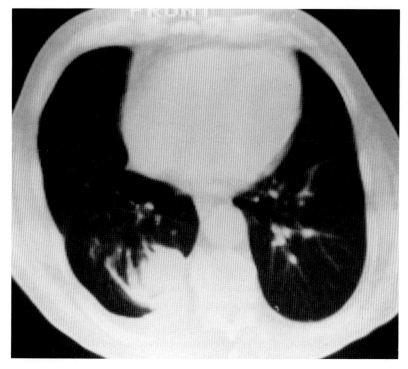

Figure 27-3

QUESTIONS 128 THROUGH 130: MARK YOUR ANSWER
SHEET TRUE (T) OR FALSE (F) FOR EACH OF THE RE-
SPONSE CHOICES.

128. Concerning bronchogenic carcinomas,

    (A) less than 50% of adenocarcinomas occur in the lung
        periphery

    (B) the "tail sign" is specific for the bronchioloalveolar cell
        type

    (C) visible calcification excludes the diagnosis

    (D) the most frequently cavitating type is small-cell
        carcinoma

    (E) a relationship to smoking is well established for all cell
        types

CASE 27 (Cont'd)

129. Concerning rounded atelectasis,

    (A) there is a correlation with asbestos exposure
    (B) the mass occurs at the site of maximum pleural thickening
    (C) the mass is composed of airless lung
    (D) calcification within the mass is common
    (E) it usually occurs at the lung apex

130. Concerning plasma cell granulomas,

    (A) there is usually a clinical history of pneumonia
    (B) they usually occur as multiple lesions
    (C) most are not calcified
    (D) transformation to multiple myeloma occurs in approximately 10% of cases
    (E) their diagnosis is readily established by percutaneous needle aspiration biopsy

CASE 28: Questions 131 through 134

This 27-year-old woman presented with pneumonia. You are shown posteroanterior (Figure 28-1) and lateral (Figure 28-2) chest radiographs and a frontal view of the abdomen (Figure 28-3) taken at another time.

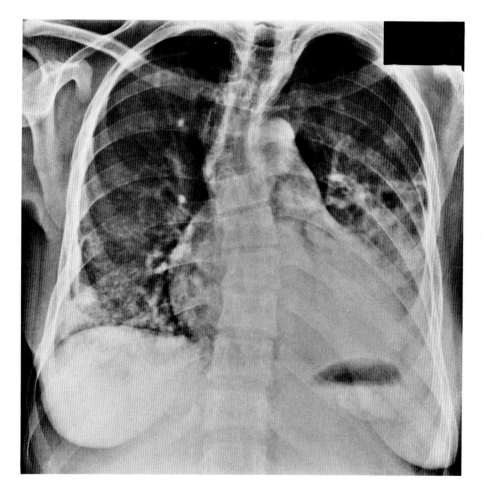

Figure 28-1

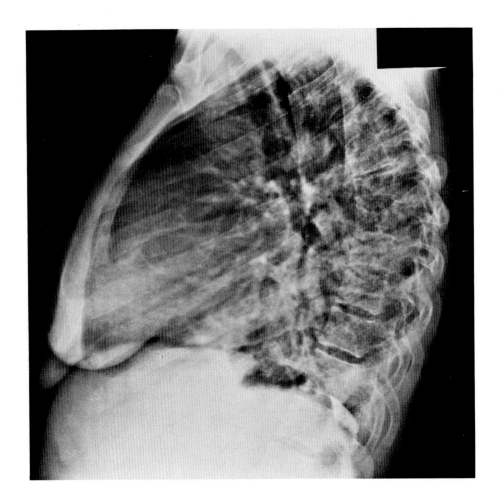

Figure 28-2

131. Which *one* of the following is the MOST likely diagnosis?

    (A) Granulomatous infection
    (B) Sickle cell disease
    (C) Cystic fibrosis
    (D) Leukemia
    (E) Lupus erythematosus

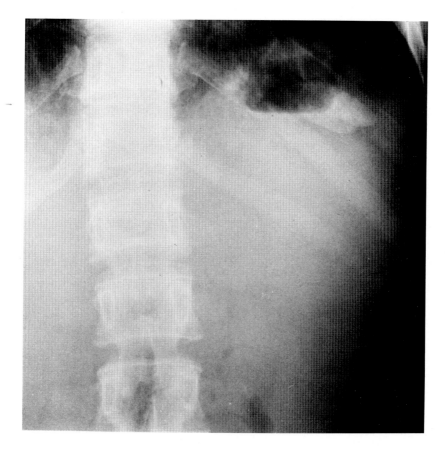

Figure 28-3

QUESTIONS 132 THROUGH 134: MARK YOUR ANSWER SHEET TRUE (T) OR FALSE (F) FOR EACH OF THE RESPONSE CHOICES.

132. Concerning patients with sickle cell disease,

(A) they have a higher incidence of pneumonia than do members of the general population
(B) they rarely develop pleural effusions
(C) the most common intrathoracic radiographic finding is cardiomegaly
(D) they have a high incidence of massive pulmonary embolism

133. Concerning cystic fibrosis,

(A) the pulmonary radiographic abnormalities occur predominantly in the lower lobes
(B) mucoid impaction is a rare radiographic feature
(C) pleural effusion is a common radiographic feature
(D) blood-streaked sputum is a common clinical sign

134. Concerning lupus erythematosus,

(A) it frequently produces a specific pneumonitis
(B) it leads to pulmonary hyperexpansion and a flat diaphragm
(C) hilar adenopathy is a common feature
(D) Libman-Sacks endocarditis frequently results in congestive heart failure

CASE 29: Questions 135 through 138

History withheld. You are shown an anteroposterior portable chest radiograph (Figure 29-1).

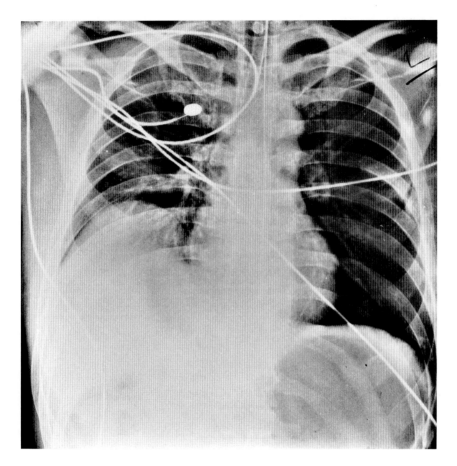

Figure 29-1

CASE 29 (Cont'd)

QUESTIONS 135 THROUGH 138: MARK YOUR ANSWER
SHEET TRUE (T) OR FALSE (F) FOR EACH OF THE RE-
SPONSE CHOICES.

135. Based on the radiographic findings alone, diagnostic possibilities include:

(A) paralysis of the right hemidiaphragm
(B) eventration of the right hemidiaphragm
(C) right subpulmonic effusion
(D) right lower lobe collapse
(E) traumatic diaphragmatic rupture

136. Concerning diaphragmatic paralysis,

(A) the affected hemidiaphragm moves upward during
sniffing
(B) at fluoroscopy, it is not easily differentiated from
eventration
(C) it indicates unresectability in patients with broncho-
genic carcinoma
(D) when bilateral it can be diagnosed easily by fluoroscopy
(E) the etiology is most often benign

137. Concerning subpulmonic effusions,

(A) they represent an uncommon distribution of pleural
fluid
(B) the apparent hemidiaphragmatic dome is shifted medially
(C) they obscure vessels normally visible through the
apparent hemidiaphragm on frontal radiographs
(D) they have a characteristic appearance on computed
tomography (CT) when they invert the hemidiaphragm
(E) the majority are loculated

138. Concerning diaphragmatic secondary to blunt trauma,

    (A) it is not diagnosed on initial radiographs in more than 50% of cases
    (B) CT is the procedure of choice for confirming the diagnosis
    (C) it occurs more commonly on the right side
    (D) delayed herniation of abdominal contents is rare
    (E) in most instances, it is an isolated injury

CASE 30: Questions 139 through 142

This 60-year-old man was evaluated for a 40-lb weight loss and anemia. You are shown a posteroanterior chest radiograph (Figure 30-1) and an anterior bone scintigram (Figure 30-2).

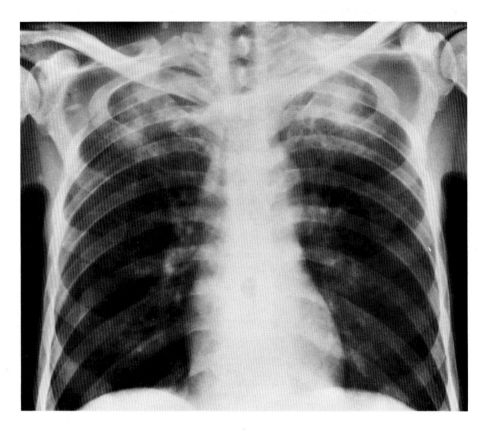

Figure 30-1

139. Which *one* of the following is the MOST likely diagnosis?

    (A) Idiopathic pulmonary ossification
    (B) Alveolar microlithiasis
    (C) Metastatic calcification
    (D) Tuberculosis
    (E) Mucinous adenocarcinoma of the stomach

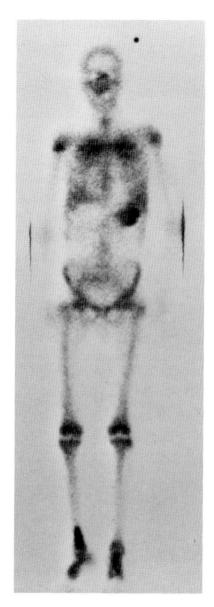

Figure 30-2

QUESTIONS 140 THROUGH 142: MARK YOUR ANSWER SHEET TRUE (T) OR FALSE (F) FOR EACH OF THE RESPONSE CHOICES.

140. Concerning idiopathic pulmonary ossification,

(A) most patients have associated interstitial fibrosis
(B) its radiographic appearance is similar to that of the ossification associated with mitral stenosis
(C) the radiographic findings are most apparent in the lower lobes
(D) bone scintigraphy demonstrates pulmonary uptake
(E) serum calcium, phosphorus, and phosphatase levels are all normal

141. Concerning metastatic calcification,

(A) the calcium is deposited in previously damaged tissues
(B) the most commonly involved pulmonary structure is the alveolar basement membrane
(C) the process is irreversible
(D) it is commonly caused by renal failure

142. In the normal upright person,

(A) the pO_2 is higher in the apex than in the base of the lung
(B) the lung apices are better ventilated than the lung bases
(C) the lung bases are better perfused than the lung apices
(D) the tissue pH is higher in the lung apex than in the lung base

These three patients have the same disease (Figures 31-1 through 31-3). You are shown posteroanterior chest radiographs.

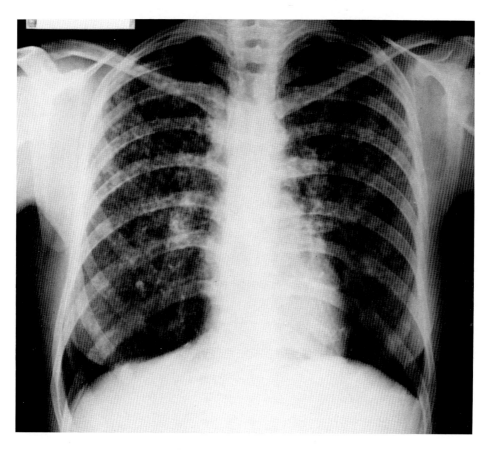

Figure 31-1

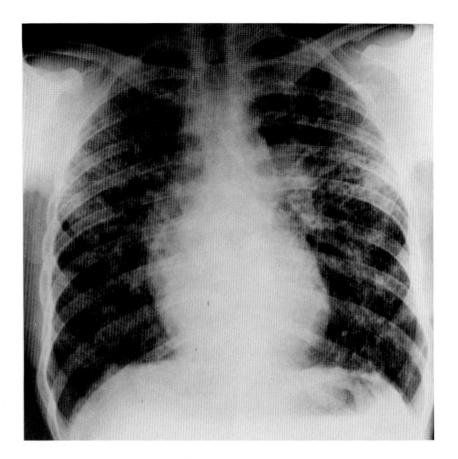

Figure 31-2

143. Which *one* of the following is the MOST likely diagnosis?

    (A) Collagen vascular disease
    (B) Asbestosis
    (C) Eosinophilic granuloma
    (D) Cystic fibrosis
    (E) Acute farmer's lung

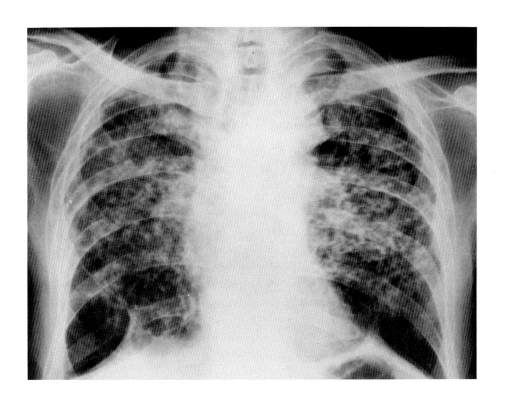

Figure 31-3

QUESTIONS 144 AND 145: MARK YOUR ANSWER SHEET TRUE (T) OR FALSE (F) FOR EACH OF THE RESPONSE CHOICES.

144. Concerning pulmonary eosinophilic granuloma,

   (A) clinical symptoms correlate well with the severity of the radiographic abnormality
   (B) upper lobe disease is characteristic
   (C) reduction of lung volume occurs early in the course of the disease
   (D) acute chest pain is usually due to rib fracture from a concomitant rib lesion
   (E) peripheral blood eosinophilia is a reliable indicator of active disease

145. Concerning farmer's lung,

   (A) peripheral eosinophilia is an important clinical finding
   (B) the etiologic agents are spores of thermophilic fungi
   (C) chronic exposure leads to hilar lymph node enlargement
   (D) the primary injury occurs in the respiratory bronchiole
   (E) end-stage pulmonary fibrosis is a result of chronic exposure

CASE 32: Questions 146 through 149

This 14-year-old boy presented with progressive dyspnea. You are shown a posteroanterior chest radiograph (Figure 32-1) and a close-up of the same radiograph (Figure 32-2).

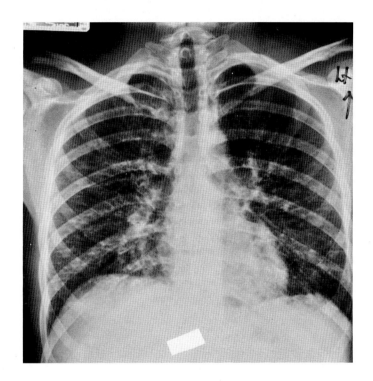

Figure 32-1

146. Which *one* of the following is the LEAST likely diagnosis?

    (A) Sclerosing mediastinitis
    (B) Pulmonary veno-occlusive disease
    (C) Left atrial myxoma
    (D) Mitral insufficiency
    (E) Cor triatriatum

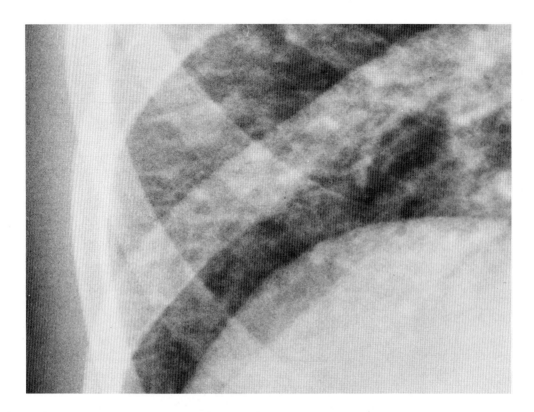

Figure 32-2

147. Swan-Ganz catheterization of this patient demonstrated a normal pulmonary capillary wedge pressure. On the basis of this additional information, which *one* of the following is the MOST likely diagnosis?

(A) Sclerosing mediastinitis
(B) Pulmonary veno-occlusive disease
(C) Left atrial myxoma
(D) Mitral insufficiency
(E) Cor triatriatum

QUESTIONS 148 AND 149: MARK YOUR ANSWER SHEET TRUE (T) OR FALSE (F) FOR EACH OF THE RESPONSE CHOICES.

148. The anatomic components of a Kerley B line include:

    (A) interlobular septum
    (B) pulmonary venule
    (C) pulmonary arteriole
    (D) pulmonary lymphatics

149. Concerning left atrial myxoma,

    (A) it is the most common primary tumor of the heart
    (B) it mimics mitral stenosis on the chest radiograph
    (C) computed tomography is preferable to echocardiography for establishing the diagnosis
    (D) the presence of calcification within the tumor allows distinction from left atrial thrombus
    (E) it most commonly arises from the left atrial appendage

This 50-year-old woman was asymptomatic. You are shown two posteroanterior chest radiographs (Figures 33-1 and 33-2) taken 1 month apart.

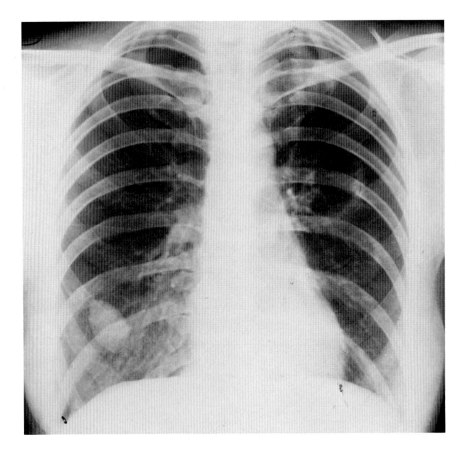

Figure 33-1

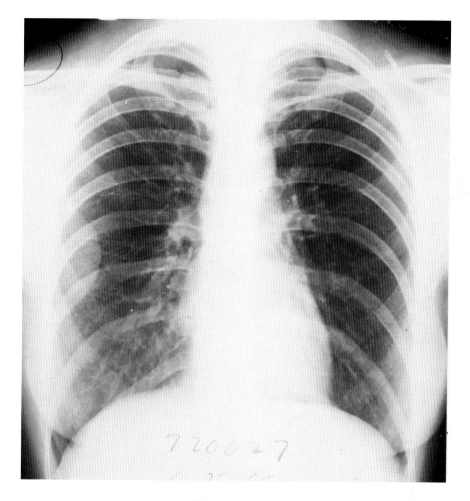

Figure 33-2

150. Which *one* of the following is the MOST likely diagnosis?

    (A) Inflammatory pseudotumor
    (B) Pleural pseudotumor (fluid)
    (C) Lipoma
    (D) Localized fibrous mesothelioma
    (E) Rounded atelectasis

QUESTIONS 151 THROUGH 153: MARK YOUR ANSWER
SHEET TRUE (T) OR FALSE (F) FOR EACH OF THE RE-
SPONSE CHOICES.

151. Concerning pleural pseudotumor (fluid),

   (A) the most common location is in the minor fissure
   (B) it resorbs spontaneously
   (C) elliptical or biconvex margins are characteristic
   (D) the most common etiology is closed chest trauma

152. Concerning intrathoracic lipoma,

   (A) it is more common in female patients
   (B) parenchymal lesions change shape with phases of
       respiration
   (C) its fat density is rarely recognized on routine radio-
       graphs
   (D) hypertrophic pulmonary osteoarthropathy occurs in
       10% of patients

153. Concerning localized fibrous mesothelioma,

   (A) it is associated with asbestos exposure
   (B) there is potential for malignancy
   (C) it arises predominantly from the parietal pleura
   (D) it is associated with hypertrophic pulmonary os-
       teoarthropathy
   (E) an apical location is characteristic

This 41-year-old foundry worker was admitted to the emergency room after a cerebrovascular accident. You are shown a portable chest radiograph (Figure 34-1) and a close-up of the same radiograph (Figure 34-2).

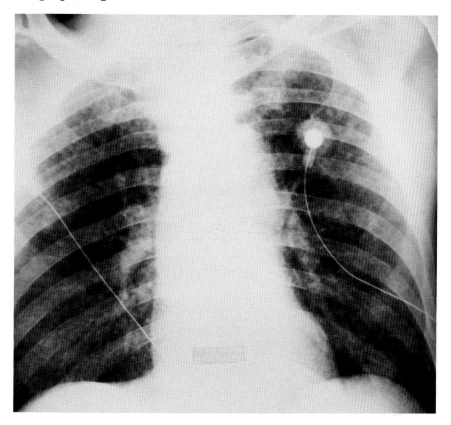

Figure 34-1

154. Which *one* of the occupational diseases listed below is the LEAST likely diagnosis?

   (A) Silicosis
   (B) Asbestosis
   (C) Coal worker's pneumoconiosis
   (D) Siderosis
   (E) Stannosis

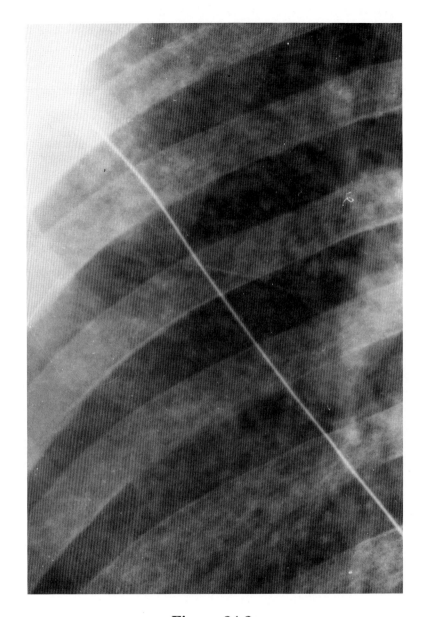

Figure 34-2

QUESTIONS 155 AND 156: MARK YOUR ANSWER SHEET TRUE (T) OR FALSE (F) FOR EACH OF THE RESPONSE CHOICES.

155. In comparing silicosis and siderosis,

   (A) pulmonary fibrosis caused by silicosis is less severe than that caused by siderosis
   (B) there are fewer clinical symptoms in siderosis
   (C) the exposure time required to produce radiographic abnormality is greater for silicosis
   (D) conglomerate masses (large opacities) are seen in both

156. Concerning coal worker's pneumoconiosis,

   (A) the unit pathologic lesion is similar to that of silicosis
   (B) lower lung zones are more frequently involved than upper zones
   (C) calcification of pulmonary nodular opacities occurs frequently
   (D) the "simple" form progresses even in the absence of further exposure
   (E) the distinction between "simple" and "complicated" forms of the disease is based on the radiographic findings

157. Which *one* of the following pulmonary structures is MOST susceptible to deposition and accumulation of inhaled dust?

   (A) Subpleural lymphatics
   (B) Interlobular septum
   (C) Alveolar wall
   (D) Terminal bronchiole
   (E) Alveolar sac

DEMOGRAPHIC DATA QUESTIONS

Please answer all of the questions below. The data you provide will be used to supply information that will allow you to compare your performance on the examination with that of others at similar levels of training and with similar backgrounds, and for purposes of planning continuing education projects. Please answer each question as accurately and as objectively as possible. Please mark the *one* BEST response for each question. Recall, of course, that we do *not* want individual names. Our analyses will reflect only categories and groups; everything will remain completely anonymous and no attempt will be made to identify any specific individual.

158. The ACR will be evaluating the questions in this examination to determine their degree of difficulty and to determine the success of the examination as an instrument of self-evaluation and continuing education. To assist the ACR, please indicate in which of the following ways you took this examination.

    (A) Used reference materials or read the syllabus portion of this book to assist in answering some portion of the examination
    (B) Did *not* use reference materials and did not read the syllabus portion of this book while taking the examination

159. How much residency and fellowship training in *Diagnostic Radiology* have you completed as of June 1989?

    (A) None
    (B) Less than 1 year
    (C) 1 year
    (D) 2 years
    (E) 3 years
    (F) 4 or more years

160. When did you *finish* your residency training in Radiology?

    (A) Prior to 1979
    (B) 1979–1983
    (C) 1984–1988
    (D) 1989
    (E) Not yet completed
    (F) Radiology is *not* my specialty

161. Have you completed residency training in a field *other than* Radiology?

    (A) Yes
    (B) No

162. Approximately how much residency training or practice experience have you had *other* than Radiology?

    (A) None
    (B) 1 year
    (C) 2 years
    (D) 3 to 5 years
    (E) More than 5 years

163. Have you been certified by the American Board of Radiology?

    (A) Yes
    (B) No

164. Approximately how much of your practice career (or residency/fellowship for current trainees) has been devoted to *Diagnostic* Radiology in *each* of the following practice categories?

    A. Community or general hospital—less than 200 beds

(A) None
(B) Less than 1 year
(C) 1 to 3 years
(D) 3 to 5 years
(E) More than 5 years

    B. Community or general hospital—200 to 499 beds

(A) None
(B) Less than 1 year
(C) 1 to 3 years
(D) 3 to 5 years
(E) More than 5 years

    C. Community or general hospital—500 or more beds

(A) None
(B) Less than 1 year
(C) 1 to 3 years
(D) 3 to 5 years
(E) More than 5 years

    D. University-affiliated hospital

(A) None
(B) Less than 1 year
(C) 1 to 3 years
(D) 3 to 5 years
(E) More than 5 years

E. Solo office practice

(A) None
(B) Less than 1 year
(C) 1 to 3 years
(D) 3 to 5 years
(E) More than 5 years

F. Office practice with 1 to 4 partners

(A) None
(B) Less than 1 year
(C) 1 to 3 years
(D) 3 to 5 years
(E) More than 5 years

G. Group: 5 or more in office practice

(A) None
(B) Less than 1 year
(C) 1 to 3 years
(D) 3 to 5 years
(E) More than 5 years

165. Which *one* of the practice categories listed in Question 164 best describes your practice in the immediate past 3 years? (For residents and fellows, in which *one* did you or will you spend the major portion of your residency and fellowship?)

(A) (B) (C) (D) (E) (F) (G)

166. In the past 3 years how much of your working time has been devoted to radiologic procedures and to the interpretation of films?

(A) Less than 25%
(B) 25 to 49%
(C) 50 to 74%
(D) 75 to 100%

167. Approximately how many hours per month (averaging over the last year) have you devoted to professional reading, study, seminars, courses, exhibits, or other types of continuing education activity?

    (A) 0 to 9 hours
    (B) 10 to 19 hours
    (C) 20 to 29 hours
    (D) 30 to 39 hours
    (E) 40 to 49 hours
    (F) 50 or more hours

168. In which *one* of the following general areas of Radiology do you consider yourself MOST expert?

    (A) Chest
    (B) Bone
    (C) Gastrointestinal
    (D) Genitourinary
    (E) Head and neck
    (F) Neuroradiology
    (G) Pediatric radiology
    (H) Cardiovascular radiology
    (I) Other

169. In which *one* of the following radiologic modalities do you consider yourself MOST expert?

    (A) General angiography
    (B) Interventional radiology
    (C) Magnetic resonance imaging
    (D) Nuclear medicine
    (E) Ultrasonography
    (F) Computed tomography
    (G) Radiation therapy
    (H) Other

Chest Disease (Fourth Series)

Table of Contents

The Table of Contents is placed in this unusual location so that the reader will not be distracted by the answers before completing the test. A detailed index of the areas considered in this syllabus is provided (beginning on p. 633) for further reference.

Chest Disease (Fourth Series)
Syllabus

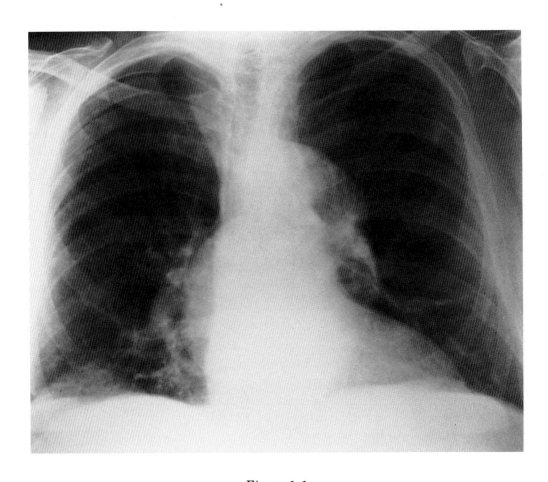

Figure 1-1
Figures 1-1 through 1-4. Routine posteroanterior (Figure 1-1) and
lateral (Figure 1-2) chest radiographs taken on this 72-year-old man
showed a mass that was later evaluated by contrast-enhanced computed
tomography (CT) (Figures 1-3 and 1-4). The CT numbers of the mass
were higher than those of water but lower than those of adjacent muscle.

Case 1: Bronchogenic Cyst

Question 1

Which *one* of the following is the MOST likely diagnosis?

(A) Teratoma
(B) Aortic aneurysm
(C) Bronchogenic cyst
(D) Achalasia
(E) Adenopathy

Posteroanterior (Figures 1-1 and 1-5) and lateral (Figures 1-2 and 1-6) chest radiographs show a large subcarinal mass projecting posteriorly and to the right. Contrast-enhanced computed tomographic (CT) scans (Figures 1-3, 1-4, 1-7, and 1-8) demonstrate a well-circumscribed low-density mass beginning superiorly in the subcarinal region and extending inferiorly, posterior to the heart and anterior to the spine. The esophagus is visible as an air-containing structure displaced to the left (Figure 1-9) by the large mass. This combination of radiographic findings is strongly suggestive of a foregut cyst, so that bronchogenic cyst is the most likely diagnosis **(Option (C) is correct).**

Teratomas (Option (A)) seldom occur in this region; rather, they occur in the mediastinum anterior to the base of the great vessels. While a large cystic component may occur in teratomas (dermoids), a soft tissue component, as well as fat and areas of calcification, is often present. Additionally, these masses tend to occur in young adults.

An aneurysm (Option (B)) is unlikely in this patient, since the mass appears separable from the descending aorta on the CT scans and shows no contrast enhancement in any portion. Magnetic resonance imaging (MRI) of the mediastinum is often helpful in demonstrating the presence or extent of an aortic aneurysm including any dissection.[4] While CT is practically limited to transverse images of the mediastinum, MRI allows studies in multiple planes (transverse, sagittal, and coronal). Flowing blood is virtually devoid of any MR signal; thus vascular structures and

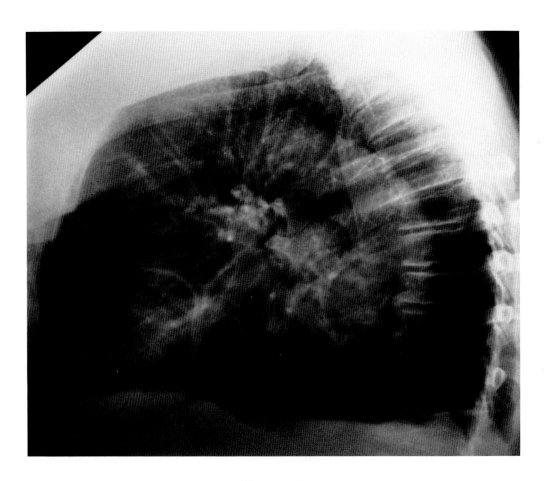

Figure 1-2

cardiac chambers appear markedly lucent (with properly chosen pulse sequences) and the need for intravenous contrast medium is eliminated. Figure 1-10 is a spin-echo MR image of a 55-year-old man with an infected gortex graft of the ascending aorta with pseudoaneurysm formation and adjacent mediastinitis. The pseudoaneurysm and its proximity to the sternum are nicely demonstrated. In this case, reoperation was necessary and the sternotomy was modified to avoid the pseudoaneurysm, which lay precariously close to the sternum. CT had not demonstrated the size and extent of the lesion as well as the MR study.

Achalasia (Option (D)) is not likely since the air-containing esophagus on the CT scan is of normal caliber and is displaced by the mass. While an esophageal smooth muscle tumor could occasionally present as a mass

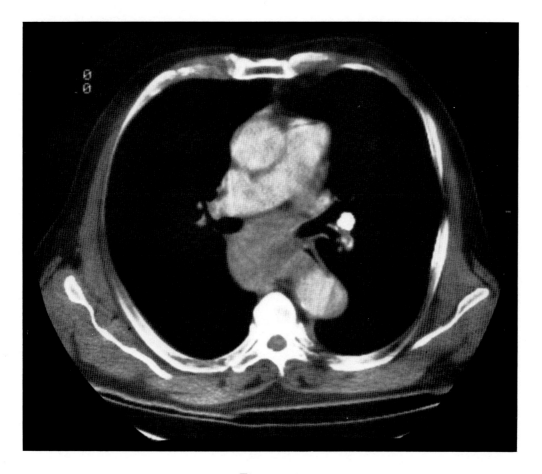

Figure 1-3

of this dimension, such masses are comparable to muscle in their attenuation characteristics. Esophageal carcinoma may present as a large mass, and administration of oral contrast medium will usually demonstrate the opacified lumen with adjacent tumor (Figure 1-11).

The remaining choice in this case is subcarinal adenopathy (Option (E)). In bronchogenic carcinoma, subcarinal metastatic nodes are often recognized on CT scans of the mediastinum when conventional radiographs and tomograms are equivocal or normal. Metastatic nodes are of soft tissue density on CT, however, and may have an infiltrative appearance. Adenopathy is therefore less likely than bronchogenic cyst.

When nodes become necrotic, they will demonstrate mixed attenuation on CT, rather than homogeneous low density. Figure 1-12 is an example of a contrast-enhanced CT scan of the mediastinum in a patient with

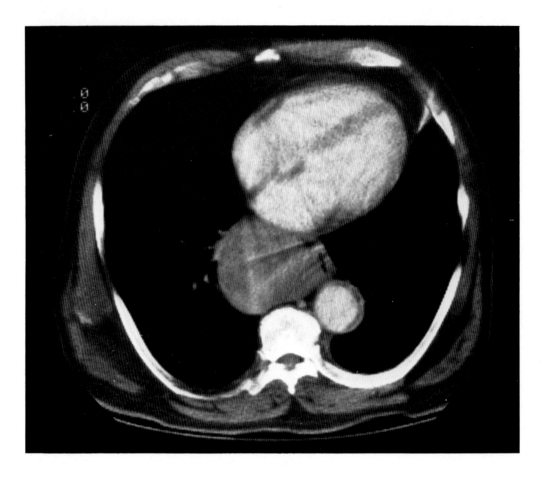

Figure 1-4

suppurative caseating granulomatous involvement of the subcarinal lymph nodes. Note the mass of mixed attenuation extending anterior to the descending aorta on the left and into the azygoesophageal recess on the right. This mass of nodes contained cystic necrotic areas in addition to a significant amount of solid tissue.

Bronchogenic cysts are congenital cystic lesions arising from the primitive foregut and are found within the lungs or mediastinum.[7,13,16,17] They are thought to be one of a spectrum of foregut malformations, which also includes esophageal cysts, gastroenteric cysts, and mediastinal cysts of undefinable origin. Some authors, who propose a unifying etiological concept for bronchopulmonary foregut malformations, also include intralobar and extralobar sequestrations, as well as sequestrations with

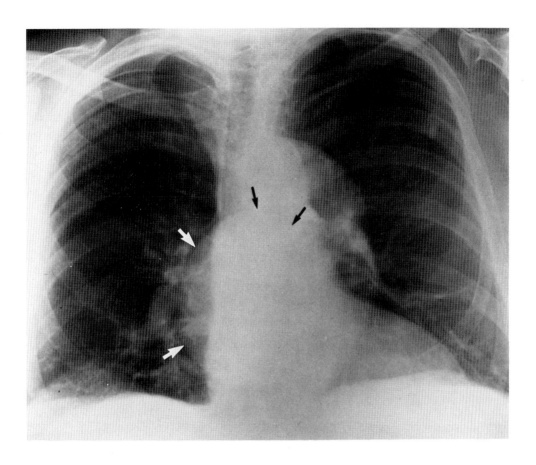

Figure 1-5
Figures 1-5 and 1-6 (Same as Figures 1-1 and 1-2, respectively). Note
the large subcarinal mass (arrows).

gastroesophageal communication and esophageal and gastric diverticula.[8]

The formation of a bronchogenic cyst is best understood embryologically. The respiratory and enteric tracts have a common origin from the
primitive foregut. A lateral septum invades from each side, forming
ventral and dorsal components, the former resulting in the respiratory
bud and the latter resulting in the esophagus, after the components have
separated from each other. Bronchogenic cysts are formed by abnormal
budding of the respiratory primordium (mediastinal cysts) or abnormal
branching of the tracheobronchial tree (parenchymal cysts). If the
connection with the tracheobronchial tree is lost, the parenchymal cyst

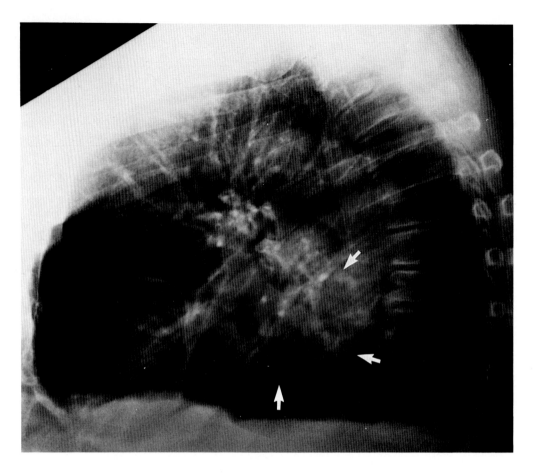

Figure 1-6

is filled with secretions of the respiratory epithelium and appears to be solid on conventional studies. When the cyst communicates with the airway, it becomes filled with air.

Mediastinal bronchogenic cysts are the most common congenital cysts of the mediastinum, accounting for 40 to 50% of all congenital mediastinal cysts. They occur in all age groups but are most frequently found in adults in the third and fourth decades. The male-female ratio is 1.5:1. Adult patients are usually asymptomatic at the time of diagnosis, although symptoms such as cough, wheezing, recurrent respiratory infection, dyspnea, and dysphagia may accompany the mass. In infancy and childhood, respiratory distress is more common. This may be due, at least in part, to less rigid, more compressible airways in childhood.

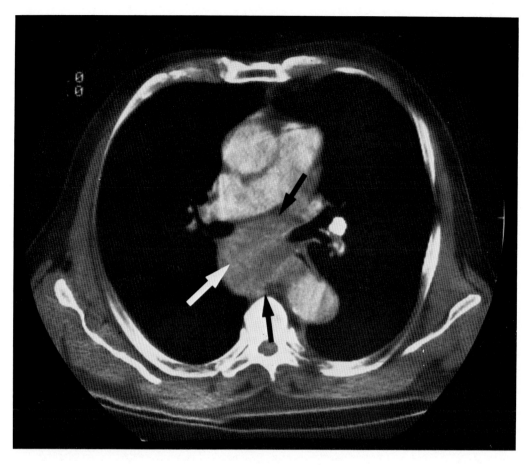

Figure 1-7
Figures 1-7 and 1-8 (Same as Figures 1-3 and 1-4, respectively). These CT scans demonstrate the mass (arrows).

Traditionally, mediastinal bronchogenic cysts have been considered more common than parenchymal cysts, although the largest series in the radiologic literature found parenchymal cysts to be twice as common as mediastinal cysts.[17]

When in the mediastinum the bronchogenic cyst classically presents as a homogeneous mass juxtaposed with the carina. The cyst is usually located subcarinally, extending posteriorly and inferiorly. More commonly, it extends to the right rather than to the left. Mediastinal cysts do not communicate with the tracheobronchial tree unless they become infected or rupture into the airway. As a result, they almost never contain air, unlike the parenchymal cysts, which more frequently contain air

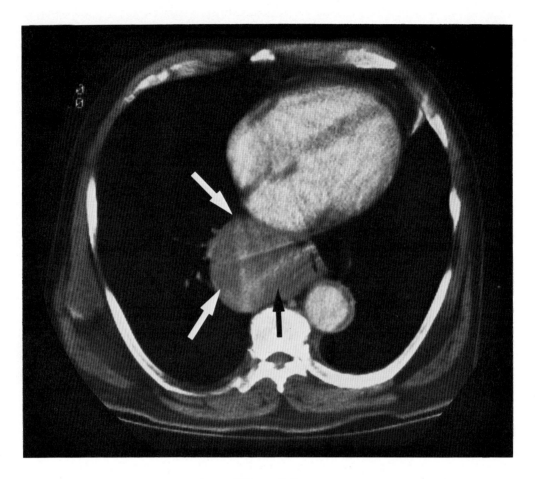

Figure 1-8

without becoming infected. While bronchogenic cysts in the mediastinum often occur subcarinally, they may be found in other locations (paratracheal, hilar, paraesophageal, etc.). Bronchogenic cysts in these locations may occasion clinical symptoms different from those associated with subcarinal ones.

Pathologically, bronchogenic cysts are usually spherical and unilocular, with a thin wall and a smooth gray outer surface. The cyst is usually filled with a white-gray mucinous material but may contain brown inspissated material resembling pus.

Histologically, the cysts consist of respiratory epithelium with a lamina propria containing bronchial glands, connective tissue, smooth muscle, and cartilage. The distinction between bronchogenic and

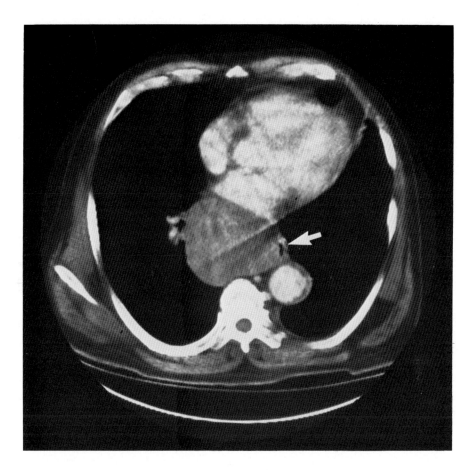

Figure 1-9. Same patient as in Figures 1-1 to 1-8. The esophagus (arrow) is displaced to the left by the mass.

esophageal cysts may be difficult because of their similar topographic distribution and morphology. The difference between the two is evident only histologically. Esophageal cysts are recognized by their histologic similarity to the esophagus. The cyst wall is lined with nonkeratinized stratified squamous epithelium and has a lamina propria with esophageal glands as well as a muscularis propria composed of two well-defined layers of smooth muscle. Some cysts, however, lack a clear histologic relationship with the airways or esophagus and cannot be accurately classified. These may have arisen in an earlier stage of embryologic development. The presence of inflammatory changes in the wall may also render a cyst wall histologically indeterminate. This occurs more commonly with parenchymal cysts than with mediastinal cysts.

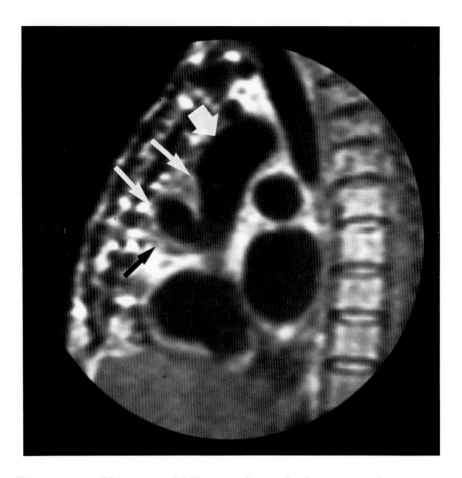

Figure 1-10. This sagittal MR scan shows the lucent pseudoaneurysm and surrounding dense inflammatory reaction (thin arrows) just behind the sternum. Note the ascending aorta (wide arrow).

Bronchogenic cysts are not associated with vertebral anomalies. However, neurenteric cysts are developmental cysts of the posterior mediastinum in patients who usually have vertebral abnormalities. Such cysts often occur in infancy. The cyst wall usually contains gastroenteric epithelium.

Radiographically, a mediastinal bronchogenic cyst usually presents as a homogeneous juxtacarinal middle mediastinal mass partially obscured by the overlying heart and great vessels. A CT scan frequently shows a circumscribed mass of water density easily separated from the great vessels. If the cyst displays attenuation values substantially lower than those of soft tissue or similar to those of water and does not enhance

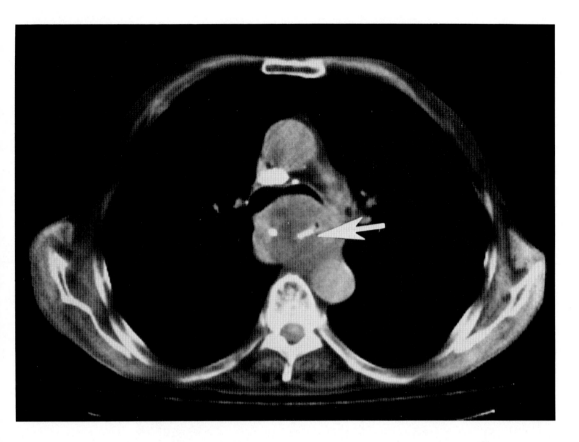

Figure 1-11. A large retrocarinal esophageal carcinoma is shown. The esophageal lumen (arrow) is partially filled with air and oral contrast material. A calcified node lies to the right of the esophageal lumen.

with contrast material, the cystic nature of the mass is confirmed. However, if it is of solid or mixed density due to hemorrhage or viscous secretions, it cannot be easily distinguished from a soft tissue mass of other etiology. Esophageal and bronchogenic cysts may share an identical appearance. While, in general, cysts of enteric origin occur above and those of bronchogenic origin occur below the carina, there is enough variation in the position of each to preclude accurate diagnosis by position alone.

Treatment of bronchogenic cysts has not been standardized. While the majority are resected, some are observed if there are no clinical symptoms while others are aspirated through a transbronchial or percutaneous approach. Infection is always a risk with the latter technique.

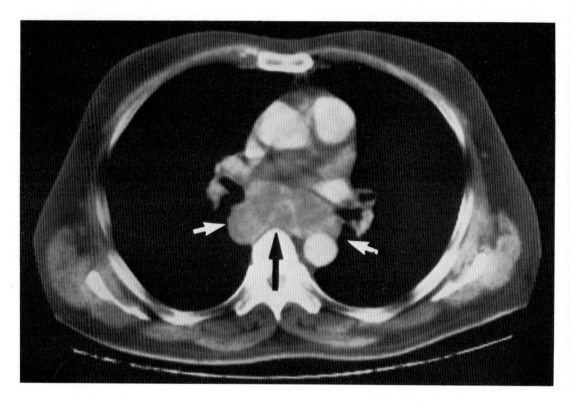

Figure 1-12. The mass of granulomatous adenopathy (arrows) shows mixed attenuation.

Question 2

Regarding CT numbers in the evaluation of mediastinal masses,

- (A) they reliably separate schwannomas from meningoceles
- (B) they reliably separate mediastinal cysts from solid lesions
- (C) they characterize fatty lesions more reliably than do conventional radiographic techniques
- (D) they detect lymph node calcification more reliably than does conventional tomography
- (E) a rise after administration of contrast medium as an intravenous drip indicates a vascular structure

Levi et al.[12] have shown in an experiment with test phantoms that the use of CT numbers as absolute values is unreliable due to individual scanner variation. CT numbers of individual tumors also vary from patient to patient. Other physical factors affect CT numbers as well. On a practical basis it is more helpful to relate the CT numbers of a given mass or abnormality to adjacent known structures such as muscle, bone, subcutaneous fat, and water-density structures (e.g., the urinary bladder). Contrast enhancement may also aid in separating vascular masses from nonvascular masses and solid lesions from cystic lesions.

Neurogenic tumors often have attenuation values significantly lower than those of adjacent muscle tissue, even following contrast enhancement.[11] CT does not always differentiate neural tumors, especially schwannomas, from meningoceles because the densities of both lesions may be similar **(Option (A) is false).** For example, lipid-rich cells and cystic accumulations of fluid have correlated with CT numbers from 5 to 25 Hounsfield units (HU) in schwannomas.[1,11] If a neurogenic tumor contains calcification or enhances with intravenous contrast medium, the correct CT diagnosis is more likely.

As experience has grown in CT scanning of the mediastinum, it has become apparent that in some cases mediastinal cysts do not yield attenuation values of water density. Marvasti et al.[14] have reported five benign mediastinal cysts with CT numbers similar to those of solid tissue. The higher-than-expected attenuation values in these cysts were probably due to the presence of thick viscous fluid in each **(Option (B) is false).**

In contrast to mediastinal cysts, fatty masses are more easily separated from those that are solid or cystic by means of their very low attenuation values (usually 50 to 100 HU below that of water).[2,3] Because of the greater sensitivity of CT as compared with conventional radiographic

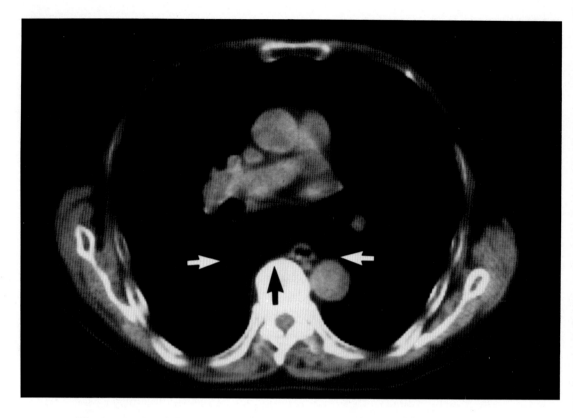

Figure 1-13. A low-density fatty mass, an omental hernia (arrows), is clearly visible on CT, whereas it appeared as a soft tissue mass on conventional studies.

techniques for detecting small changes in attenuation values of tissues, fatty lesions appear as low-density masses on CT (Figure 1-13) **(Option (C) is true).** They will usually be of the same density as other mediastinal structures with conventional radiographic techniques.

Siegelman et al.[18] have shown that calcification within pulmonary nodules may be more accurately detected by CT than by conventional radiography. Similarly, calcification within hilar or mediastinal lymph nodes is more easily detected by CT **(Option (D) is true).** This fact is sometimes helpful in separating granulomatous from neoplastic lymph nodes, although a small amount of calcification located eccentrically within large nodes may represent a calcified node engulfed by or immediately adjacent to a tumor.

While dynamic CT with bolus injections of contrast material has proven helpful in distinguishing vascular lesions from nonvascular lesions in the lung and mediastinum, most solid masses will show some opacification with the intravenous drip administration of contrast agent **(Option (E) is false)**. Occasionally, highly vascular solid masses of the hilum or mediastinum, such as some metastatic hypernephromas and vascular thymomas, will become densely opacified with contrast material and become difficult to distinguish from vascular structures. Godwin and Webb[5] have shown that time-density curves are often helpful in the separation of vascular structures from highly vascular masses.

Question 3

Concerning middle mediastinal masses in adults,

   (A) they are most commonly benign
   (B) they are more likely to be a cause of respiratory distress in adults than in children
   (C) partial calcification favors a neoplastic etiology
   (D) they are more easily delineated by CT than by conventional radiography
   (E) following detection by chest radiography, biopsy is the diagnostic procedure of choice

Enlarged lymph nodes involved with lymphoma or metastatic disease constitute the majority of middle mediastinal masses in adults. Approximately 90% of lesions in the middle mediastinum are malignant[10] **(Option (A) is false)**.

Mediastinal masses are more likely to cause compression of the airways with respiratory distress in an infant or child than in an adult **(Option (B) is false)**. This difference is especially evident with foregut cysts in the middle mediastinum. While they are often asymptomatic in the adult, they often cause severe respiratory symptoms in infants and can present as surgical emergencies. In a literature review of 40 cases of bronchogenic cysts of the mediastinum in the pediatric age group, Grafe et al.[6] emphasized that a bronchogenic cyst of the mediastinum should be considered in the differential diagnosis of acute and chronic respiratory illnesses in childhood.

Two of the most common etiologies for calcification within the middle mediastinum are calcified or partially calcified lymph nodes (due to previous granulomatous infection) and calcium in the wall of an atherosclerotic aorta. Benign calcification within lymph nodes may be accompanied by a significant soft tissue component. This type of calcium is usually very dense and occurs in large coarse aggregates.[15] When an atherosclerotic aneurysm of the aorta develops, a helpful diagnostic clue to its etiology is the presence of curvilinear calcification within its walls. While some primary and secondary neoplasms of the mediastinum will occasionally contain some calcification, calcification is more common in teratomas and thyroid masses of the anterior mediastinum **(Option (C) is false)**.

The advantages of CT of the middle mediastinum in comparison with conventional radiography reflect the ability of CT to distinguish an abnormal mass from the surrounding vessels, to define its contour and extent, and in many cases to predict whether it is cystic, solid, or fatty. Because of the cross-sectional view obtained with CT, the mass is more easily distinguished from the great vessels and heart than by conventional radiography[2,9] **(Option (D) is true)**.

Homogeneous fatty masses in the mediastinum are benign and do not warrant surgery or biopsy for diagnosis. Aortic aneurysms of the proximal thoracic aorta require special surgical management (e.g., bypass surgery, prosthetic valves, and grafts). There is a small but definite risk of hemorrhage in percutaneous biopsy of an aneurysm. For these reasons, once a mass in the middle mediastinum is discovered by conventional radiography, it is wise to try to further characterize its nature by CT, MRI, or angiography prior to biopsy or surgery **(Option (E) is false)**.

SUGGESTED READINGS

1. Aughenbaugh GL. Thoracic manifestations of neurocutaneous diseases. Radiol Clin North Am 1984; 22:741–756
2. Crowe JK, Brown LR, Muhm JR. Computed tomography of the mediastinum. Radiology 1978; 128:75–87
3. Gale ME. Bochdalek hernia: prevalence and CT characteristics. Radiology 1985; 156:449–452
4. Geisinger MA, Risius B, O'Donnell JA, et al. Thoracic aortic dissections: magnetic resonance imaging. Radiology 1985; 155:407–412
5. Godwin JD, Webb WR. Dynamic computed tomography in the evaluation of vascular lung lesions. Radiology 1981; 138:629–635
6. Grafe WR, Goldsmith EI, Redo SF. Bronchogenic cysts of the mediastinum in children. J Pediatr Surg 1966; 1:384–393
7. Gwinn JL, Lee FA. Radiological case of the month. Am J Dis Child 1975; 129:953–954

8. Heithoff KB, Shashikant MS, Williams HJ, et al. Bronchopulmonary foregut malformations: a unifying etiological concept. AJR 1976; 126:46–55

9. Heitzman ER, Goldwin RL, Proto AV. Radiologic analysis of the mediastinum utilizing computed tomography. Radiol Clin North Am 1977; 15:309–329

10. Joseph WL, Murray JF, Mulder DG. Mediastinal tumors—problems in diagnosis and treatment. Dis Chest 1966; 50:150–160

11. Kumar AJ, Kuhajda FP, Martinez CR, Fishman EK, Jezic DV, Siegelman SS. Computed tomography of extracranial nerve sheath tumors with pathological correlation. J Comput Assist Tomogr 1983; 7:857–865

12. Levi C, Gray JE, McCullough EC, Hattery RR. The unreliability of CT numbers as absolute values. AJR 1982; 139:443–447

13. Marchevsky AM, Kaneko M. Surgical pathology of the mediastinum. New York: Raven Press; 1984:217–233

14. Marvasti MA, Mitchell GE, Burke WA, Meyer JA. Misleading density of mediastinal cysts on computerized tomography. Ann Thorac Surg 1981; 31:167–170

15. McLeod RA, Brown LR, Miller WE, DeRemee RA. Evaluation of the pulmonary hila by tomography. Radiol Clin North Am 1976; 14:51–84

16. Reed JC, Sobonya RE. Morphologic analysis of foregut cysts in the thorax. AJR 1974; 120:851–860

17. Rogers LF, Osmer JC. Bronchogenic cyst. A review of 46 cases. AJR 1964; 91:273–283

18. Siegelman SS, Khouri NF, Scott WW Jr, Leo FP, Zerhouni EA. Computed tomography of the solitary pulmonary nodule. Semin Roentgenol 1984; 19:165–172

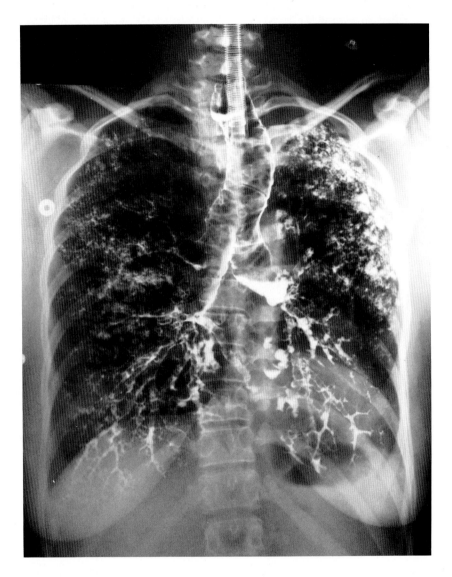

Figure 2-1. This 29-year-old woman presented with a history of recurrent respiratory infections since childhood. She had previously undergone a lobectomy for bronchiectasis. You are shown an anteroposterior bronchogram.

Case 2: Mounier-Kuhn Syndrome

Question 4

Which *one* of the following is the MOST likely diagnosis?

(A) Tracheopathia osteochondroplastica
(B) Chronic relapsing polychondritis
(C) The Mounier-Kuhn syndrome
(D) Hypogammaglobulinemia
(E) The Kartagener syndrome

In Figure 2-1, a bilateral bronchogram, the most important radiographic finding is marked dilatation of the trachea and main bronchi. This is characteristic of tracheobronchomegaly or the Mounier-Kuhn syndrome **(Option (C) is the most likely diagnosis)**. Additional radiographic features include protrusion of redundant nonmuscular membranous tissue between the dilated cartilaginous rings to form multiple tracheal and bronchial diverticula, bronchiectasis, and a tracheal diameter exceeding 3 cm[1,3,9,10] (Figures 2-2 and 2-3).

Tracheopathia osteochondroplastica (Option (A)) typically causes some degree of airway narrowing, rather than dilatation, and therefore is not likely.

Chronic relapsing polychondritis (Option (B)) is characterized by inflammatory changes of cartilaginous structures throughout the body, including the larynx, trachea, and bronchi. When the cartilages of the airway are involved, the airway characteristically becomes narrowed due initially to edema and finally to cicatrization.[3,7,11,12] Figures 2-4 and 2-5 show advanced involvement of the trachea and left main bronchus in a case of relapsing polychondritis. Owing to laryngeal involvement as well, a tracheostomy tube was required. Airway involvement occurs in about half of cases and is the most common cause of death in patients with this disease. Conventional radiographs and tomograms of the airways are often helpful in detecting early narrowing, an important finding since many cases will respond to steroid treatment. These findings are all

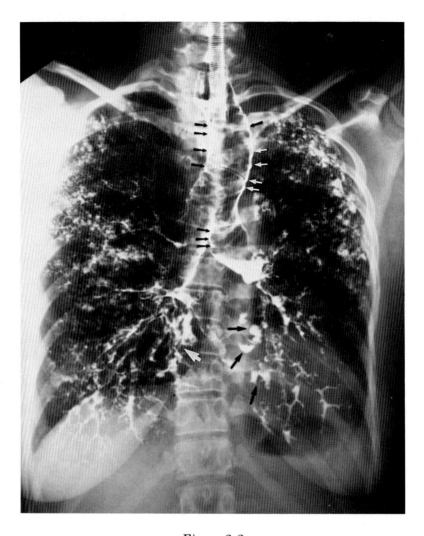

Figure 2-2
Figures 2-2 and 2-3. Figure 2-2 is the same illustration as Figure 2-1.
Anteroposterior (Figure 2-2) and lateral (Figure 2-3) bronchograms show
radiographic features of the Mounier-Kuhn syndrome, or tracheobronchomegaly, in two patients: shallow diverticula (small arrows) protruding
between cartilaginous rings, bronchiectasis (large arrows), and an
increased tracheal diameter.

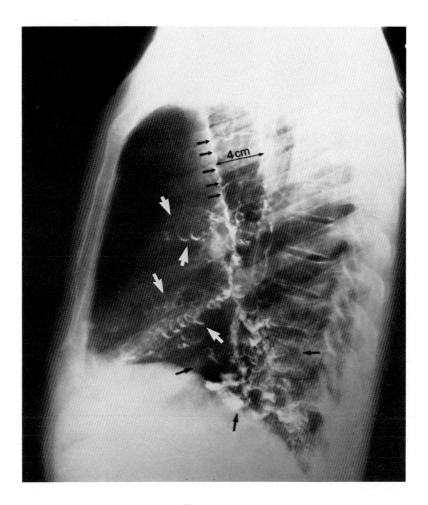

Figure 2-3

inconsistent with those visible in Figure 2-1; thus, chronic relapsing polychondritis is untenable.

Hypogammaglobulinemia (Option (D)) is characterized by chronic recurrent infections due to altered immunity. Recurrent bronchitis and pneumonia may eventually lead to pulmonary fibrosis, air trapping, bronchial wall thickening, and bronchiectasis. However, the diameter of the major airways remains relatively unaffected; thus, hypogammaglobulinemia is unlikely.

The syndrome of chronic sinusitis, bronchiectasis, and situs inversus (Option (E)) was first described by Kartagener and therefore bears his name (Figures 2-6 to 2-8). The tracheal caliber is normal. The Kartagener

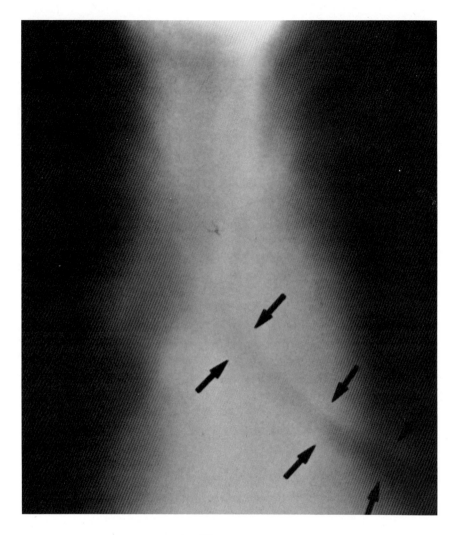

Figure 2-4
Figures 2-4 and 2-5. Anteroposterior (Figure 2-4) and lateral (Figure 2-5) linear tomograms show diffuse narrowing of the left main bronchus (arrows, Figure 2-4) and trachea (arrows, Figure 2-5) due to relapsing polychondritis.

syndrome is now recognized as one manifestation of the immotile cilia syndrome, a disorder characterized by specific genetically determined defects of the respiratory cilia.[12] Such genetically transmitted structural defects cause ciliary dysfunction, leading not only to lack of mucociliary clearance of respiratory irritants and organisms but also to recurrent respiratory infection and chronic obstructive pulmonary disease. Situs

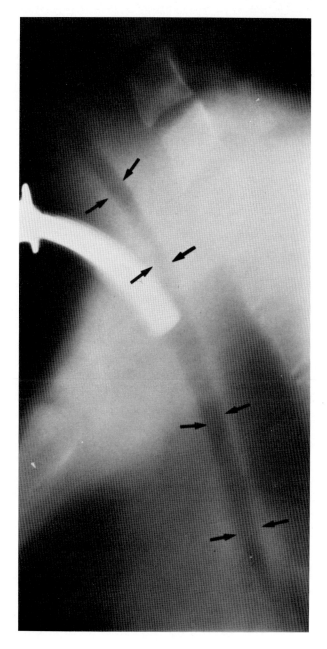

Figure 2-5

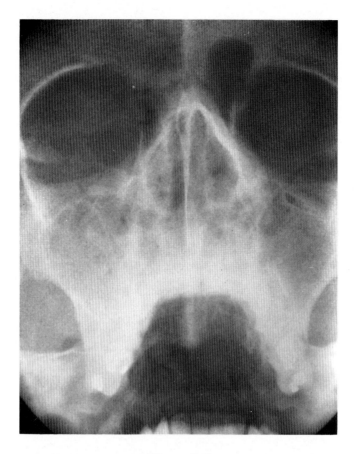

Figure 2-6
Figures 2-6 through 2-8. In this patient with the Kartagener syndrome, a view of the sinuses (Figure 2-6) shows maxillary clouding, a finding consistent with chronic sinusitis. The posteroanterior chest radiograph (Figure 2-7) shows situs inversus totalis and peribronchial thickening at the right lung base. On the anteroposterior bronchogram (Figure 2-8), basilar cylindrical bronchiectasis (arrows) is demonstrated.

inversus is present in 50% of cases. It is theorized that the immotility of the cilia during embryonic development results in random distribution of the body organs. Clinical manifestations of the immotile cilia syndrome include respiratory infections, sinusitis, nasal polyposis, recurrent otitis media, and male sterility. Chest radiographic findings include bronchial wall thickening, atelectasis, bronchiectasis, and hyperinflation. These findings are inconsistent with those visible in Figure 2-1; thus, the Kartagener syndrome is also unlikely.

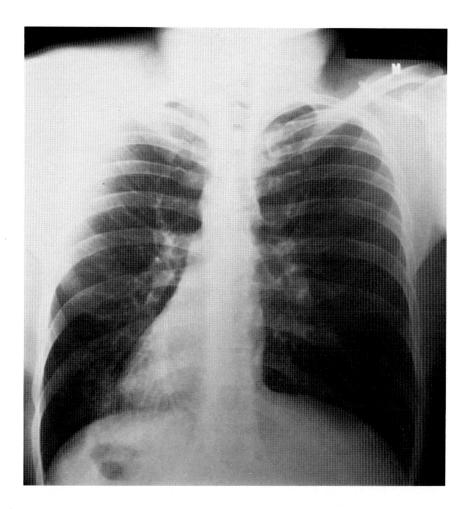

Figure 2-7

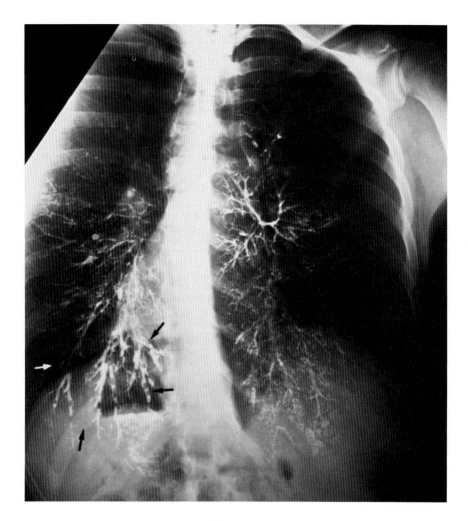

Figure 2-8

Question 5

Concerning tracheopathia osteochondroplastica,

    (A) it is frequently associated with tracheal diverticulosis
    (B) it is a premalignant condition
    (C) it is associated with mucosal ulcerations in the tracheobronchial tree
    (D) it is characterized by osteocartilaginous masses along the inner anterolateral surfaces of the trachea
    (E) it typically involves a short segment of the trachea or main bronchi

Tracheopathia osteochondroplastica is a benign condition consisting of multiple submucosal osteocartilaginous masses found primarily along the inner anterolateral walls of the trachea and main bronchi[3,8,15] **(Option (D) is true)**. The nodular inner contour of the narrowed airway is caused by protrusion of these submucosal masses into the airway lumen (Figure 2-9), rather than by redundant tissue forming diverticula **(Option (A) is false)**. The mucosa overlying the nodular masses is intact **(Option (C) is false)**. There typically is involvement of a long segment of the airway **(Option (E) is false)**. Although in one reported instance a bronchogenic carcinoma arose from an osteocartilaginous mass of a bronchus, tracheopathia osteochondroplastica typically is not a premalignant condition[4] **(Option (B) is false)**.

Tracheopathia osteochondroplastica affects men more often than women (3 to 1), and the average age is over 50 years. The etiology is unknown. Histologically, there are submucosal islands of hyaline cartilage with areas of lamellar bone. Native cartilage may play a role in the pathogenesis. The nodular masses frequently contain calcification, which at times may be visualized on conventional radiographs and tomograms. The presence of calcification may help separate this entity from others that involve a long segment of the airway, such as tracheobronchial papillomatosis, amyloidosis, lymphoma, and relapsing polychondritis. Computed tomography may be helpful in demonstrating such calcification.[2]

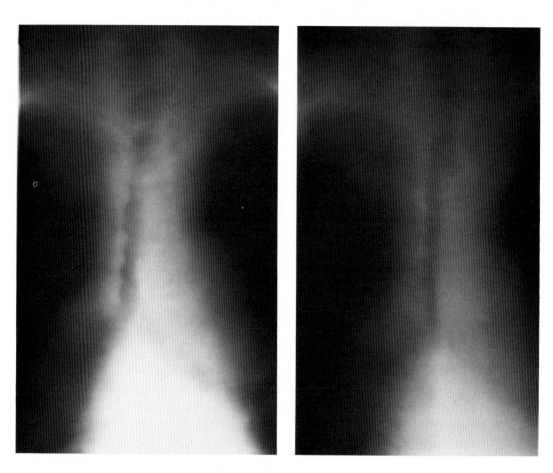

Figure 2-9. Two contiguous 1-cm anteroposterior tomograms show diffuse nodular submucosal masses and narrowing of the trachea in this patient with tracheopathia osteochondroplastica.

Question 6

Concerning the Mounier-Kuhn syndrome,

    (A) it is frequently associated with bronchiectasis
    (B) it is characterized by congenital diverticula of the trachea and bronchi
    (C) it radiographically resembles tracheobronchial amyloidosis
    (D) it usually occurs secondary to chronic recurrent infections

Tracheobronchomegaly, or the Mounier-Kuhn syndrome,[1,3,9,10] was first described by Czyhlarz in 1897, and Mounier-Kuhn published the first clinical description of the syndrome in 1932. The principal feature is dilatation of the trachea and main bronchi. Pathologically, a defect of elastic and muscle fibers is present. Since the syndrome sometimes occurs in childhood, the defect is probably congenital. A familial occurrence has been demonstrated in one series **(Option (D) is therefore false).**

With tracheobronchomegaly there is proportionate enlargement of both cartilaginous and membranous portions of the involved airway. The majority of patients have bronchiectasis, which may be cylindrical or saccular **(Option (A) is true).** It is thought that bronchiectasis is a secondary phenomenon probably related to faulty clearing of bronchial secretions, resulting in chronic infection. A strong argument for this is the later onset of the associated bronchiectasis. Virtually all patients show other types of postinflammatory pulmonary processes, such as diffuse emphysema, chronic bronchitis, pulmonary fibrosis, and bronchiolectasis. While these other pulmonary processes are seen with some frequency in the general population, the Mounier-Kuhn syndrome is rare. This provides further evidence that the Mounier-Kuhn syndrome is not an acquired disease.

The radiographic findings in tracheobronchomegaly are characteristic, as already described. The trachea and main bronchi show dilatation rather than the narrowing one sees in tracheobronchial amyloidosis **(Option (C) is false).** On the lateral chest radiograph, the trachea may have an anteroposterior diameter of 3 cm or more (or wider than the adjacent vertebral body). The airways manifest a corrugated appearance. This eventually results from protrusion of redundant nonmuscular membranous tissue between the enlarged cartilaginous rings to form diverticulum-like structures that pool contrast material. These diverticula are not congenital, however **(Option (B) is false).** In children, fluoroscopy of the airway during inspiration, expiration, quiet breathing, and phonation may be diagnostic; thus bronchography can be avoided.

Other examples of tracheal widening are found in patients with the Ehler-Danlos syndrome (isolated reports) and cutis laxa, both of which have additional clinical manifestations that allow their diagnosis.[3]

Question 7

Concerning diverticula of the trachea and bronchi,

    (A) rudimentary bronchus is a type
    (B) the congenital type arises from the distal bronchi
    (C) the acquired type results from chronic irritation or infection
    (D) tracheocele is a type that develops from high levels of intratracheal pressure
    (E) redundant nonmuscular membranous tissue is a cause

Tracheobronchial diverticula typically include any type of outpouching from the lumina of the trachea or bronchi. Neilsen,[13] using this broad definition, separated diverticula into three types.

(1) Rudimentary or supernumerary bronchi are usually short and cylindrical **(Option (A) is true).** This type, which is congenital and arises from the right aspect of the trachea above the carina **(Option (B) is false),** contains all the structural elements of the tracheal wall. Clinically, the patient is usually asymptomatic.

(2) Acquired diverticula, ranging in size from a few millimeters to 3 cm or more, are due to postinflammatory dilatations following drainage of pus-filled bronchial and tracheal mucous glands **(Option (C) is true).** At bronchography they present as flask-shaped diverticula with narrow necks,[5] as seen with chronic bronchitis.

(3) Diverticulum-like protrusions of redundant nonmuscular segments of membrane may occur between the transverse bands of muscle fibers and cartilage. On bronchography, these diverticula present as multiple shallow, wide-mouthed outpouchings protruding from the walls of the dilated airways. They constitute one of the major bronchographic findings in the Mounier-Kuhn syndrome **(Option (E) is true).**

An additional type of outpouching is the tracheocele, also known as "tracheal hernia."[6,14] This is a single, large, air-containing sac with a wide mouth that communicates with the lumen of the trachea. The tracheocele usually develops from a localized weakness in the right posterior tracheal wall, often as a result of prolonged increased intratracheal pressure **(Option (D) is true).** Classically, this occurs in musicians (especially those playing wind instruments), drill sergeants, and patients predisposed to violent episodes of prolonged coughing. Radiographically, the tracheocele is a paratracheal or superior mediastinal air cavity, with or without an air-fluid level due to retained secretions. It is easily outlined with contrast material.

SUGGESTED READINGS

1. Bateson EM, Woo-Ming M. Tracheobronchomegaly. Clin Radiol 1973; 24:354–358
2. Bottles K, Nyberg DA, Clark M, Hinchcliffe WA. CT diagnosis of tracheobronchopathia osteochondroplastica. J Comput Assist Tomogr 1983; 7:324–327
3. Choplin RH, Wehunt WD, Theros EG. Diffuse lesions of the trachea. Semin Roentgenol 1983; 18:38–50
4. Dalgaard JB. Tracheopathia chondro-osteoplastica. A case elucidating the problems concerning development and ossification of elastic cartilage. Acta Pathol Microbiol Scand 1947; 24:118–134
5. Ettman IK, Keel DT. Tracheal diverticulosis. Radiology 1962; 78:187–190
6. Gronner AT, Trevino RJ. Tracheocele. Br J Radiol 1971; 44:979–981
7. Horns JW, O'Loughlin BJ. Tracheal collapse in polychondritis. AJR 1962; 87:844–846
8. Howland WJ Jr, Good CA. The radiographic features of tracheopathia osteoplastica. Radiology 1958; 71:847–850
9. Johnston RF, Green RA. Tracheobronchomegaly. Report of five cases and demonstration of familial occurrence. Am Rev Respir Dis 1965; 91:35–50
10. Katz I, LeVine M, Herman P. Tracheobronchomegaly. The Mounier-Kuhn syndrome. AJR 1962; 88:1084–1094
11. Kilman WJ. Narrowing of the airway in relapsing polychondritis. Radiology 1978; 126:373–376
12. Nadel HR, Stringer DA, Levison H, Turner JA, Sturgess JM. The immotile cilia syndrome: radiological manifestations. Radiology 1985; 154:651–655
13. Nielsen K. A case of multiple tracheal diverticula. Acta Radiol 1948; 29:331–334
14. Surprenant EL, O'Loughlin BJ. Tracheal diverticula and tracheobronchomegaly. Dis Chest 1966; 49:345–351
15. Young RH, Sandstrom RE, Mark GJ. Tracheopathia osteoplastica: clinical, radiologic, and pathologic correlations. J Thorac Cardiovasc Surg 1980; 79:537–541

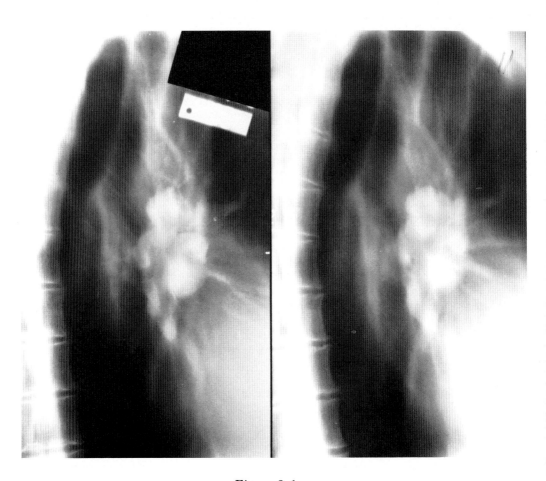

Figure 3-1

Case 3: 55° Oblique Hilar Tomography

Questions 8 through 12

For each of the numbered 55° oblique hilar tomograms shown (Figures 3-1 through 3-5), select the *one* lettered structure or diagnosis (Option A, B, C, D, or E) MOST closely associated with it. Each lettered structure or diagnosis may be selected once, more than once, or not at all.

  8. Figure 3-1. Left hilar tomogram
  9. Figure 3-2. Left hilar tomogram
 10. Figure 3-3. Left hilar tomogram
 11. Figure 3-4. Right hilar tomogram
 12. Figure 3-5. Left hilar tomogram

    (A) Hilar adenopathy
    (B) Superior pulmonary vein
    (C) Bronchogenic carcinoma with metastases
    (D) Endobronchial obstructive lesion
    (E) Prominent venous confluence

An understanding of normal anatomy (as presented in the discussion for Question 14) is important in diagnosing abnormalities of the hilum in the 55° oblique position.

Figure 3-1 shows 55° oblique tomograms of the left hilum at 10 and 11 cm above the tabletop. In this instance there are multiple convex masses in the bronchial angles with extension posteromedial to the left main bronchus, all consistent with left hilar adenopathy (Figure 3-6) **(Option (A) is the correct response to Question 8).** The adenopathy was due to sarcoidosis and was present bilaterally.

Normal hilar nodes are too small to be recognized as separate structures on oblique hilar tomograms.[4] Enlarged lymph nodes, on the other hand, may be recognized and differentiated from vessels in the bronchial angles and parabronchial areas.[1,8] Vascular structures occasionally confused with adenopathy in the upper and lower hilum are the superior and inferior pulmonary veins, respectively.[2,5] When these

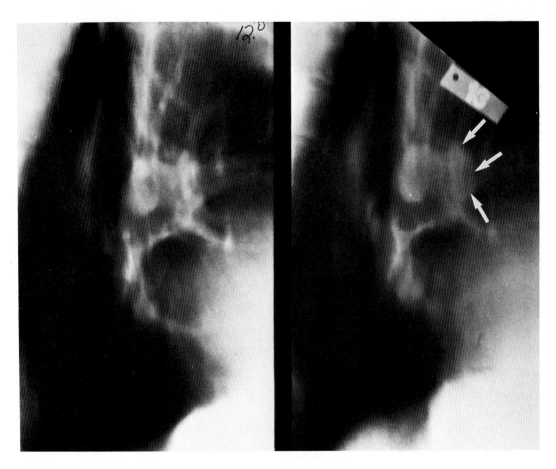

Figure 3-2

pulmonary veins are prominent, their branching pattern helps confirm their vascular nature. Enlarged lymph nodes have convex margins and appear dense, whereas vascular structures more frequently have straight margins and tend to be less dense. Vascular structures do not deform or alter the position of the bronchi, whereas lymph nodes, especially when large or infiltrative, may do so.

Often an enlarged node will be visible on only one tomographic level, so that careful inspection of all levels is mandatory. When nodes are only minimally enlarged, they may be obscured by overlying vascular shadows. For this reason, tomography in two projections should be considered a more complete study of the hilum. Computed tomography (CT) of the hilum with bolus intravenous administration of contrast

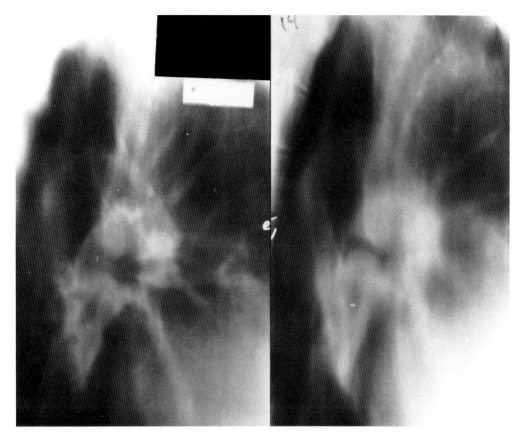

Figure 3-3

material may clearly differentiate confusing vascular shadows from enlarged nodes when necessary.

The presence of multiple enlarged hilar lymph nodes suggests several etiological possibilities. Bilateral symmetric hilar adenopathy, particularly when associated with paratracheal adenopathy, should strongly suggest sarcoidosis, especially if the patient is only mildly symptomatic or asymptomatic. The enlarged nodes tend to be of relatively uniform size in this disease. In only 5% of cases is the hilar adenopathy of sarcoidosis unilateral. On occasion, the bilateral adenopathy will be asymmetric. In such instances, differentiation from neoplasm is more difficult. Significant hilar node calcification occurs in approximately 5% of patients with sarcoidosis.

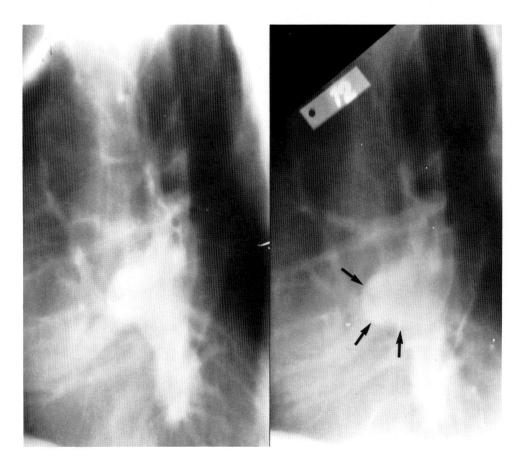

Figure 3-4

Metastasis, primary lung cancer (especially small-cell carcinoma), lymphoma, infection (most often granulomatous), and some pneumoconioses represent other etiologies of hilar adenopathy. The enlarged nodes in lung cancer frequently demonstrate indistinct margins and bronchial distortion due to tumor extension. If bilateral and due to lung cancer, lymphoma, or metastasis, the adenopathy is often asymmetric. Inflammatory adenopathy of granulomatous origin is more frequently unilateral. If long-standing, such adenopathy may calcify.

For comparison with the abnormal study shown in Figure 3-1, Figure 3-7 is an example of a normal right hilum seen with 55° oblique tomography at 11 and 12 cm above the tabletop. In this view, the bronchi are easily visualized framing the vascular complex of the right superior pulmonary vein and right pulmonary artery. Note that the bronchial

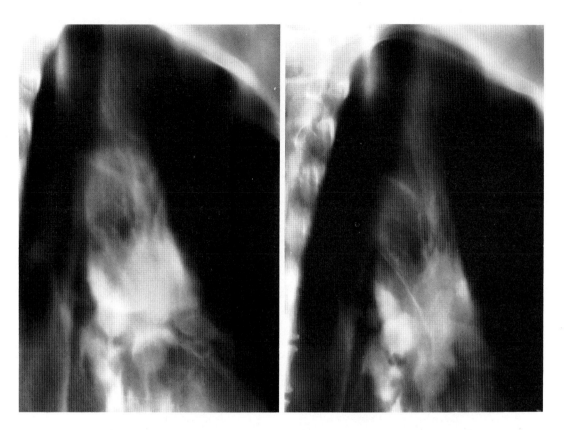

Figure 3-5

angles are empty and that the branching vascular structures are smooth, unlike the nodes that partially obscured vessels and occupied the bronchial angles in Figure 3-6.

The arrows in Figure 3-2 point to a portion of the left superior pulmonary vein as it courses along the apical-posterior segment of the left upper lobe bronchus **(Option (B) is the correct response to Question 9).** The branching nature of this shadow is better appreciated on the adjacent section.

Figures 3-8 and 3-9 are drawings of the 55° oblique left and right hilum, respectively. They illustrate the usual position of each superior pulmonary vein with respect to the ipsilateral pulmonary artery and bronchi. Dilated or prominent superior pulmonary veins, as they course along the hilum, may easily be confused with enlarged lymph nodes. On the left, the superior pulmonary vein arches anterior and lateral to the left upper lobe bronchus. Tomographically, the vein is usually not

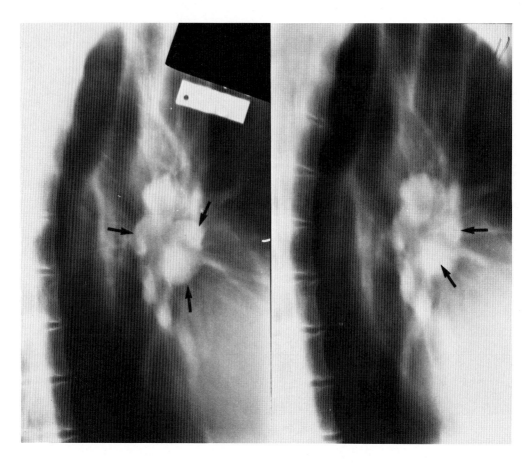

Figure 3-6 (Same as Figure 3-1). These two tomograms show multiple enlarged lymph nodes in the bronchial angles (arrows).

visualized beyond the junction of the left upper lobe bronchus with the left lower lobe bronchus. The vein is most often confused with an enlarged node: (1) lateral to the upper division of the left upper lobe bronchus; (2) in the angle between the upper and lower (lingular) divisions of the left upper lobe bronchus; and (3) sometimes in the angle between the left upper and left lower lobe bronchi.

On the right, the superior pulmonary vein arches along and overlaps the anterolateral margin of the right pulmonary artery. The vein and artery form a vascular complex, the lateral margin of which represents the vein. The complex is framed by the upper, intermediate, and middle lobe bronchi. The inferior aspect of the superior pulmonary vein, along with the middle lobe vein, may form a prominent confluence easily

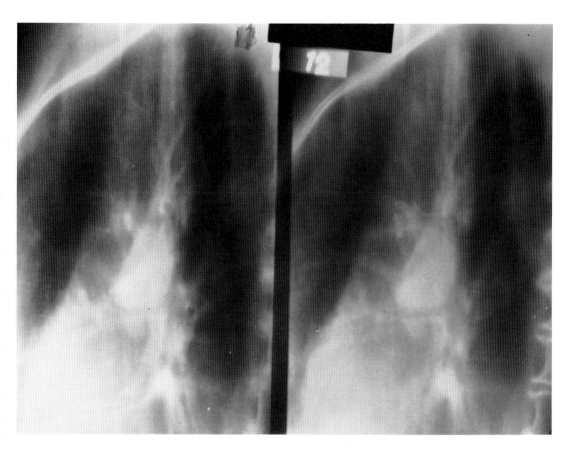

Figure 3-7. Normal 55° oblique tomograms of the right hilum. See text for description.

mistaken for a mass. At times this confluence will overlap the angle between the middle and lower lobe bronchi. The vascular complex formed by the right pulmonary artery and right superior pulmonary vein cannot be separated into its arterial and venous components where the vessels make contact. However, the identities of the artery and vein may be inferred from the direction and position of the respective branches of each. Careful attention to the branching nature of prominent vascular structures, as well as the use of at least one additional projection, will in most instances eliminate false-positive errors when searching for enlarged hilar nodes.

Figure 3-3 shows two 55° oblique tomographic levels of the left hilum, at 13 and 14 cm above the tabletop. In this case, there is an endobronchial

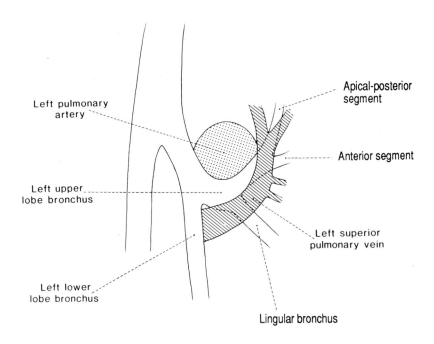

LEFT

Apical-posterior segment

Anterior segment

Left pulmonary artery

Left superior pulmonary vein

Left upper lobe bronchus

Left lower lobe bronchus

Lingular bronchus

Figure 3-8. This drawing of the left hilum in the 55° oblique position emphasizes the course of the left superior pulmonary vein and its relationship to the ipsilateral pulmonary artery and upper lobe bronchi. The arterial and bronchial anatomy have been simplified to focus attention on the vein.

carcinoid tumor obstructing the left lower lobe bronchus (Figure 3-10) **(Option (D) is the correct response to Question 10).** The tumor mass has a smooth, convex superior border and has caused left lower lobe collapse (Figure 3-11). A CT scan from the same patient shows that the mass protrudes into the distal left main bronchus (Figure 3-12).

A carcinoid tumor is by far the most common slowly growing neoplasm of the bronchi. It accounts for 80 to 90% of what were formerly termed bronchial adenomas and arises from cells of neuroectodermal origin. The majority of bronchial carcinoid tumors are found in the major bronchi and, as in this case, the carcinoid may present as a central endobronchial mass with lobar collapse or consolidation.[6] Approximately 10% of the time the tumor presents as a peripheral pulmonary nodule. Hilar tomograms are especially helpful in patients with "atypical" asthma, since an endobronchial lesion may be uncovered before it would become

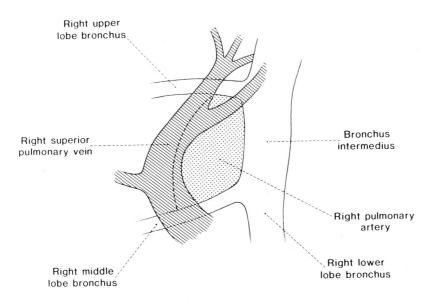

Figure 3-9. This drawing of the right hilum in the 55° oblique position emphasizes the course of the right superior pulmonary vein. Other structures have been simplified, as in Figure 3-8. Note the vascular complex of vein and artery as the vein passes lateral to the artery.

visible on a chest radiograph. Once peripheral infiltration, consolidation, or collapse has occurred, it is more difficult to visualize and characterize the obstructing lesion.[4]

Figure 3-4 shows two 55° oblique tomograms of the right hilum. The arrows indicate a prominent confluence formed by the right superior pulmonary vein and the middle lobe vein **(Option (E) is the correct response to Question 11).** The vascular nature of this structure may be ascertained by its branching characteristics on the adjacent tomographic level. While this confluence is somewhat more prominent than usual, the right superior pulmonary vein may normally become somewhat bulbous as it receives the middle lobe vein.

Figure 3-5 (55° oblique left hilar tomograms) demonstrates a large spiculated mass occupying the superior aspect of the left hilum and obstructing the apical-posterior bronchus of the left upper lobe. The mass bulges into the remaining visible portion of the left upper lobe bronchus

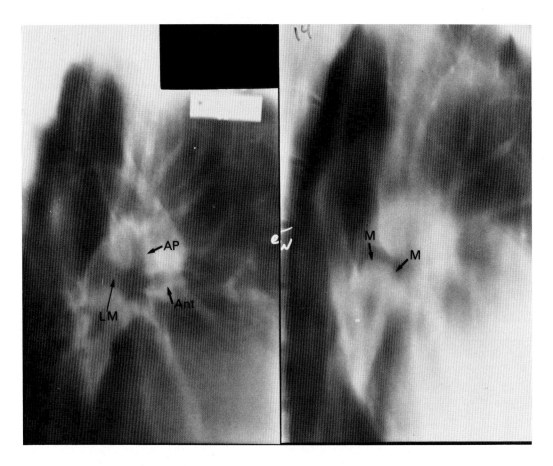

Figure 3-10. Same patient as in Figure 3-3. These two 55° oblique tomograms of the left hilum demonstrate the upper margin of an endobronchial mass (M) occluding the left lower lobe bronchus. The patent apical-posterior segmental bronchus (AP) and anterior segmental bronchus (Ant) of the left upper lobe bronchus are also visible. LM = left main bronchus.

(Figure 3-13). There are enlarged metastatic lymph nodes distorting the left main bronchus and occupying the angle between the left upper and lower lobe bronchi. The irregular nature of the mass, the enlarged adjacent nodes, and bronchial distortion and obstruction are all characteristic of bronchogenic carcinoma with metastases **(Option (C) is the correct response to Question 12).**

In the author's experience, approximately 25% of carcinomas at the hilum will present with a spiculated appearance similar to the

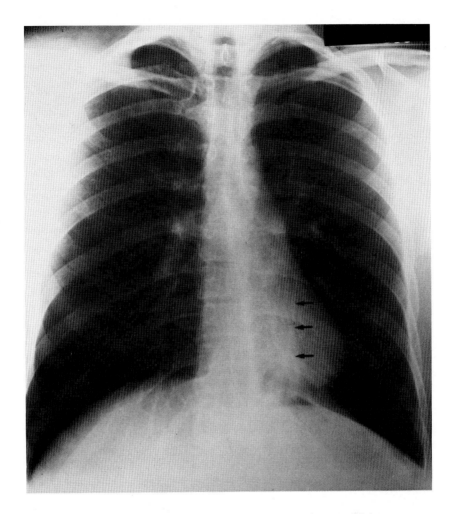

Figure 3-11. Same patient as in Figures 3-3 and 3-10. This posteroanterior chest radiograph shows left lower lobe collapse (arrows).

appearance of a scirrhous malignant neoplasm of the breast on a mammogram. Additionally, 75% of cases will demonstrate some abnormality of the tracheobronchial tree. A complete bronchial obstruction, with a tapered or "rat-tail" configuration, is highly suggestive of primary carcinoma. More commonly there are irregular narrowing and distortion of the affected bronchus. When such distortion occurs, it becomes difficult to evaluate for complete obstruction owing to the altered position of the bronchus.

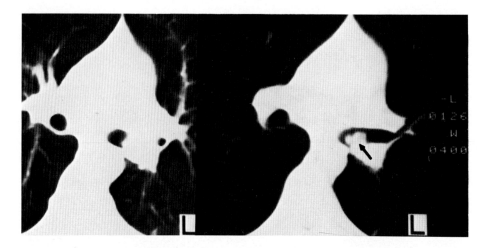

Figure 3-12. Same patient as in Figures 3-3, 3-10, and 3-11. The left lower lobe endobronchial mass (arrow) protrudes into the distal left main bronchus on the CT examination.

When a smooth rounded mass at a bronchial angle is diagnosed as carcinoma, it is more likely to be metastatic involvement of a node than a primary malignancy. The presence of enlarged nodes accompanying a malignant hilar mass is good evidence of regional metastases and is helpful in determining the stage of the neoplasm. Careful observation of the adjacent lung parenchyma during interpretation of hilar tomograms may reveal a primary mass that was not detected on posteroanterior and lateral conventional radiographs.

In the author's experience, nearly 40% of primary carcinomas at the hilum will contain some calcification, usually a few scattered flecks. These may be the result of engulfment of previously existing calcium by tumor. Any sparsely calcified hilar mass, particularly one that has a large soft tissue component, is potentially malignant.

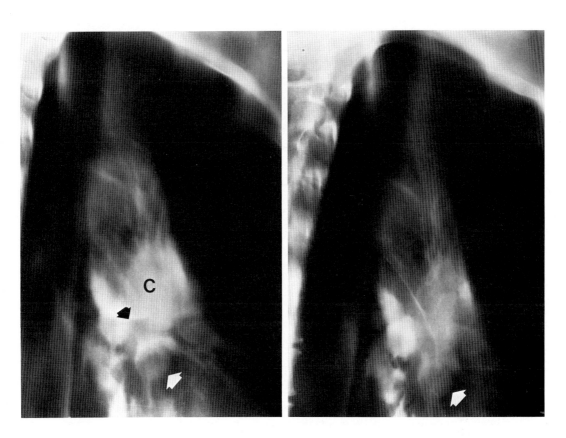

Figure 3-13 (Same as Figure 3-5). Two consecutive tomograms from a left 55° oblique hilar study show a spiculated bronchogenic carcinoma (C) obstructing the apical-posterior division (black arrowhead) of the left upper lobe bronchus. The rounded structures in the bronchial angles represent metastatic lymph nodes (white arrowheads).

Question 13

Concerning 55° oblique hilar tomography,

    (A) to study the left hilum, the patient's left side is closest to the tabletop
    (B) the x-ray tube is angled 55° posteriorly
    (C) the paramediastinal areas are well evaluated
    (D) a wedge filter is usually helpful in obtaining good-quality studies
    (E) the presence of a few flecks of calcium within a hilar mass excludes malignancy
    (F) nonvisualization of a bronchus indicates obstruction

Figure 3-14 illustrates the proper positioning for a 55° oblique tomogram of the left hilum. To study the left hilum, the patient's left side is closest to the tabletop **(Option (A) is true)**. The angle of 55° refers to the angle of the patient with respect to the horizontal line of the tabletop. The x-ray tube is not angled **(Option (B) is false)**. Ideally, each part of the lung and bronchial tree requires a different degree of positioning and angulation for optimal radiographic visualization. However, 55° of angulation represents a compromise and incorporates most of the pertinent anatomy. An additional tomographic projection (usually anteroposterior) is necessary for adequate evaluation of the paramediastinal areas **(Option (C) is false)** and other anatomic structures that superimpose with each other on the 55° oblique tomogram.

Technically, the 55° of angulation required for hilar tomograms is most consistently achieved by the construction of a 55° plywood block that is positioned under the patient (Figure 3-14). Linear rather than pluridirectional motion is preferred, primarily because structures such as bronchi and vessels outside the plane of focus are not totally blurred, allowing further appreciation of the relationship of hilar structures to each other.[7] If the anteroposterior projection is used for tomography, an aluminum wedge filter is of help (Figure 3-15). This apparatus allows sufficient exposure of the mediastinum while preventing overexposure of the adjacent lung and lateral hilar borders. It is not used in oblique hilar tomography **(Option (D) is false)**.

As discussed in relation to Question 12, the presence of a few flecks of calcium within a hilar mass does not exclude malignancy **(Option (E) is false)**.

Nonvisualization of a bronchus is not always evidence of obstruction. When markedly altered in caliber or position by tumor or inflammation, the bronchus may appear totally obstructed when in fact its lumen is patent at bronchoscopy **(Option (F) is therefore false)**.

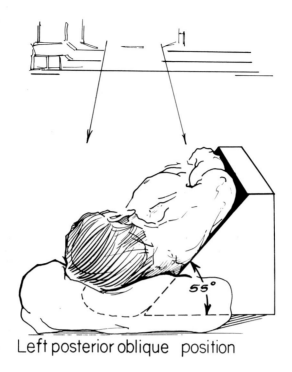

Left posterior oblique position

Figure 3-14. This diagram demonstrates the proper positioning for a 55°
left oblique hilar tomogram.

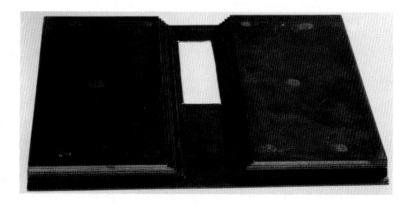

Figure 3-15. Aluminum wedge filter used for anteroposterior tomography.

Question 14

Concerning normal anatomy in 55° oblique hilar tomography,

    (A) the left pulmonary artery is located above the left upper lobe bronchus
    (B) the right inferior pulmonary vein is located anterior to the right hilum
    (C) the left superior pulmonary vein is located anterior to the left upper lobe bronchus
    (D) multiple large rounded structures in the bronchial angles represent arteries and veins
    (E) the middle lobe bronchus is usually too small to be visualized
    (F) major fissures are usually visualized
    (G) the azygos vein is less visible than on anteroposterior tomography

Genereux[5] describes the hilum as an imprecisely defined area between the mediastinum medially and the lung laterally. Through the hilum pass the bronchi, pulmonary and systemic arteries and veins, nerves, lymphatics, and lymph nodes. The main structures that are visible, however, are the bronchi and the pulmonary arteries and pulmonary veins.

In the usual situation, the main pulmonary artery branches at about the level of the carina into a shorter left pulmonary artery and a longer right pulmonary artery (Figure 3-16). The left pulmonary artery enters the hilum as a single vessel and arches over the left upper lobe bronchus. It gives rise to two or more small branches to the upper lobe and then descends as the interlobar and lower lobe arteries lateral to the left lower lobe bronchus. When the patient is turned into the 55° oblique position for left hilar tomography, the left pulmonary artery is visible above the left main and upper lobe bronchi (Figure 3-17). It is framed by the left upper lobe bronchus below it, the left main bronchus medial to it, and the apical-posterior bronchus lateral to it **(Option (A) is true).** This normal relationship in the left hilum is important to understand, since other rounded structures may be abnormal. The superior margin of the left pulmonary artery is smooth and round. On the right the pulmonary artery divides, before entering the hilum, into a smaller truncus anterior branch to the right upper lobe and a larger interlobar branch that descends along the lateral aspect of the bronchus intermedius. In the 55° right oblique position, the hilar right pulmonary artery is framed by the upper lobe bronchus superiorly, the intermediate bronchus medially, and the middle lobe bronchus inferiorly (Figures 3-7 and 3-18). The right hilar "pulmonary artery" appears oval.

As illustrated in Figure 3-8, the left superior pulmonary vein passes anterior to the left upper lobe bronchus **(Option (C) is true)** and

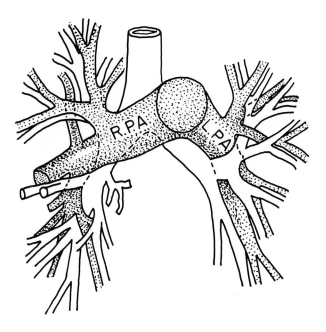

Figure 3-16. The normal pulmonary arteries and their relation to the tracheobronchial tree are illustrated in this diagram. R.P.A. = right pulmonary artery; L.P.A. = left pulmonary artery.

terminates near the angle between the left upper and lower lobe bronchi. The right superior pulmonary vein is visible primarily as a convexity along the lateral margin of the right pulmonary artery (Figure 3-9). The vein forms part of the vascular complex on the right (artery-vein) and cannot be easily separated from the right pulmonary artery. In fact, early drawings of this complex did not show the superior pulmonary vein.[1,4,8] Chasen is credited with describing the significant contribution of the superior pulmonary veins to the vascular shadows of each hilum.[2]

The left and right inferior pulmonary veins are positioned inferior and somewhat posterior to the main hilar structures on the 55° oblique hilar tomogram. They are seen almost end-on as bulbous structures (Figures 3-17 and 3-18) **(Option (B) is false).** When prominent, the inferior pulmonary vein may be mistaken for a mass.

The bronchial angles are usually clear. The presence of multiple large, rounded structures in these angles is good evidence of hilar adenopathy **(Option (D) is false).** As previously mentioned, hilar nodes of normal size are not visible on oblique tomography. Prominent veins visible in

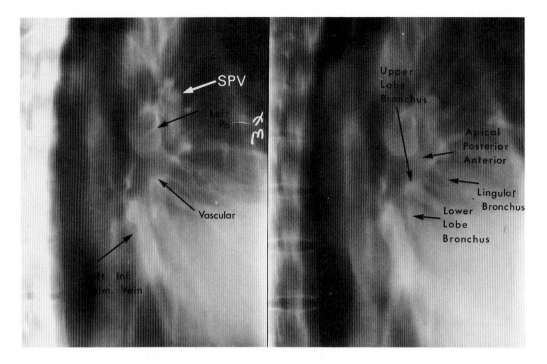

Figure 3-17. These two contiguous tomograms show normal 55° oblique left hilar anatomy. SPV = left superior pulmonary vein; Left Pa = left pulmonary artery; Left Inf. Pulm. Vein = left inferior pulmonary vein.

the bronchial angles on some sections undergo branching on adjacent sections, a helpful clue in distinguishing them from enlarged nodes.

The larger proximal bronchi, including the middle lobe bronchus, are easily visualized on 55° oblique hilar tomograms **(Option (E) is false).** On sections closer to the tabletop, a portion of the major fissure is usually visible **(Option (F) is true).**[4] This is helpful in localizing an area of pulmonary parenchymal abnormality, such as a nodule or an infiltrate, to the proper lobe. While the azygos vein may be seen on 55° oblique tomography, its size and position are more easily determined on the anteroposterior tomogram owing to removal of overlapping vascular shadows **(Option (G) is true).**

In evaluating the normal anatomy and pathology of the hilum, CT has become a popular technique often used instead of, or in addition to, hilar tomography. Each technique has its proponents.[1,4,5,8,9,11,12] Magnetic resonance imaging (MRI) recently also has been shown useful for detecting hilar and mediastinal adenopathy.[3] The advantage of CT over

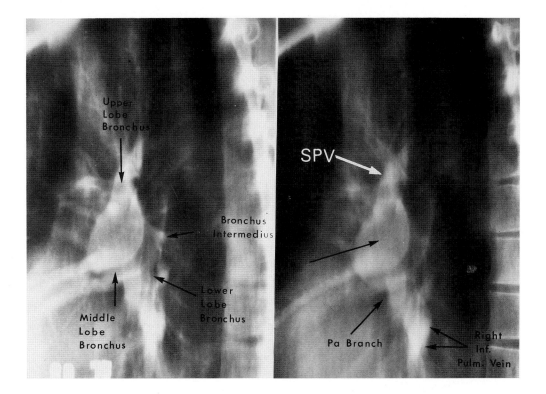

Figure 3-18. These two contiguous tomograms show normal 55° oblique right hilar anatomy. SPV = right superior pulmonary vein; Pa = right hilar pulmonary artery; Right Inf. Pulm. Vein = right inferior pulmonary vein.

oblique tomography lies in its ability to evaluate the mediastinum while studying the hilar structures. Disadvantages include the extra expense and time required for CT, as well as the small but definite risk of an intravenous contrast material reaction (contrast material is usually required for CT evaluation of the hila). Oblique tomography is inexpensive, requires no contrast material, and is easily adaptable to any radiologic practice. It is not as accurate as CT for evaluating the mediastinum, however.[10] With MRI, hilar and mediastinal vascular structures are easily differentiated from surrounding soft tissue structures. An added advantage of MRI is that sagittal, coronal, and transverse images may be easily obtained. Determination of the most accurate method of hilar evaluation is a topic of ongoing investigation.

SUGGESTED READINGS

1. Brown LR, DeRemee RA. 55° oblique hilar tomography. Mayo Clin Proc 1976; 51:89–95

2. Chasen MH, Yrizarry JM. Tomography of the pulmonary hili. Anatomical reassessment of the conventional 55° posterior oblique. Radiology 1983; 149:365–369

3. Cohen AM, Creviston S, LiPuma JP, Bryan PJ, Haaga JR, Alfidi RJ. NMR evaluation of hilar and mediastinal lymphadenopathy. Radiology 1983; 148:739–742

4. Favez G, Willa C, Heinzer F. Posterior oblique tomography at an angle of 55° in chest roentgenology. AJR 1974; 120:907–915

5. Genereux GP. Conventional tomographic hilar anatomy emphasizing the pulmonary veins. AJR 1983; 141:1241–1257

6. Greene R, McLoud TC, Stark P. Other malignant tumors of the lung. Semin Roentgenol 1977; 12:225–237

7. Matalon TA, Sakowicz BA, Mintzer RA, Panella JS, Lin P-JP, Claycamp HG. Pluridirectional versus linear motion in 55° oblique tomography of the pulmonary hilus. Appl Radiol 1982; 11(4):49–58

8. McLeod RA, Brown LR, Miller WE, DeRemee RA. Evaluation of the pulmonary hila by tomography. Radiol Clin North Am 1976; 14:51–84

9. Naidich DP, Khouri NF, Stitik FP, McCauley DI, Siegelman SS. Computed tomography of the pulmonary hila: 2. Abnormal anatomy. J Comput Assist Tomogr 1981; 5:468–475

10. Osborne DR, Korobkin M, Ravin CE, et al. Comparison of plain radiography, conventional tomography, and computed tomography in detecting intrathoracic lymph node metastases from lung carcinoma. Radiology 1982; 142:157–161

11. Sone S, Higashihara T, Morimoto S, et al. CT anatomy of hilar lymphadenopathy. AJR 1983; 140:887–892

12. Webb RW, Glazer G, Gamsu G. Computed tomography of the normal pulmonary hilum. J Comput Assist Tomogr 1981; 5:476–484

Notes

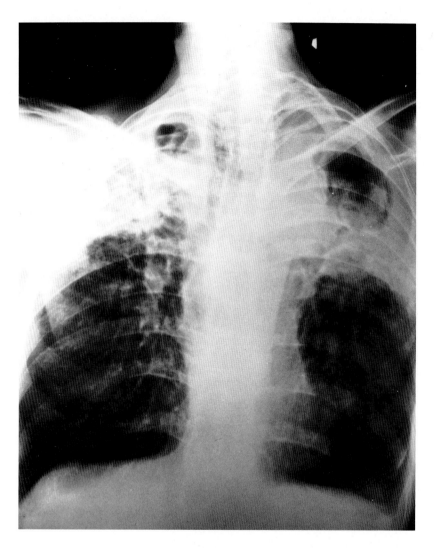

Figure 4-1
Figures 4-1 and 4-2. This 60-year-old man has a history of recurrent pneumonias. You are shown posteroanterior (Figure 4-1) and lateral (Figure 4-2) chest radiographs.

Case 4: Ankylosing Spondylitis

Question 15

The constellation of radiographic findings seen in Figures 4-1 and 4-2 is BEST explained by which *one* of the following?

(A) Sarcoidosis
(B) Atypical mycobacterial infection
(C) Silicosis
(D) Collagen vascular disease
(E) Semi-invasive aspergillus infection

Figures 4-1 and 4-2 demonstrate a variety of radiographic abnormalities. The upper lobes are retracted, with hilar elevation, and show bullous changes. There is an appearance of a left upper lobe cavity with surrounding pleural thickening. A mass lies within this cavity; this was confirmed on an anteroposterior tomogram (Figure 4-3). There are bony changes of the thoracic spine, visible on the lateral radiograph, consistent with ankylosing spondylitis (Figure 4-2). This combination of radiographic findings (pulmonary and thoracic bony changes of long-standing ankylosing spondylitis, a collagen vascular disease, complicated by a fungus ball) makes collagen vascular disease the best answer **(Option (D) is correct).** Sarcoidosis (Option (A)), atypical mycobacterial infection (Option (B)), silicosis (Option (C)), and semi-invasive aspergillus infection (Option (E)) are all examples of diseases which may share one or more of the radiographic findings shown in Figures 4-1 and 4-2. However, with the bony changes of ankylosing spondylitis, none of these other options is the best choice.

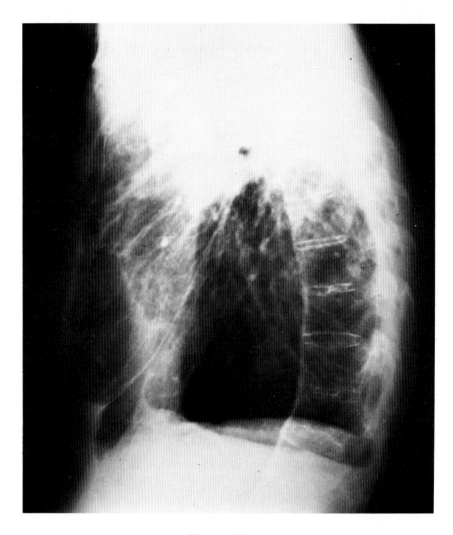

Figure 4-2

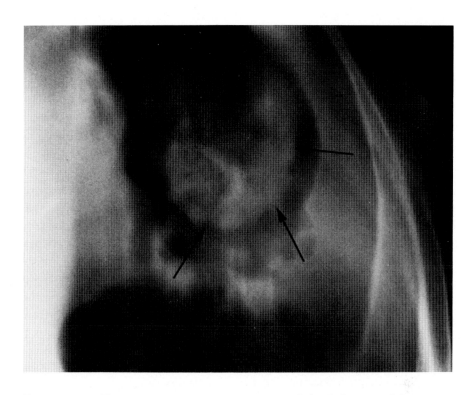

Figure 4-3. This anteroposterior tomogram of the left upper lobe cavity demonstrates an intracavitary mass (fungus ball) (arrows).

Question 16

Regarding cystic and fibrobullous changes in the upper lobes,

(A) progressive adjacent pleural thickening usually indicates complicating malignancy

(B) hemoptysis is common in uncomplicated cases

(C) allergic bronchopulmonary aspergillosis is a common complication

(D) tomography is frequently helpful in the diagnosis of mycetomas

Fibrobullous cystic changes in the upper lobes are an irreversible process resulting from destruction of lung parenchyma and subsequent fibrous repair. The hila are often retracted superiorly, and there is reduction in upper lung volume. Such findings are most commonly due to healed or healing granulomatous infections caused by typical or atypical mycobacteria or fungi. Other, more common noninfectious processes include chronic pulmonary sarcoidosis and ankylosing spondylitis.

Residual cysts or cavities in the upper lobes frequently harbor one or more intracavitary mycetomas (fungus balls), which grow in a noninvasive saprophytic manner. Mycetomas most commonly are caused by *Aspergillus fumigatus*,[13] although other fungi are occasionally responsible.[12] The appearance of progressive pleural thickening adjacent to residual cysts or cavities often accompanies or precedes the development of an intracavitary fungus ball.[14] Thus, any new pleural thickening should be regarded as suggestive of early mycetoma rather than malignancy **(Option (A) is false)**. Hemoptysis (potentially fatal) is a feature of an intracavitary fungus ball complicating a residual cavity or cyst in the upper lobes. While hemoptysis may occasionally occur secondary to upper lobe bronchiectasis with fibrobullous changes, it is more commonly associated with the complication of mycetoma **(Option (B) is false)**.

Allergic bronchopulmonary aspergillosis is a hypersensitivity disease of the lungs and is not considered a complication of upper lobe fibrobullous/cystic disease **(Option (C) is therefore false)**.

While mycetomas may be visible with conventional radiography, tomography is often helpful in demonstrating an air ring or meniscus around the fungus ball to confirm the diagnosis **(Option (D) is true)**. An additional helpful radiographic clue to mycetoma is the change in position of the intracavitary mass with changes in the patient's position (e.g., decubitus views).

Question 17

Concerning silicosis,

- (A) most small opacities are found in the mid- and lower lung zones
- (B) radiographically, it is classified as "complicated" only if an opacity larger than 3 cm is detected
- (C) cavitation due to infection of a conglomerate mass is most often caused by fungal disease
- (D) a diffuse bilateral alveolar pattern on the chest radiograph indicates the advanced chronic form
- (E) conglomerate masses begin centrally and migrate peripherally

Silicosis results when the inhalation of silica over a prolonged period of time, or in high enough concentration, produces fibrotic lung disease. In the simple form of the disease, "small rounded opacities" are the major radiographic feature. They are found predominantly in the upper lung zones[19] **(Option (A) is false)**. The small rounded opacities have been classified arbitrarily into three sizes on the basis of their diameter. The "p" opacities are up to 1.5 mm in diameter, the "q" opacities are 1.5 to 3 mm in diameter, and the "r" opacities are 3 to 10 mm in diameter.[9] These opacities constitute what is termed "simple" pneumoconiosis. If any opacity becomes larger than 1 cm, the pneumoconiosis is termed "complicated" **(Option (B) is false)**. Infrequently, silicosis may show "small irregular opacities" ("s", "t", and "u"), but these are seen more commonly in asbestosis, where they are predominantly found in the lower lung zones.

The massive fibrotic lesions (conglomerate masses) of silicosis usually develop within the upper lung zones. They incorporate the small rounded opacities and also contain obliterated blood vessels and bronchi.[19] These conglomerate masses appear as large (greater than 1 cm) homogeneous areas of opacity. As they enlarge, they migrate from the periphery of the lung toward the hila centrally **(Option (E) is false)**. Their medial margin tends to be unsharp, while their lateral margin is sharply etched by adjacent emphysematous lung. Conglomerate masses may cavitate, owing to infection or ischemia. Infection is the most common cause of cavitation and is usually the result of tuberculosis[7] **(Option (C) is false)**.

Acute silicosis results from exposure to high concentrations of silica, usually in confined spaces. The disease develops quickly, within a year or two of exposure. Pathologically, the alveolar walls are thickened by fibrous tissue, while the alveolar spaces are filled with an acidophilic alveolar fluid containing desquamated cells and fine granules. The intra-alveolar fluid is rich in lipids and proteins and gives a strongly positive periodic acid-Schiff reaction. This has led some observers to term this process alveolar silicolipoproteinosis. The principal radiographic feature is the presence of a diffuse alveolar pattern resembling alveolar proteinosis. This pattern is, therefore, not characteristic of *chronic* silicosis **(Option (D) is false).** Acute silicosis is usually fatal.[4]

Question 18

Concerning semi-invasive aspergillosis,

(A) it usually is preceded by cavities
(B) mycetomas are a feature
(C) it is associated with mild immunosuppression
(D) mucoid impaction is a common feature

Pulmonary aspergillosis may occur in several forms: (1) A noninvasive saprophytic form in which mycetomas (fungus balls) populate pre-existing cystic or cavitary spaces (Figure 4-3) primarily found in the upper lobes. (2) An invasive primary form in which aspergillus pneumonitis develops in an otherwise immunocompetent and healthy individual. This is a rare manifestation of the disease characterized by a necrotizing, frequently fatal pneumonitis. Massive exposure to aspergillus spores has been reported in several of the cases.[16] (3) An invasive secondary form which is a serious, often fatal, infection occurring in patients on immunosuppressive therapy or with chronic malignant or nonmalignant debilitating disease. (4) An allergic bronchopulmonary aspergillosis form characterized by asthma, blood and sputum eosinophilia, mucous plugs, proximal bronchiectasis, mucoid impaction, and allergic pneumonitis. These patients manifest immunologic reactivity to the aspergillus antigen.

It has recently been recognized that in addition to the above traditional classification, pulmonary aspergillosis may also exist in a form intermediate between the saprophytic and invasive ones. This form, termed semi-invasive pulmonary aspergillosis, results from aspergillus infection that produces lung necrosis despite the lack of vascular invasion.[3,8] This process often shows pulmonary consolidation early in the disease, followed by a well-developed cavity with or without the subsequent formation of an intracavitary mycetoma **(Option (B) is**

true). The absence of previous cavitation allows the distinction from the saprophytic form **(Option (A) is false)**.

In the cases reported by Gefter et al.,[8] semi-invasive pulmonary aspergillosis occurred in the clinical setting of mild immunosuppression or fibrotic noncavitary underlying pulmonary disease. Clinical conditions included malignancy, diabetes mellitus, noncavitary sarcoidosis, low-dose steroid therapy, and radiation fibrosis **(Option (C) is true)**. Mucoid impaction is not a manifestation of this form of aspergillosis, unlike the allergic bronchopulmonary form **(Option (D) is therefore false)**.

Other unusual reported manifestations of aspergillosis include allergic bronchopulmonary aspergillosis and fungus balls terminating in disseminated aspergillosis and an allergic bronchopulmonary aspergillosis-like syndrome consequent to aspergilloma.[1,6]

Discussion

Ankylosing spondylitis, an arthropathy of unknown cause, predominantly affects the synovial joints of the spine, including the articulating facets of the vertebrae and the costovertebral and sacroiliac joints. Ossification of the spinal ligaments is a major feature of the disease. Peripheral joint disease occurs in 20 to 35% of cases. Extra-articular manifestations include cor pulmonale, cardiomegaly, pericarditis, aortitis, iritis, and amyloidosis in chronic cases.[2,5]

Pleuropulmonary involvement is a less well known but important extraskeletal expression of this disease. The frequency of pleuropulmonary involvement in ankylosing spondylitis varies from 0 to 30% in published reports. In a review of the records of 2,080 patients with ankylosing spondylitis seen at the Mayo Clinic between 1966 and 1975, Rosenow et al.[17] reported that 28 (1.3%) had pleuropulmonary manifestations. All 28 patients were men, and the mean age was 60 years. The average interval between onset of disease and the radiographic appearance of pleuropulmonary involvement was 21 years. Spondylitis always preceded the development of pleuropulmonary disease, by which time the spondylitis was usually inactive. Chest expansion was decreased, implying bony ankylosis of the costovertebral articulations of the thoracic spine. In the series by Chakera et al.[5] there was a striking correlation between the radiographic extent of spinal involvement and pulmonary fibrotic changes.

The etiology of the pleuropulmonary disease is not known. Hamilton,[10] who first described the association in 1949, concluded that impaired respiratory mechanisms (especially an ineffective cough mechanism) predisposed these patients to nonspecific infections that, in some cases, eventually produced fibrosis and destruction of the upper lobes. While infectious organisms have been suspected as causing the pulmonary disease, none has been found. The association of the histocompatibility antigen HLA-B27 in nearly 90% of patients with ankylosing spondylitis provides evidence for a genetic predisposition to the disease.[18] It is unknown whether this genetic predisposition extends to the extra-articular manifestations of the disease as well.[15]

The most common pleuropulmonary radiographic finding in ankylosing spondylitis is the presence of fibrobullous changes in the upper lobes (26 of 28 patients in the Mayo Clinic series).[17] It is thought that initially there is a fibronodular appearance with pleural thickening at one or both apices. Later, small cysts or bullae form; these sometimes are visible only on tomography. The cysts may enlarge, and the upper lobes may become fibrotic with upward displacement of the hila. This process may progress or may remain stable for many years.

The upper lobe fibrous and bullous/cystic findings are often asymptomatic, unless complicated by mycetomas. Secondary involvement of the cystic spaces with aspergillus or, occasionally, with other organisms may occur. In the case of mycetoma formation, often both pleural thickening adjacent to the cystic cavity and thickening of the cavity wall herald the onset of fungus ball development within. Hemoptysis may imply development of an intracavitary mycetoma. In the series by Rosenow et al.,[17] 5 of 28 patients had mycetomas.

Other occasional manifestations of pleuropulmonary disease in ankylosing spondylitis include pleural effusion and pneumothorax. The histologic features of the pleuropulmonary disease, according to Jessamine,[11] consist of interalveolar fibrosis obliterating alveoli along with foamy macrophages in the persisting alveoli. Fragmentation of elastic tissue, degeneration of collagen, areas of hyalinization, and foci of lymphocytic infiltration occur within the lung.

Since the fibrobullous changes are often asymptomatic, treatment for uncomplicated upper lobe disease is usually not necessary. The treatment of mycetomas has not been standardized. In cases of severe hemoptysis, surgery is often necessary but may frequently be complicated by bronchopleural fistulas. Other forms of treatment consist of systemic or intracavitary antifungal drugs or systemic steroids. These agents have been used with mixed success.

SUGGESTED READINGS

1. Anderson CJ, Craig S, Bardana EJ Jr. Allergic bronchopulmonary aspergillosis and bilateral fungal balls terminating in disseminated aspergillosis. J Allergy Clin Immunol 1980; 65:140–144
2. Appelrouth D, Gottlieb NL. Pulmonary manifestations of ankylosing spondylitis. J Rheumatol 1975; 2:446–453
3. Binder RE, Faling LJ, Pugatch RD, Mahasaen C. Chronic necrotizing pulmonary aspergillosis: a discrete clinical entity. Medicine 1982; 60:109–124
4. Buechner HA, Ansari A. Acute silicoproteinosis: a new pathological variant of acute silicosis in sandblasters, characterized by histologic features resembling alveolar proteinosis. Dis Chest 1969; 55:274–284
5. Chakera TM, Howarth FH, Kendall MJ, Lawrence DS, Whitfield AG. The chest radiograph in ankylosing spondylitis. Clin Radiol 1975; 26:455–459
6. Ein ME, Wallace RJ Jr, Williams TW Jr. Allergic bronchopulmonary aspergillosis-like syndrome consequent to aspergilloma. Am Rev Respir Dis 1979; 119:811–820
7. Fraser RG, Paré JAP. Diagnosis of diseases of the chest, 2nd ed. Philadelphia: WB Saunders; 1978:1484–1502
8. Gefter WB, Weingrad TR, Epstein DM, Ochs RH, Miller WT. "Semi-invasive" pulmonary aspergillosis: a new look at the spectrum of aspergillus infections of the lung. Radiology 1981; 140:313–321
9. Guidelines for the use of ILO international classification of radiographs of pneumoconiosis. Occupational Safety and Health Series (No. 22). Geneva: International Labor Office, 1980:1–48
10. Hamilton KA. Pulmonary disease manifestations of ankylosing spondylarthritis. Ann Intern Med 1949; 31:216–227
11. Jessamine AG. Upper lung lobe fibrosis in ankylosing spondylitis. Can Med Assoc J 1968; 98:25–29
12. Katz AS, Naidech HJ, Malhotra P. The air meniscus as a radiographic finding: a review of the literature and presentation of nine unusual cases. CRC Crit Rev Diagn Imaging 1978; 11:167–183
13. Klein DL, Gamsu G. Thoracic manifestations of aspergillosis. AJR 1980; 134:543–552
14. Libshitz HI, Atkinson GW, Israel HL. Pleural thickening as a manifestation of aspergillus superinfection. AJR 1974; 120:883–886
15. Luthra HS. Extra-articular manifestations of ankylosing spondylitis (Editorial). Mayo Clin Proc 1977; 52:655–656
16. Roselle GA, Kauffman GA. Case report: invasive pulmonary aspergillosis in a nonimmunosuppressed patient. Am J Med Sci 1978; 276:357–361
17. Rosenow E, Strimlan CV, Muhm JR, Ferguson RH. Pleuropulmonary manifestations of ankylosing spondylitis. Mayo Clin Proc 1977; 52:641–649
18. Schlosstein L, Terasaki PI, Bluestone R, Pearson CM. High association of an HL-A antigen, W27, with ankylosing spondylitis. N Engl J Med 1973; 288:704–706
19. Ziskind M, Jones RN, Weill H. Silicosis. Am Rev Respir Dis 1976; 113:643–665

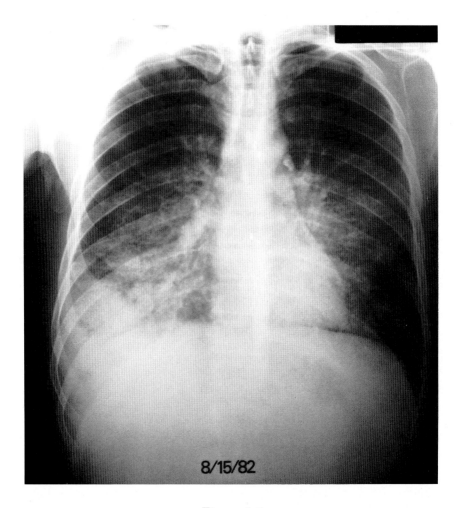

8/15/82

Figure 5-1
Figures 5-1 through 5-3. This 20-year-old man had a 6-month history of mild dyspnea on exertion. No specific treatment was given. You are shown a series of posteroanterior chest radiographs.

Case 5: Alveolar Proteinosis

Question 19

Which *one* of the following is the MOST likely diagnosis?

(A) Bronchioloalveolar cell carcinoma
(B) Hydrostatic pulmonary edema
(C) Lymphoma
(D) Alveolar proteinosis
(E) Pulmonary hemorrhage

The initial chest radiograph of 15 August 1982 (Figure 5-1) demonstrates a diffuse, poorly marginated, bilateral perihilar and right lower lobe process. Close-up views of the right and left bases (Figures 5-4 and 5-5, respectively) from the same study show a fluffy parenchymal abnormality on either side, an area of consolidation at the right costophrenic angle, and air bronchograms. These findings are consistent with a predominantly alveolar or air-space process. Follow-up radiographs approximately 1 and 3 months later (Figures 5-2 and 5-3, respectively) demonstrate slow but definite resolution of the abnormality. The long duration is consistent with a chronic alveolar process, and the resolution without treatment favors a benign condition. Of the choices offered in Question 19, only alveolar proteinosis would most likely demonstrate all of these features (**Option (D) is the most likely diagnosis**).

A chronic, predominantly alveolar pattern may be seen in several disease states. Some common ones, in addition to alveolar proteinosis, are bronchioloalveolar cell carcinoma, lymphoma, and sarcoidosis. Other, less common entities that are chronic and that may have somewhat of an alveolar appearance, although they may or may not primarily involve the air spaces pathologically, include alveolar microlithiasis, desquamative interstitial pneumonitis, lymphocytic interstitial pneumonitis, hair spray pneumonia, mineral oil and lipoid pneumonia, tuberculosis, and fungal disease.[5,8,20]

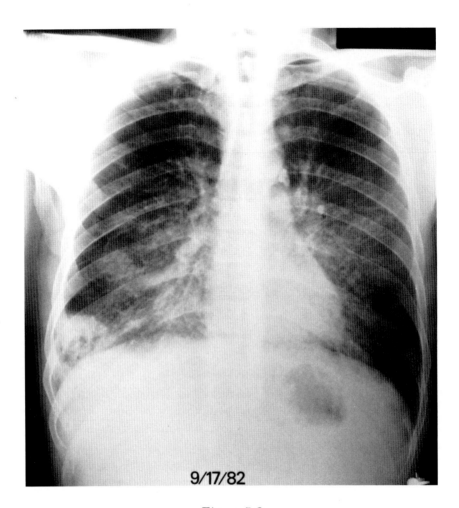

9/17/82

Figure 5-2

Bronchioloalveolar cell carcinoma has a varied appearance. It may present as a single nodule, multiple ill-defined nodules, a focal alveolar process, or a multifocal alveolar process. The radiographic manifestations of the disseminated form reflect its natural history, which consists of a progression from nodules that coalesce to simulate areas of air-space consolidation.[2] While bronchioloalveolar cell carcinoma could conceivably have an appearance identical to that in Figure 5-1, the subsequent improvement of the alveolar process without treatment (Figures 5-2 and 5-3) excludes the possibility of this diagnosis (Option (A) is, therefore, not likely).

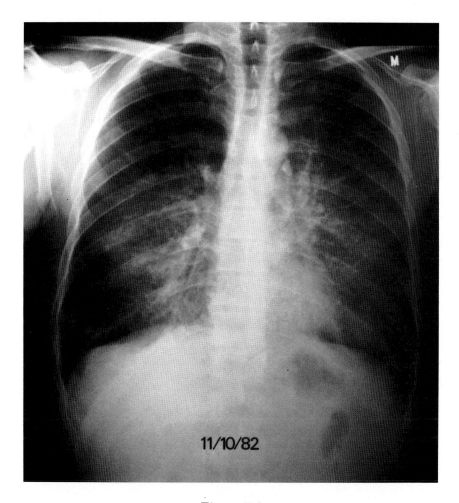

11/10/82

Figure 5-3

Of the choices offered in Question 19, hydrostatic pulmonary edema is the most common cause of a widespread alveolar process. However, it would be unlikely in a young patient without cardiomegaly but with a long-term history. Therefore, hydrostatic pulmonary edema (Option (B)) is not the most likely diagnosis. Primary pulmonary lymphoma, pathologically interstitial in location, may appear radiographically as an alveolar process. Here again, however, regression without treatment makes lymphoma (Option (C)) an unlikely diagnosis.

Pulmonary hemorrhage, like hydrostatic pulmonary edema, is an acute alveolar process. Blood floods the alveoli and small airways. Radiographically, the process waxes and wanes much more rapidly than the example

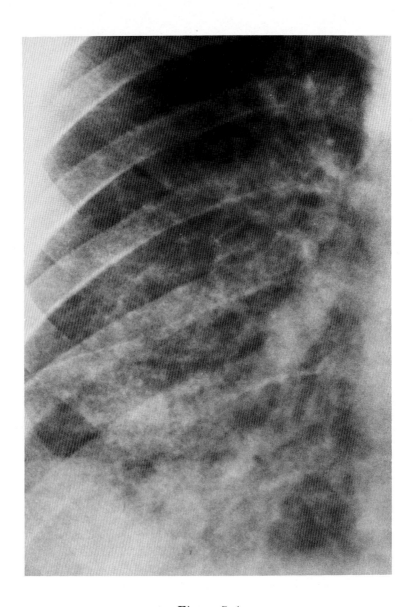

Figure 5-4
Figures 5-4 and 5-5. Close-up views of the right (Figure 5-4) and left
(Figure 5-5) bases of the patient in Figure 5-1. The findings indicate an
alveolar (air-space) process (see text for description).

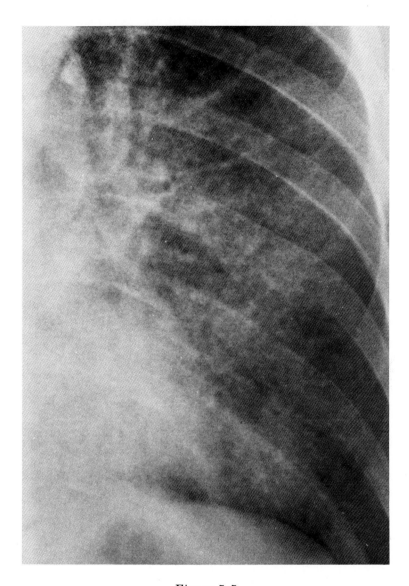

Figure 5-5

shown in Figures 5-1 to 5-3. Therefore, pulmonary hemorrhage (Option (E)) is unlikely.

While all of the conditions listed in Question 19 may manifest a diffuse bilateral alveolar pattern, a knowledge of additional clinical information and the natural history of each disease is very helpful in distinguishing the various disorders. In chronic alveolar processes, lung biopsy may be necessary to obtain a definitive diagnosis.

Question 20

Conditions that can appear alveolar but primarily involve the interstitium include:

    (A) microlithiasis
    (B) lobar pneumonia
    (C) sarcoidosis
    (D) primary pulmonary lymphoma

Of the four options listed in Question 20, the pathologic abnormalities of sarcoidosis and primary pulmonary lymphoma are primarily interstitial in location, although radiographically they may appear alveolar **(Options (C) and (D) are therefore true)**. Pulmonary alveolar microlithiasis is a rare disease, of unknown etiology, in which calcium phosphate microliths are deposited throughout the lungs in the alveolar spaces with sparing of the interstitium[14] **(Option (A) is false)**. Lobar pneumonia in the classic sense is an acute bacterial infection, most often pneumococcal in origin, with involvement of a large portion of a lobe or an entire lobe. It consists of a widespread exudate filling alveoli, with resultant radiographic consolidation. It is primarily an alveolar process pathologically **(Option (B) is false)**.

With regard to alveolar sarcoidosis, an air-space pattern with air bronchograms may be seen in approximately 5% of patients who exhibit parenchymal abnormalities. Interstitial noncaseating granulomas become densely packed and extensive enough to crowd the distal air spaces while leaving adjacent bronchi patent, producing air bronchograms. Obstruction of distal airways with secretions may also cause alveolar filling and result in an alveolar pattern radiographically.[18]

Primary pulmonary lymphoma is thought to arise within lymphoid aggregates of the pulmonary interstitium. It is, therefore, a purely interstitial process pathologically. As the interstitial neoplastic process expands, it replaces broad areas of pulmonary parenchyma and, thus, may radiographically appear as an air-space process. Lymphoma, when extensive, may cause cellular debris within the alveolar spaces.[1,7,10,21]

It is apparent from the above discussion that, in some cases, recognition of an interstitial disease that radiographically simulates air-space disease may be difficult. Hence, when an alveolar-appearing process slowly progresses, a chronic advanced interstitial process, such as sarcoidosis or primary pulmonary lymphoma, must be considered.

Question 21

Hallmarks of an alveolar pattern on the chest radiograph include:

    (A) ill-defined vessels
    (B) air bronchograms
    (C) fluffy margins
    (D) segmental or lobar distribution
    (E) small irregular shadows

Felson[6] has described the typical radiographic signs of alveolar disease. These include fluffy margins, early coalescence, segmental or lobar distribution, butterfly or bat-wing pattern, air bronchograms or air alveolograms, and rapid timing **(Options (B), (C), and (D) are therefore true)**. While there may be an alveolar component to an interstitial process, ill-defined pulmonary vessels and small irregular shadows are generally recognized as indicative of an interstitial process **(Options (A) and (E) are false)**.

Ziskind et al.[22] have described the acinar "nodule" in alveolar disease. The acinus is a unit of lung made up of a terminal bronchiole and all that is distal to it, including several orders of respiratory bronchioles, alveolar ducts, atria, alveolar sacs, and alveoli. The presence of acinar filling creates a radiographic "nodule" with fluffy margins (the acinar nodule). Some authors have suggested that the radiographic acinar nodule represents a focal peribronchiolar exudate, not acinar filling.[17]

While a diffuse, purely alveolar process can usually be recognized, the alveolar pattern in some pulmonary processes coexists with other patterns. An example is pulmonary edema secondary to congestive heart failure. Initially, the interstitial edema is manifested by Kerley lines and other well-known radiographic signs of interstitial disease. Later, combined interstitial and alveolar edema may be evident. When alveolar edema is "full-blown," the interstitial pattern may be masked by the superimposed air-space edema, since air is not present in the air spaces to outline the thickened interstitial structures.

Question 22

Concerning alveolar proteinosis,

    (A) the infiltrate consists primarily of intra-alveolar red blood cells and a variable number of chronic inflammatory cells

    (B) the infiltrate is caused by an antigen-antibody reaction in the pulmonary capillary

    (C) the severity of the radiographic appearance correlates closely with the clinical condition of the patient

    (D) the radiographic appearance is identical in adults and children

    (E) the radiographic appearance changes rapidly

Alveolar proteinosis is a chronic disease of the lungs characterized by the deposition, within the lumina of the distal air spaces, of periodic acid–Schiff-positive granular and floccular proteinaceous material rich in lipids. Little if any inflammatory reaction is associated, and red blood cells are not a characteristic component of the intra-alveolar material[19] **(Option (A) is false).** No identifiable etiology has been demonstrated **(Option (B) is also false).** Many authors believe that the disease represents a nonspecific response of the lung to an exogenous or endogenous insult.

The radiographic findings correlate quite poorly with the severity of respiratory impairment or the presence or absence of respiratory symptoms[16] **(Option (C) is therefore false).**

While in adults the radiographic appearance is usually that of a diffuse alveolar process, in children it is usually that of a reticulonodular, interstitial, or miliary process.[12,16] However, the disease is rare in childhood. McCook et al.[12] report that these small nodular opacities represent acini filled with periodic acid–Schiff-positive eosinophilic material. They postulate that the gradual increase in acinar size from birth to maturity may explain why small miliary nodules and a reticulonodular pattern are seen in children as opposed to the air-space or "pulmonary edema" pattern present in adulthood **(Option (D) is therefore false).**

All patterns of alveolar proteinosis are chronic in nature. Resolution occurs slowly over a period of weeks to months **(Option (E) is false).**

Question 23

Concerning pulmonary hemorrhage,

(A) when it occurs in the idiopathic form, it frequently results in marked, radiographically visible chronic interstitial changes
(B) when it occurs in the Goodpasture syndrome, hemoptysis is a frequent feature
(C) it occurs infrequently in patients given anticoagulants
(D) it is found as a manifestation of lupus erythematosus

Pulmonary hemorrhage is another type of acute air-space disease. In fact, the three main categories of acute air-space disease are infection, pulmonary edema, and pulmonary hemorrhage. When diffuse, the three cannot be separated solely on radiographic grounds.

The etiologies of pulmonary hemorrhage are extremely diverse and difficult to classify. Among the more common ones are lung contusion and laceration; aspiration of blood from large airway lesions; pulmonary embolism; hemorrhagic diatheses; granulomatous lesions, such as tuberculosis and fungal disease; neoplasms; and congestive heart failure. Less common etiologies include the Goodpasture syndrome, idiopathic pulmonary hemosiderosis, collagen vascular disease, and pulmonary vasculitis.[9]

Radiographically, diffuse hemorrhage often results in confluent, poorly marginated air-space disease often associated with air bronchograms, air alveolograms, acinar nodules, and a butterfly or bat-wing appearance. The process tends to wax and wane relatively rapidly. Pathologically, there is a massive accumulation of red blood cells in the alveolar spaces. The red blood cells are cleared by macrophages, which migrate to the interstitium. If hemorrhage is recurrent, this process will frequently result in mild interstitial fibrosis.

Determination of the etiology of pulmonary hemorrhage, once diagnosed, may be aided by the clinical history if from one of the more common causes. On the other hand, the etiology of diffuse microvascular pulmonary hemorrhage in immune and idiopathic disorders (i.e., the "alveolar hemorrhage syndromes") may be difficult to determine. Leatherman et al.[11] have described examples of these disorders, which include: (1) anti-basement membrane antibody disease (the Goodpasture syndrome), (2) idiopathic pulmonary hemorrhage, (3) systemic lupus erythematosus, and (4) several of the systemic vasculitides.

Anti-basement membrane antibody disease is probably the most common of the alveolar hemorrhage syndromes. The antibody binds specifically to basement membrane antigens of the alveolus, glomerulus, renal tubule, and choroid plexus. The disease occurs most often between 16 and 30 years of age and is twice as common in male patients as in female patients. The main clinical features are pulmonary hemorrhage and glomerulonephritis, and patients usually present because of their lung involvement. Hemoptysis is common, occurring in 80% of cases **(Option (B) is true)**. Other symptoms and signs include exertional dyspnea, anemia, and pulmonary infiltrates. Early in the course of the disease, if glomerulitis is minor or absent, a misdiagnosis of diffuse pneumonia may be made.

Histopathologically, the dominant feature in the lung is alveolar hemorrhage with hemosiderin-laden macrophages. Immunofluorescence studies reveal linear deposits of IgG and the third component of complement along alveolar septa and in glomeruli. Diagnosis is made by clinical examination, by the detection of circulating serum anti-basement membrane antibody, and, in those cases with concomitant glomerulonephritis, by renal biopsy. Alveolar hemorrhage in patients with this disease may be precipitated or worsened by smoking. The prognosis is variable. Current treatment consists of high-dose steroids, plasma exchange, and immunosuppressive drugs.

Idiopathic pulmonary hemorrhage refers to alveolar hemorrhage that occurs in the absence of hemodynamic abnormality, infection, coagulopathy, or systemic disorders, such as anti-basement membrane antibody, lupus erythematosus, and vasculitis. Its etiology remains obscure. Children and young adults are predominantly affected. Repetitive alveolar hemorrhage is the hallmark of this disease. Repeated episodes of hemorrhage frequently lead to interstitial fibrosis, but this is usually mild **(Option (A) is false)**. Dyspnea, clubbing, and right heart failure are also complications. Iron deficiency anemia is almost always present, and the serum IgA concentration is frequently elevated.

The diagnosis is made from the demonstration of alveolar hemorrhage by the finding of hemosiderin-laden macrophages in the sputum or gastric washings or by bronchoalveolar lavage, measurement of carbon monoxide uptake, or lung biopsy. Other etiologies must be excluded. Recent treatments have included high-dose corticosteroids, plasmapheresis, and azathioprine. There is a tendency for spontaneous remission and exacerbation. The prognosis is variable.

Diffuse alveolar hemorrhage is the most serious form of lung disease in lupus erythematosus[11] **(Option (D) is true)**. However, such hemorrhage is rarely the initial manifestation of the disease. Typically, there is other evidence of active disease, such as fever, arthritis, and glomerulonephritis. The alveolar hemorrhage is usually extensive and carries a grave prognosis.

Alveolar hemorrhage, while not common, is nevertheless a complication of the systemic vasculitides. Occasionally, it is the primary manifestation of the disease. The alveolar hemorrhage associated with this category of disease is thought to arise from diffuse injury of the capillary wall, rather than from sites of necrotizing vasculitis in the lung.

Other causes of the alveolar hemorrhage syndrome as listed by Leatherman et al.[11] include rapidly progressive glomerulonephritis and exogenous agents, such as D-penicillamine, lymphographic contrast material, and trimellitic anhydride. While bleeding into the pulmonary parenchyma occurs as a complication of anticoagulants, it is rare **(Option (C) is false)**.[14]

Discussion

Alveolar proteinosis was first described by Rosen et al. in 1958.[19] It is an uncommon disease of worldwide distribution. It is usually seen in the fourth or fifth decade of life and is predominantly a disease of male patients, with a male-female ratio of 3:1. As previously mentioned, the etiology is obscure. Exposure to various types of dusts, fumes, or industrial products has been reported. Among these are wood and wood products, broken fluorescent light tubes, various forms of silica dust, petroleum products, and cigarette smoke.[3,8] Claypool et al. have suggested that the disease may result from an alteration of normal surfactant reprocessing in relation to alveolar type II pneumocytes.[23]

Clinically, alveolar proteinosis is an insidious disease. In most cases it is difficult to establish its exact time of onset. Almost 50% of patients will manifest a premonitory febrile illness, usually considered to be pneumonitis. Progressive dyspnea and productive cough often are found. Physical signs are remarkably few. Alveolar capillary block is the principal physiologic abnormality and is characterized by: (1) hyperventilation at rest; (2) a normal or slightly reduced peripheral arterial oxygen level at rest, with a fall to abnormal levels with exercise; and (3) a normal partial pressure of carbon dioxide in the blood.

Lung preparations stained with hematoxylin and eosin show a granular and floccular acidophilic material occupying the alveoli, with sparing of the interalveolar areas.[19] Cellular debris is scattered within this acidophilic material. The intra-alveolar material, probably a combination of serum transudate and degenerating alveolar cells, has a high lipid content.[4] While not a common characteristic of this disease, an interstitial component is occasionally found and consists of lympho-cytes and macrophages along with thickening of the alveolar septa.[13] Interstitial fibrosis may occasionally develop. It has been suggested that interstitial changes occur when the disease has been present for many years.

The findings on chest radiographs are consistent with an alveolar process. Initial descriptions of alveolar proteinosis were those of a fine, diffuse perihilar or vaguely nodular infiltrate resembling the butterfly pattern of pulmonary edema. While this is the typical appearance, the radiographic distribution may vary. In our experience, a perihilar and basilar distribution, as shown in Figure 5-1, is common. The process may appear in one lobe while it is disappearing from another. While peripheral clearing is the rule, at times central clearing may result in an impressive peripheral distribution of opacity. Areas of hyperinflation and atelectasis have been described.[16] Unilateral involvement has been reported. If the disease progresses, massive consolidation may be seen.

Hilar adenopathy, cardiac failure, and pleural effusions are not characteristic of alveolar proteinosis. If any of these features are present, an alternative or additional diagnosis should be suspected.

Complications, such as interstitial fibrosis with subsequent ventricular failure, are rare. The major complication is infection. While various infecting organisms may be seen (viruses, staphylococci, and gram-negative bacteria), the most remarkable feature is the frequency of fungal invasion. Nocardiosis, aspergillosis, cryptococcosis, and candidiasis have all been reported as secondary infections. A radiographic appearance of cavitation, rapidly increasing infiltrate, or pleural effusion is probably due to infection. Clinical signs of fever, sepsis, or increasing shortness of breath frequently accompany secondary infection. In fact, the area of consolidation at the right costophrenic angle in Figure 5-1 was thought to be secondary to infection, but a specific organism was not isolated. Adult alveolar proteinosis may also occur in association with hematologic malignancy and silicosis.

While some investigators have established the diagnosis of alveolar proteinosis by examination of the sputum or pulmonary washings, lung biopsy is usually necessary for a definite diagnosis. Bronchopulmonary lavage has proved to be a successful treatment method. Refractory or life-threatening cases may require several repeat irrigations. Following lavage, large amounts of alveolar material may yet remain in the lung so that progressive radiographic clearing might not become apparent for 2 to 3 weeks.[15]

SUGGESTED READINGS

1. Baron MG, Whitehouse WM. Primary lymphosarcoma of the lung. AJR 1961; 85:294–308

2. Berkmen YM. The many faces of bronchiolo-alveolar carcinoma. Semin Roentgenol 1977; 12:207–214

3. Davidson JM, Macleod WM. Pulmonary alveolar proteinosis. Br J Dis Chest 1969; 63:13–28

4. Divertie MB, Brown AL, Harrison EG. Pulmonary alveolar proteinosis. Am J Med 1966; 40:351–359

5. Felson B. The roentgen diagnosis of disseminated pulmonary alveolar diseases. Semin Roentgenol 1967; 2:3–21

6. Felson B. Chest roentgenology. Philadelphia: WB Saunders; 1973:288–306

7. Felson B. A new look at pattern recognition of diffuse pulmonary disease. AJR 1979; 133:183–189

8. Greenspan RH. Chronic disseminated alveolar disease of the lungs. Semin Roentgenol 1967; 2:77–97

9. Heitzman ER. The lung: radiologic pathologic correlations, 2nd ed. St Louis: CV Mosby; 1984:189–192

10. Heitzman ER, Markarian B, DeLise CT. Lymphoproliferative disease of the thorax. Semin Roentgenol 1975; 10:73–81

11. Leatherman JW, Davies SF, Hoidal JR. Alveolar hemorrhage syndromes: diffuse microvascular lung hemorrhage in immune and idiopathic disorders. Medicine 1984; 63:343–361

12. McCook TA, Kirks DR, Merten DF, Osborne DR, Spock A, Pratt PC. Pulmonary alveolar proteinosis in children. AJR 1981; 137:1023–1027

13. Miller PA, Ravin CE, Smith GJ, Osborne DR. Pulmonary alveolar proteinosis with interstitial involvement. AJR 1981; 137:1069–1071

14. Prakash UB, Barham SS, Rosenow EC III, Brown ML, Payne WS. Pulmonary alveolar microlithiasis. A review including ultrastructural and pulmonary function studies. Mayo Clin Proc 1983; 58:290–300

15. Ramirez J. Alveolar proteinosis: importance of pulmonary lavage. Am Rev Respir Dis 1971; 103:666–678

16. Ramirez J. Pulmonary alveolar proteinosis. A roentgenologic analysis. AJR 1964; 92:571–577

17. Recavarren S, Benton C, Gall EA. The pathology of acute alveolar disease of the lung. Semin Roentgenol 1967; 2:22–32

18. Reed JC, Madewell JE. The air bronchogram in interstitial disease of the lungs. Radiology 1975; 116:1–9

19. Rosen SH, Castleman B, Liebow AA. Pulmonary alveolar proteinosis. N Engl J Med 1958; 258:1123–1142

20. Sahn SA, Schwarz MI, Lakshminarayan S. Sarcoidosis: the significance of an acinar pattern on chest roentgenogram. Chest 1974; 65:684–687

21. Saltzstein SL. Pulmonary malignant lymphomas and pseudolymphomas: classification, therapy, and prognosis. Cancer 1963; 16:928–955

22. Ziskind MM, Weill H, Payzant AR. The recognition and significance of acinus-filling processes of the lungs. Am Rev Respir Dis 1963; 87:551–559

ADDITIONAL READING

23. Claypool WD, Rogers RM, Matuschak GM. Update on the clinical diagnosis, management, and pathogenesis of pulmonary alveolar proteinosis (phospholipidosis). Chest 1984; 85:550–558

Notes

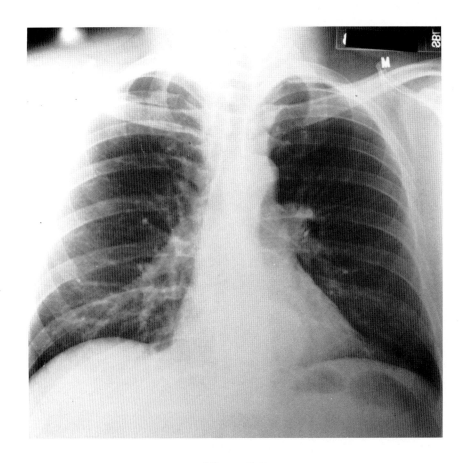

Figure 6-1
Figures 6-1 and 6-2. This 46-year-old patient had a routine chest
radiograph (Figure 6-1) and a subsequent computed tomographic (CT)
examination (Figure 6-2).

Case 6: Lateral Meningocele

Question 24

Diseases that should be considered in the differential diagnosis include:

(A) lateral meningocele
(B) neurofibroma
(C) extramedullary hematopoiesis
(D) neurenteric cyst
(E) pheochromocytoma

Figure 6-1, a routine posteroanterior chest radiograph, shows a left lower paraspinal mass, which was barely visible on the lateral view (not shown). A representative CT scan demonstrates the mass and its extension into the spinal canal (Figure 6-2). The left pedicle is eroded, and the density of the mass appears to be lower than that of the adjacent skeletal musculature or liver. Overall, the radiographic features are very consistent with a neurogenic tumor of the posterior mediastinum involving the spinal canal **(Option (B) is true)**. Although the density of the mass appears higher than that of water, as was the case when measured, a lateral meningocele cannot be excluded **(Option (A) is also true)**. In fact, a preoperative myelogram shows that the mass is a lateral meningocele (Figure 6-3). During the clinical work-up, the patient was found to have cafe-au-lait spots; thus, the final diagnosis was neurofibromatosis with associated lateral meningocele.

Extramedullary hematopoiesis (Option (C)) is a condition in which lobulated bone marrow-like masses form in the mid- to lower thoracic paraspinal areas, usually in response to a chronic anemia such as thalassemia or hereditary spherocytosis. Typically there is no bony erosion, and often the masses are multiple and bilateral[12] **(Option (C) is therefore false)**.

Neurenteric cyst is a rare, purely cystic malformation associated with vertebral anomalies rather than with bony erosion **(Option (D) is false)**. Such cysts are due to incomplete or delayed obliteration of the

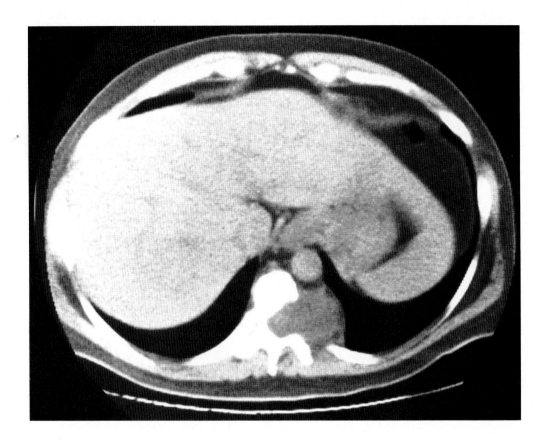

Figure 6-2

neurenteric canal. Cord anomalies, such as localized dilatation, tethering, patent fistula, and intradural cyst, may be present. Vertebral anomalies include scoliosis, spina bifida, hemivertebrae, and fused vertebrae. These anomalies may not be at the same level as the cyst. Neurenteric cyst is more commonly diagnosed in the pediatric age group.

Pheochromocytoma (Option (E)) is quite rare in the thorax and, when present, only occasionally occurs in a paravertebral location. Hypertension, diaphoresis, palpitation, and headache due to catecholamine release are accompanying features. Bony erosion is not a characteristic feature of intrathoracic pheochromocytoma **(Option (E) is false).**

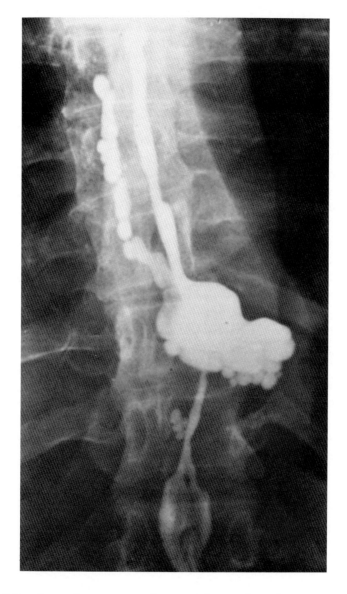

Figure 6-3. A pantopaque myelogram shows that the mass fills with contrast material and represents a lateral meningocele.

Questions 25 through 28

For each of the numbered masses listed below (Questions 25 through 28), select the *one* lettered characteristic (A, B, C, D, or E) MOST closely associated with it. Each lettered characteristic may be selected once, more than once, or not at all.

25. Neuroblastoma
26. Ganglioneuroma
27. Schwannoma
28. Neurofibroma

    (A)   occurs most commonly in the third and fourth decades
    (B)   is a round cell tumor arising from sympathetic ganglia
    (C)   occurs most commonly early in the third decade
    (D)   is associated with localized congenital vertebral abnormalities
    (E)   age of peak occurrence is over 65

Neuroblastoma is a round cell tumor arising from sympathetic ganglion cells **(Option (B) is therefore the correct answer for Question 25).** It is malignant and occurs much more frequently than the other neurogenic ganglion tumors. It is usually found in children under 2 years of age. Ganglioneuroma, the benign counterpart of neuroblastoma, occurs most commonly in early adulthood, with a peak incidence in the early twenties[11,19,20] **(Option (C) is therefore the correct response for Question 26).** The benign nerve sheath tumor, schwannoma, affects patients of both sexes in their third and fourth decades[17] **(Option (A) is therefore the correct choice for Question 27).** Similarly, the related tumor, neurofibroma, arising from the nerve itself, occurs most frequently in the third and fourth decades[17] **(Option (A) is the correct response for Question 28 as well).**

Question 29

Concerning schwannomas (neurilemmomas),

    (A) they are tumors arising from both sheath and nerve cells
    (B) they are the most common posterior mediastinal tumors
    (C) most are elongated and oriented vertically
    (D) they are the most common tumors in neurofibromatosis
    (E) on CT, they are frequently denser than adjacent skeletal muscle

Schwannomas are neurogenic tumors derived from the sheath of Schwann, which forms the connective tissue component of the nerve root. The schwannoma is a slow-growing, benign, well-encapsulated tumor that contains no nerve cells **(Option (A) is false).** It is the most common posterior mediastinal mass, accounting for one-third of thoracic neural tumors[22] **(Option (B) is therefore true).** When visible on the posteroanterior chest radiograph or anteroposterior tomogram, its shape is most often round and it is well circumscribed **(Option (C) is therefore false).** This is in contradistinction to the ganglioneuroma, which often presents as an elongated paraspinal mass.[22]

In neurofibromatosis, neurofibromas often arise in multiple locations and are found more frequently than schwannomas **(Option (D) is false).** CT has not reliably differentiated neurofibroma from schwannoma. Both lesions are usually of lower density than adjacent skeletal muscle. Some neurofibromas are of the same density as muscle.[2] Neither lesion is of higher density than adjacent skeletal muscle **(Option (E) is therefore false).**

Question 30

Concerning neurofibromatosis,

   (A) when the lung is involved, cystic air collections are often present
   (B) scoliosis spanning the upper 7 to 10 thoracic vertebral bodies is characteristic of thoracic spine involvement
   (C) associated middle mediastinal masses represent mediastinal adenopathy
   (D) patients with the central, rather than peripheral, form seldom have mediastinal neurofibromas

The reported involvement of the pulmonary parenchyma in neurofibromatosis varies from common[18,23] to rare.[5] When it occurs, thin-walled cystic air collections are found in the upper lobes[2,18,23] **(Option (A) is therefore true).** Interstitial fibrosis that may progress to honeycombing is a frequent finding in some series. A common thoracic skeletal abnormality in neurofibromatosis is scoliosis, with or without kyphosis.[14] Short-segment scoliosis of less than six vertebral bodies is usual and occurs in the lower thoracic spine[13] **(Option (B) is therefore false).** In the patient with neurofibromatosis, the presence of multiple lobulated masses in the middle mediastinum extending from the thoracic inlet to the hila usually represents plexiform neurofibromatous change of the vagus nerves rather than adenopathy[2,17] **(Option (C) is therefore false).**

Histologically, plexiform neurofibromas consist of multiple enlarged tortuous nerve fibers admixed with a loose connective tissue stroma containing Schwann cells and fibroblasts. They produce thick convoluted masses that have been likened to a "bag of worms."[17] Figure 6-4 shows neurofibromatous lesions extensively involving the posterior and middle mediastinum and intercostal nerves in a patient with neurofibromatosis. Figure 6-5 is from a pelvic CT scan in a patient with neurofibromatosis. Multiple low-density neurofibromatous lesions are present in the iliac, psoas, and gluteus muscles.

Neurofibromatosis is a hereditary autosomal dominant disorder that involves all the germ cell layers but more commonly the ectoderm and mesoderm. It can affect virtually any organ and occurs in 1 of every 3,000 births.[6] Spontaneous mutation accounts for 50% of cases, and penetrance approaches 100%.[2] Neurofibromatosis can be classified into two forms: peripheral (or neurofibromatosis 1) and central (or neurofibromatosis 2).[24,25] These two variants do not usually overlap in a patient or in members of a family affected by the disorder. Patients with central neurofibromatosis present with nervous system tumors, including schwannomas, astrocytomas, meningiomas, and/or ependymomas. The

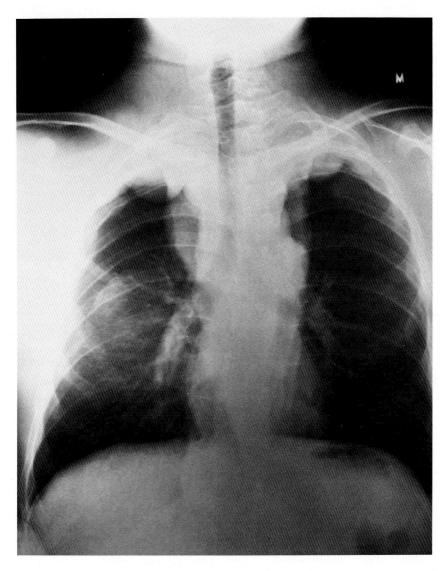

Figure 6-4. In this posteroanterior radiograph of a patient with neurofibromatosis, multiple masses of neurofibromatous tissue involve the middle and posterior mediastinum and intercostal nerves.

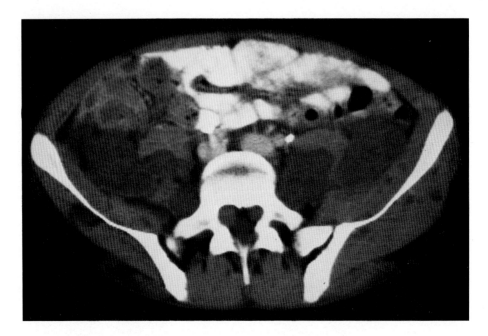

Figure 6-5. A pelvic CT scan of a patient with neurofibromatosis demonstrates multiple low-density masses consistent with neurofibromas.

hallmark of this disorder is bilateral acoustic neuromas. Patients with neurofibromatosis 2 seldom have peripheral abnormalities or mediastinal neurofibromas[9,17] **(Option (D) is therefore true).** Mediastinal neurofibromas are associated, instead, with the peripheral form of neurofibromatosis.

Extrathoracic findings in the peripheral form of neurofibromatosis include skin pigmentation (cafe-au-lait spots), multiple neurofibromas, congenital bowing of bones with pseudoarthroses, orbital malformations, megacolon, vascular lesions, pheochromocytomas, lipoma, medullary carcinoma of the thyroid, and other systemic abnormalities. Thoracic findings include meningoceles, pulmonary interstitial and cystic changes, scoliosis, and rib deformities, as well as benign and sometimes malignant neural tumors.

Discussion

Felson describes the posterior mediastinum as that compartment behind an imaginary line drawn 1 cm posterior to the anterior margins of the thoracic vertebral bodies.[10] Tumors of neurogenic origin are the most common masses found in the posterior compartment. These tumors arise from peripheral nerves, sympathetic ganglia, and paraganglia. Common tumors of peripheral nerves include schwannoma, neurofibroma, and the malignant schwannoma (malignant tumor of nerve sheath origin). Ganglionic tumors consist of the benign ganglioneuromas and the related malignant tumors (the neuroblastoma and the "differentiating neuroblastoma" or so-called ganglioneuroblastoma). Paraganglionic tumors are paraganglioma and pheochromocytoma. Both are rare in the thorax.[17] The most common neurogenic tumor is the benign schwannoma (neurilemmoma). Prior to 1955, distinction between this tumor and the neurofibroma was not made; both were called "neurofibroma."

Histologically, the two tumors differ, however. Schwannomas are derived from the sheath of Schwann and do not contain nerve cells. They develop as slowly growing, well-encapsulated tumors forming a lateral mass on the parent nerve. Schwannomas affect both sexes equally and occur most commonly in the third and fourth decades of life. In most instances, patients with schwannomas are asymptomatic, although compression of the involved nerve can elicit neurological symptoms and signs suggestive of a malignant process. These benign tumors are cured by surgical excision.

Neurofibromas are the second most common neurogenic tumor of the mediastinum.[17] They may occur as solitary masses or in association with neurofibromatosis. Neurofibromas result from the proliferation of perineural fibroblasts, Schwann cells, and nerve cells. They usually grow within the nerve of origin, resulting in a fusiform mass. The age and sex distributions, as well as the clinical signs and symptoms, are identical to those of schwannomas. An important pathologic variant of this tumor is the benign plexiform neurofibroma associated almost exclusively with neurofibromatosis. This is composed of normal nerve cell elements that are bizarrely arranged to form a network of fusiform enlargements that often infiltrate and incorporate adjacent soft tissues.[2]

Radiographically, schwannoma and solitary neurofibroma are identical. Each usually presents as a small to medium-sized round or oval mass in a paravertebral location. A small percentage of such tumors will contain calcification, although calcification is more common in the sympathetic ganglionic and paraganglionic tumors.[22] A variety of bony abnormalities occur in association with all types of neurogenic tumors, even neurofibroma and schwannoma. These abnormalities include spreading, erosion, and destruction of adjacent ribs. Enlargement of a neural foramen indicates possible extension of the mass into the spinal canal. Such a complication is more common in benign nerve root tumors but can occur with malignant ones as well. More slowly growing tumors, such as schwannomas, tend to erode bone, whereas malignant ones invade and destroy bone.

Lesions that extend into the spinal canal require special surgical management. About 10% of mediastinal neurogenic tumors will extend through an intervertebral foramen. Approximately 40% of these "dumbbell" tumors will be unassociated with neurological symptoms. Intraspinal extension should be suspected if conventional radiographs of the spine or CT scans demonstrate pedicle erosion or adjacent enlargement of an intervertebral foramen. Myelographic studies can be done to determine whether a dumbbell lesion is present.[1] The absence or presence of intraspinal extension can also be determined by CT scanning after the injection of water-soluble contrast material into the subarachnoid space. However, magnetic resonance imaging (MRI) currently provides a noninvasive technique for analyzing spinal and paraspinal neurogenic tumor involvement.[4]

Schwannomas, isolated neurofibromas, plexiform neurofibromas, and lateral meningoceles all frequently appear as masses of low density on CT scanning. Kumar et al. performed CT on 15 patients with extracranial neurogenic tumors, including neurofibromas, schwannomas, plexiform neurofibromas, and neurofibrosarcomas.[15] Of the 15 lesions, 11 had attenuation values lower than that of muscle. Four lesions had attenuation values within the range of muscle. Others have reported similar findings.[3,7] The low density in these tumors is due to the presence of lipid material in some instances and cystic spaces or cystic degeneration in others.[15] Some nerve sheath tumors will show enhancement of a portion or all of the mass with the administration of intravenous contrast material. Enhancement, if present, is helpful in distinguishing solid tumors from lateral meningoceles. MRI T1 and T2 characteristics afford further distinction between solid tumors and lateral meningoceles.[4]

Lateral meningocele may occur as an isolated lesion, but 85% of lateral meningoceles are associated with neurofibromatosis. The mass is a saccular diverticulum of the meninges and has the capability of producing marked bone erosion.[16] The erosion is due to pulsation of the meninges.

Protrusion through and enlargement of an intervertebral foramen commonly occurs. Rib erosion, localized scoliosis, and displacement of adjacent pleura also occur. In neurofibromatosis, a discrete mass in the intrathoracic paravertebral region is more likely to be a lateral meningocele than a neurogenic tumor.[2] Multiple meningoceles may be present. Only 17% of patients will have associated neurological abnormalities. As discussed in Question 29, CT does not always differentiate a low-density nerve sheath tumor from a meningocele, especially when there is no contrast enhancement of the former. While myelography is diagnostic in the case of a meningocele, demonstrating filling of the mass with contrast material as in Figure 6-3, MRI provides a less invasive technique for making this diagnosis.[4] This differentiation of meningocele from nerve sheath tumor is important since surgery on meningoceles is sometimes complicated by serious postoperative spinal fluid leaks.[8]

Benign tumors of autonomic ganglia are usually ganglioneuromas. These typically occur in young adults. Pathologically, they are well-circumscribed, encapsulated, firm tumors with a whorled surface. Histologically, they are composed of Schwann cells, nerve fibers, and large ganglion cells. On the chest radiograph, the ganglioneuroma tends to be larger than the schwannoma or neurofibroma and typically has a somewhat elongated appearance. Calcification in the ganglionic series of neurogenic tumors is more common than in those of nerve sheath origin.

Neuroblastoma is the most common malignant tumor of early childhood and involves 1 in every 10,000 live births. It is much more common than ganglioneuroma or ganglioneuroblastoma. One-half of patients with neuroblastoma are under 2 years of age, and 90% of cases are discovered before the age of 5 years. Neuroblastomas usually arise from the adrenal gland but involve the mediastinum in about 15% of cases. They may be congenital and are presumed to be of neural crest origin.

Patients may present with signs and symptoms of spinal cord or nerve involvement as well as encephalopathy, myoclonus-ataxia-opsoclonus, or chronic diarrhea. Pathologically, neuroblastomas are usually large, lobulated, and encapsulated masses composed of multiple small round cells with dark-staining nuclei. Radiographically, they tend to present as large, elongated, vertically oriented posterior mediastinal masses. They often have tapered superior and inferior margins. Spine and rib destruction is not uncommon. Calcification, usually stippled in appearance, is often present and may be better demonstrated by CT scanning.

Intraspinal extension is not rare. Although neuroblastoma is malignant, it has a favorable prognosis when diagnosed in a patient under 1 year of age.[21]

Ganglioneuroblastomas show features of mature sympathetic elements histologically, but clinically they act as malignant lesions. Ganglioneuroblastomas tend to occur in patients younger than those with ganglioneuromas. Ganglioneuroblastomas may be metabolically active, as may neuroblastomas.

The paraganglionic tumors, paraganglioma and pheochromocytoma, are both quite rare in the mediastinum. Paraganglioma has no particular distinguishing characteristics. Pheochromocytoma is usually distinguished by clinical symptoms and signs secondary to catecholamine production.

Non-neurogenic masses may also be found in the posterior mediastinum, either in the area where neurogenic tumors are found or slightly anterior to that area. These masses include extramedullary hematopoiesis, duplication cysts, malignant and benign adenopathy, tuberculous abscess, aneurysm, pancreatic pseudocyst, and mediastinal varices.

SUGGESTED READINGS

1. Akwari OE, Payne WS, Onofrio BM, Dihes DE, Muhm JR. Dumbbell neurogenic tumors of the mediastinum. Diagnosis and management. Mayo Clin Proc 1978; 53:353–358
2. Aughenbaugh GL. Thoracic manifestations of neurocutaneous diseases. Radiol Clin North Am 1984; 22:741–756
3. Biondetti PR, Vigo M, Fiore D, De Faveri D, Ravasini R, Benedetti L. CT appearance of generalized von Recklinghausen neurofibromatosis. J Comput Assist Tomogr 1983; 7:866–869
4. Burk DL, Brunberg JA, Kanal E, Latchaw RE, Wolf JL. Spinal and paraspinal neurofibromatosis: surface coil MR imaging at 1.5 T. Radiology 1987; 162:797–801
5. Casselman ES, Miller WT, Shu Ren Lin, Mandell GA. Von Recklinghausen's disease: incidence of roentgenographic findings with a clinical review of the literature. CRC Crit Rev Diagn Imaging 1977; 9:387–419
6. Crowe FW, Schull WJ, Neel JV. A clinical, pathological and genetic study of multiple neurofibromatosis. Springfield, IL: Charles C Thomas; 1956
7. Daneman A, Mancer K, Sonley M. CT appearance of thickened nerves in neurofibromatosis. AJR 1983; 141:899–900
8. Edeiken J, Lee KF, Libshitz H. Intrathoracic meningocele. AJR 1969; 106:381–384

9. Enzinger FM, Weiss SW. Soft tissue tumors. St Louis: CV Mosby; 1983:606–624
10. Felson B. Chest roentgenology. Philadelphia: WB Saunders; 1973:419
11. Gale AW, Jelihovsky T, Grant AF, Leckie BD, Nicks R. Neurogenic tumors of the mediastinum. Ann Thorac Surg 1974; 7:434–443
12. Heitzman ER. The mediastinum. Radiologic correlations with anatomy and pathology. St Louis: CV Mosby; 1977:205
13. Holt JF. 1977 Edward B. D. Neuhauser lecture: neurofibromatosis in children. AJR 1978; 130:615–639
14. Hunt JC, Pugh DG. Skeletal lesions in neurofibromatosis. Radiology 1961; 76:1–20
15. Kumar AJ, Kuhajda FP, Martinez CR, Fishman EK, Jezic DV, Siegelman SS. Computed tomography of extracranial nerve sheath tumors with pathological correlation. J Comput Assist Tomogr 1983; 7:857–865
16. Loop JW, Akeson WH, Clawson DK. Acquired abnormalities in neurofibromatosis. AJR 1965; 93:416–424
17. Marchevsky AM, Kaneko M. Surgical pathology of the mediastinum. New York: Raven Press; 1984:256–280
18. Massaro D, Katz S. Fibrosing alveolitis: its occurrence, roentgenographic, and pathologic features in von Recklinghausen's neurofibromatosis. Am Rev Respir Dis 1966; 93:934–942
19. Oosterwijk WM, Swierenga J. Neurogenic tumors with an intrathoracic localization. Thorax 1968; 23:374–384
20. Pachter MR, Lattes R. Neurogenous tumors of the mediastinum: a clinicopathologic study based on 50 cases. Dis Chest 1963; 44:79–87
21. Putman CE. Pulmonary diagnosis: imaging and other techniques. New York: Appleton-Century-Crofts; 1981:282
22. Reed JC, Hallet KK, Feigin DS. Neural tumors of the thorax: subject review from the AFIP. Radiology 1978; 126:9–17
23. Webb WR, Goodman PC. Fibrosing alveolitis in patients with neurofibromatosis. Radiology 1977; 122:289–293

ADDITIONAL READINGS

24. Martuza RL, Eldridge R. Neurofibromatosis 2 (bilateral acoustic neurofibromatosis). N Engl J Med 1988; 318:684–688
25. Riccardi VM. Von Recklinghausen neurofibromatosis. N Engl J Med 1981; 305:1617–1627

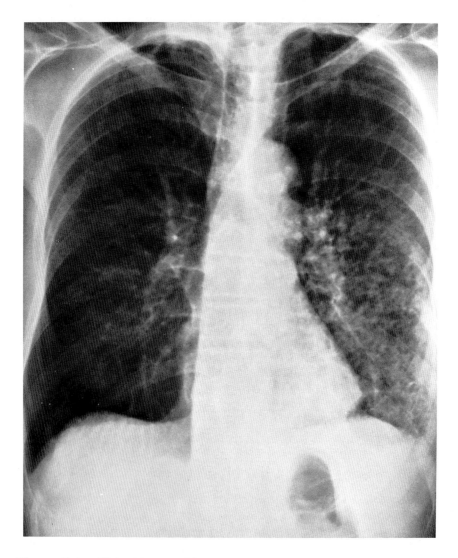

Figure 7-1. This 66-year-old man with known poorly differentiated granulocytic leukemia presented with pleuritic left chest pain. You are shown the posteroanterior chest radiograph taken on the day of admission.

Case 7: Pulmonary Infiltration Complicating Leukemia

Question 31

Which *one* of the following is the MOST likely diagnosis?

(A) Infectious pneumonia
(B) Leukemic infiltration of the lung
(C) Amyloidosis
(D) Hemorrhage
(E) Drug reaction

The chest radiograph (Figure 7-1) shows an ill-defined parenchymal infiltrate in the left lower lung; otherwise, the lungs are clear. There is no enlargement of hilar or mediastinal lymph nodes. Because of the localized nature of the parenchymal infiltrate, and considering the relative frequencies of the disease processes offered as options, an infectious pneumonia is the most likely diagnosis **(Option (A) is correct).**

Patients with the conditions listed in the other options usually present with bilateral infiltrates, and these other options should not be primary considerations in patients with localized disease. Leukemic infiltration of the lung (Option (B)) most often results in accentuation of vascular or peribronchial shadows or a diffuse reticular pattern. Amyloidosis (Option (C)) likewise results in a bilateral reticular infiltrate that has a basilar predominance. Pulmonary nodules may be present with either leukemia or amyloidosis and are usually bilateral in distribution. When amyloidosis is localized, it usually has the appearance of a mass. Pulmonary hemorrhage (Option (D)) occurs frequently in patients with leukemia and is most often associated with an infectious pneumonia when focal. In patients with massive pulmonary hemorrhage, diffuse alveolar damage is usually present and the infiltrates are diffuse. Drug reactions in the lung (Option (E)) almost always manifest as bilateral infiltrates.

Antineoplastic agents may result in pulmonary fibrosis with predominant involvement of the lower lobes. Methotrexate toxicity has rarely started as a focal infiltrate but almost always progresses to a diffuse process. Since the other options listed above usually present as bilateral processes, none of them would probably cause the left lower lobe infiltrate.

The development of pulmonary infiltration in a patient with leukemia represents a difficult problem in differential diagnosis for the radiologist. Diagnostic categories that must be considered include the following: (1) an extension of the primary disease process, (2) an effect of treatment, (3) an infectious complication of the disease process or its treatment, and (4) an unrelated process. In sorting these out it is helpful to know whether the patient is presenting for the first time, whether the infiltrate is localized or diffuse, what antineoplastic chemotherapy is being administered, whether a fever is present, and whether the patient has a low platelet count with a bleeding diathesis.

In a study of pulmonary infiltrates in patients with leukemia, Tenholder and Hooper reviewed records of 139 patients seen between 1973 and 1978.[35] In 87 of these patients, 98 episodes of pulmonary infiltration were categorized as either localized or diffuse on chest radiographs. A cause could be established in 86% (84 of 98) of these episodes. In the 17 patients with infiltrates at initial presentation, 66% of the localized infiltrates were the result of infection. On the other hand, none of the 5 patients with diffuse infiltrates had infections. Eighty-one instances of pulmonary infiltration occurred in the remaining 70 patients during their treatment. Of the localized infiltrates developing in these patients, 82% were infectious, whereas only 35% of diffuse infiltrates were infectious. Gram-negative bacterial pneumonias accounted for the majority of infections. The noninfectious causes of infiltrates included pulmonary hemorrhage, congestive heart failure, pulmonary fibrosis, and leukemia.

As part of an autopsy study of 113 leukemia patients seen between 1971 and 1981, Maile et al. reviewed records of 60 patients for whom a chest radiograph had been taken within 5 days of death.[23] In 54 patients (90%) the radiographs showed infiltrates, and in 28 patients (46%) the infiltrates were bilateral. An end-airspace consolidation pattern was present in 50% of patients; an interstitial pattern was present in 20% of patients. These infiltrates could be attributed to a single etiology in 33 patients. Sixty-six percent (22 of 33) were caused by infection, the most common etiologic agent being gram-negative bacterial pneumonia. Pulmonary hemorrhage was responsible in 4 cases (12%), pulmonary edema was responsible in 2 cases (6%), and leukemia was responsible in 1 case (3%). Multiple causes were responsible in 13 patients (24%). The most frequent combinations were infection plus pulmonary hemorrhage and pulmonary edema plus pulmonary hemorrhage. Pulmonary hemorrhage plus leukemic infiltration accounted for only 1 case (8%). In the 8 remaining cases, the cause of the predominant radiographic infiltrate in the lungs could not be determined.

Pulmonary hemorrhage is a frequent autopsy finding in patients with leukemia, and massive pulmonary hemorrhage accounts for 2 to 3% of all deaths from leukemia.[7] In the study by Maile et al., 74% (83 of 113) of the patients had some degree of pulmonary hemorrhage at autopsy, yet bleeding was the sole cause of infiltrate noted on the chest radiograph in only 4 of 33 patients.[23] In most patients, the hemorrhage was associated with some other abnormality, most frequently infectious pneumonia. Smith and Katzenstein examined three patients with massive pulmonary hemorrhage in leukemia and found evidence of diffuse alveolar damage in all three.[31] They suggested that, in addition to a low platelet count, an episode of alveolar injury is necessary for the hemorrhage to occur. Patients with moderate to severe pulmonary hemorrhage have dyspnea, fever, hypoxemia, and pulmonary infiltrates. Hemoptysis is unusual but may suggest the diagnosis when present. Demonstration of hemosiderin-laden macrophages in sputum or bronchoalveolar lavage fluid indicates that hemorrhage has occurred.[12] The infiltrates in pulmonary hemorrhage are usually diffuse (Figure 7-2).

Although infection is the most likely cause of infiltrates in a patient with leukemia, the case shown (Figure 7-1) is actually an example of leukemic infiltration of the lung. The patient was afebrile, and multiple cultures of both sputum and blood were negative. Multiple transbronchial lung biopsies showed leukemic infiltration without evidence of infection. Leukemic infiltration of the lung may be diagnosed from pathologic specimens when extravascular collections of leukemic cells are detected without other apparent cause for their presence. The infiltration usually occurs in the peribronchial/perivascular interstitial space and is present in 20 to 40% of patients with leukemia. Although the infiltration may be present in any form of the disease, it is most frequent in chronic myelogenous leukemia. Most patients are asymptomatic, but respiratory symptoms may develop if infiltration is extensive. While leukemic infiltration is not rare, it is an unusual cause of *radiographically visible* infiltrates in the lung. Patterns that have been noted in association with

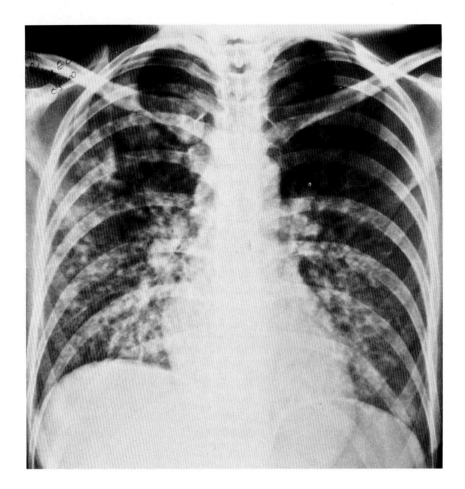

Figure 7-2. Pulmonary hemorrhage in leukemia. A 27-year-old woman with acute promyelocytic leukemia had an episode of pneumococcal sepsis. Her initial chest radiograph (not shown) was normal. Two days later she developed hemoptysis and a decreased hematocrit, with a platelet count of 62,000/μL. Her chest radiograph now showed diffuse nodular infiltrates due to hemorrhage, which cleared over the next 4 days.

such infiltration include accentuation of vascular and peribronchial markings, diffuse reticular infiltrates, pulmonary nodules, and pulmonary edema.[1,19,20,23,35]

Question 32

Which one of the following is the MOST likely etiologic agent to be isolated in leukemic patients with infectious pneumonia?

(A) A gram-negative bacillus
(B) A fungus
(C) A gram-positive coccus
(D) *Pneumocystis carinii*
(E) A virus

Infections are the major cause of morbidity and mortality in leukemic patients, accounting for approximately 75% of reported deaths in the acute leukemias.[9,29] Defects in phagocytosis, cellular immunity, or humoral immunity commonly result from either the disease process or its treatment. In addition, anatomic barriers are often violated by intravenous lines and urinary and intestinal catheters and as a result of mucosal injury by antineoplastic agents.[3,13] Although the lung is the most commonly affected single organ, 75% of the infections in these patients will disseminate. The etiologic agents have changed over the past three decades, but bacteria continue to be the leading cause of these infections. Prior to 1960, *Staphylococcus aureus* was the agent most frequently isolated. After development of antistaphylococcal penicillins, gram-negative bacilli became the most frequent agents **(Option (A) is the correct answer)** and continue to be more likely etiologic agents today than fungi (Option (B)), gram-positive cocci (Option (C)), *Pneumocystis carinii* (Option (D)), and viruses (Option (E)). A large variety of unusual bacterial organisms have been reported in isolated instances. The incidence of fungal infections has also increased in the past decade,[8] most commonly due to *Candida* and *Aspergillus* species. Comparatively speaking, *P. carinii* pneumonia is responsible for relatively few infections in adult patients with leukemia, but it does represent a major problem at some children's medical centers.[18]

Although many attempts have been made to suggest an etiologic diagnosis from the radiographic appearance of the infiltrates, so much overlap is present that these attempts have been unsuccessful.[13,21] Since the etiology of such infiltrates is so difficult to determine and since these pneumonias are life-threatening, biopsy (percutaneous, transbronchial, or open-lung) is often performed when the patient is able to tolerate the procedure.[14,34,36]

Question 33

Leukemic involvement of the thorax produces:

(A) mediastinal and hilar lymph node enlargement
(B) pneumothorax
(C) ill-defined lung infiltrates
(D) pleural effusion
(E) lung nodules

While the infectious complications of leukemia cause the majority of abnormalities visible on the chest radiograph, the disease process itself may have a variety of radiographic manifestations. Ill-defined lung infiltrates and lung nodules may be seen, as already mentioned **(Options (C) and (E) are true)**. Enlargement of mediastinal and/or hilar lymph nodes (Figure 7-3) is radiographically apparent in 5 to 15% of patients, a considerably lower frequency than the 40 to 50% involvement described in autopsy series **(Option (A) is true)**. Microscopic invasion of lymph nodes of normal size is the primary reason for the discrepancy. Pleural effusions (Figure 7-4) are present in about 40% of patients and are seen both on the chest radiograph and at autopsy **(Option (D) is true)**. Pneumothorax has not been described as a complication of leukemia in the thorax **(Option (B) is false)**. Two other thoracic manifestations that are occasionally identified are pleural thickening and rib involvement (Figure 7-5).[26,30]

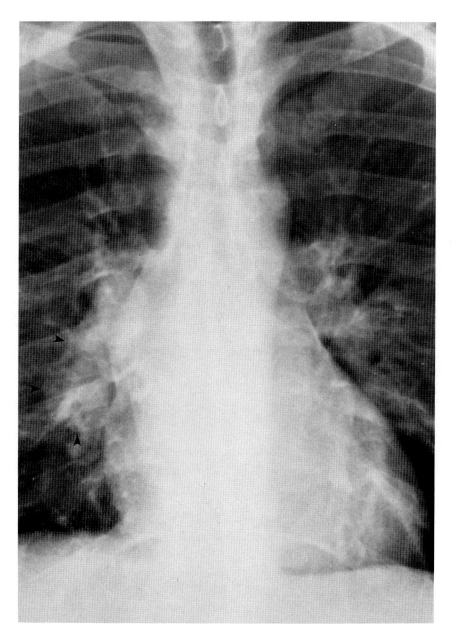

Figure 7-3. Hilar lymph node enlargement in leukemia. The patient is a 19-year-old man presenting with acute lymphocytic leukemia. The frontal chest radiograph shows a lobulated right hilar mass (arrowheads).

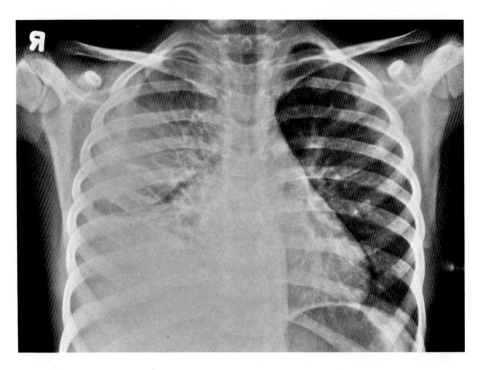

Figure 7-4. Pleural effusion in leukemia. An 8-year-old boy with right chest pain and low-grade fever for 1 week was found to have acute myelogenous leukemia. His frontal chest radiograph showed a large right pleural effusion which consisted of fluid and leukemic cells.

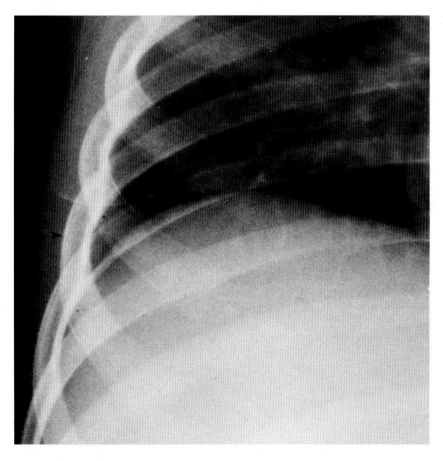

Figure 7-5. Rib involvement in leukemia. A 1½-year-old boy presented with acute lymphocytic leukemia. The frontal chest radiograph shows rib periostitis (arrowheads).

Question 34

Which *one* of the following is the LEAST likely radiographic pattern to be associated with thoracic amyloidosis?

(A) Cardiomegaly
(B) Pulmonary nodules
(C) Hilar and mediastinal lymph node enlargement
(D) Pleural plaques
(E) Reticular lung infiltrate

Amyloid is a proteinaceous material that can infiltrate various organs and lead to their dysfunction. Biochemically, there are a number of different amyloid proteins. While disorders resulting from amyloidosis are often classified as primary and secondary, there is considerable overlap in their clinical and pathological manifestations.[11] The heart and lungs, either separately or together, are involved in approximately 25% of patients.[6,15,17,38] A pattern of cardiomegaly (Option (A)) and basilar interstitial infiltration may mimic congestive heart failure. A clue to the correct diagnosis is persistence of the chest radiographic pattern despite attempts at diuresis. Alternatively, the heart may be of normal size and the lungs may be involved with reticular infiltrate (Option (E)), which is almost always bilateral.

Single or multiple pulmonary nodules (Option (B)) ranging in size from 2 mm to 6 cm may result from amyloid deposition. These nodules may cavitate or show stippled calcification. Hilar and mediastinal lymph node enlargement (Option (C)) occurs, but in fewer than 20% of cases (Figure 7-6). The lymph nodes may also calcify with either an amorphous or an eggshell pattern.[16,28] Pleural plaques have not been described as a manifestation of thoracic amyloidosis and thus are least likely **(Option (D) is correct).** Finally, amyloid involvement of the tracheobronchial tree may cause diffuse narrowing of the trachea, lobar atelectasis, obstructive hyperinflation, or recurrent pneumonias. This type of amyloidosis frequently presents without other manifestations of systemic disease.[28]

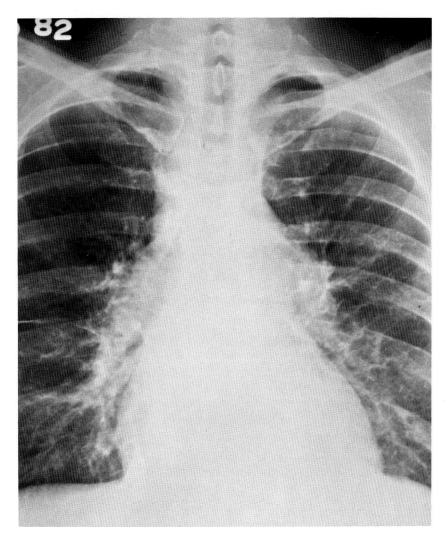

Figure 7-6. Lymph node enlargement in amyloidosis. This 52-year-old man presented with fatigue, weight loss, and adenopathy of 4 years' duration. His frontal chest radiograph shows bilateral mediastinal and left hilar adenopathy. Rectal biopsy and mediastinal lymph node biopsy showed amyloidosis. (Case courtesy of Peter G. Herman, M.D., Long Island Jewish Medical Center, Long Island, N.Y.)

Question 35

Which of the following drugs used in the treatment of leukemia may result in pulmonary toxicity?

(A) Busulfan
(B) Prednisone
(C) Methotrexate
(D) Daunorubicin
(E) Vincristine

Pulmonary toxicity results from many of the antineoplastic drugs used in modern antileukemic chemotherapy.[2,10,27,33] When considering drug toxicity, it is important to know how long the patient has been taking the drug, whether the reaction is dose-dependent, the cumulative dose, the patient's age, and concomitant therapy, if any, with other drugs or radiation. Drugs commonly used in the treatment of leukemia and associated with pulmonary toxicity include busulfan, methotrexate, cyclophosphamide, chlorambucil, melphalan, and cytosine arabinoside **(Options (A) and (C) are true; Options (B), (D), and (E) are false).**

Mechanisms of pulmonary injury from these drugs vary. Many cause injury to the capillary endothelial cells, with subsequent formation of interstitial edema and inflammation. The pneumocytes may also experience injury and slough into the alveolar space. Hyaline membranes may form, and a proliferative phase may ensue with progression to fibrosis. In other instances, allergic reactions or immune responses may result in eosinophilic infiltration, as well as interstitial fibrosis. Additionally, otherwise unexplained pulmonary edema may develop during drug therapy.

Busulfan (Myleran®), an alkylating agent used to treat patients with chronic myelogenous leukemia, causes pulmonary fibrosis in 2 to 11% of patients.[4,22] Onset occurs as early as 1 year after treatment begins but in most instances is delayed for 4 or more years. The problem usually develops while the patient is taking the drug, but it may begin after the drug has been discontinued. Symptoms usually include fever and dyspnea. Addisonian-like hyperpigmentation of the skin may develop. The development of fibrosis is not strictly dose-dependent, but the fact that it rarely occurs in patients receiving a total dose of less than 500 mg suggests that there is a threshold for development. Pathologically, the lungs demonstrate a diffuse alveolitis with large, bizarre type II pneumocytes and an organizing fibrinous edema. There may also be bronchial epithelial dysplasia, and drug-related pulmonary injury may be diagnosed from cytological preparations of sputum. As physicians have become aware of the pulmonary toxicity, total doses have been reduced or the alternative drug melphalan (Alkeran®) has been used instead.

The pulmonary fibrosis associated with busulfan may be potentiated by radiation therapy. A diffuse reticular pattern develops, reflecting the fibrotic process (Figures 7-7 to 7-9). In one report, a patient's lungs showed diffusely increased uptake on Ga-67 scintigraphy at a time when the chest radiograph appeared normal.[24]

Methotrexate is an antimetabolite most commonly used in the treatment of acute lymphocytic leukemia. The exact incidence of pulmonary toxicity related to this drug is uncertain but has been reported in up to 7% of patients.[5,32] The reaction may occur after oral, intravenous, or intrathecal administration of the drug but does not appear to be dose-dependent. It has occurred as early as 12 days and as late as 5 years after initiation of treatment. Histopathological analysis shows alveolitis with interstitial mononuclear infiltrates and, occasionally, fibrosis similar to that seen with busulfan. Poorly formed, noncaseating granulomas may also be present and are associated almost exclusively with methotrexate toxicity. Prodromal headache and malaise, followed by cough and tachypnea, are common, and fever may reach 40.5°C. Skin eruptions appear in 17% of patients, and eosinophilia is present in 40%. Chest radiographs may show reticular, nodular, or end-airspace consolidation or mixed patterns (Figures 7-10 and 7-11). The parenchymal disease is almost always diffusely distributed, although it may be focal at the outset. Lymph node enlargement and pleural effusions have been noted in some patients. Resolution occurs within 1 to 4 weeks and may be hastened by prednisone treatment. Interestingly, resolution is seen in some patients on continued therapy. On the other hand, a few patients have progressed to pulmonary fibrosis.

Prednisone has no direct toxic pulmonary effect, although its immunosuppressive properties may increase patients' susceptibility to opportunistic infections.

Daunorubicin has no pulmonary toxicity but is toxic to the heart.[37] Relatively high doses result in degeneration of myocardial cells, loss of contractile substance, and mitochondrial swelling. Patients sometimes develop cardiomegaly or congestive heart failure, either of which may occur months after cessation of drug therapy. This complication is fatal up to 75% of the time. The frequency of congestive heart failure is higher in children than in adults and is dose-dependent. At doses of 550 mg/m²,

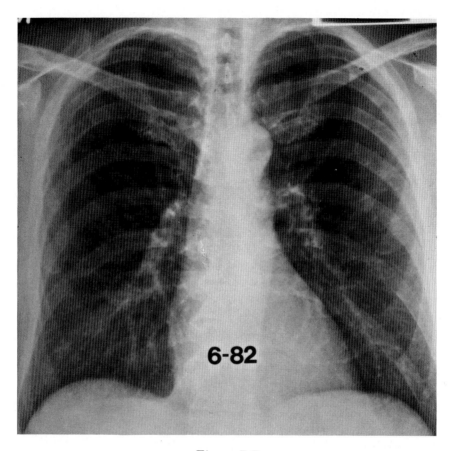

Figure 7-7

Figures 7-7 to 7-9. Busulfan toxicity. A 61-year-old man had chronic myelocytic leukemia and was given busulfan for 24 months. After the drug was stopped, he had low-grade intermittent fevers and developed a rapidly progressive diffuse pulmonary fibrosis from which he died 4 months later. A frontal chest radiograph before treatment began (Figure 7-7) was normal. A study taken 3 months after discontinuation of busulfan (Figure 7-8) shows a subtle interstitial pattern, particularly at the lung bases. One month later (Figure 7-9), diffuse lung disease has supervened. Lung biopsy showed diffuse pulmonary fibrosis consistent with busulfan toxicity.

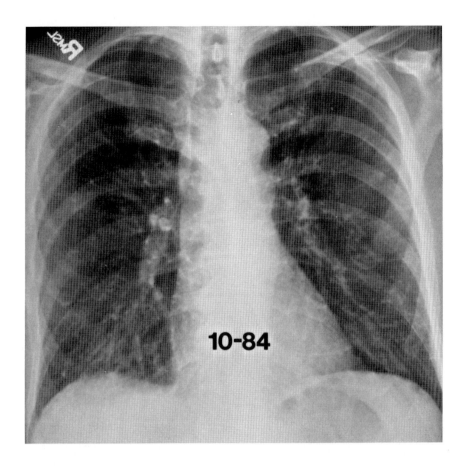

Figure 7-8

the frequency is about 6% for children and 1.3% for adults and progressively increases at doses above that level.

Vincristine is toxic primarily to the peripheral nervous system, and neuropathies represent the major toxic effect. No pulmonary complications are known to result from its administration.

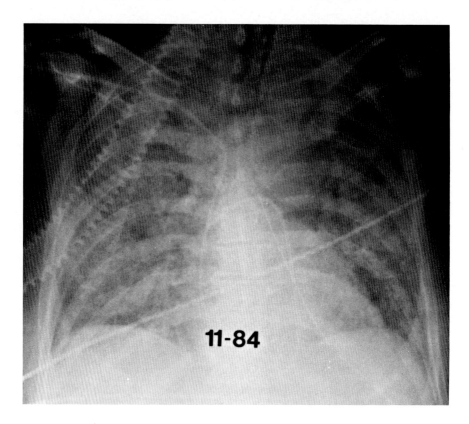

Figure 7-9

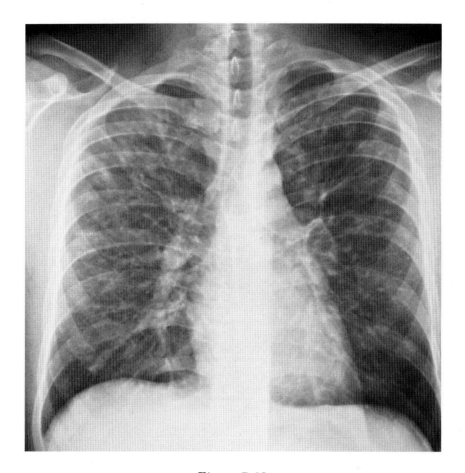

Figure 7-10

Figures 7-10 and 7-11. Methotrexate toxicity. A 19-year-old man presented with acute lymphocytic leukemia and was placed on a multiple drug regimen, which included methotrexate. After 8 months of therapy, he developed fever to 38.9°C and pleuritic chest pain. A frontal chest radiograph (Figure 7-10) and close-up view (Figure 7-11) of the upper lobes from the same study show ill-defined infiltrates primarily in the upper zones of both lungs. Transbronchial biopsy showed diffused interstitial pneumonitis. Although the patient continued to receive methotrexate, the infiltrates cleared spontaneously.

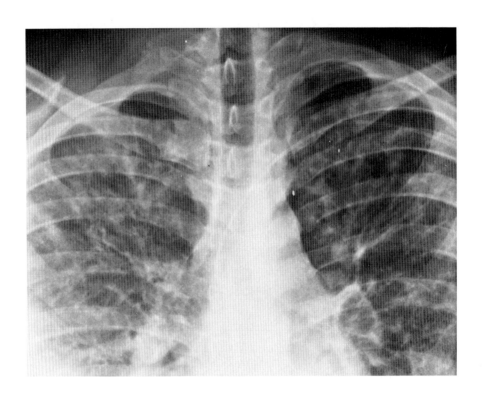

Figure 7-11

Question 36

Which *one* of the following is the LEAST likely radiographic pattern to result from cytotoxic drug-induced pulmonary injury?

    (A) Ill-defined peripheral infiltrates
    (B) Central "butterfly" infiltrates
    (C) Localized parenchymal infiltrates
    (D) Bilateral basilar reticular infiltrates
    (E) Bilateral apical reticular infiltrates

The least likely radiographic pattern to result from cytotoxic drug-induced pulmonary injury is that of localized parenchymal infiltrates **(Option (C) is correct).**[25] A localized infiltrate that progressed to diffuse involvement has been described in one patient with methotrexate toxicity.[5] Otherwise, infiltrates resulting from chemotherapy have been diffusely distributed and have included all of the varieties offered as options (Options (A), (B), (D), and (E)).

SUGGESTED READINGS

1. Armstrong P, Dyer R, Alford BA, O'Hara M. Leukemic pulmonary infiltrates: rapid development mimicking pulmonary edema. AJR 1980; 135:373–374
2. Batist G, Andrews JL Jr. Pulmonary toxicity of antineoplastic drugs. JAMA 1981; 246:1449–1453
3. Bodey GP, Bolivar R, Fainstein V. Infectious complications in leukemic patients. Semin Hematol 1982; 19:193–226
4. Burns WA, McFarland W, Matthews MJ. Busulfan-induced pulmonary disease. Report of a case and review of the literature. Am Rev Respir Dis 1970; 101:408–413
5. Case Records of the Massachusetts General Hospital. Case 6–1985. N Engl J Med 1985; 312:359–369
6. Celli BR, Rubinow A, Cohen AS, Brody JS. Patterns of pulmonary involvement in systemic amyloidosis. Chest 1978; 74:543–547
7. Chang H-Y, Rodriguez V, Narboni G, Bodey GP, Luna MA, Freireich EJ. Causes of death in adults with acute leukemia. Medicine 1976; 55:259–268
8. DeGregorio MW, Lee WM, Linker CA, Jacobs RA, Ries CA. Fungal infections in patients with acute leukemia. Am J Med 1982; 73:543–548
9. Estey EH, Keating MJ, McCredie KB, Bodey GP, Freireich EJ. Causes of initial remission induction failure in acute myelogenous leukemia. Blood 1982; 60:309–315
10. Ginsberg SJ, Comis RL. The pulmonary toxicity of antineoplastic agents. Semin Oncol 1982; 9:34–51

11. Glenner GG. Amyloid deposits and amyloidosis. The β-fibrilloses. N Engl J Med 1980; 302:1283–1292, 1333–1343

12. Golde DW, Drew WL, Klein HZ, Finley TN, Cline MJ. Occult pulmonary haemorrhage in leukaemia. Br Med J 1975; 2:166–168

13. Greene R. Opportunistic pneumonias. Semin Roentgenol 1980; 15:50–72

14. Greenman RL, Goodall PT, King D. Lung biopsy in immunocompromised hosts. Am J Med 1975; 59:488–496

15. Gross BH. Radiographic manifestations of lymph node involvement in amyloidosis. Radiology 1981; 138:11–14

16. Gross BH, Schneider HJ, Proto AV. Eggshell calcification of lymph nodes: an update. AJR 1980; 135:1265–1268

17. Himmelfarb E, Wells S, Rabinowitz JG. The radiologic spectrum of cardiopulmonary amyloidosis. Chest 1977; 72:327–332

18. Hughes WT, Rivera GK, Schell MJ, Thornton D, Lott L. Successful intermittent chemoprophylaxis for *Pneumocystis carinii* pneumonitis. N Engl J Med 1987; 316:1627–1632

19. Klatte EC, Yardley J, Smith EB, Rohn R, Campbell JA. The pulmonary manifestations and complications of leukemia. AJR 1963; 89:598–609

20. Kumar R. Multiple pulmonary nodules in leukemia. J Can Assoc Radiol 1980; 31:71–72

21. Libshitz HI, Shuman LS, Gresik MV, Heaston DK. Pneumonia in hairy-cell leukemia. Radiology 1981; 139:19–24

22. Littler WA, Kay JM, Hasleton PS, Heath D. Busulphan lung. Thorax 1969; 24:639–655

23. Maile CW, Moore AV, Ulreich S, Putman CE. Chest radiographic-pathologic correlation in adult leukemia patients. Invest Radiol 1983; 18:495–499

24. Manning DM, Strimlan CV, Turbiner EH. Early detection of busulfan lung: report of a case. Clin Nucl Med 1980; 5:412–414

25. Morrison DA, Goldman AL. Radiographic patterns of drug-induced lung diseases. Radiology 1979; 131:299–304

26. Nixon GW, Gwinn JL. The roentgen manifestations of leukemia in infancy. Radiology 1973; 107:603–609

27. Rosenow EC III. The spectrum of drug-induced pulmonary disease. Ann Intern Med 1972; 77:977–991

28. Rubinow A, Celli BR, Cohen AS, Rigden BG, Brody JS. Localized amyloidosis of the lower respiratory tract. Am Rev Respir Dis 1978; 118:603–611

29. Sickles EA, Young VM, Greene WH, Wiernik PH. Pneumonia in acute leukemia. Ann Intern Med 1973; 79:528–534

30. Siegel MJ, Shackelford GD, McAlister WH. Pleural thickening. An unusual feature of childhood leukemia. Radiology 1981; 138:367–369

31. Smith LJ, Katzenstein AL. Pathogenesis of massive pulmonary hemorrhage in acute leukemia. Arch Intern Med 1982; 142:2149–2152

32. Sostman HD, Matthay RA, Putman CE, Smith GJ. Methotrexate-induced pneumonitis. Medicine 1976; 55:371–388

33. Sostman HD, Putman CE, Gamsu G. Review: diagnosis of chemotherapy lung. AJR 1981; 136:33–40

34. Springmeyer SC, Silvestri RC, Sale GE, et al. The role of transbronchial biopsy for the diagnosis of diffuse pneumonias in immunocompromised marrow transplant recipients. Am Rev Respir Dis 1982; 126:763–765

35. Tenholder MF, Hooper RG. Pulmonary infiltrates in leukemia. Chest 1980; 78:468–473
36. Toledo-Pereyra LH, DeMeester TR, Kinealey A, MacMahon H, Churg A, Golomb H. The benefits of open lung biopsy in patients with previous non-diagnostic transbronchial lung biopsy. A guide to appropriate therapy. Chest 1980; 77:647–650
37. Von Hoff DD, Layard M. Risk factors for development of daunorubicin cardiotoxicity. Cancer Treat Rep 1981; 65(Suppl 4):19–23
38. Wilson SR, Sanders DE, Delarue NC. Intrathoracic manifestations of amyloid disease. Radiology 1976; 120:283–289

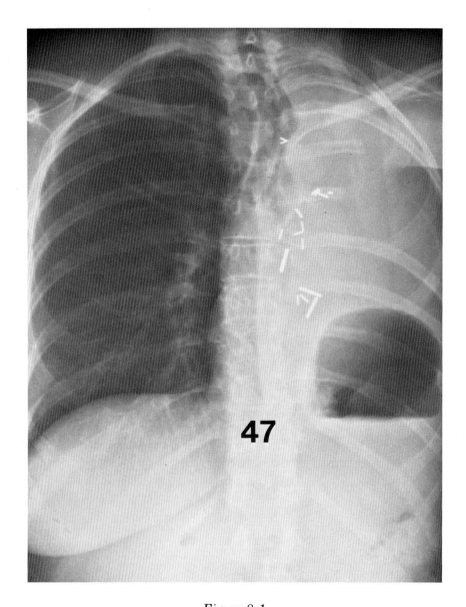

Figure 8-1
Figures 8-1 and 8-2. This woman had a pneumonectomy for metastatic breast carcinoma at age 45 years. Five years later, she developed dyspnea and orthopnea. You are shown chest radiographs taken at ages 47 and 50 years.

Case 8: Recurrent Tumor after Pneumonectomy

Question 37

Diagnoses that should be considered at age 50 years (Figure 8-2) include:

(A) normal postpneumonectomy appearance
(B) bronchopleural fistula
(C) empyema
(D) recurrent carcinoma
(E) bronchoesophageal fistula

The radiograph at age 47 (Figure 8-1), 2 years postpneumonectomy, shows absence of the left breast, left fifth and sixth rib resections, an opaque left hemithorax, and surgical clips in the mediastinum. The left hemidiaphragm is elevated, as shown by the position of the stomach, and the mediastinum has shifted to the left. At age 50 (Figure 8-2), the mediastinum has shifted to the right. Note that the right lung is normal on both examinations and that there are no air collections in the left hemithorax.

Since the appearance of the chest radiograph after pneumonectomy normally includes shift of the mediastinum and hemidiaphragm toward the postpneumonectomy space, any shift in the opposite direction should suggest a space-occupying process within the postpneumonectomy space. In view of the mediastinal shift back toward the midline at age 50, the later radiograph cannot represent a normal postpneumonectomy appearance **(Option (A) is false)**. Both bronchopleural fistula and bronchoesophageal fistula would be suggested by the reappearance of air in the postpneumonectomy space, but no air is visible in Figure 8-2 **(Options (B) and (E) are therefore false)**. Recurrence of carcinoma or empyema developing in the postpneumonectomy space may result in shift of the mediastinum back toward the midline, as is visible in Figure 8-2 **(Options (C) and (D) are therefore true)**.

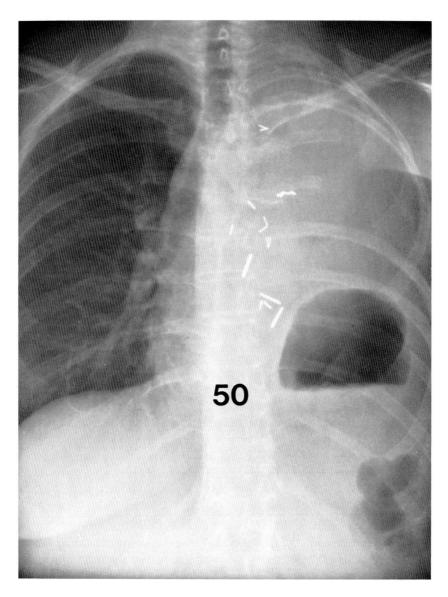

Figure 8-2

To properly assess chest radiographs of postpneumonectomy patients, it is important to understand the alterations expected.[16,25,44] In the immediate postoperative period, chest radiographs show an air-filled ipsilateral hemithorax, which then gradually fills with fluid (Figures 8-3 to 8-5). Complete opacification occurs as early as 3 weeks after surgery or may be delayed as long as 7 months. Rarely, an air collection remains permanently. Opacification is said to occur slightly earlier on the left than on the right and in patients operated upon for benign rather than malignant disease.

In the immediate postoperative period, the mediastinum ideally should remain midline to avoid respiratory compromise of the contralateral lung or decreased venous blood return to the heart. Thereafter, the mediastinum gradually shifts toward the side of pneumonectomy, and the ipsilateral hemidiaphragm rises. Any subsequent reversal of this mediastinal shift (shift away from the side of pneumonectomy) (Figure 8-2) should suggest an abnormality, such as bronchopleural fistula, empyema, hemothorax, or recurrent carcinoma. The final appearance of the chest is dependent upon the compliance of the mediastinum, the remaining lung, and the hemidiaphragm and ranges from one of relatively minimal shift to one of extreme mediastinal shift (Figures 8-6 and 8-7).

When assessing mediastinal shift, the depth of inspiration and the site of mediastinal shift must be taken into account. In one study of postpneumonectomy patients evaluated with inspiratory/expiratory radiographs, the heart shifted away from the side of pneumonectomy during expiration in 15 of 16 patients.[50] The average shift was 20 mm in the early postoperative period (3 to 11 days) and 13.4 mm in the later postoperative period (46 days or more). On the other hand, contralateral tracheal shift during expiration occurred in only 9 of 16 patients. Of five patients in the late postoperative period, the trachea shifted contralaterally with expiration in only one. Thus, the trachea may be a more reliable indicator of a space-occupying process on the side of pneumonectomy, especially in the late postoperative period.

Bronchopleural fistula developing after a pneumonectomy is an uncommon event that occurs in 6 to 12% of patients.[12,20,54] It is a serious complication, with mortality rates ranging from 25 to 50%. The majority of patients present within the first 3 months after surgery. There may be an acute onset of cough productive of large amounts of brown fluid and with flooding of the contralateral lung. Alternatively, the patient may undergo a slow wasting process associated with fever and slight cough. Rarely, the patient remains asymptomatic. These fistulas are more

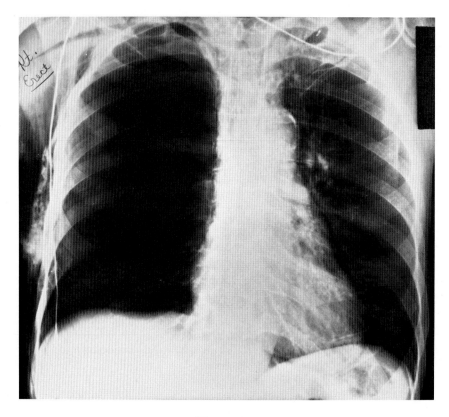

Figure 8-3

Figures 8-3 through 8-7. Normal postpneumonectomy appearances. Figures 8-3 to 8-6 are from one patient, and Figure 8-7 is from another; both patients had pneumonectomy for squamous cell carcinoma. On postoperative day 1 (Figure 8-3), the right hemithorax is air-filled and the mediastinum is midline. On postoperative day 10 (Figure 8-4), there is partial filling of the hemithorax with fluid, while the mediastinum remains virtually midline. On postoperative day 77 (Figure 8-5), the amount of fluid has increased and loculated air-fluid collections are visible. The mediastinum has begun to shift to the right. Complete opacification had occurred by 11 months (not shown). Eleven years postoperatively (Figure 8-6), the hemithorax is opaque and calcification has developed in the pleural space (arrows). There is a moderate shift of the mediastinum and minimal compensatory hyperexpansion of the left lung across the midline (arrowheads). On the other hand, another patient (Figure 8-7) shows extreme mediastinal shift 2 years after pneumonectomy. The two vertical lung margins projecting within the left hemithorax reflect anterior and posterior compensatory hyperexpansion of the right lung.

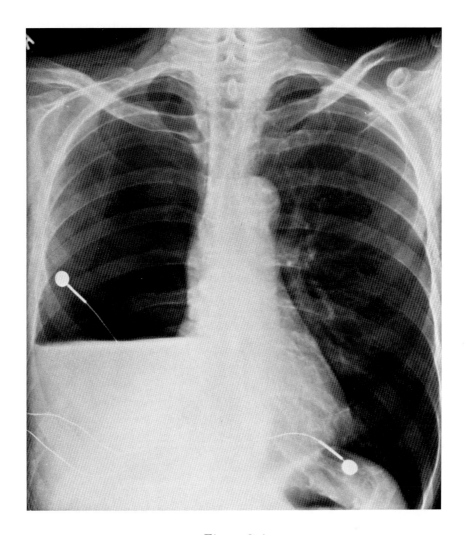

Figure 8-4

common on the right than on the left. Risk factors for their development relate to an infection in the pleural space, a long residual bronchial stump, and the type of bronchial closure. Recurrence of neoplasm at the bronchial stump is a relatively uncommon cause of bronchopleural fistula.

In the early postoperative period, the radiographic finding most suggestive of bronchopleural fistula is a fall in the air-fluid level of more than 2 cm. Lesser decreases in the fluid level may be due to technical factors or to presumed small bronchopleural fistulas, which are of no

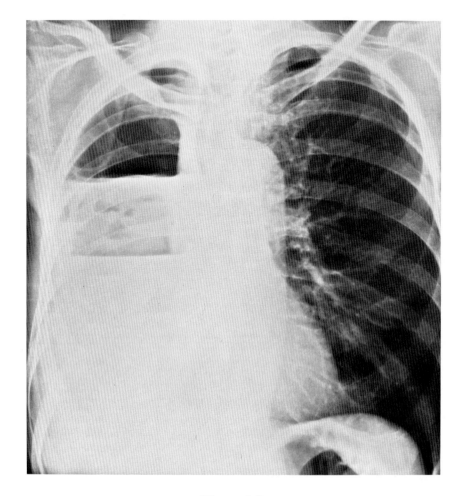

Figure 8-5

clinical consequence.[8] Occasionally, patients will exhibit complete disappearance of fluid, remain asymptomatic, and eventually obliterate the pleural space.[35] Other signs suggesting bronchopleural fistula include air bubbles persisting in or developing in the pleural fluid (Figures 8-8 to 8-11), reappearance of air in a previously opacified hemithorax (Figures 8-12 and 8-13), progressive chest wall or mediastinal emphysema, or persistent pneumothorax in the early postoperative period.

Bronchopleural fistula may be confirmed by bronchoscopy, by instillation of methylene blue into the trachea with its subsequent appearance in the pleural fluid, or by bronchography. Rarely, when these methods

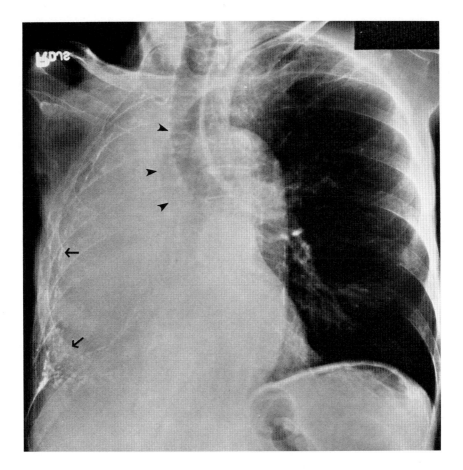

Figure 8-6

have been negative, the fistula has been confirmed by ventilation scintigraphy with [133]Xe.[56]

Bronchoesophageal fistula after pneumonectomy is most often associated with esophagopleural fistula, with the latter occurring alone more commonly than the former.[42,43,44] However, an esophagopleural fistula after pneumonectomy is a rare event; it is seen in fewer than 1% of patients. Eighty percent of esophagopleural fistulas occur after a right pneumonectomy. Presumably, the descending aorta on the left protects the esophagus from operative injury or inflammatory erosion. Patients with esophagopleural fistulas always have symptoms and signs of empyema.

When esophagopleural fistulas occur in the early postoperative period, they are almost always associated with a difficult dissection involving

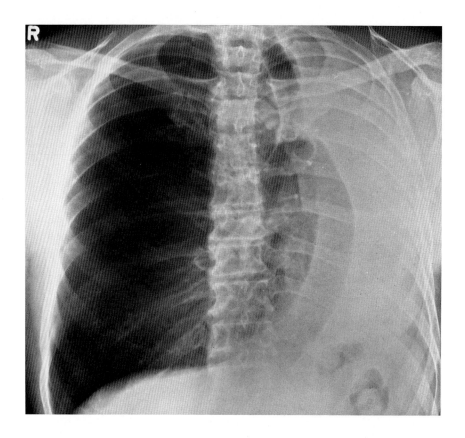

Figure 8-7

the lower mediastinum. The esophagus has a segmental blood supply which is poorest from the level of the carina inferiorly, and fistulas during the early period are probably related to ischemia. In the late postoperative period, a bronchopleural fistula or empyema is commonly present prior to the esophagopleural fistula, and presumably these perforate into the esophagus. Recurrent carcinoma rarely causes esophagopleural fistula.

The radiographic signs of bronchoesophageal or esophagopleural fistula are similar to those of bronchopleural fistula, as already described. If a bronchoesophageal fistula is present, parenchymal disease from aspiration may appear in the remaining lung. Esophagopleural fistulas are confirmed either by demonstration of food particles or ingested methylene blue in the empyema drainage or by barium swallow. In the test case, since air is not visible in the left hemithorax in Figure 8-2, and

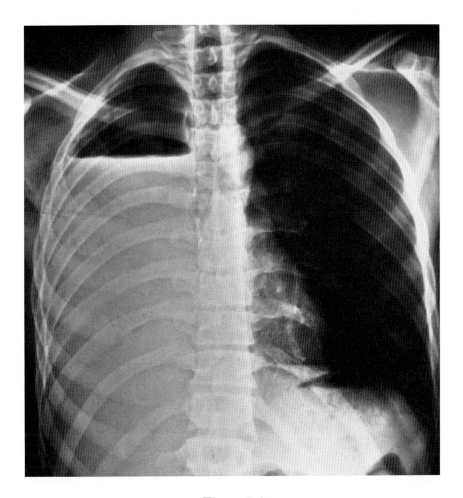

Figure 8-8

Figures 8-8 through 8-11. Postpneumonectomy bronchopleural fistula/empyema. Right pneumonectomy was performed for a lung abscess that had resulted from a gunshot wound. On postoperative day 12 (Figure 8-8), the hemithorax had partially filled with fluid and the mediastinum remained midline. Pleural fluid cultures were negative at this time. On postoperative day 16 (Figure 8-9), multiple loculated air-fluid collections had developed. Since the patient was clinically improving, a small bronchopleural fistula was suspected rather than infection. No specific treatment was undertaken. On postoperative day 46 (Figure 8-10), the hemithorax had filled further with fluid but air-fluid collections remained. The patient continued to have no clinical evidence of infection. On postoperative day 65 (Figure 8-11), a large air collection had reappeared, concurrent with drainage of fluid through the thoracotomy incision. The patient had had a fever for 24 hours. Further drainage was subsequently established via a lower rib resection. A bronchopleural fistula was found at bronchoscopy.

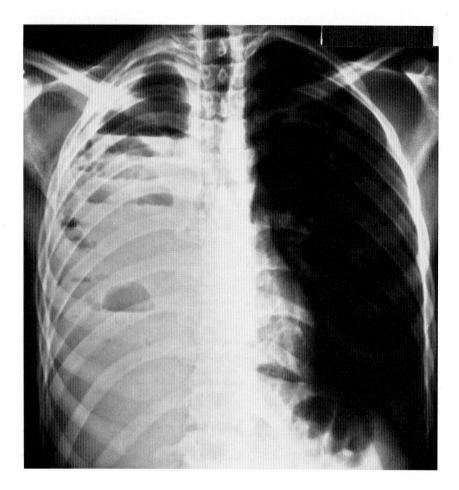

Figure 8-9

since there is no parenchymal disease in the right lung, a bronchoesophageal fistula is unlikely.

Postoperative empyema is an uncommon complication of pneumonectomy.[23,24,27,33] It occurs after 2 to 4% of pneumonectomies performed for carcinoma but may occur in as many as 45% of patients with inflammatory disease and preexisting empyema. Most of these infections occur in the early postoperative period and result from contamination at the time of surgery or from development of bronchopleural or esophagopleural fistulas. The organism most frequently isolated is *Staphylococcus aureus*, although gram-negative bacteria or fungi are identified at times.[28] Empyema developing in the late period is relatively rare and may result from a bronchopleural fistula, an esophagopleural

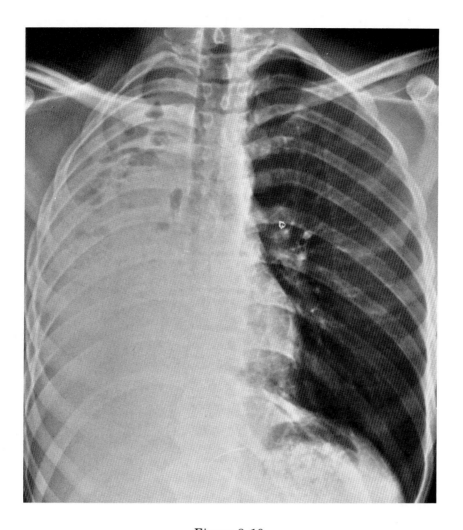

Figure 8-10

fistula, or hematogenous dissemination. Patients with bronchopleural fistulas usually have cough productive of sputum, which may be copious and may increase in amount when the patient is in the contralateral decubitus position. On the other hand, a patient with empyema, but without a fistula, may have minimal symptoms except for not feeling well. Illness may persist for months before the diagnosis is established, usually due to empyema necessitatis. Unfortunately, most patients with late onset of empyema show no radiographic clues, although shift of the mediastinum away from the side of pneumonectomy should suggest the diagnosis (Figures 8-14 and 8-15). In one report, four of five patients with

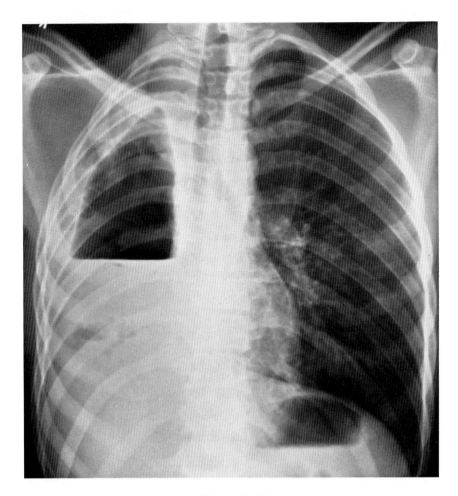

Figure 8-11

late-onset empyemas without fistulas had no mediastinal (tracheal) shift. The patient who demonstrated shift did so only after experiencing gradual deterioration with illness for 1 year.[23]

For patients who have had lobectomy or pneumonectomy, recurrence of carcinoma is most likely to occur in the mediastinum or ipsilateral hemithorax.[17,46] Prior to the advent of computed tomography, shift of the trachea toward the midline and away from the side of pneumonectomy was the most sensitive radiographic sign of recurrent carcinoma.[13]

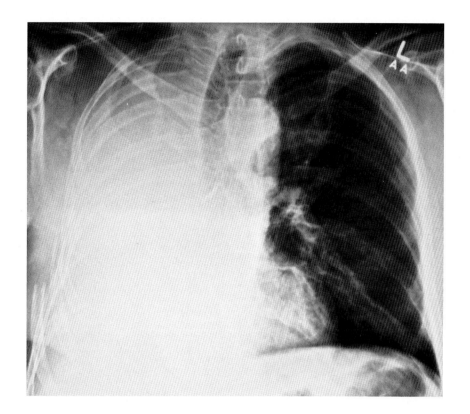

Figure 8-12

Figures 8-12 and 8-13. Postpneumonectomy bronchopleural fistula. Right pneumonectomy was performed for squamous cell carcinoma with gross tumor remaining in the mediastinum. Radiation therapy was administered postoperatively. On postoperative day 13 (Figure 8-12), the right hemithorax was opacified and the mediastinum had shifted to the right, suggesting a normal postoperative appearance. On postoperative day 57 (Figure 8-13), air was present in the right hemithorax, although the patient remained asymptomatic. Culture of the fluid grew *S. aureus*, and the patient was treated with rib resection and open drainage as well as antibiotics. Residual tumor was subsequently demonstrated.

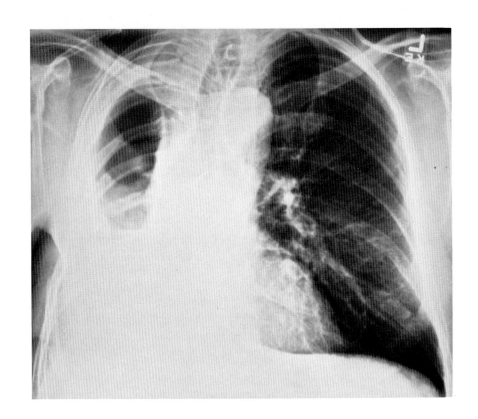

Figure 8-13

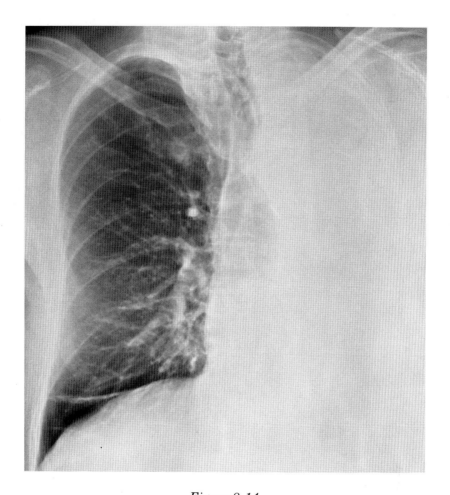

Figure 8-14

Figures 8-14 and 8-15. Postpneumonectomy empyema. Left pneumonectomy was performed for squamous cell carcinoma. By postoperative day 61 (Figure 8-14), the left hemithorax was opacified and the mediastinum had shifted to the left. By postoperative day 106 (Figure 8-15), the mediastinum had shifted away from the side of pneumonectomy, suggesting a space-occupying process on the left. An empyema without carcinomatous recurrence was subsequently proven.

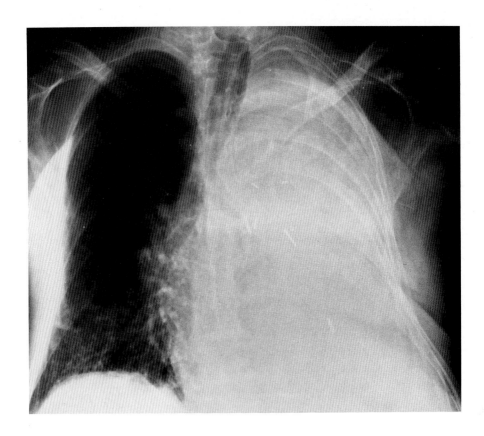

Figure 8-15

Question 38

Which *one* of the following would be the next MOST effective imaging study?

(A) Conventional tomography
(B) Computed tomography
(C) Ga-67 scintigraphy
(D) Barium esophagram
(E) Tc-99m methylene diphosphonate (MDP) scintigraphy

A number of tests are available to help distinguish between an empyema and recurrent carcinoma (the two true options from Question 37). While conventional tomography (Option (A)) may demonstrate small amounts of air or gas, which suggest a fistulous connection or empyema, respectively, its limited soft tissue discrimination does not detect recurrent carcinomatous masses or non-gas-producing empyemas. Scintigraphy with Ga-67 (Option (C)) has shown uptake in patients with either lung cancer or empyema, both before and after pneumonectomy.[24] While a positive scan would help confirm the presence of a space-occupying neoplastic or inflammatory process, it would not reliably differentiate between recurrent tumor and empyema. Diffuse uptake of a Tc-99m-labeled bone seeker may occur in the normal postpneumonectomy space, and therefore Tc-99m MDP scintigraphy (Option (E)) would not be helpful.[38] A barium esophagram (Option (D)) would confirm the position of the esophagus but is not likely to yield further discriminatory information. Almost all patients with postpneumonectomy esophagopleural or bronchoesophageal fistulas have had air readily demonstrated in the postoperative space, and the esophagram has been used to confirm and localize the fistula.

Computed tomography (CT) may best identify and characterize abnormalities in the postpneumonectomy space **(Option (B) is correct).** Postpneumonectomy recurrence of carcinoma has been identified as a mass adjacent to the bronchial stump, as a mass projecting into postpneumonectomy fluid, or as mediastinal lymph node enlargement.[15,36] The patient shown in Figures 8-1 and 8-2 had recurrent tumor demonstrated in the left hemithorax by CT (Figure 8-16).

CT has also demonstrated empyema in the postpneumonectomy space.[18] In addition to shift away from the side of pneumonectomy, there may be alteration in the contour of the interface between the mediastinum and pneumonectomy space. Normally, this interface is straight or concave on the side of the pneumonectomy space. As the pneumonectomy space fills, the contour reverses and becomes convex

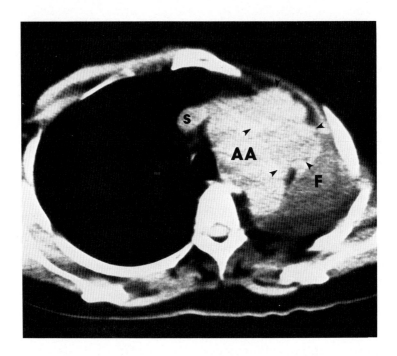

Figure 8-16. Same patient as in Figures 8-1 and 8-2. Postpneumonectomy carcinoma recurrence. CT at the level of the aortic arch (AA) shows recurrent tumor in mediastinal lymph nodes (arrowheads). S = superior vena cava; F = postpneumonectomy pleural fluid.

(Figures 8-17 and 8-18). While recurrent neoplasm with an accompanying increase in pleural fluid could produce a similar appearance, the absence of other radiographic evidence of recurrence or a clinical setting suggesting empyema should lead to the correct diagnosis.

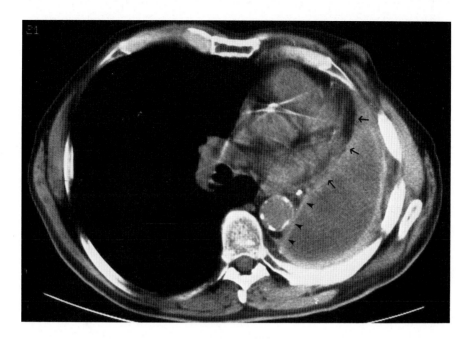

Figure 8-17

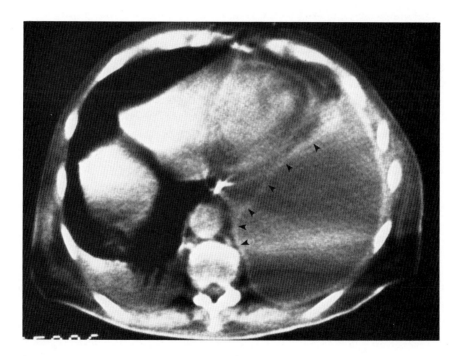

Figure 8-18
Figures 8-17 and 8-18. Postpneumonectomy empyema. Two patients
with previous pneumonectomies for carcinoma. CT of a normal postpneumonectomy space (Figure 8-17) shows that the mediastinum/pneu-
monectomy space contour is straight (arrowheads) or slightly concave
(arrows) on the pneumonectomy space side. CT in a patient with
empyema (Figure 8-18; same patient as in Figures 8-14 and 8-15) shows
shift of the heart and descending aorta to the right and a convex contour
(arrowheads) on the pneumonectomy space side.

Question 39

Concerning the postpneumonectomy patient,

    (A) the aortic arch undergoes rotation to a more sagittal orientation after a right pneumonectomy

    (B) fluid is completely resorbed from the pleural space within 1 year

    (C) compensatory lung growth by formation of new alveoli takes place in a patient who undergoes a pneumonectomy at age 12 years

    (D) chronic overdistention of the remaining lung results in emphysema with destruction of alveolar walls

    (E) the risk of respiratory failure is high when the predicted postoperative forced expiratory volume in 1 second (FEV_1) is less than 1.0 L

A number of anatomic and physiologic changes take place in the thorax after a pneumonectomy has been performed. As previously described, the mediastinum shifts toward the side of pneumonectomy during the late postoperative period. As part of this shift, the heart and aorta undergo rotation around the fixed axis of the descending aorta.[3] After a right pneumonectomy, the aortic arch rotates into a more coronal plane, while after a left pneumonectomy it rotates into a more sagittal plane (Figures 8-19 and 8-20) **(Option (A) is false).** In addition to the rotational changes, the remaining lung undergoes compensatory hyperinflation. Although this has been referred to as herniation, it is not a true hernia since the mediastinal pleura remains intact and the lung simply moves along with the mediastinum. After a right pneumonectomy, this hyperinflation occurs almost exclusively anteriorly (Figure 8-21). After a left pneumonectomy, nearly one-half of the patients have lung hyperinflation posteriorly as well (Figure 8-22).

Early after removal of a lung, the postpneumonectomy space is filled with fluid and air. The amount of fibrin-rich fluid gradually increases until it entirely fills the hemithorax. During the late postoperative period, this fluid organizes with ingrowth of fibroblasts and development of granulation tissue. While some older reports suggested that the entire thorax eventually becomes fibrous, a brown or amber-colored pleural fluid, with a density on CT near that of water, remains permanently in the majority of patients **(Option (B) is false).**[3,48] There is more thickening of the parietal pleura along the chest wall than along the mediastinum. The postpneumonectomy space is totally obliterated in only 23 to 40% of patients, and in these, extreme shift of the mediastinum and elevation of the hemidiaphragm occur.

After a pulmonary resection, the remaining lung grows in volume, weight, and cell number but does not reach a state equivalent to the

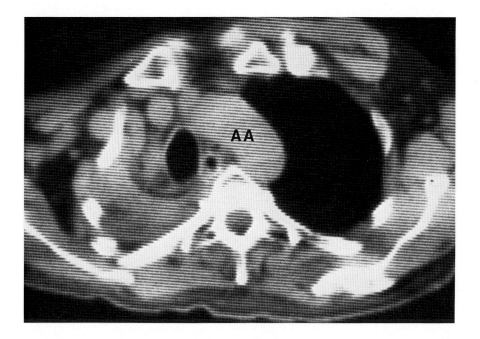

Figure 8-19
Figures 8-19 through 8-22. Figures 8-19 and 8-21, same patient as in Figures 8-12 and 8-13; Figures 8-20 and 8-22, same patient as in Figure 8-7. Postpneumonectomy CT appearances. CT at the level of the aortic arch shows its relatively coronal orientation after a right pneumonectomy (Figure 8-19) and sagittal orientation after a left pneumonectomy (Figure 8-20). CT at the level of the main pulmonary artery shows compensatory hyperinflation of the left lung anteriorly (Figure 8-21) with a right pneumonectomy. With a left pneumonectomy, the right lung hyperinflates anteriorly and posteriorly (Figure 8-22). Note also the ascending and descending aorta in these last two images. AA = aortic arch; A = ascending aorta; D = descending aorta; P = main/proximal right pulmonary artery; F = postpneumonectomy pleural fluid; T = tumor recurrence.

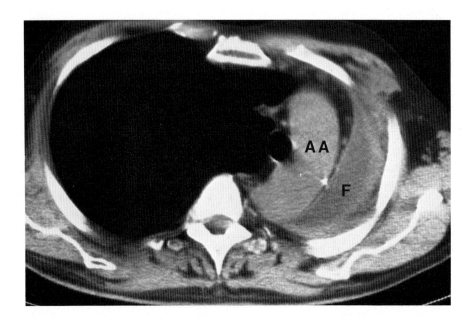

Figure 8-20

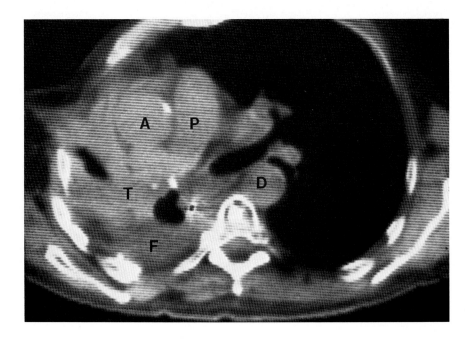

Figure 8-21

140 / *Chest Disease IV*

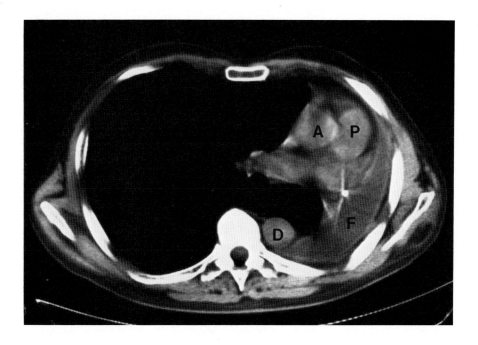

Figure 8-22

original one.[6,39] In adult patients having pneumonectomy, lung volumes increase during the first 1 to 2 years and then plateau. In patients without significant disease in the remaining lung, these volumes may approach but do not actually reach normal predicted or preoperative ones. Patients are usually asymptomatic and have minimal exercise limitation. On the other hand, patients with preoperative disease in the remaining lung are more often symptomatic and do not approach their preoperative states as closely as do patients without preoperative disease. Children undergoing pulmonary resection usually closely approach their predicted lung volumes when they reach adulthood. The earlier the resection occurs in childhood, the more likely that normal volumes will be present in adulthood.[30,37]

Alveoli normally continue to form in the lungs of infants and young children, the 20 million alveoli present at birth increasing to the adult number of about 300 million. Although early studies suggested that this process continues up to about age 8 years, more recently it has been suggested that the process is complete by age 2 years in boys and by age 4 years in girls **(Option (C) is false)**.[9,11,49] Controversy has existed over whether postresectional compensatory lung growth in children is accomplished by the dilatation of existing alveoli or by the addition of new ones. A number of studies with laboratory animals have suggested that pneumonectomy performed at an early age stimulates alveolar multiplication, implying that the compensation is by the addition of new alveoli. Other studies have been unable to confirm this alveolar multiplication. A recent study of beagles undergoing pneumonectomy as puppies and followed to adulthood found that resection does stimulate alveolar multiplication, but the final number of alveoli per lobe is that which would be present in the absence of resection.[10] This suggests that pneumonectomy accelerates the maturation process but does not affect the absolute number of alveoli per lobe present in adults.

Although the remaining postpneumonectomy lung may undergo considerable hyperexpansion, this does not cause a true destructive emphysema **(Option (D) is false)**.[45] Pulmonary function studies show relatively normal values unless the patient had emphysema preoperatively. In a study of patients having resection for lung carcinoma and subsequently undergoing autopsy, emphysema was demonstrated in the remaining lung in 8 of 14 patients.[14] Most of these patients also had emphysema in the previously resected lung, suggesting that it was a preexisting disorder and not a result of the pneumonectomy.

While the majority of patients with lung cancer may undergo resectional surgery without difficulty, chronic obstructive pulmonary disease is of sufficient severity in about 10 to 20% of patients to influence the decision regarding surgery. When the forced expiratory volume in 1 second (FEV_1) falls below 1.0 L, exercise tolerance decreases. There is a concomitant increased frequency of carbon dioxide retention and mortality from respiratory insufficiency (10% per year) **(Option (E) is true)**.[7] Since pneumonectomy always results in some decrease in pulmonary function, it is important to know the contribution to overall function of the lung that will remain so as to avoid chronic respiratory insufficiency. Moreover, in patients with marginal pulmonary reserve, the 30-day mortality rate from any cause is 15% after pneumonectomy.[4]

Routine pulmonary function tests unfortunately do not reflect the regional distribution of lung abnormality. Quantitative scintigraphic techniques have been developed to evaluate regional ventilation and perfusion and have been used to predict the postoperative FEV_1. Both ^{133}Xe ventilation imaging and Tc-99m macroaggregated albumin perfusion scintigraphy have been used to predict postoperative FEV_1.[34,52] In general, calculation of the predicted postoperative value involves multiplying the preoperative FEV_1 by the scintigraphically measured percentage of function contributed by the lung that will remain. In a follow-up study of 38 high-risk patients (predicted postoperative FEV_1, 0.86 to 1.69 L), 5 patients (13%) died of respiratory insufficiency. Four of the five deaths occurred more than 1 year postoperatively. Although this figure suggests considerable risk, it must be considered in the light of an otherwise fatal disease (lung cancer). In the same group of 38 patients, 5 (13%) survived for 5 years.[4]

Question 40

Which *one* of the following is the LEAST likely cause of acquired bronchoesophageal fistula?

(A) Mediastinal neoplasm
(B) Mediastinal granuloma
(C) Tuberculosis
(D) Trauma
(E) Wegener's granulomatosis

Acquired fistulas between the tracheobronchial tree and the esophagus are uncommon. The majority of these communications result from neoplasia, such as lymphoma and carcinoma of the esophagus, lung, and trachea (Option (A)).[29,31,47] Most benign fistulas result from infection or trauma.[1,21,22,32,53,55] The most common infectious agents include tuberculosis (Option (C)), syphilis, actinomycosis, histoplasmosis, and esophageal candidiasis. In tuberculosis, histoplasmosis, and syphilis, the fistula results from granulomatous mediastinal inflammation in adjacent paratracheal or subcarinal lymph nodes. Mediastinal granuloma (Option (B)) is thus a cause of bronchoesophageal fistula. It should be pointed out, however, that bronchoesophageal fistula is an uncommon manifestation of mediastinal granuloma, which more commonly narrows the airways or esophagus. Trauma (Option (D)) responsible for fistula formation may be blunt or penetrating, relate to ingestion of foreign bodies or caustic substances, or result from endotracheal intubation or esophageal dilatation or may be secondary to irradiation for carcinoma.[19,41,55] Wegener's granulomatosis involves the sinuses and lungs but rarely involves the larynx or proximal trachea. As of this writing, no instances of bronchoesophageal or tracheoesophageal fistula have been reported in this disorder (**Option (E) is therefore least likely and the correct answer**).

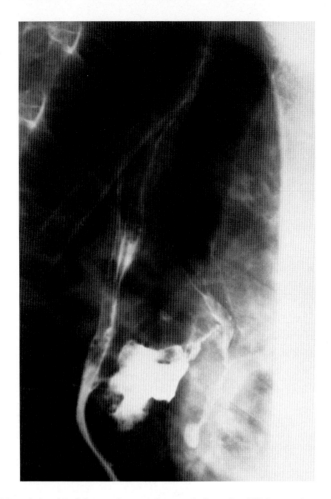

Figure 8-23. Acquired bronchoesophageal fistula. This patient, treated with radiation 1 year previously for adenocarcinoma of the lung, had noted coughing associated with swallowing. His barium examination shows a bronchoesophageal fistula traversing enlarged subcarinal lymph nodes.

Patients with bronchoesophageal fistulas have cough (especially with ingestion of liquids), hemoptysis, or recurrent pneumonias.[40] These symptoms may be intermittently present for years. Chest radiography is unrevealing except when pneumonia occurs. A contrast examination will demonstrate the fistula in nearly all patients (Figure 8-23). In a few patients, repeated examinations with thin barium sulfate suspensions will be necessary to demonstrate the fistula. Care must be taken to perform the examination in multiple positions, and it may be helpful to ask the patient whether there is a position in which the symptoms may be precipitated. CT may demonstrate these but is usually not required.[2]

Question 41

Which *one* of the following is LEAST likely to cause an empyema?

(A) *Mycobacterium tuberculosis*
(B) Anaerobic bacilli
(C) Fungi
(D) *Streptococcus pneumoniae* (pneumococci)
(E) *Pneumocystis carinii*

Empyema is a collection of pus in the pleural space. The features of postpneumonectomy empyema have been previously discussed. Empyemas occurring in other settings are most often associated with underlying pneumonia, recent surgery (thoracic or upper abdominal, most commonly), or trauma with hemothorax.[27,28,51] Patients may have fever, an elevated leukocyte count, and pleuritic chest pain.

In the preantibiotic era, *Streptococcus pneumoniae* (Option (D)) was the most common cause of empyema. In the 1950s and 1960s, *Staphylococcus aureus* was the most common cause. Currently, anaerobic bacilli (Option (B)) are the most commonly identified organisms, although both *S. pneumoniae* and *S. aureus* continue to be isolated. The most commonly encountered empyemas are postpneumonic or postoperative, and multiple organisms are isolated in 65% of these. These organisms include gram-positive and gram-negative anaerobic and aerobic bacteria. In contrast, a single organism is isolated in 70% of patients with posttraumatic empyemas.

A variety of other organisms have been identified as etiologic agents in empyema. Fungi (Option (C)) include *Aspergillus* species, *Blastomyces dermatitidis*, *Coccidioides immitis*, *Cryptococcus neoformans*, and *Histoplasma capsulatum*. *Mycobacterium tuberculosis* (Option (A)) is yet another etiologic agent. *Pneumocystis carinii* is a parasite responsible for pulmonary infections in immunocompromised hosts, particularly patients with acquired immunodeficiency syndrome, transplants, or hematologic malignancy. Although the lung infection may be severe, pleural effusions and empyema are extraordinarily rare **(Option (E) is least likely and the correct answer).**[5]

SUGGESTED READINGS

1. Anderson RP, Sabiston DC Jr. Acquired bronchoesophageal fistula of benign origin. Surg Gynecol Obstet 1965; 121:261–266

2. Berkmen YM, Auh YH. CT diagnosis of acquired tracheoesophageal fistula in adults. J Comput Assist Tomogr 1985; 9:302–304

3. Biondetti PR, Fiore D, Sartori F, Colognato A, Ravasini R, Romani S. Evaluation of the post-pneumonectomy space by computed tomography. J Comput Assist Tomogr 1982; 6:238–242

4. Boysen PG, Harris JO, Block AJ, Olsen GN. Prospective evaluation for pneumonectomy using perfusion scanning: follow-up beyond one year. Chest 1981; 80:163–166

5. Burke BA, Good RA. *Pneumocystis carinii* infection. Medicine 1973; 52:23–51

6. Burrows B, Harrison RW, Adams WE, Humphreys EM, Long ET, Reimann AF. The postpneumonectomy state: clinical and physiologic observations in thirty-six cases. Am J Med 1960; 28:281–297

7. Burrows B, Strauss RH, Niden AH. Chronic obstructive lung disease III: interrelationships of pulmonary function data. Am Rev Respir Dis 1965; 91:861–868

8. Christiansen KH, Morgan SW, Karich AF, Takaro T. Pleural space following pneumonectomy. Ann Thorac Surg 1965; 1:298–304

9. Davies G, Reid L. Growth of the alveoli and pulmonary arteries in childhood. Thorax 1970; 25:669–681

10. Davies P, McBride J, Murray GF, Wilcox BR, Shallal JA, Reid L. Structural changes in the canine lung and pulmonary arteries after pneumonectomy. J Appl Physiol 1982; 53:859–864

11. Dunnill MS. Postnatal growth of the lung. Thorax 1962; 17:329–333

12. Forrester-Wood CP. Bronchopleural fistula following pneumonectomy for carcinoma of the bronchus: mechanical stapling versus hand suturing. J Thorac Cardiovasc Surg 1980; 80:406–409

13. Fraser RG, Paré JA. Diagnosis of diseases of the chest, 2nd ed. Philadelphia: WB Saunders; 1979:1619–1623

14. Fry WA, Archer FA, Adams WE. Long-term clinical-pathologic study of the pneumonectomy patient. Dis Chest 1967; 52:720–726

15. Glazer HS, Aronberg DJ, Sagel SS, Emami B. Utility of CT in detecting postpneumonectomy carcinoma recurrence. AJR 1984; 142:487–494

16. Goodman LR. Postoperative chest radiograph. II. Alterations after major intrathoracic surgery. AJR 1980; 134:803–813

17. Green N, Kern W. The clinical course and treatment results of patients with postresection locally recurrent lung cancer. Cancer 1978; 42:2478–2482

18. Heater K, Revzani L, Rubin JM. CT evaluation of empyema in the postpneumonectomy space. AJR 1985; 145:39–40

19. Hishikawa Y, Tanaka S, Miura T. Esophageal fistula associated with intracavitary irradiation for esophageal carcinoma. Radiology 1986; 159:549–551

20. Hoier-Madsen K, Schulze S, Moller-Pedersen V, Halkier E. Management of bronchopleural fistula following pneumonectomy. Scand J Thorac Cardiovasc Surg 1984; 18:263–266

21. Hutchin P, Lindskog GE. Acquired esophagobronchial fistula of infectious origin. J Thorac Cardiovasc Surg 1964; 48:1–10

22. Judd DR, Dubuque T Jr. Acquired benign esophagotracheobronchial fistula. Dis Chest 1968; 54:237–240

23. Kerr WF. Late-onset post-pneumonectomy empyema. Thorax 1977; 32:149–154

24. Kutty CP, Varkey B. Empyema seven years after pneumonectomy. Detection by gallium 67 scan. JAMA 1979; 242:2322–2324

25. La Cour Andersen J, Egedorf J, Stougoard J. The pleural space succeeding pneumonectomy. A roentgenological and clinical study of 167 cases of bronchogenic carcinoma. Scand J Thorac Cardiovasc Surg 1968; 2:70–73

26. Lams P. Radiographic signs in postpneumonectomy bronchopleural fistula. J Can Assoc Radiol 1980; 31:178–180

27. Le Roux BT, Mohlala ML, Odell JA, Whitton ID. Suppurative diseases of the lung and pleural space. Part I: empyema thoracis and lung abscess. Curr Probl Surg 1986; 23:1–89

28. Light RW. Pleural diseases. Philadelphia: Lea & Febiger; 1983:101–139

29. Little AG, Ferguson MK, DeMeester TR, Hoffman PC, Skinner DB. Esophageal carcinoma with respiratory tract fistula. Cancer 1984; 53:1322–1328

30. Martini N, Goodner JT, D'Angio GJ, Beattie EJ Jr. Tracheoesophageal fistula due to cancer. J Thorac Cardiovasc Surg 1970; 59:319–324

31. McBride JT, Wohl ME, Strieder DJ, et al. Lung growth and airway function after lobectomy in infancy for congenital lobar emphysema. J Clin Invest 1980; 66:962–970

32. Obrecht WF Jr, Richter JE, Olympio GA, Gelfand DW. Tracheoesophageal fistula: a serious complication of infectious esophagitis. Gastroenterology 1984; 87:1174–1179

33. Odell JA, Henderson BJ. Pneumonectomy through an empyema. J Thorac Cardiovasc Surg 1985; 89:423–427

34. Olsen GN, Block AJ, Tobias JA. Prediction of postpneumonectomy pulmonary function using quantitative macroaggregate lung scanning. Chest 1974; 66:13–16

35. O'Meara JB, Slade PR. Disappearance of fluid from the postpneumonectomy space. J Thorac Cardiovasc Surg 1974; 67:621–628

36. Peters JC, Desai KK. CT demonstration of postpneumonectomy tumor recurrence. AJR 1983; 141:259–262

37. Peters RM, Wilcox BR, Schultz EH Jr. Pulmonary resection in children: long-term effect on function and lung growth. Ann Surg 1964; 159:652–659

38. Ravin CE, Hoyt TS, De Blanc H. Concentration of 99m technetium polyphosphate in fibrothorax following pneumonectomy. Radiology 1977; 122:405–408

39. Reid LM. Lung growth in health and disease. Br J Dis Chest 1984; 78:113–134

40. Sacks RP, Du Bois JJ, Geiger JP, Severance RC. The esophagobronchial fistula. Case report and review of the literature. AJR 1967; 99:204–209

41. Schmitz GL. Acquired tracheoesophageal fistula. Otolaryngol Clin North Am 1979; 12:823–827

42. Sethi GK, Takaro T. Esophagopleural fistula following pulmonary resection. Ann Thorac Surg 1978; 25:74–81

43. Shama DM, Odell JA. Esophagopleural fistula after pneumonectomy for inflammatory disease. J Thorac Cardiovasc Surg 1985; 89:77–81

44. Sharma R, Fulkerson LL, Stein E, Guzman LG. Persistent pneumothorax after pneumonectomy. J Thorac Cardiovasc Surg 1973; 66:588–591
45. Spencer H. Pathology of the lungs, 4th ed. Oxford: Pergamon Press; 1985:566
46. Spjut HJ, Mateo LE. Recurrent and metastatic carcinoma in surgically treated carcinoma of lung. Cancer 1965; 18:1462–1466
47. Stark P. Bronchoenteric fistulae in lymphoma. AJR 1981; 136:615–617
48. Suarez J, Clagett T, Brown AL Jr. The postpneumonectomy space: factors influencing its obliteration. J Thorac Cardiovasc Surg 1969; 57:539–542
49. Thurlbeck WM. Postnatal human lung growth. Thorax 1982; 37:564–571
50. Wechsler RJ, Goodman LR. Mediastinal position and air-fluid height after pneumonectomy: the effect of the respiratory cycle. AJR 1985; 145:1173–1176
51. Wehr CJ, Adkins RB Jr. Empyema thoracis: a ten-year experience. South Med J 1986; 79:171–176
52. Wernly JA, DeMeester TR, Kirchner PT, Myerowitz PD, Oxford DE, Golomb HM. Clinical value of quantitative ventilation-perfusion lung scans in the surgical management of bronchogenic carcinoma. J Thorac Cardiovasc Surg 1980; 80:535–543
53. Wigley FM, Murray HW, Mann RB, Saba GP, Kashima H, Mann JJ. Unusual manifestation of tuberculosis: TE fistula. Am J Med 1976; 60:310–314
54. Williams NS, Lewis CT. Bronchopleural fistula: a review of 86 cases. Br J Surg 1976; 63:520–522
55. Wychulis AR, Ellis FH Jr, Andersen HA. Acquired nonmalignant esophagotracheobronchial fistula. Report of 36 cases. JAMA 1966; 196:117–122
56. Zelefsky MN, Freeman LM, Stern H. A simple approach to the diagnosis of bronchopleural fistula. Radiology 1977; 124:843–844

Notes

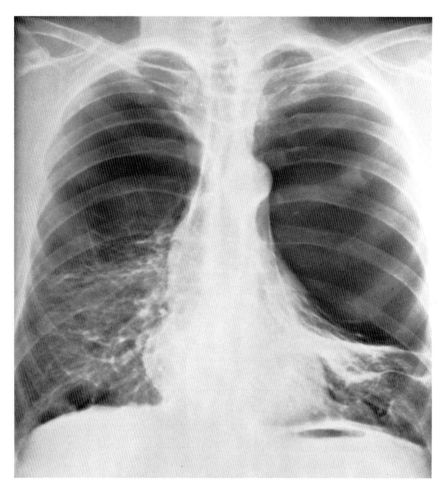

Figure 9-1. This 48-year-old man had progressively increasing dyspnea and wheezing for 1 year. A posteroanterior chest radiograph was taken at the time of a hand injury. Note that the opacity at the level of the left third anterior rib is an artifact.

Case 9: Giant Bullous Cysts

Question 42

Which *one* of the following is the MOST likely diagnosis?

(A) Bilateral pneumothorax
(B) Bilateral lower lobe atelectasis
(C) The Swyer-James syndrome
(D) Giant bullous cysts
(E) Alpha-1-antitrypsin deficiency

The chest radiograph (Figure 9-1) shows increased lucency in each upper hemithorax and increased opacity in each lower one. Vascular markings are absent in the areas of increased lucency, with a few linear strands projecting upward at the mid right hemithorax. On the left, the increased lucency is sharply demarcated and is convex toward the hilum. The heart and mediastinal structures are normal.

Abnormal lucencies are often visible on the chest radiograph. Careful analysis of the characteristics of a lucency with regard to its position, shape, degree of lucency, and associated findings will usually lead to the correct diagnosis. Entities to be considered in the differential diagnosis include abnormalities of the lung and chest wall, pneumothorax, and technical artifacts. Due to the combination of lucency and the absence of vascular markings in Figure 9-1, abnormalities of the lung and pneumothorax are the primary considerations.

Bilateral pneumothorax (Option (A)) is visible as bilateral apical increased lucencies in the erect patient. A pneumothorax is distributed peripherally with regard to the lung, the margin of which is often visible as a thin white curvilinear line (the visceral pleura) nearly parallel to the chest wall (Figure 9-2). Unless there is considerable collapse of the lung or one of its lobes, normal parenchymal density remains, especially in the upper lobes. As the lung collapses further, vessels are crowded into a smaller space but continue to show an arborizing pattern. As complete collapse of the lung occurs, increased opacity is visible, as is loss of

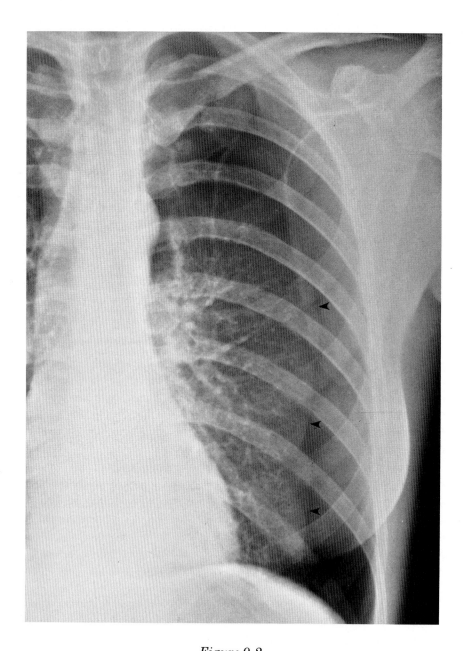

Figure 9-2
Figures 9-2 and 9-3. Pneumothorax. A small to moderate-sized pneumothorax is visible on the left, peripheral to the lung margin (arrowheads), in Figure 9-2. The pulmonary vasculature arborizes but is crowded into a smaller lung volume. With a large right pneumothorax (Figure 9-3), the lucency is more dramatic. The lung has shrunken to a small volume, and the upper lobe appears opaque, with pulmonary vessels being obscured for the most part. Air bronchograms are suggested. Pulmonary vessels are partially visible in the lower lobe.

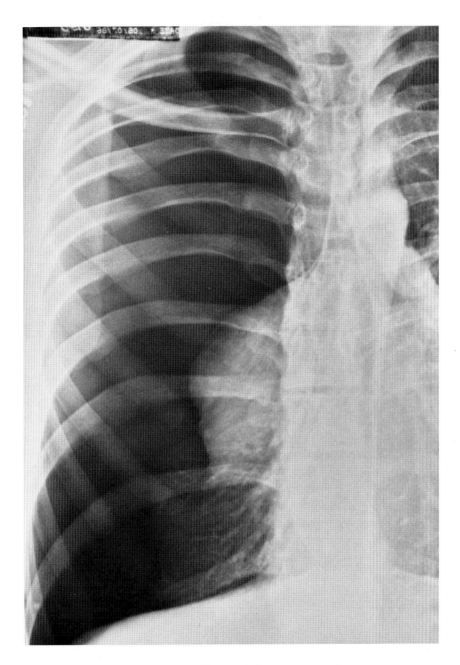

Figure 9-3

definition of the pulmonary vessels (Figure 9-3). Air bronchograms may also be noted.

Except in trauma, simultaneous bilateral pneumothoraces are rare, occurring in fewer than 3% of patients with spontaneous pneumothorax.[14] In patients with underlying lung disease, pneumothorax is almost always unilateral. Bilateral pneumothorax is unlikely in the test patient, since a clear demarcation between lung and pneumothorax is not visible on the right in Figure 9-1. Moreover, on the left the lucency is convex toward the hilum. While a tension pneumothorax with pleural adhesions might conceivably produce such an appearance, the patient's relatively minimal to moderate respiratory symptoms would argue against it.

Bilateral lower lobe atelectasis (Option (B)) is most frequently seen in postsurgical hospitalized patients. Upper zone lucency reflects compensatory hyperexpansion of the upper lobe, in which pulmonary vessels are still visible but spread apart. Pulmonary vessels are absent in the bilateral upper zone lucencies shown in Figure 9-1, and thus atelectasis is an unlikely explanation.

The Swyer-James (Swyer-James-Macleod) syndrome (Option (C)) is a disorder in which abnormal lucency in one lung is the classical characteristic feature.[20,25] The abnormality is due to an obliterative bronchiolitis, which is somewhat patchily distributed throughout the affected lung. The radiographic diagnosis may be confidently made with inspiratory/expiratory views of the chest (Figures 9-4 to 9-6). In addition to being lucent, the affected lung and hemithorax are small or normal in size on inspiration. On expiration, however, the abnormal lung remains lucent and traps air so that the mediastinum shifts contralaterally and the affected hemithorax is relatively large compared with the opposite one. The hilum on the affected side is small, as are the pulmonary vessels, which appear somewhat attenuated but have a relatively normal arborization pattern. Since these findings are not present in our test case (Figure 9-1), Swyer-James syndrome is not likely. Although the patients described by Swyer and James and later by Macleod had abnormalities confined to one lung, other authors have described patients with lobar, rather than entire lung, involvement.[11,24] Findings at bronchography, angiography, and ventilation-perfusion scintigraphy have been described; however, such studies are not considered necessary for the diagnosis in most cases.

Giant bullous cysts (Option (D)) are subpleural air spaces in the lung that have undergone extreme enlargement and may be 10 cm or more in diameter. The radiographic findings vary considerably, depending upon the amount of associated emphysema and the position of the cyst(s) (see

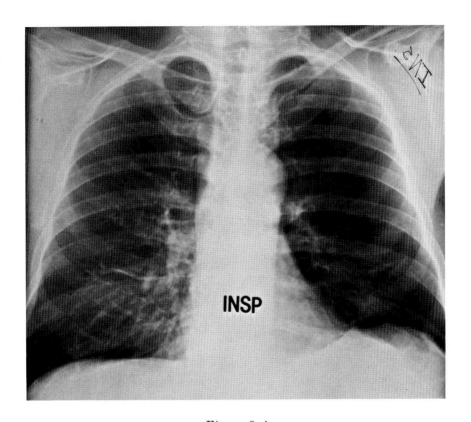

INSP

Figure 9-4

Figures 9-4 through 9-6. The Swyer-James syndrome. The left hemithorax is relatively lucent in comparison to the right on the inspiratory view (Figure 9-4). On the close-up image of the left lung from the same view (Figure 9-5), the left hilum is small and the pulmonary vessels are attenuated but still arborize. On the expiratory view (Figure 9-6), the left hemithorax remains lucent with mediastinal shift to the right, indicating air-trapping in the left lung.

below). When giant bullous cysts occur alone, they are most often confined to the upper lobes. Essentially devoid of any significant structure, the cysts are very lucent. Remnants of pulmonary vasculature may be seen as thin branching lines surrounding the bullous cysts (Figure 9-7). As a cyst enlarges, the displaced pulmonary vessels assume a curvilinear course along its margin. The walls of these bullous cysts may be visualized as thin opaque lines that tend not to parallel the chest wall, unlike the visceral "pleural" line seen with pneumothorax. The appearance shown in Figure 9-1 is consistent with such findings; thus, giant bullous cysts are most likely **(Option (D) is the correct answer).**

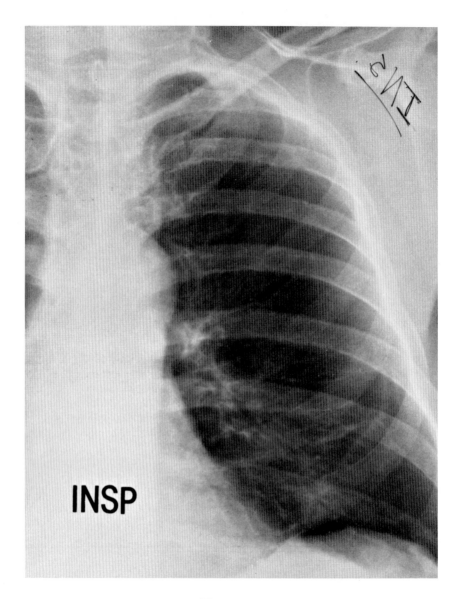

Figure 9-5

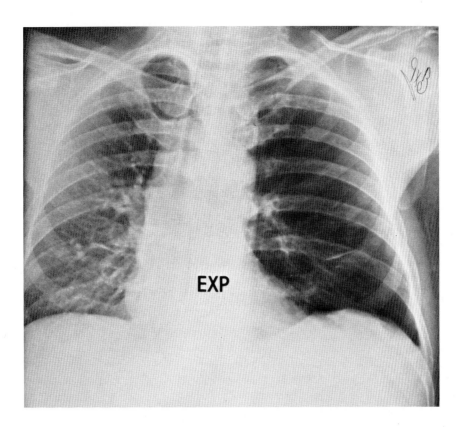

Figure 9-6

Alpha-1-antitrypsin deficiency (Option (E)) is a genetic disorder resulting in pulmonary emphysema, which has a particular affinity for the *lower* lung zones.[17] In the early stages of the disorder, the lungs may be hyperinflated; however, abnormal lucency is not usually noted. In the later stages, the lung becomes abnormally lucent. Pulmonary vessels appear straightened and attenuated, and bullae form (Figure 9-8). Because of its predilection for the lower zones, alpha-1-antitrypsin deficiency is an unlikely explanation for the findings in Figure 9-1, where the disease is centered in the upper zones.

The subject of bullous disease of the lung is confusing because of differences in terminology and because of the incompletely understood association of bullous disease with emphysema. The CIBA Guest Symposium of 1959 defined a "bulla" as an emphysematous space in the lung with a diameter of more than 1 cm in the distended state.[9] In current usage, the term "bullae" refers to subpleural air cysts, which are located

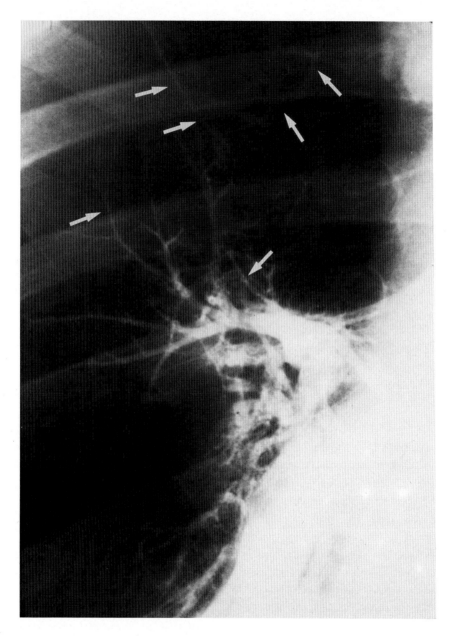

Figure 9-7. Giant bullous cysts. A close-up view from a pulmonary arteriogram shows vascular remnants (arrows) surrounding upper zone bullae.

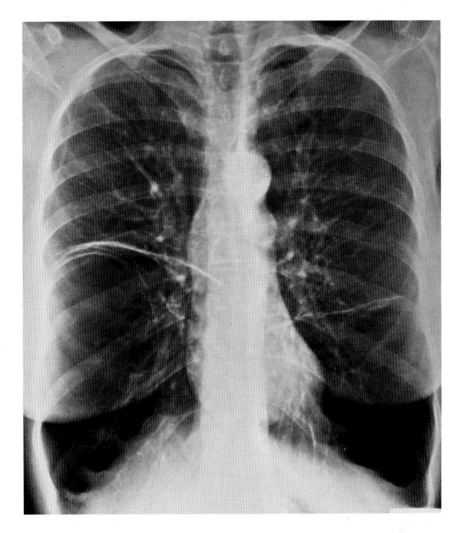

Figure 9-8. Alpha-1-antitrypsin deficiency. Both lower lung zones are involved with bullae around which pulmonary vessels are displaced. The vessels to the upper zones are larger than normal, reflecting redistribution of blood flow due to the lower zonal abnormality.

immediately beneath the pleura and are distributed in the lung apex, along the anterior free margins of the upper lobes, adjacent to the azygoesophageal recess, and on the diaphragmatic surfaces of the lower lobes.[19,24] These cysts result from dissolution of alveolar walls with enlargement of air spaces. The wall is composed of flattened compressed alveolar tissue without an epithelial lining. The interior of the cyst is traversed by remnants of the pulmonary vasculature and interlobular septa. Bullae may be found as isolated abnormalities in otherwise normal lungs or in association with some form of emphysema. Whether bullae represent an exaggerated form of emphysema or a separate pathological process is not currently understood.

The clinical presentation of bullous disease varies markedly and largely depends upon the extent of associated bronchitis and emphysema. In many patients who are asymptomatic, the disease is discovered at routine chest radiography. Other patients, such as the man whose chest radiograph is shown in Figure 9-1, have gradually increasing dyspnea, which develops as the relatively normal lung is compressed by bullae. Dyspnea and cough may be related to associated bronchitis and emphysema, and bullae contribute an additional burden only if they enlarge rapidly. A very high percentage of patients with bullae are cigarette smokers.

Spontaneous pneumothorax is a frequent and serious problem in patients with bullous disease. It occurs in about 15% of such patients, in contradistinction to a 0.3% occurrence in patients with chronic obstructive lung disease.[3,12] Pneumothorax is a serious complication since it results in additional respiratory compromise for lungs already diseased. Persistent air leak is common, since the visceral pleura overlying a bulla has an inadequate underlying support to seal the rupture. In one series, 15 of 84 patients (18%) operated on for bullous disease underwent surgery due to repeated episodes of pneumothorax.[3]

Radiographic identification of pneumothorax in patients with bullous disease may be difficult since the walls of bullae and the visceral pleura in pneumothorax both appear as thin white lines. One must rely upon the shape of the line, its position in the thorax, change from previous studies, and variations in the position of the white line with changes in patient positioning or at fluoroscopy (Figures 9-9 and 9-10). Since bullae most often occur in the subpleural lung, normal lung density and normal arborizing pulmonary vessels may not be present on the parenchymal side of the visceral pleural line when pneumothorax is present. The white line with pneumothorax may be distinguished from a bullous wall by virtue of its projection relatively parallel to the chest wall, mediastinum, or hemidiaphragm in almost all cases. The line with pneumothorax may also be recognized when seen as a new line in comparison to recent prior studies. Fluoroscopy may be helpful in positioning the patient for optimal demonstration of the "pleural" line and its respiratory excursion with pneumothorax. Bullae, on the other hand, show little respiratory

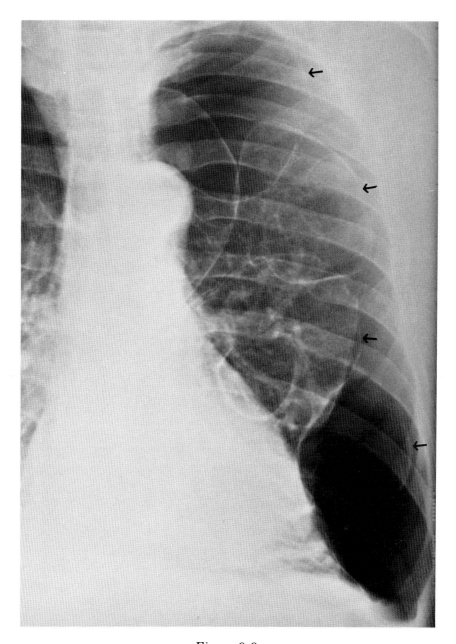

Figure 9-9

Figures 9-9 and 9-10. Bullous disease with pneumothorax. With pneumothorax (Figure 9-9), the visceral "pleura" appears as a thin white line with lucency on either side of it. Since multiple cysts project from the lung surface, the visceral pleural contour is polycyclic (arrows) but generally parallel to the chest wall. When the pneumothorax resolves (Figure 9-10), the walls of the bullae are visible as lines that are convex (arrowheads) or concave (arrows) towards the chest wall.

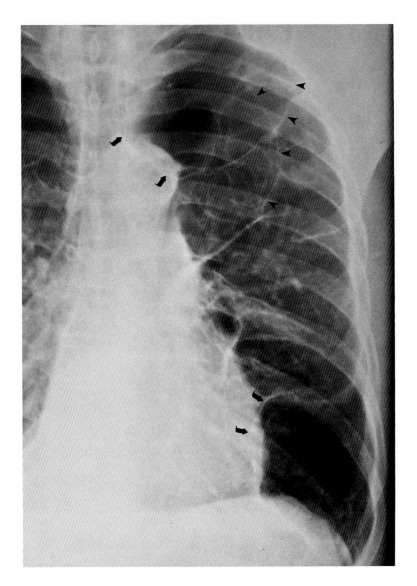

Figure 9-10

excursion. When the distinction cannot otherwise be made, computed tomography (CT) may be needed.

The assessment of patients for bullectomy to relieve dyspnea may be aided by radiographic examinations. The most important factor predicting the success of surgery is the state of the underlying lung with regard to concomitant emphysema. Fluoroscopy, inspiratory/expiratory radiographs, angiography, and CT have all been used to help elucidate the presence or absence of emphysema.[12] When fluoroscopy or inspiratory/ expiratory radiographs are employed, it is important to note the degree of opacification of lung parenchyma surrounding the bullae. Maintenance of lucency and a large volume in the surrounding parenchyma indicate emphysema, suggest that symptoms are only partially related to the bullae, and suggest that a poor surgical outcome is likely. Pulmonary arteriography showing crowded but otherwise normally branching pulmonary arteries suggests that little underlying emphysema is present and that the patient may expect a good response to surgery (Figure 9-11).[2] Recently, CT has been used to detect and categorize areas of emphysema (Figure 9-12).[1,10,12,21] As more experience is gained with CT, it may become the preferred method of assessment. The patient shown in Figure 9-1 underwent fluoroscopy, which suggested a relatively normal but compressed lung. Bulla plication was performed and resulted in an increase in vital capacity and a near normal appearance of the postoperative chest radiograph (Figure 9-13).

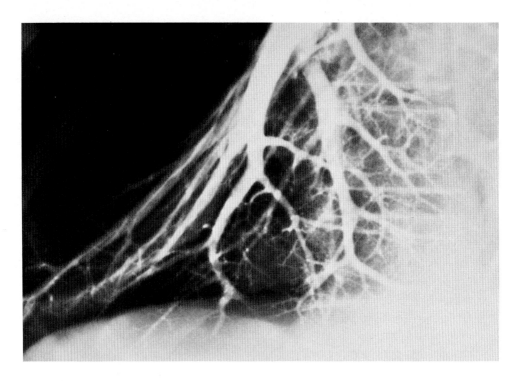

Figure 9-11. Arteriography in bullous disease. A close-up view shows bullous disease displacing and crowding pulmonary arteries. Side branches of the smaller vessels are relatively normal, suggesting little emphysema.

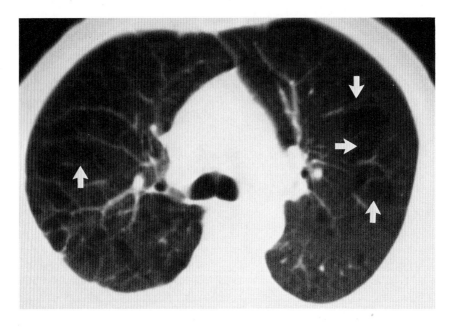

Figure 9-12. CT in emphysema. A section taken at the level of the carina shows emphysematous areas as irregular lucencies (arrows) asymmetrically distributed throughout both upper lobes.

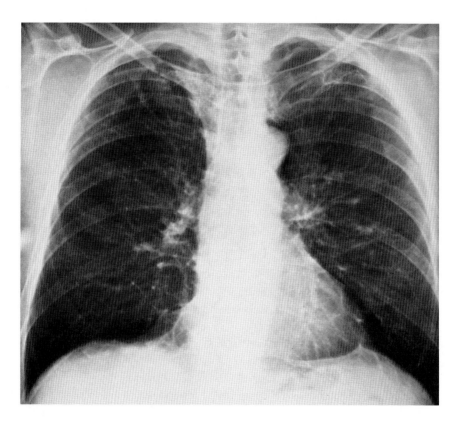

Figure 9-13. Same patient as in Figure 9-1. Bulla plication. Note the marked improvement in appearance after bulla plication. The patient's vital capacity increased from 1.63 to 4.71 L.

Questions 43 through 46

For each of the conditions listed below (Questions 43 through 46), select the *one* histopathologic designation (A, B, C, D, or E) MOST closely associated with it. Each histopathologic designation may be used once, more than once, or not at all.

43. The Swyer-James syndrome
44. Giant bullous cysts
45. Alpha-1-antitrypsin deficiency
46. "Smoker's lung"

    (A) Paraseptal emphysema
    (B) Centrilobular emphysema
    (C) Panacinar emphysema
    (D) Alveolar overdistention without alveolar wall disruption
    (E) Subpleural fibrosis with focal emphysema

The Swyer-James syndrome is an obliterative bronchiolitis thought to result from a serious respiratory infection in infancy. Respiratory syncytial virus, influenza virus, or adenovirus infections that occur while the lung is still growing probably account for most of these episodes of infection. The infection damages the terminal bronchioles, which subsequently undergo fibrosis. Acinar units supplied by these obliterated airways become scarred. Alternatively, these units may remain aerated, via collateral ventilation, with resultant overdistention. Since this process occurs in a somewhat random fashion, the final appearance of the lung is that of a patchwork of scarred and overdistended acinar units.[24,27] In contradistinction to other types of emphysema, destruction of the alveolar walls does not occur with this syndrome **(Option (D) is the correct answer to Question 43).**

Emphysema is divided by pathologists into four major types: paraseptal, panacinar (panlobular), centrilobular (centriacinar), and paracicatricial.[4,9,16,24,26] Each of these types has a characteristic gross morphologic appearance. Moreover, each type tends to be different in its distribution in the lung and in its associated disease processes. It is important to note, however, that there is considerable overlap in these associations and that more than one type of emphysema is usually present in any given lung.

As discussed above, giant bullous cysts may occur as an isolated abnormality or in association with emphysema. In the latter situation, the emphysema is usually paraseptal **(Option (A) is the correct answer to Question 44).**[5,12] This form of emphysema involves the acinar periphery with sparing of the acinar central area. Subpleural regions and those adjacent to interlobular septa are favored sites, as opposed to deeper regions of the lung parenchyma. The emphysematous spaces are distributed in the apices and along the free margins of the upper and middle lobes, sometimes creating a row of small cysts along the lung edge. The cystic spaces range from a few millimeters to several centimeters in diameter. The underlying lung may be normal, although other types of emphysema frequently coexist.

Panacinar emphysema is most frequently associated with alpha-1-antitrypsin deficiency **(Option (C) is the correct answer to Question 45).** In this type of emphysema, there are dilatation and destruction of both the respiratory bronchioles and the alveoli. Although panacinar emphysema is relatively uniformly distributed throughout the entire lung, the lower zones are affected to a slightly greater degree than the upper zones. The affected regions of lung show their normal alveoli and respiratory bronchioles to be replaced by large, thin-walled airspaces. In contrast to the usual findings in centrilobular (centriacinar) emphysema (see below), there is no evidence of inflammation unless the patient has had a terminal pneumonia.

Centrilobular emphysema is most closely associated with "smoker's lung" and is the most common form of emphysema **(Option (B) is the correct answer to Question 46).** There are dilatation and destruction of the first- and second-order respiratory bronchioles with relative sparing of the peripheral acinar alveoli. Peribronchiolar polymorphonuclear leukocytic and lymphocytic infiltration of the supplying terminal bronchiole is present. The emphysema is nonuniformly distributed and affects the upper lung zones more frequently than the lower ones.

"Focal dust emphysema" is a term that has been applied to a morphologic appearance similar to that of centrilobular emphysema but in workers exposed to carbon dust. In addition to the emphysematous changes, carbon particles are deposited adjacent to the respiratory bronchioles. While it has been suggested that this disorder may occur in the absence of smoking, the issue is controversial. Since the morphologic appearance is identical to that of centrilobular emphysema, except for the presence of carbon particles, Dunnill has suggested elimination of the term "focal dust emphysema."[4] He suggests that all cases be classified as centrilobular emphysema with or without carbon dust deposition.

Question 47

Which *one* of the following is the LEAST likely to be associated with lower lobe atelectasis?

    (A) Depression of the ipsilateral interlobar pulmonary artery
    (B) Development of an ipsilateral juxtaphrenic peak
    (C) Obscuration of the ipsilateral posterior hemidiaphragm on the lateral view
    (D) Vertical orientation of the ipsilateral lower lobe bronchus
    (E) Mediastinal shift toward the atelectatic side

Signs of atelectasis include rearrangement of anatomic structures and opacity of the involved lobe. The exact appearance of these signs depends upon the amount of volume loss and whether it is lobar, segmental, or subsegmental. In addition, the presence of disease in other regions of the thorax and its contiguous structures may alter appearances. Depression of the ipsilateral interlobar pulmonary artery (Option (A)), vertical orientation of the ipsilateral lower lobe bronchus (Option (D)), mediastinal shift toward the atelectatic side (Option (E)), and obscuration of the ipsilateral posterior hemidiaphragm on the lateral view (Option (C)) are all signs expected with lower lobe atelectasis (Figures 9-14 to 9-16).[7,23]

Hilar arterial alteration is an important sign of atelectasis. The interlobar portion of the right or left pulmonary artery courses in the major fissure before it actually enters the lung parenchyma. As a lower lobe loses volume, the interlobar hilar pulmonary artery shifts to a more inferior and medial position. As the volume of the lower lobe decreases further, lower lobe opacity increases. A small portion of the lateral margin of the interlobar artery may remain visible owing to its contact with the adjacent aerated lung.[23]

The bronchi to the lower lobes and the right and left main bronchi have relatively oblique orientations, pointing toward the lateral costophrenic angles in the normal state. As lower lobe volume loss occurs, these bronchi shift toward the midline, assuming a more vertical orientation.[23]

The mediastinum shifts toward the side of atelectasis when the atelectasis is unilateral. With bilateral atelectasis, the mediastinum may remain midline. Similarly, the hemidiaphragm elevates slightly on the same side as the atelectatic lobe.

As the lower lobe loses volume, the major fissure shifts posteriorly and its lateral aspect rotates into a more sagittal orientation. This lobe is attached to the mediastinum by the hilum and the inferior pulmonary ligament. A totally collapsed lower lobe is a flattened structure lying

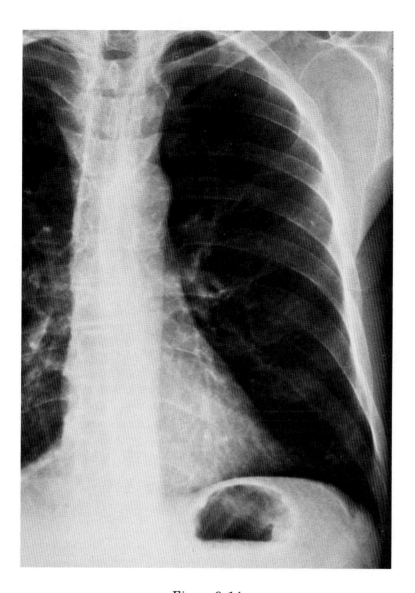

Figure 9-14
Figures 9-14 through 9-16. Lower lobe atelectasis. Note the normal
appearance of the left lower lobe in Figure 9-14. With left lower lobe
atelectasis (Figure 9-15), the left interlobar pulmonary artery has shifted
inferiorly and medially while the proximal portion of the left lower lobe
bronchus (arrow) is more vertically oriented. The mediastinum has
shifted ipsilaterally. On the lateral view (Figure 9-16), there is abnormal
opacity over the lower thoracic spine along with left hemidiaphragmatic
obscuration.

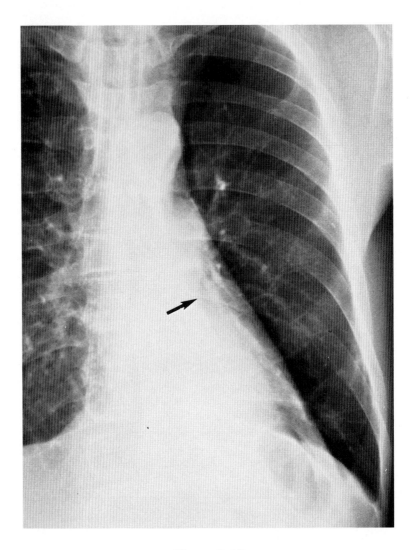

Figure 9-15

adjacent to the lower posterior mediastinum/paravertebral gutter. On the frontal view, the lateral margin of the triangular opaque lobe represents the major fissure in its rearranged position. On the lateral view, the juxtaposition of the opaque lobe with its hemidiaphragm posteriorly causes obscuration of that portion of the hemidiaphragm.

The juxtaphrenic peak sign is one described with upper lobe atelectasis (Figure 9-17) **(Option (B) is least likely).**[15] The juxtaphrenic peak is a triangular opacity of variable size located at or near the dome of the

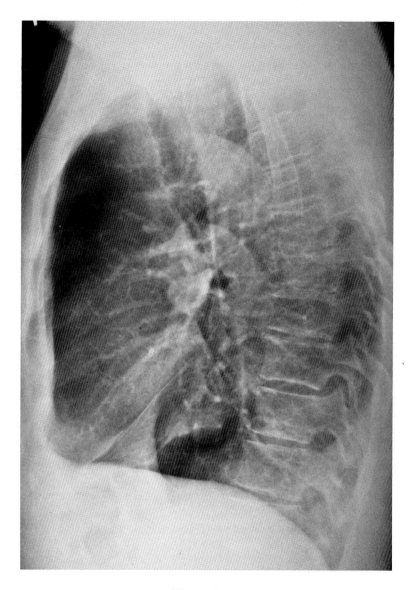

Figure 9-16

ipsilateral hemidiaphragm. It may be seen on either the frontal or the lateral view. The exact mechanism by which this opacity develops is uncertain. The triangle may vary in size from 1 to 3 cm along its base and may reach 4 cm in height. It may develop with volume loss from any etiology and may disappear if the lobe reexpands. It should be differentiated from the small triangle often seen with an inferior accessory fissure, hemidiaphragmatic "tenting" in otherwise normal individuals, and an occasional bulla. Other signs of upper lobe volume

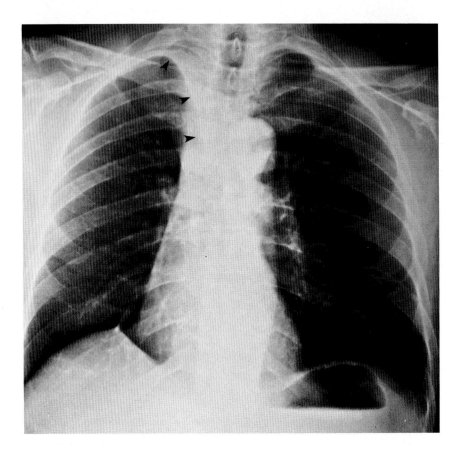

Figure 9-17. Juxtaphrenic peak sign. The right hemidiaphragm has an abnormal contour with a peak at its dome. The opaque triangle (arrowheads) represents the collapsed right upper lobe.

loss (e.g., elevated position of the ipsilateral interlobar pulmonary artery, opaque upper lobe, horizontal orientation of the main bronchus, and cephalad displacement of the minor fissure) make the differentiation relatively easy.[23]

Question 48

Concerning alpha-1-antitrypsin deficiency,

- (A) adult heterozygous patients are at high risk of developing emphysema even in the absence of smoking
- (B) severe emphysema will develop in almost all homozygous patients, even in the absence of smoking
- (C) cirrhosis of the liver is present in the majority of adult patients
- (D) hilar enlargement results from the associated lymphadenopathy

The pathogenesis of emphysema has been greatly clarified in the last two decades.[13,18] A protease/antiprotease theory, which is widely accepted, suggests that destructive changes in the walls of alveoli result from inadequate inactivation of protease by the antiprotease system of the lung. The cause of the problem may sometimes be known, as it is for alpha-1-antitrypsin deficiency; however, more often the cause is unknown.

Alpha-1-antitrypsin (also known as alpha-1-antiprotease inhibitor) is the major protein of the alpha globulin class and the only antiprotease important in the protease/antiprotease system of the lower respiratory tract. Synthesis of this protein is controlled by a pair of genes found in chromosome 14. More than 25 alleles of the gene have been described and are designated by letters. These variants are transmitted by simple Mendelian inheritance. Over 90% of people are homozygous for the alpha-1-antitrypsin MM phenotype, have 150 to 300 mg of the inhibitor per dL of serum, and are normal. Most patients with alpha-1-antitrypsin deficiency associated with severe lung disease have the alpha-1-antitrypsin ZZ phenotype and have only 10 to 15% of the normal level of inhibitor. Fewer than 1% of subjects in the populations studied have the ZZ phenotype. The most common heterozygous phenotypes are MS and MZ. Individuals with one of these phenotypes have levels of the inhibitor that are 50 to 60% of normal.[22] Since alpha-1-antitrypsin levels must fall below 35% of normal for the balance to shift in favor of the protease, adult heterozygous patients are not at high risk of developing emphysema unless they smoke **(Option (A) is false).**

While the initially described patients with alpha-1-antitrypsin deficiency all had severe degrees of emphysema, recent reports have indicated that many patients with the deficiency may live essentially normal lives if they avoid smoking and occupations with adverse respiratory consequences. A recent study from Sweden has shown that only about one-half of the homozygous patients with ZZ alpha-1-

antitrypsin deficiency will develop symptomatic emphysema **(Option (B) is false).**[6]

Alpha-1-antitrypsin is a protein synthesized by hepatocytes. It is normally transported through the endoplasmic reticulum and Golgi apparatus, where it is glycosylated and secreted. In ZZ homozygous patients, the protein is not properly processed and accumulates in the hepatocyte endoplasmic reticulum in an underglycosylated form. It may be detected there as periodic acid-Schiff (PAS)-positive granules. Increased incidences of both cirrhosis and primary liver cancer have been identified in patients with alpha-1-antitrypsin deficiency, although the associations achieve statistical significance only for male patients. At the worst, these disorders occur in no more than 25% of homozygous patients **(Option (C) is false).**[6]

Patients with alpha-1-antitrypsin deficiency who develop hilar enlargement do so late in the course of their emphysema. The hilar enlargement results from pulmonary hypertension secondary to the emphysema (Figures 9-18 and 9-19). Alpha-1-antitrypsin deficiency does not lead to lymph node enlargement in any organ **(Option (D) is false).**

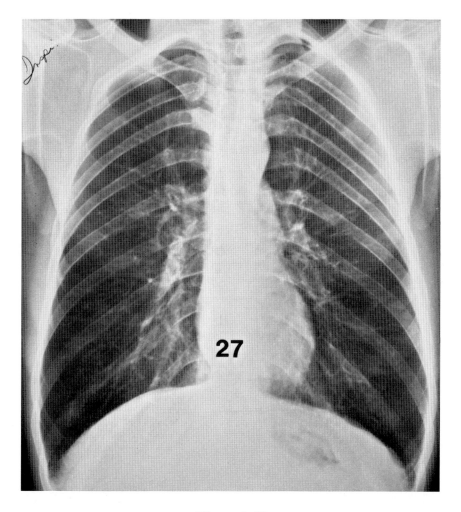

Figure 9-18

Figures 9-18 and 9-19. Hilar enlargement in alpha-1-antitrypsin deficiency. A frontal chest radiograph at age 27 (Figure 9-18) shows hyperinflation with a heart of normal size and normal hilar pulmonary arteries. At age 35 (Figure 9-19), the heart and hilar pulmonary arteries have enlarged as cor pulmonale has developed.

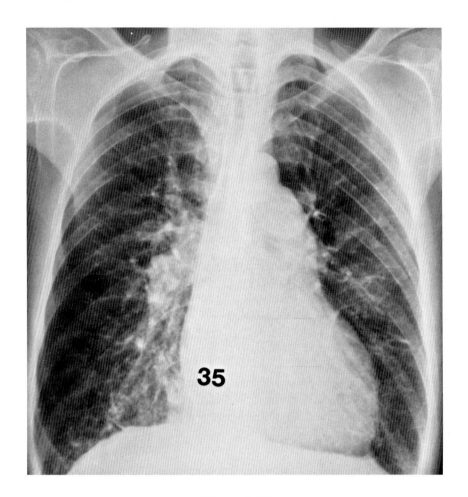

Figure 9-19

SUGGESTED READINGS

1. Bergin CJ, Muller NL, Miller RR. CT in the qualitative assessment of emphysema. J Thorac Imaging 1986; 1:94–103
2. Delarue NC, Woolf CR, Sanders DE, et al. Surgical treatment for pulmonary emphysema. Can J Surg 1977; 20:222–231
3. Dines DE, Clagett OT, Payne WS. Spontaneous pneumothorax in emphysema. Mayo Clin Proc 1970; 45:481–487
4. Dunnill MS: Pulmonary pathology. Edinburgh: Churchill Livingstone; 1982:81–112
5. Edge J, Simon G, Reid L. Peri-acinar (paraseptal) emphysema: its clinical, radiological, and physiological features. Br J Dis Chest 1966; 60:10–18
6. Eriksson S, Carlson J, Velez R. Risk of cirrhosis and primary liver cancer in alpha-1-antitrypsin deficiency. N Engl J Med 1986; 314:736–739
7. Felson B. Chest roentgenology. Philadelphia: WB Saunders; 1973:92–142
8. FitzGerald MX, Keelan PJ, Cugell DW, Gaensler EA. Long-term results of surgery for bullous emphysema. J Thorac Cardiovasc Surg 1974; 68:566–587
9. Fletcher CM, Gilson JG, Hugh-Jones P, Scadding JG. Terminology, definitions, and classification of chronic pulmonary emphysema and related conditions: a report of the conclusions of a CIBA guest symposium. Thorax 1959; 14:286–299
10. Foster WL Jr, Pratt PC, Roggli VL, Godwin JD, Halvorsen RA Jr, Putnam CE: Centrilobular emphysema: CT-pathologic correlation. Radiology 1986; 159:27–32
11. Fraser RG, Paré JA. Diagnosis of diseases of the chest, vol 3. Philadelphia: WB Saunders; 1979:1431–1443
12. Gaensler EA, Jederlinic PJ, FitzGerald MX. Patient work-up for bullectomy. J Thorac Imaging 1986; 1:75–93
13. Garver RI Jr, Mornex JF, Nukiwa T, et al. Alpha-1-antitrypsin deficiency and emphysema caused by homozygous inheritance of non-expressing alpha-1-antitrypsin genes. N Engl J Med 1986; 314:762–766
14. Greene R, McLoud TC, Stark P. Pneumothorax. Semin Roentgenol 1977; 12:313–325
15. Kattan KR, Eyler WR, Felson B. The juxtaphrenic peak in upper lobe collapse. Semin Roentgenol 1980; 15:187–193
16. Katzenstein AA, Askin FB. Surgical pathology of non-neoplastic lung disease. Philadelphia: WB Saunders; 1982:387–392
17. Kueppers F, Black LF. Alpha-1-antitrypsin and its deficiency. Am Rev Respir Dis 1974; 110:176–194
18. Kuhn C III. The biochemical pathogenesis of chronic obstructive pulmonary diseases: protease-antiprotease imbalance in emphysema and diseases of the airways. J Thorac Imaging 1986; 1:1–6
19. Laurenzi GA, Turino GM, Fishman AP. Bullous disease of the lung. Am J Med 1962; 32:361–378
20. Macleod WM. Abnormal transradiancy of one lung. Thorax 1954; 9:147–153
21. Morgan MD, Strickland B. Computed tomography in the assessment of bullous lung disease. Br J Dis Chest 1984; 78:10–25

22. Morse JO, Lebowitz MD, Knudson RJ, Burrows B. Relation of protease inhibitor phenotypes to obstructive lung diseases in a community. N Engl J Med 1977; 296:1190–1194
23. Proto AV, Tocino I. Radiographic manifestations of lobar collapse. Semin Roentgenol 1980; 15:117–173
24. Spencer H. Pathology of the lung. Oxford: Pergamon Press; 1985:557–594
25. Swyer PR, James GC. A case of unilateral pulmonary emphysema. Thorax 1953; 8:133–146
26. Thurlbeck WM. Chronic airflow obstruction in lung disease. Philadelphia: WB Saunders; 1976:96–234
27. Wohl ME, Chernick V. State of the art: bronchiolitis. Am Rev Respir Dis 1978; 118:759–781

Notes

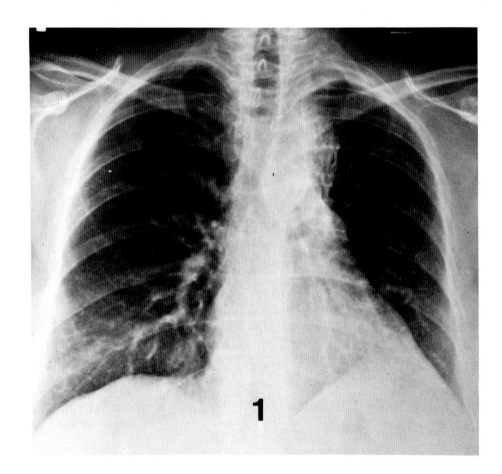

Figure 10-1

Case 10: Pulmonary Radiation Injury

Questions 49 through 53

For each of the numbered posteroanterior chest radiographs (Figures 10-1 through 10-5), select the *one* lettered description (A, B, C, D, or E) MOST closely associated with it. Each statement may be used once, more than once, or not at all.

49. Figure 10-1
50. Figure 10-2
51. Figure 10-3
52. Figure 10-4
53. Figure 10-5

   (A) Acute-phase radiation effect; port for treatment of lung carcinoma
   (B) Acute-phase radiation effect; mantle port for treatment of lymphoma
   (C) Acute-phase radiation effect; port for treatment of breast carcinoma
   (D) Fibrotic-phase radiation effect; port for treatment of lung carcinoma
   (E) Fibrotic-phase radiation effect; mantle port for treatment of lymphoma

Figure 10-1 shows consolidation of the upper medial portion of the left lung with resultant obscuration of the aortic knob. Note also the pleura-like opacity at the left apex. Left upper lobe volume loss is indicated by a more horizontal orientation of the left main bronchus and elevation of the left hemidiaphragm. The right lung is clear. These findings are consistent with the fibrotic phase of radiation effect as might be seen in a portal area for treatment of lung carcinoma **(Option (D) is the correct answer to Question 49).**

Figure 10-2 shows elevation of both hila, elevation of the minor fissure, and blurring of normal upper mediastinal contours bilaterally (e.g., the outlines of the aortic arch and azygos vein are not visible). These findings are consistent with the fibrotic phase of radiation effect as might be seen in a mantle portal area for treatment of lymphoma **(Option (E) is the correct answer to Question 50).**

Figure 10-3 shows diffuse, inhomogeneous opacity projecting at the right hemithorax. The right pulmonary vessels continue to be visible

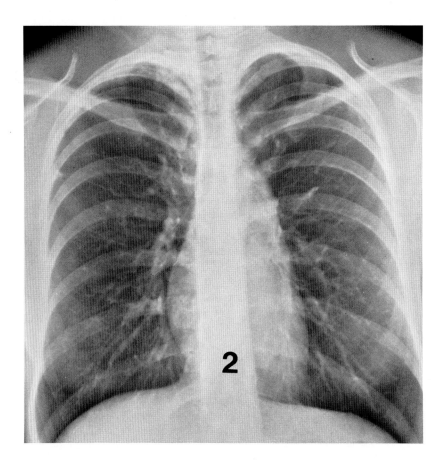

Figure 10-2

through the opacity, there is no volume loss, the mediastinal contours are normal, and the costophrenic angle is preserved. Two surgical clips are visible in the right axilla. These findings are consistent with the acute phase of radiation effect as might be seen in a portal area for treatment of breast carcinoma **(Option (C) is the correct answer to Question 51).**

Figure 10-4 shows opacity in the upper medial portions of the lungs bilaterally. The margins of the hila are blurred, but the aortic knob and right paratracheal stripe are relatively well defined. There is no volume loss. These findings are consistent with the acute phase of radiation effect as might be seen in a mantle portal area for treatment of lymphoma **(Option (B) is the correct answer to Question 52).**

Figure 10-5 shows inhomogeneous opacity of the right lateral mid-lung zone. The opacity has relatively straight margins, is nonsegmental, and

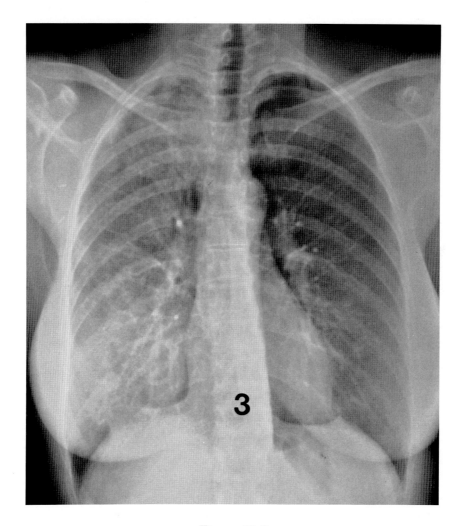

Figure 10-3

crosses the minor fissure. The right hilar vessels are partially obscured, but mediastinal borders are otherwise normal. The left lung is clear. These findings are consistent with the acute phase of radiation effect as might be seen in a portal area for treatment of lung carcinoma **(Option (A) is the correct answer to Question 53).**

Development of parenchymal opacities as a result of radiation therapy is a common occurrence. The two most important factors that should be assessed to help determine whether these opacities are most likely due to radiation or to some other pleuropulmonary process are as follows: (1)

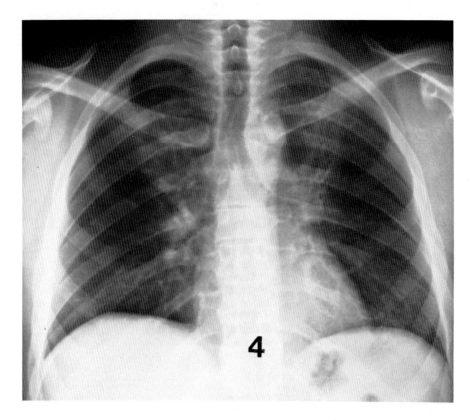

Figure 10-4

the shape of the opacities and (2) the time interval since the completion of radiotherapy.

Knowledge of commonly used radiotherapy ports may be of considerable assistance in the differential diagnosis of opacities occurring in the postradiotherapy patient. Patients with lung carcinoma, breast carcinoma, and lymphoma account for the majority of those receiving such therapy to the thorax. Typical ports used for treating these three malignancies are shown in Figures 10-6 and 10-7. The actual ports used for the patients shown in Figures 10-1 through 10-5 are illustrated in Figures 10-8 through 10-12, respectively.

Radiotherapy is generally given through opposing portals, with the beam traversing the patient first in one direction and then in the other. The ports for palliative treatment have contours that are more angular than those for cure. Such ports for palliation are simple to fashion, and the radiotherapy doses are smaller, with sparing of normal tissue being

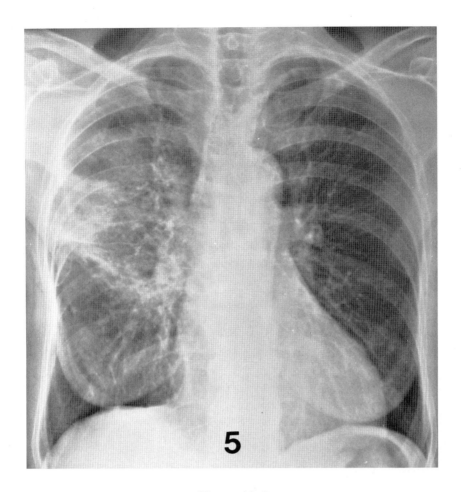

Figure 10-5

less critical. For curative higher-dose treatments, individually tailored curvilinear ports are cut from styrofoam and used as molds in forming the radiation blocks (Figure 10-13).

To understand both the timing and the radiographic appearance of radiation effects, it is helpful to review the underlying pathologic process.[27] This process is traditionally divided into an early exudative phase and a late fibrotic phase. The early phase lasts until about 6 months after completion of radiotherapy, and the fibrotic phase spans the next 12 months. Occurrences during the early phase include capillary obstruction with platelets and fibrin, endothelial cell damage, intimal proliferation, and collection of lipid-laden macrophages subintimally. The alveolar septa are thickened by edema and a mononuclear cell

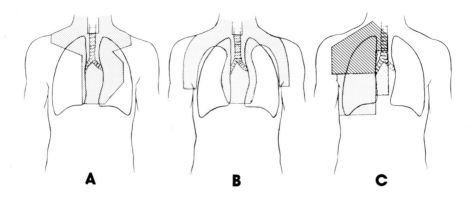

A   **B**   **C**

Figure 10-6. Diagram of commonly used ports for radiotherapy. Port A (stippled) is for treatment of lung carcinoma at the left hilum and includes the tumor, mediastinum, and supraclavicular areas. Port B (stippled) is for treatment of lymphoma and includes the mediastinum, hila, and supraclavicular and axillary areas. Port C is for treatment of breast carcinoma and includes a combination of three ports: internal mammary lymph nodes (cross-hatched), supraclavicular lymph nodes (diagonal lines), and chest wall (stippled).

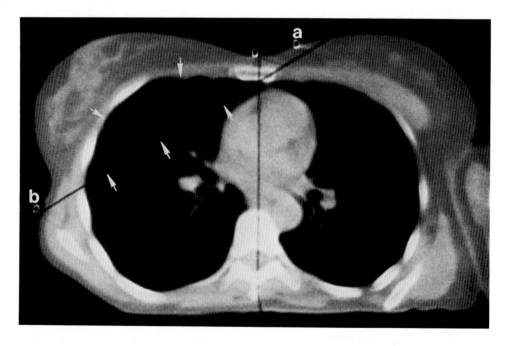

Figure 10-7. Chest wall port. The chest wall port is tangential to the body and includes a thin strip of lung anteriorly (between arrows). This port may be used to treat the chest wall in patients who have had a mastectomy or may be slightly modified to treat the breast in patients having lumpectomy and radiation therapy. Metallic markers (a and b) are used in setting up the port (see Figure 10-10).

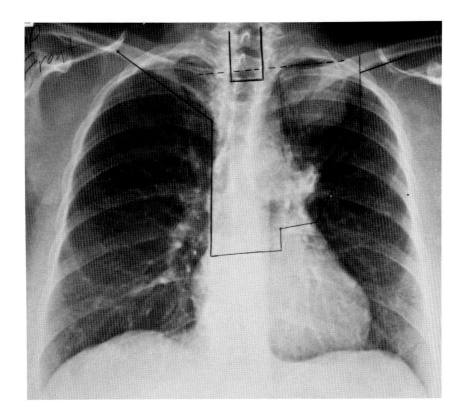

Figure 10-8. The port shown was used for the patient in Figure 10-1 and encompasses the mass in the left upper lobe, a large amount of lung, and the ipsilateral hilum. Note the near approximation of the right port margin to the mediastinum, a finding in contrast to the port used for lymphoma (Figure 10-9).

infiltrate. Alveolar epithelial cells, which show atypia and hyperplasia, desquamate into the alveolar space. Hyaline membranes form within the alveolar spaces. This process may resolve or evolve into a variable degree of interstitial fibrosis. When the late fibrotic phase supervenes, the alveolar walls show a reduced number of capillaries and are thickened by dense fibrosis. As the fibrosis matures, the irradiated portion of the lung loses volume and compensatory overinflation occurs in the nonaffected portions of the lung. Cicatrization bronchiectasis occurs within the area of fibrosis.

The most important radiographic sign in either the early or late phase is limitation of the findings to the radiation portals.[11,16] Early-phase radiation effects range from blurring of normal vascular markings to

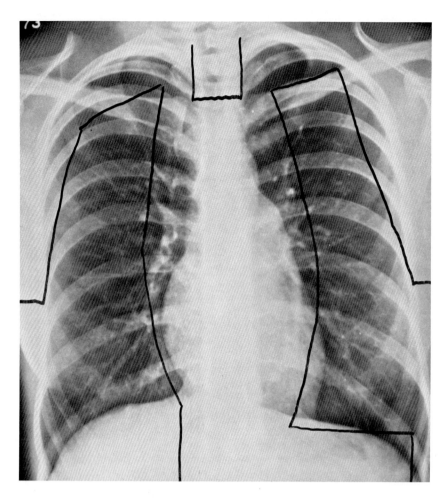

Figure 10-9. The port shown was used for the patient in Figure 10-2 and encompasses a wider right mediastinal margin than is used in patients with lung cancer. This wider margin is necessary to include any contiguously involved nodes and accounts for the greater amount of paramediastinal pulmonary fibrosis in such patients. Note the differences in the position and sharpness of anatomic structures in comparison to Figure 10-2.

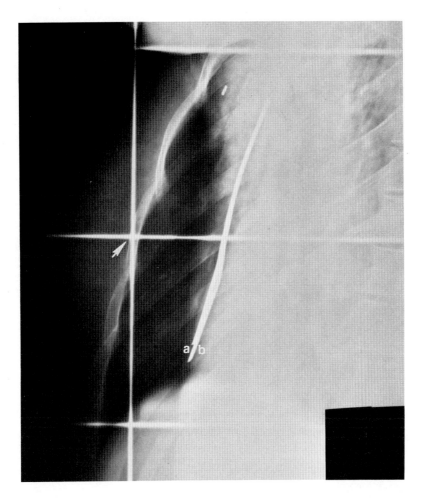

Figure 10-10. The port shown was used for the patient in Figure 10-3 (the same patient as in Figure 10-7). In this right posterior oblique view, the radiation beam is centered at the cross-hatch (arrow). The treatment port extends posteriorly to the superimposed markers (a and b).

dense consolidation with air bronchograms. The abnormality is nonsegmental and may be patchy or confluent. An important feature is maintenance of normal lung volume. Early-phase parenchymal disease *conforms to the shape of the radiotherapy portal* and has straight, polygonal, or curvilinear outlines. Its margins are often serrated or blurred. Although computed tomographic (CT) scans may demonstrate parenchymal disease somewhat earlier than conventional radiographs, the disease will still maintain the characteristics just described (Figures

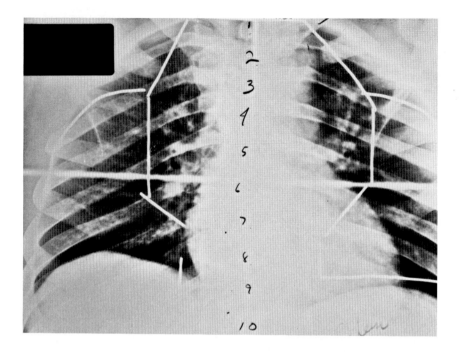

Figure 10-11. The port shown was used for the patient in Figure 10-4. Note that the parenchymal opacities in Figure 10-4 are located within and conform to the outlines of the port.

10-14 and 10-15).[21] The early-phase abnormality may resolve with relatively little residuum or may merge into patterns seen in the late fibrotic phase.

Late-phase radiation effects consist of linear shadows, loss of normal anatomic contours due to adjacent fibrosis, and volume loss in the affected regions. Dense consolidations may result from the combination of volume loss and fibrosis (Figure 10-1). The effects of the scarring process are confined to the radiation portal, and they may evolve from early-phase parenchymal disease or may be seen without antecedent abnormality. In the late phase, any enlargement of a previously shrunken area is suspicious for recurrent neoplasm (Figure 10-16). Occasionally, however, continued maturation of the fibrotic process may retract more tissue into an area and appear to enlarge it, thus incorrectly suggesting recurrent neoplasm (Figures 10-17 and 10-18).[14]

Glazer et al. have described the utility of magnetic resonance imaging (MRI) in distinguishing radiation fibrosis from recurrent neoplasm.[8,9] Most patients with fibrosis had areas of low signal intensity on both

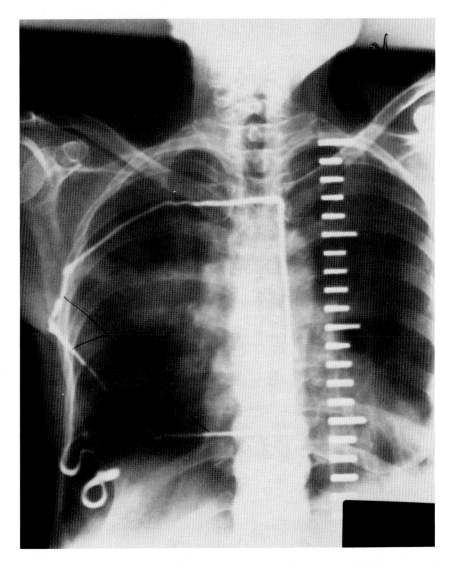

Figure 10-12. The port shown was used for the patient in Figure 10-5. Note that the right mid-lung opacity in Figure 10-5 conforms to the port.

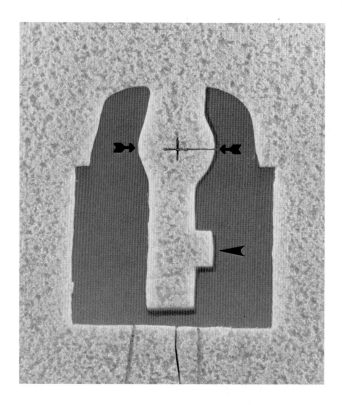

Figure 10-13. Styrofoam mold for lymphoma port. The styrofoam has been cut with a hot wire in a configuration to include the desired areas. The bulge centrally (arrows) is for treatment of the hila. The projection below (arrowhead) is for treatment of the splenic pedicle.

T1-and T2-weighted images. The signal intensity of tumor, on the other hand, was high on the T2-weighted images (Figures 10-19 through 10-22). Unfortunately, Glazer et al. were unable to distinguish persistent or recurrent tumor from acute radiation pneumonitis, infection, or pulmonary hemorrhage. Moreover, in a few patients, regions of fibrosis had high signal intensity on T2-weighted images. Further studies will be needed to clarify the role of MRI in this setting.

The differential diagnosis for parenchymal disease in either phase includes infections, persistent or recurrent tumor, and radiation effect. As already stated, an important radiographic finding is limitation of the affected area to the radiation portal, but this finding must be considered in the context of the time elapsed since radiation therapy was completed. For example, patchy nonsegmental opacity without associated volume

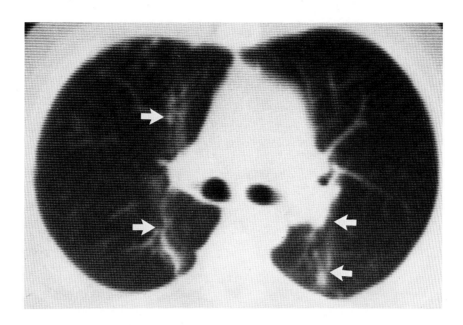

Figure 10-14

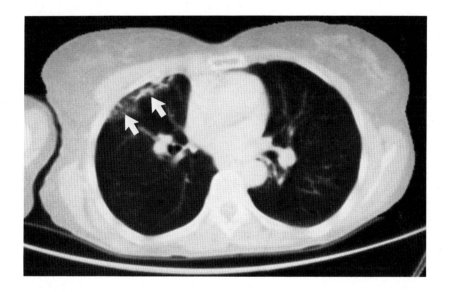

Figure 10-15

Figures 10-14 and 10-15. CT appearance of radiation-induced parenchymal disease. CT (Figure 10-14; same patient as in Figure 10-4) through the upper mediastinum shows opacity in the medial portions of the lungs bilaterally. Note the *straight* distributional margins (arrows), which conform to the edges of the anterior and posterior radiation ports in this patient with lymphoma. CT (Figure 10-15; same patient as in Figure 10-3) through the upper right breast region shows opacity in the anterolateral right lung with a *straight* distributional margin (arrows) conforming to the chest wall port for treatment of breast carcinoma.

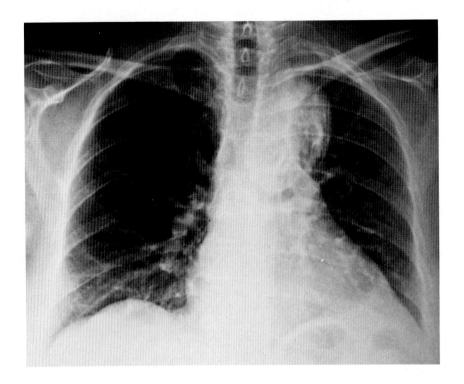

Figure 10-16. Recurrence of carcinoma within the radiation port. A follow-up radiograph at 3 years of the patient shown in Figures 10-1 and 10-8 reveals enlargement of the consolidated shrunken lung previously noted (compare with Figure 10-1).

loss appearing during the late phase suggests an infection or recurrent neoplasm, since the late-phase fibrosis is almost always associated with volume loss. Alternatively, opacity developing very soon after completion of radiation therapy most probably represents a superimposed infection or worsened neoplasm. When cultures and sputum examination cannot clarify the radiographic appearances, biopsy may be necessary to establish the correct diagnosis if a period of watchful waiting is deemed unwise.

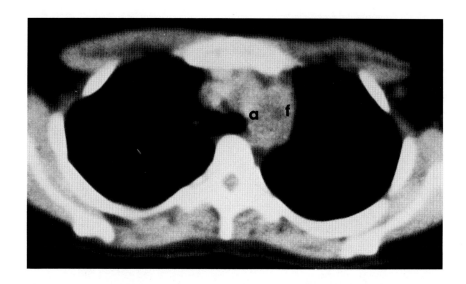

Figure 10-17

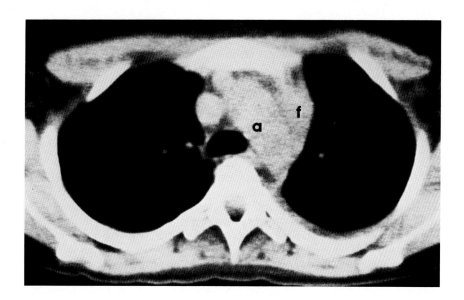

Figure 10-18
Figures 10-17 and 10-18. Late-phase enlargement of fibrosis. CT (Figure 10-17) performed 18 months after radiotherapy in a 21-year-old woman with Hodgkin's disease shows residual soft tissue (f) just lateral to the aortic arch (a). The appearance had been stable for 6 months. A scan obtained 5 months later (Figure 10-18) shows enlargement of the soft tissue (f) lateral to the arch (a), as well as pleural thickening posteriorly. At surgery, a large fibrous plaque was present with no evidence of recurrence.

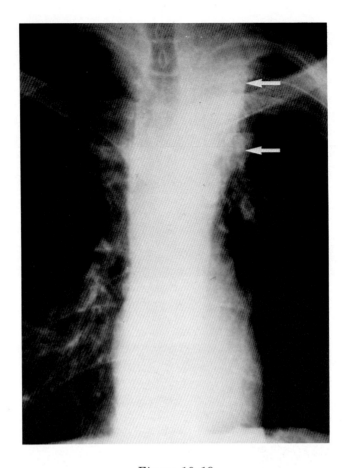

Figure 10-19

Figures 10-19 to 10-22. Differentiation of tumor from fibrosis by MRI. A posteroanterior radiograph (Figure 10-19) 2½ years after radiation treatment shows interval widening of the left upper mediastinum (arrows), a finding that is highly suggestive of recurrent tumor. A CT scan (Figure 10-20) shows the mass (arrows) as well as the left common carotid artery (C), the left subclavian artery (S), and the left brachio-cephalic vein (V). Figure 10-21 is a T1-weighted MR scan (SE 300/30) at the same level as Figure 10-20 that shows the mass (arrows) to be of much lower intensity than the adjacent white mediastinal fat. Note also the left subclavian artery (s), the trachea (T), and the esophagus (e). Figure 10-22 is a T2-weighted MR scan (SE 1,500/90) at the same level as Figure 10-21 that shows that the mass has a high-intensity component laterally (white arrows) and a low-intensity component medially (black arrows). Surgical biopsy of the high-intensity component indicated recurrent tumor, while biopsy of the low-intensity component revealed radiation fibrosis. (Reprinted with permission from Glazer et al. [9].)

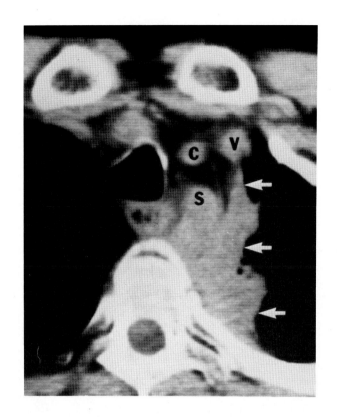

Figure 10-20

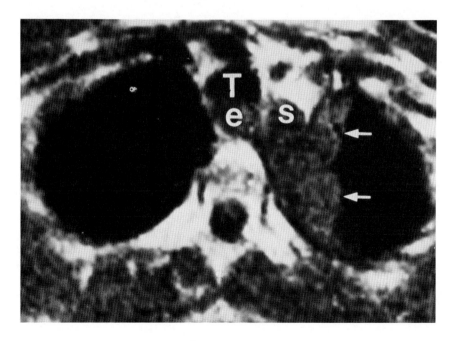

Figure 10-21

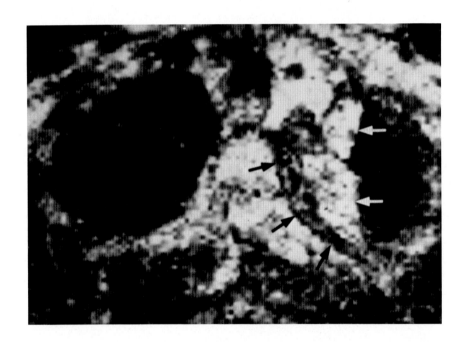

Figure 10-22

Question 54

Which *one* of the following is the LEAST likely effect of radiation therapy?

(A) Pleural effusion
(B) Pericardial effusion
(C) Pulmonary opacities
(D) Superior vena cava obstruction
(E) Regional volume loss

The frequency of radiation effects developing in the lungs has been reported to be from 0 to 100%. As pointed out by Gross,[11] this wide variation probably reflects differences in awareness of the problem, in equipment and treatment schedules, and in methods of reporting (inclusion of only symptomatic patients versus inclusion of all patients with parenchymal disease). Despite this variability, parenchymal opacities (Option (C)) and regional volume loss (Option (E)) are the most frequently encountered effects of radiotherapy in the thorax and may be expected in 5 to 15% of patients.[6,11]

The frequency of radiation effects involving thoracic structures other than the lungs is lower. Pleural effusions (Option (A)) have been noted in 4 to 6% of patients irradiated for breast carcinoma.[3] These effusions usually develop from 3 to 6 months after completion of therapy and are almost always accompanied by an early-phase parenchymal opacity. The effusions are freely mobile and usually small to moderate in size (Figure 10-23). They usually resolve spontaneously over several months but may last for up to 3 years. Similar pleural effusions may occur in patients irradiated for lung carcinoma or lymphoma. Pleural effusions developing later than 6 months after completion of therapy are usually malignant. In either case, cytological examination of the fluid may help in the differentiation.

Early-phase pericardial effusions (Option (B)) have been reported in 7 to 30% of patients irradiated for Hodgkin's disease.[24] In approximately one-half of these patients, the effusion leads to a limitation of activity or necessitates pericardiectomy. Late-phase studies have demonstrated clinically evident or occult constrictive pericarditis in a similar percentage.[2,25] Additional cardiac effects of radiotherapy include an abnormal hemodynamic response to a fluid challenge, coronary artery disease, and right or left ventricular dysfunction.[1,2,25]

Superior vena cava obstruction due to mediastinal radiation is unusual. Whitcomb and Schwarz described a single patient with mediastinal fibrosis and superior vena cava obstruction 15 months after

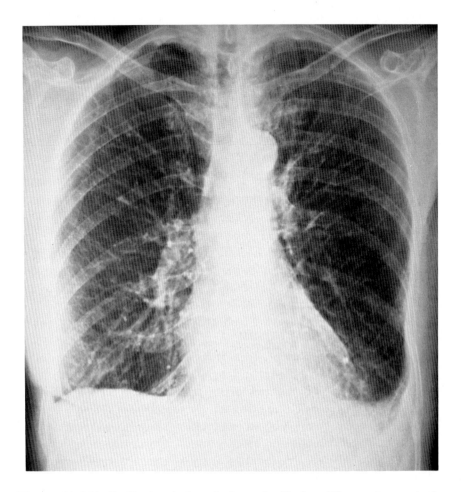

Figure 10-23. Radiation-induced pleural effusion. The posteroanterior radiograph shows a small left pleural effusion which developed 3½ months after completion of radiotherapy as primary treatment for breast carcinoma. The pleural fluid cytology was negative for tumor cells, and the effusion resolved spontaneously at 7 months.

mediastinal irradiation.[29] Radiotherapy-induced superior vena cava obstruction occurred in only 1 of 86 patients seen at the Mayo Clinic between 1960 and 1979.[22] In another series of 16 patients with benign causes of superior vena cava obstruction seen at the Cleveland Clinic, radiation therapy was not listed **(Option (D) is least likely and the correct answer).**[17] Other late-phase abnormalities due to radiotherapy include pneumothorax, mediastinal hematoma, atrophy of a pulmonary artery, subclavian or carotid artery stenosis, esophageal stenosis, and osteoradionecrosis.[5,7,12,13,15,18,20]

Question 55

After the completion of radiation therapy, patients who develop symptomatic radiation pneumonitis most commonly present within:

(A) 1 to 5 weeks
(B) 3 to 6 months
(C) 6 to 12 months
(D) 12 to 18 months
(E) 18 to 24 months

The usual starting date for assessing the effects of radiation therapy is the date of treatment completion.[11] The intervals given below are to be used as guidelines for when specific changes may be expected to appear. Although some exceptions will occur, abnormalities arising outside of these time frames should not be attributed to radiation effect until other possibilities have been excluded.

The early phase for radiation effects is the first 6 months after completion of therapy. Frequently, parenchymal opacities develop within the irradiated area, although the patient remains asymptomatic. Such opacities should be termed radiation effects, whereas the term radiation pneumonitis should be restricted to those patients developing symptoms and signs associated with the radiation-induced opacities. Of patients developing radiation pneumonitis, 90% will do so during the first 6 months; most present at 3 to 6 months **(Option (B) is correct).** When radiation pneumonitis develops, the symptoms are usually insidious in onset. Patients may have a nonproductive cough, dyspnea, fever, and pleuritic chest pain. The chest physical examination is usually normal. A mild leukocytosis and increase in sedimentation rate occur. Most of the patients developing this constellation of findings will recover within 1 to 4 weeks. Although some patients develop parenchymal opacities before 3 months, the narrower the interval between therapy completion and presentation, the more likely it is that the patient has developed a superimposed infection or worsened neoplasm. Goldman and Enquist have reported a single case as an example of hyperacute radiation pneumonitis occurring on day 8 of radiation therapy.[10] Although the parenchymal opacities did occur within the radiation therapy port, they could have alternatively been explained by bronchial mucosal edema and mucus plugging of the airways with a "drowned" lung appearance.

The late phase for radiation effects begins 6 months after therapy completion. Beyond this time it is unusual for patients to develop either symptomatic parenchymal opacities or clinical radiation pneumonitis. This phase is characterized by maturation of the fibrotic process that was initiated in the early phase. The maturation takes place over the subsequent 6 to 18 months so that the findings on the chest radiograph have stabilized by 12 to 24 months after completion of treatment. Although most patients do not have symptoms as a result of radiation fibrosis, those with limited pulmonary reserve may develop respiratory failure if enough areas of the lung have been damaged.

Question 56

Which *one* of the following is NOT a risk factor for developing radiation pneumonitis?

    (A) Large lung volume irradiated
    (B) Short radiation delivery time
    (C) Concomitant chemotherapy
    (D) Concomitant pneumonia
    (E) Previous radiation therapy

Although some degree of lung damage probably takes place whenever radiation therapy is given, a number of factors increase the likelihood that clinically significant disease will develop: large lung volume irradiated (Option (A)), large radiation dose, and short radiation delivery time (Option (B)).[28] In general, radiographic evidence of disease is rare below a total dose of 3,000 rad, while it is almost always seen at doses above 4,000 rad.[16] Concomitant chemotherapy (Option (C)) with the antineoplastic drugs dactinomycin, cyclophosphamide, vincristine, and busulfan potentiates the effects of radiation therapy.[11,26] In addition, a previously present radiation pneumonitis may be reactivated by subsequent administration of adriamycin or actinomycin.[19] Withdrawal of corticosteroids may precipitate latent early-phase postradiation reactions.[23] Patients who have had previous radiotherapy to the thorax (Option (E)) are at increased risk of developing clinical radiation pneumonitis.

Although it has been suggested that a concomitant pneumonia will predispose to development of radiation pneumonitis because of increased x-ray absorption, no studies done in the antibiotic era have demonstrated that this is a significant risk factor **(Option (D) is not a risk factor and is the correct answer).**[4]

SUGGESTED READINGS

1. Annest LS, Anderson RP, Li W, Hafermann MD. Coronary artery disease following mediastinal radiation therapy. J Thorac Cardiovasc Surg 1983; 85:257–263

2. Applefeld MM, Wiernik PH. Cardiac disease after radiation therapy for Hodgkin's disease: analysis of 48 patients. Am J Cardiol 1983; 51:1679–1681

3. Bachman AL, Macken K. Pleural effusions following supervoltage radiation for breast carcinoma. Radiology 1959; 72:699–709

4. Bennett DE, Million RR, Ackerman LV. Bilateral radiation pneumonitis, a complication of the radiotherapy of bronchogenic carcinoma. Cancer 1969; 23:1001–1018

5. Bethancourt B, Pond GD, Jones SE, Grogan T, Wasserman P. Mediastinal hematoma simulating recurrent Hodgkin disease during systemic chemotherapy. AJR 1984; 142:1119–1120

6. Carmel RJ, Kaplan HS. Mantle irradiation in Hodgkin's disease. An analysis of technique, tumor eradication, and complications. Cancer 1976; 37:2813–2825

7. Chabora BM, Hopfan S, Wittes R. Esophageal complications in the treatment of oat cell carcinoma with combined irradiation and chemotherapy. Radiology 1977; 123:185–187

8. Glazer HS, Lee JK, Levitt RG, et al. Radiation fibrosis: differentiation from recurrent tumor by MR imaging. Radiology 1985; 156:721–726

9. Glazer HS, Levitt RG, Lee JK, Emami B, Gronemeyer S, Murphy WA. Differentiation of radiation fibrosis from recurrent pulmonary neoplasm by magnetic resonance imaging. AJR 1984; 143:729–730

10. Goldman AL, Enquist R. Hyperacute radiation pneumonitis. Chest 1975; 67:613–615

11. Gross NJ. Pulmonary effects of radiation therapy. Ann Intern Med 1977; 86:81–92

12. Hekali P, Halttunen P, Korhola O, Rauste J. Occlusion of the right pulmonary artery: a rare, late complication of radiation therapy. Ann Clin Res 1982; 14:7–10

13. Hughes WF, Carson CL, Laffaye HA. Subclavian artery occlusion 42 years after mastectomy and radiotherapy. Am J Surg 1984; 147:698–700

14. Lever AM, Henderson D, Ellis DA, Corris PA, Gilmartin JJ. Radiation fibrosis mimicking local recurrence in small cell carcinoma of the bronchus. Br J Radiol 1984; 57:178–180

15. Libshitz HI, Banner MP. Spontaneous pneumothorax as a complication of radiation therapy to the thorax. Radiology 1974; 112:199–201

16. Libshitz HI, North LB. Lung. In: Libshitz HI (ed), Diagnostic roentgenology of radiotherapy change. Baltimore: Williams & Wilkins; 1979:33–49

17. Mahajan V, Strimlan V, Ordstrand HS, Loop FD. Benign superior vena cava syndrome. Chest 1975; 68:32–35

18. McCready RA, Hyde GL, Bivins BA, Mattingly SS, Griffen WO Jr. Radiation-induced arterial injuries. Surgery 1983; 93:306–312

19. McInerney DP, Bullimore J. Reactivation of radiation pneumonitis by adriamycin. Br J Radiol 1977; 50:224–227

20. Meyer JE. Thoracic effects of therapeutic irradiation for breast carcinoma. AJR 1978; 130:877–885

21. Pagani JJ, Libshitz HI. CT manifestations of radiation-induced change in chest tissue. J Comput Assist Tomogr 1982; 6:243–248

22. Parish JM, Marschke RF Jr, Dines DE, Lee RE. Etiologic considerations in superior vena cava syndrome. Mayo Clin Proc 1981; 56:407–413

23. Parris TM, Knight JG, Hess CE, Constable WC. Severe radiation pneumonitis precipitated by withdrawal of corticosteroids: a diagnostic and therapeutic dilemma. AJR 1979; 132:284–286

24. Ruckdeschel JC, Chang P, Martin RG, et al. Radiation-related pericardial effusions in patients with Hodgkin's disease. Medicine 1975; 54:245–259

25. Slanina J, Musshoff K, Rahner T, Stiasny R. Long-term side effects in irradiated patients with Hodgkin's disease. Int J Radiat Oncol Biol Phys 1977; 2:1–19

26. Soble AR, Perry H. Fatal radiation pneumonia following subclinical busulfan injury. AJR 1977; 128:15–18

27. Spencer H. Pathology of the lung, 4th ed. Oxford: Pergamon Press; 1985:511–517

28. Wara WM, Phillips TL, Margolis LW, Smith V. Radiation pneumonitis: a new approach to the derivation of time-dose factors. Cancer 1973; 32:547–552

29. Whitcomb ME, Schwarz MI. Pleural effusion complicating intensive mediastinal radiation therapy. Am Rev Respir Dis 1971; 103:100–107

Notes

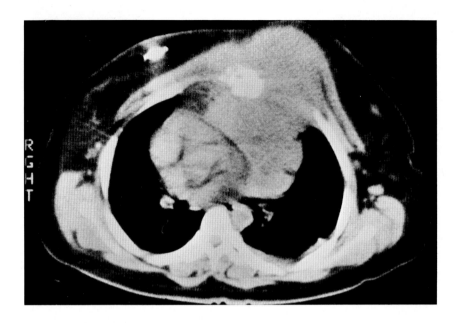

Figure 11-1

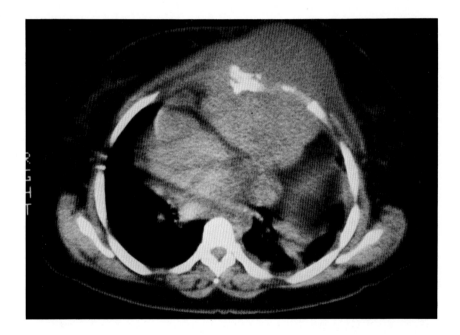

Figure 11-2
Figures 11-1 and 11-2. This 60-year-old woman developed swelling of the chest wall. You are shown scans from her computed tomographic (CT) examination.

Case 11: Lymphoma

Question 57

Which *one* of the following is the MOST likely diagnosis?

(A) Actinomycosis
(B) Malignant mesothelioma
(C) Lymphoma
(D) Candidiasis
(E) Invasive thymoma

The computed tomographic (CT) scans (Figures 11-1 and 11-2) show a large anterior mediastinal mass (wide black arrows, Figures 11-3 and 11-4) that displaces the heart to the right and extends through the anterior chest wall. Lytic destruction of a left anterior rib is present (thin black arrows, Figure 11-4). There is minimal left lower lobe consolidation (white arrowheads, Figure 11-4), and it does not appear contiguous with the mediastinal or chest wall mass. Minimal pleural thickening or effusion is present posteriorly on the left. Although the breasts are not shown in their entirety, the chest wall in these figures is cranial to them and the visualized breast tissue appears to be normal.

Chest wall masses may arise from the bones or soft tissues of the thoracic wall or may result from the contiguous spread of nearby pulmonary, mediastinal, or pleural disease. When more than one region is involved, identification of the predominant region of involvement usually is a clue to the correct differential diagnosis.

Actinomycosis (Option (A)) is an infectious disorder caused by the various types of *Actinomyces* organisms. Although these organisms are higher bacteria, the infections they cause resemble, and are frequently classified with, fungal infections. Thoracic actinomycosis is predominantly a pulmonary infection that extends by contiguous spread to involve the pleura and chest wall secondarily (Figures 11-5 to 11-7). Mediastinal involvement, when present, is almost always due to contiguous spread from the lung as well. Since the lung disease shown

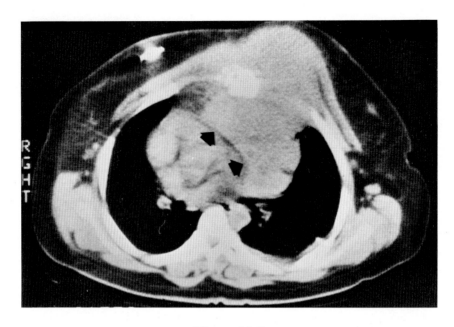

Figure 11-3

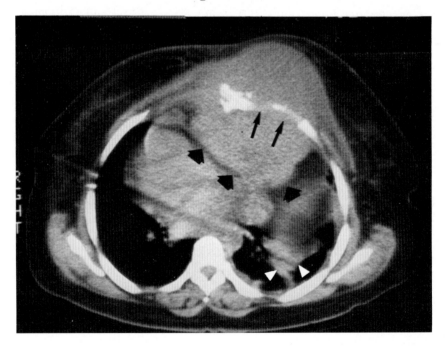

Figure 11-4
Figures 11-3 and 11-4 (Same as Figures 11-1 and 11-2, respectively).
Note the mediastinal mass (wide black arrows) displacing the heart to
the right in both figures. Left anterior chest wall extension is also seen,
along with rib destruction (thin black arrows) and minimal left lower
lobe consolidation (white arrowheads Figure 11-4).

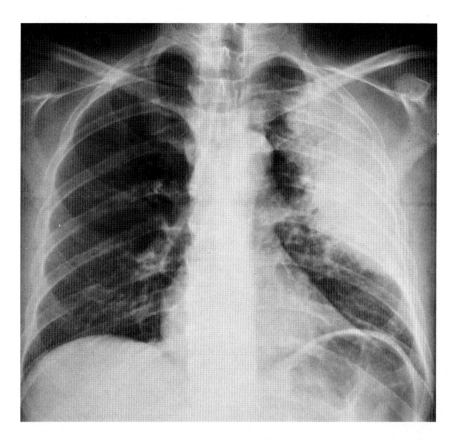

Figure 11-5

Figures 11-5 to 11-7. Actinomycosis. This 51-year-old man had chest pain, cough, and weight loss. His frontal chest radiograph (Figure 11-5) shows peripheral consolidation on the left, but a pleural component is difficult to confirm. CT scans through the upper thorax (Figures 11-6 and 11-7) show the parenchymal disease with contiguous extension into the soft tissues of the chest wall (arrows), as well as a small loculated effusion (arrowheads). (Courtesy of Lawrence Goodman, M.D., Milwaukee, Wisconsin.)

(Figures 11-2 and 11-4) does not appear to be contiguous with either the mediastinal or chest wall mass, actinomycosis is an unlikely explanation for the radiographic findings.

Malignant mesothelioma (Option (B)) is a primary pleural tumor that may involve the chest wall or mediastinum by contiguous spread. Although this tumor has a spectrum of radiographic appearances, the predominant feature is that of pleural effusion and/or pleural mass (see

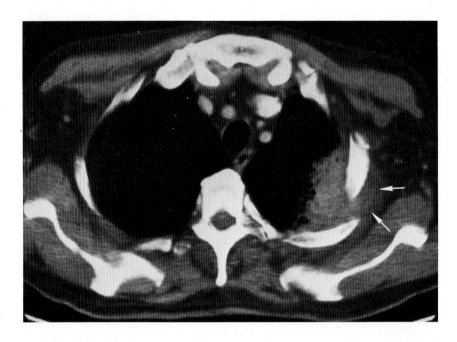

Figure 11-6

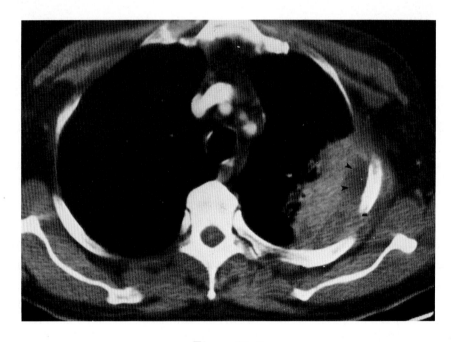

Figure 11-7

below). Owing to the minimal amount of pleural disease and the marked amount of anterior chest wall/mediastinal mass in our test case, malignant mesothelioma is an unlikely diagnosis.

Candida pneumonia and mediastinitis (Option (D)) are usually found in immunocompromised hosts, but involvement of the chest wall is very unusual. In a recent series of 20 patients with *Candida* pneumonia, the chest wall was not involved in any patient.[7] The parenchymal disease appeared as either airspace or mixed airspace/interstitial opacities, which were bilateral and nonsegmental in 8 of the 20 patients. The remaining 12 patients showed a mixture of unilateral/bilateral, lobar/segmental opacities.[7] *Candida* infections of the costochondral junction and sternal osteomyelitis have been described rarely,[12,17] but a large chest wall/ mediastinal mass has not been a feature in any of these patients.

Invasive thymoma (Option (E)) is a relatively uncommon tumor that develops from thymic epithelium. Fewer than 500 cases occur each year in the United States.[41] Because these tumors may be difficult to classify into benign and malignant varieties on the basis of histologic criteria alone, many investigators avoid these terms and prefer to call them localized or invasive.[29,31] The localized tumors make up two-thirds of the group, are well encapsulated, behave in a clinically benign fashion, and may be removed easily at surgery or autopsy. Invasive tumors involve the mediastinum, pericardium, pleura, or lung by direct extension. A few patients with invasive tumors develop bloodborne metastases, which may affect the lungs or nonthoracic organs (see below).[19]

Thymomas present as round or oval mediastinal masses adjacent to the junction of the heart and great vessels (Figures 11-8 and 11-9). Pleural spread of the tumor may produce an appearance of peripheral pleura-based masses (Figure 11-10). Invasion into the anterior chest wall is unusual; it has seldom been described. However, in a recent series of 22 patients with invasive thymoma evaluated by CT, chest wall involvement was seen in 2 patients (9%).[42] Since invasive thymoma is not a common tumor and since it does not commonly involve the chest wall, it is not the most likely explanation for the findings seen in Figures 11-1 and 11-2; thus, invasive thymoma is not correct.

The thorax is involved at some time during the course of illness in approximately 20 to 50% of patients with lymphoma.[14] Mediastinal and hilar lymph node enlargement is the most common thoracic manifestation in both Hodgkin's and non-Hodgkin's lymphomas. While involvement of the anterior chest wall with lymphoma has been thought to be rare, two recent studies using CT have found it in 24 of 250 patients (9.6%) and in 17 of 123 patients (13.8%) with any type of lym-

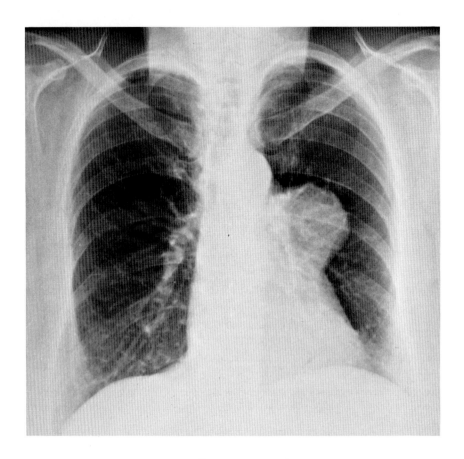

Figure 11-8
Figures 11-8 and 11-9. Thymoma. The frontal and lateral chest radiographs of a 74-year-old woman with chest pain show a smoothly marginated mass in the left anterior mediastinum adjacent to the main pulmonary artery.

phoma.[11,13,27,39] Of those patients with anterior chest wall involvement, 15 to 50% have direct extension from bulky anterior mediastinal disease. It is estimated that 33,800 new cases of lymphoma are diagnosed each year in the United States, and 450 to 2,500 cases of anterior chest wall invasion may be expected. In view of the large anterior mediastinal mass, the associated chest wall involvement, and the relative frequency of lymphoma compared with that of invasive thymoma, lymphoma is the most likely diagnosis **(Option (C) is correct)**. The patient shown in Figures 11-1 and 11-2 had Hodgkin's disease and had refused treatment until the tumor became quite extensive.

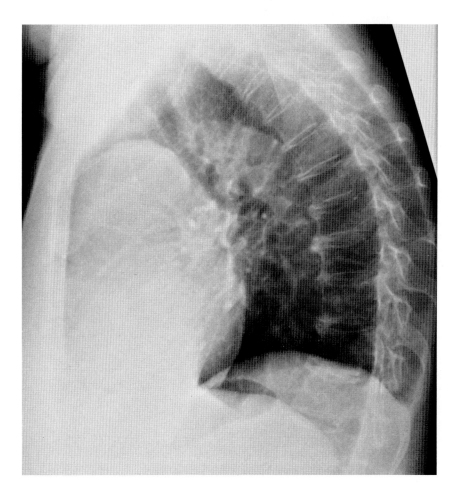

Figure 11-9

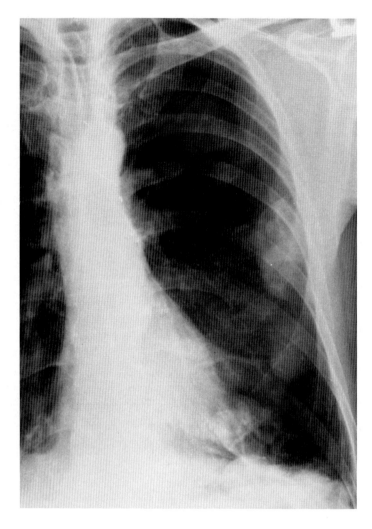

Figure 11-10. Invasive thymoma. This 51-year-old man was seen for follow-up of thymoma first diagnosed at age 25. His frontal radiograph shows multiple peripheral tumor masses in the left hemithorax.

Question 58

When a disease process arises in the thorax, abdominal CT is LEAST likely to provide additional information for which *one* of the following?

(A) Blastomycosis
(B) Malignant mesothelioma
(C) Lymphoma
(D) Candidiasis
(E) Invasive thymoma

Many disease processes that originate in the thorax may have secondary manifestations in abdominal organs. Conversely, many primary abdominal processes may appear to present with thoracic disease. CT of the abdomen, therefore, may complement the assessment of many disease processes affecting the thorax. An understanding of the clinical behavior of these various disease processes suggests when abdominal CT may be of benefit.

Malignant mesothelioma (Option (B)) arises in the pleural space in approximately two-thirds of cases and in the peritoneum or pericardium in the remaining one-third. The tumor may spread by direct contiguity or by hematogenous or lymphatic dissemination. Even when mesotheliomas originate in the pleural space, the upper abdomen is frequently involved by extension of the tumor through a diaphragmatic hiatus or by direct penetration of the diaphragm. At autopsy, metastatic disease is present in the peritoneum, liver, spleen, upper gastrointestinal tract, kidneys, retroperitoneal lymph nodes, or adrenals in 30 to 50% of patients.[2,5,15,16,26,30] In a recent series of 9 patients studied with CT, tumor was demonstrated in the upper abdomen in 5 patients (55%).[24] Abdominal involvement, therefore, is relatively common in malignant mesothelioma.

Most patients with non-Hodgkin's lymphoma and approximately 30% of patients with Hodgkin's lymphoma (Option (C)) have abdominal involvement at initial presentation.[14] While this involvement usually consists of retroperitoneal or mesenteric lymph node enlargement, the spleen, liver, kidneys, and bowel may be involved in individual instances. Abdominal CT demonstrated its value in the assessment of patients with lymphoma soon after its introduction and is now used routinely in determining the extent of disease both at initial presentation and in follow-up.

Renal, hepatic, or splenic abscesses are present at autopsy in more than one-half of patients dying of systemic candidiasis (Option (D)).[21,25]

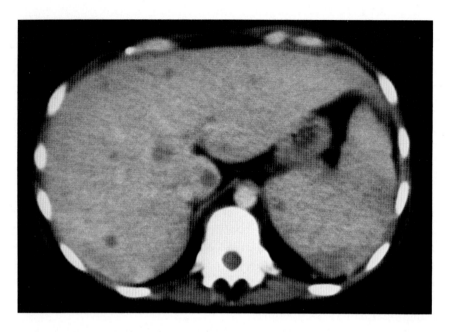

Figure 11-11. Hepatosplenic candidiasis. This 44-year-old woman had leukemia and multiple episodes of sepsis. Her CT scan shows multiple small lucent defects in the liver and spleen.

These abscesses are often small (1 to 3 cm) and multiple and usually do not result in specific symptoms. On CT, they appear as lucent areas with either smooth or irregular borders (Figure 11-11).[9] The lesions may be difficult to detect. Since *Candida* species are difficult to culture, percutaneous needle biopsy may be negative. Open biopsy has been suggested as the procedure of choice to ensure early diagnosis and institution of proper therapy.[37] Involvement of upper abdominal organs, then, is not uncommon in candidiasis, and CT is likely to aid in the diagnosis of such involvement.

While invasive thymomas (Option (E)) predominantly invade structures of the thorax, they may also disseminate to the abdomen hematogenously or by direct extension. In order of decreasing frequency, the abdominal sites of involvement are the liver, retroperitoneal lymph nodes, kidneys, adrenals, peritoneum, and spleen (Figures 11-12 and 11-13).[19,23] In a recent series of 20 patients studied by CT, 7 (35%) demonstrated involvement of an upper abdominal organ or of the retroperitoneal lymph nodes.[42]

Blastomycosis (Option (A)) is a fungal infection caused by *Blastomyces dermatitidis*. Although the fungus is thought to reside in soil, it is not

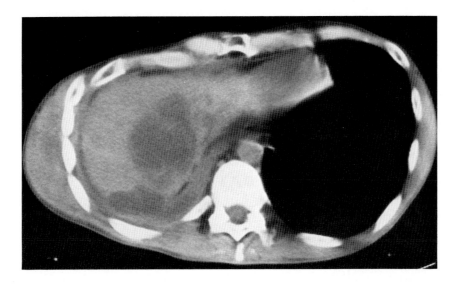

Figure 11-12

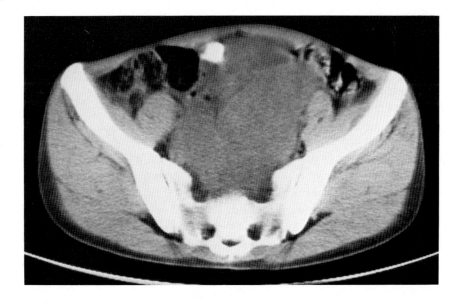

Figure 11-13
Figures 11-12 and 11-13. Invasive thymoma. This 38-year-old man had
a thymoma resected 17 years earlier. CT scans show multiple lucent
defects in the liver (Figure 11-12) and a large pelvic soft tissue mass
(Figure 11-13). Needle biopsy of the pelvic mass showed metastatic
thymoma.

easily cultured and its exact habitat is not clearly understood. As determined from clinical cases in the United States, the disease is endemic to the southeast, upper midwest, and southwest areas of the country. Blastomycosis is predominantly a respiratory tract disease; involvement of other organs is almost always the result of dissemination from the lungs. The organs or systems most frequently involved by disseminated disease include the lungs, skin, bone, male reproductive organs (prostate, epididymis, and testicles), liver, spleen, adrenal glands, and central nervous system.[8,32,35] The last four are involved in fewer than 5% of patients. Hence, abdominal CT is less likely to be useful in blastomycosis than in the other four diseases listed **(Option (A) is the correct answer).**

Question 59

On imaging studies, which *one* of the following is LEAST likely to result from malignant mesothelioma?

    (A) Pleural mass
    (B) Hilar mass
    (C) Opaque hemithorax
    (D) Pericardial thickening
    (E) Chest wall invasion

While numerous patients with mesothelioma have been reported, radiographic findings have often been discussed in general terms. Careful tabulation of specific radiographic findings has been limited to a relatively small number of patients.[1,20,22,28,36,38]

Thoracic mesotheliomas present as localized masses or as more diffuse disease in the hemithorax. Most of the localized tumors behave in a clinically benign fashion, while the diffuse variety behaves as a malignancy. Benign mesotheliomas range in size from 5 to 18 cm (Figures 11-14 and 11-15). Pleural effusions are usually small and occur in fewer than 20% of these patients. Resection of such lesions is usually curative.

Malignant mesothelioma is usually distributed diffusely within the hemithorax at the time of presentation.[20] Of patients with malignant mesothelioma, 60% have a visible pleural mass at presentation and almost all develop one during the course of the illness (Option (A) is not least likely).[38,40] The masses are usually multilobulated and situated in the inferior and lateral pleural space. A clue to the presence of a pleural

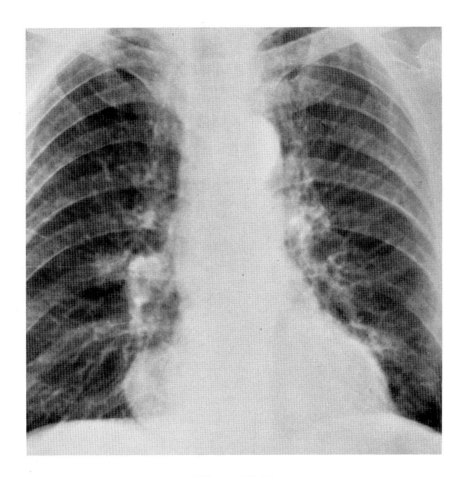

Figure 11-14

Figures 11-14 and 11-15. Benign mesothelioma. This routine frontal chest radiograph (Figure 11-14) of a 66-year-old man shows the mass at the right cardiophrenic angle. Note the mass anteriorly on the lateral view (Figure 11-15). (Courtesy of the Armed Forces Institute of Pathology, AFIP negatives 56-11435 and 56-11436, respectively.)

mass underlying a pleural effusion is a lobulated margin convex toward the lung (Figures 11-16 and 11-17).

A hilar mass (Option (B)) in patients with malignant mesothelioma is not least likely because it occurred in 6 of 23 patients (25%) in one series (Figure 11-18).[38] The most common reason for the hilar mass is believed to be growth of the tumor along the hilum as it spreads along the mediastinal pleural surface and begins to encase the lung. Metastatic

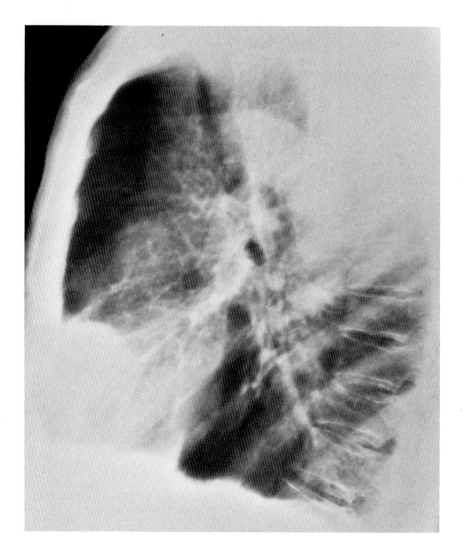

Figure 11-15

disease of the hilar and mediastinal lymph nodes is present at autopsy in 35 to 50% of cases.[33]

Pericardial thickening from mesothelioma (Option (D)) is present in as many as 40% of patients at autopsy.[33] Although it has not been described on conventional chest radiographs, it has been demonstrated by CT in three of nine patients (33%) in one series and is certainly not least likely.[24]

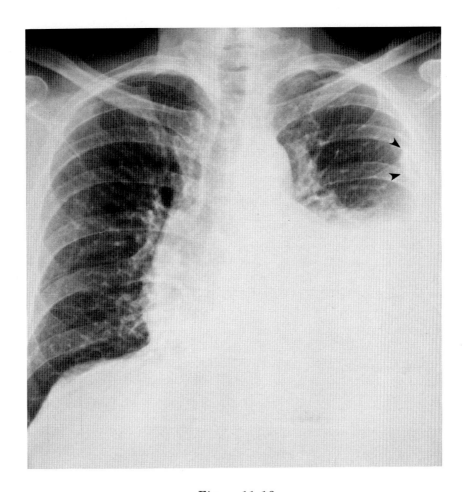

Figure 11-16

Figures 11-16 and 11-17. Malignant mesothelioma. This 70-year-old man had cough, dyspnea, and weight loss. His initial chest radiograph (Figure 11-16) shows a large left pleural effusion. Note the soft tissue opacity (arrowheads, Figure 11-16) with margins convex toward the lung. The lobulated tumor mass and its extent are more easily identified after thoracentesis (arrowhead, Figure 11-17).

Invasion of the chest wall (Option (E)) is also not least likely because it occurs in as many as 40% of patients with malignant mesothelioma.[33] It is particularly likely to occur late in the disease, often at the site of previous biopsies (Figure 11-19). Rib destruction was observed in 18% of patients in one series.[40]

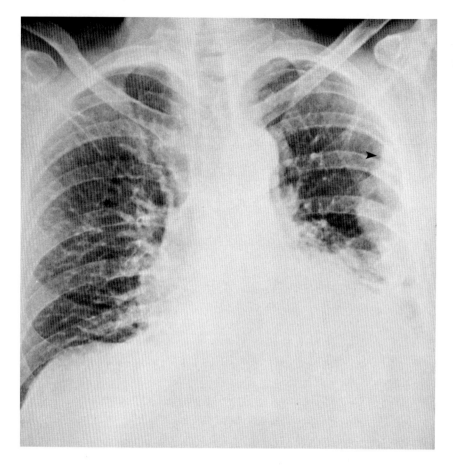

Figure 11-17

Pleural effusion is extremely common in patients with malignant mesothelioma,[10] existing at presentation in 40 to 60% of patients and at some time during their illness in as many as 94% of patients. Although the size of the effusion varies from patient to patient, it is usually moderate to large and fills one-third to two-thirds of the hemithorax (Figure 11-16).[20] On the other hand, pleural effusions massive enough to opacify an entire hemithorax occur in only 10 to 15% of patients (Figure 11-20); therefore, opaque hemithorax is least likely **(Option (C) is correct).** Even when the entire hemithorax is opacified, the mediastinum is usually not significantly shifted contralaterally. The tumor tends to result in fixation as its spread causes encasement (Figure 11-21). As the

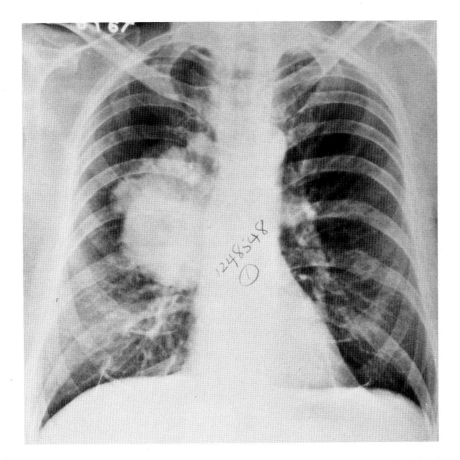

Figure 11-18. Malignant mesothelioma. This 71-year-old man had right chest pain for 1 year. His frontal chest radiograph shows a large lobulated mass that abuts the right posterior hilum. (Courtesy of the Armed Forces Institute of Pathology, AFIP negative 67-8011.)

disease progresses, however, there is usually contraction; thus, ipsilateral mediastinal shift may occur (Figures 11-22 and 11-23).[22,28]

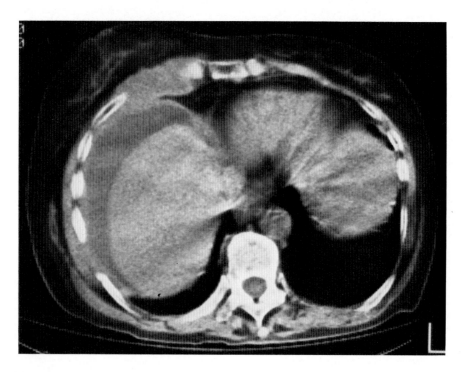

Figure 11-19. Malignant mesothelioma. This 71-year-old woman developed a right anterior chest wall mass at the site of a previous biopsy showing malignant mesothelioma.

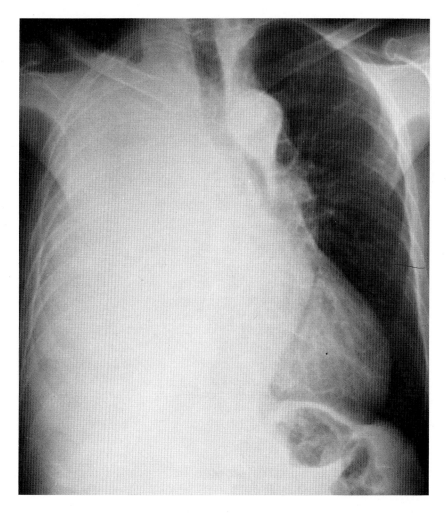

Figure 11-20. Malignant mesothelioma. This 70-year-old man had a chest radiograph because of progressive dyspnea and weight loss. Note the complete opacification of the right hemithorax with contralateral mediastinal shift, an unusual finding with malignant mesothelioma.

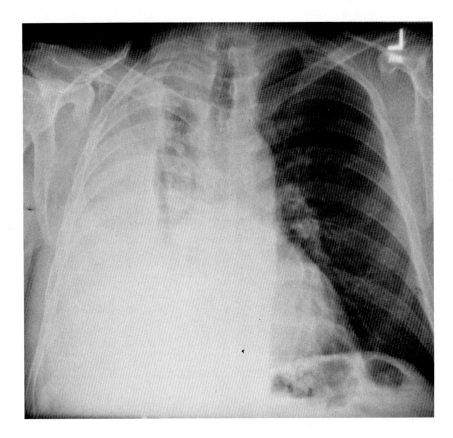

Figure 11-21. Malignant mesothelioma. This 65-year-old man had cough and right flank pain. A large right pleural effusion is present, without significant mediastinal shift (compare with Figure 11-20).

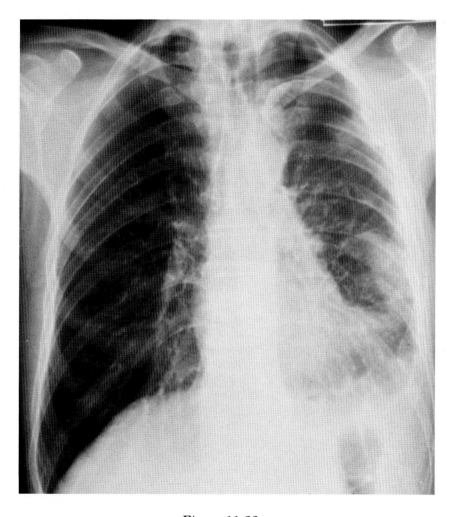

Figure 11-22
Figures 11-22 and 11-23. Malignant mesothelioma. This 49-year-old man had left chest pain for 5 months. Frontal radiographs taken 10 months apart (Figures 11-22 and 11-23) show progressive volume loss and tumor growth in the left hemithorax. The mediastinal shift in Figure 11-23 is greater than that expected for the amount of patient rotation.

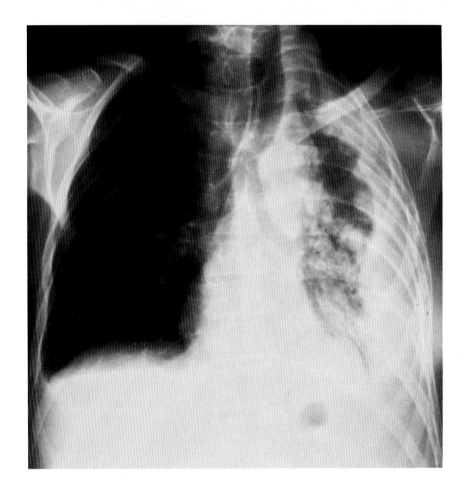

Figure 11-23

Question 60

Concerning actinomycosis,

(A) the most commonly involved site is the thorax

(B) when extension occurs across normal anatomic boundaries, it is due to elaboration of proteolytic enzymes

(C) the left lung is more frequently involved than the right one

(D) sulfur granules contain the responsible organism

Actinomycosis, historically an uncommon disease, is probably becoming even rarer, for reasons that are not completely understood. Improvements in hygiene and the widespread use of antibiotics may be playing a role, however. The disease occurs in three clinical forms: cervicofacial, thoracic, and abdominal.[4,6] Although the forms may occur concomitantly, they usually arise independently. Disseminated actinomycosis is very rare. In nearly all series, cervicofacial actinomycosis is the most frequently encountered form; it is seen in 40 to 50% of patients **(Option (A) is false).** The remaining cases are almost equally divided between the thoracic and abdominal forms, each of which has been reported as the second most commonly involved site.

In any of these sites, a brief period of acute inflammation is followed by the development of a hard granulomatous mass, which enlarges by contiguous spread.[6] A thick, densely fibrotic periphery surrounds central purulent loculi, which average 4.4 mm in diameter and contain the characteristic sulfur granules and neutrophils. Sulfur granules are round or oval masses of *Actinomyces* organisms **(Option (D) is true).** One to fifty sulfur granules are present in each loculus.

In many cases, the inflammation leads to sinus tract formation with drainage through the skin, a situation probably more common in the pre-antibiotic era than it is today. When extension of the infection occurs, it does so without regard for normal anatomic boundaries because the organisms elaborate potent proteolytic enzymes **(Option (B) is true).**[34] Because of this propensity, an infectious process that crosses pleural fissures or invades the chest wall via contiguous spread should suggest actinomycosis.

Actinomycosis may involve virtually any region of the lung.[3,18] The infection may present as a mass, a chronic end-airspace opacity, or upper-lobe fibrocavitary disease. The lower lobes have been said to be involved more often than the upper lobes; in recent series, however, involvement has been equal in both. There is, moreover, a marked preponderance of right lung involvement. In one recent series, 11 of 13 cases (84%) involved the right lung **(Option (C) is false).**[4] This right lung preponderance is cited as evidence that thoracic actinomycosis results from aspiration of oropharyngeal material.

While thoracic actinomycosis begins as a parenchymal process, pleural extension with either pleural thickening or pleural effusion has been described in 40 to 80% of patients. Large pleural effusions have been recorded. However, the infection usually extends across the pleural space to invade the chest wall, with only pleural thickening or small pleural effusions developing. Compared with the frequency reported in older series, the frequency of pleural involvement may be decreasing; it did not occur in one recent series of 13 patients.[4]

SUGGESTED READINGS

1. Alexander E, Clark RA, Colley DP, Mitchell SE. CT of malignant pleural mesothelioma. AJR 1981; 137:287–291
2. Antman KH. Clinical presentation and natural history of benign and malignant mesothelioma. Semin Oncol 1981; 8:313–320
3. Bates M, Cruickshank G. Thoracic actinomycosis. Thorax 1957; 12:99–124
4. Bennhoff DF. Actinomycosis: diagnostic and therapeutic considerations and a review of 32 cases. Laryngoscope 1984; 94:1198–1217
5. Brenner J, Sordillo PP, Magill GB, Golbey RB. Malignant mesothelioma of the pleura: review of 123 patients. Cancer 1982; 49:2431–2435
6. Brown JR. Human actinomycosis. A study of 181 subjects. Hum Pathol 1973; 4:319–330
7. Buff SJ, McLelland R, Gallis HA, Matthay R, Putnam CE. *Candida albicans* pneumonia: radiographic appearance. AJR 1982; 138:645–648
8. Busey JF, Baker R, Birch L, et al. Blastomycosis. I. A review of 198 collected cases in Veterans Administration hospitals. Am Rev Respir Dis 1964; 89:659–672
9. Callen PW, Filly RA, Marcus FS. Ultrasonography and computed tomography in the evaluation of hepatic microabscesses in the immunosuppressed patient. Radiology 1980; 136:433–434
10. Chahinian AP, Pajak TF, Holland JF, Norton L, Ambinder RM, Mandel EM. Diffuse malignant mesothelioma. Prospective evaluation of 69 patients. Ann Intern Med 1982; 96:746–755
11. Cho CS, Blank N, Castellino RA. Computerized tomography evaluation of chest wall involvement in lymphoma. Cancer 1985; 55:1892–1894
12. Collignon PJ, Sorrell TC. Disseminated candidiasis: evidence of a distinctive syndrome in heroin abusers. Br Med J 1983; 287:861–862
13. DeBeer R, Friedfeld L, Kabakow B. Complete sternal collapse associated with lymphomatous involvement of the bony thorax—case report and review of the literature. Clin Oncol 1977; 3:331–338

14. DeVita VT Jr, Jaffe ES, Hellman S. Hodgkin's disease and the non-Hodgkin's lymphomas. In: DeVita VT Jr, Hellman S, Rosenberg SA (eds), Cancer. Principles and practice of oncology, 2nd ed. Philadelphia: Lippincott; 1985:1623–1709

15. Edge JR, Choudhury SL. Malignant mesothelioma of the pleura in Barrow-in-Furness. Thorax 1978; 33:26–30

16. Elmes PC, Simpson JC. The clinical aspects of mesothelioma. Q J Med 1976; 16:427–449

17. Estrov Z, Resnitzky P, Shenker Y, Berrebi A, Hurwitz N. Candidemia and sternal *Candida albicans* osteomyelitis in a patient with chronic lymphatic leukemia. Isr J Med Sci 1984; 20:711–714

18. Flynn MW, Felson B. The roentgen manifestations of thoracic actinomycosis. AJR 1970; 110:707–716

19. Gravanis MB. Metastasizing thymoma. Report of a case and review of the literature. Am J Clin Pathol 1968; 49:690–696

20. Heller RM, Janower ML, Weber AL. The radiological manifestations of malignant pleural mesothelioma. AJR 1970; 108:53–59

21. Hughes WT. Systemic candidiasis: a study of 109 fatal cases. Pediatr Infect Dis 1982; 1:11–18

22. Kendall-Smith IM. Pulmonary encasement: a sign of advanced malignant diffuse mesothelioma. Australas Radiol 1979; 23:24–29

23. Lemaitre L, Gosselin B, Smith M, et al. [Abdominal localization of invasive thymomas. Contribution of tomodensitometry.] J Radiol 1982; 63:485–494

24. Mirvis S, Dutcher JP, Haney PJ, Whitley NO, Aisner J. CT of malignant pleural mesothelioma. AJR 1983; 140:665–670

25. Myerowitz RL, Pazin GJ, Allen CM. Disseminated candidiasis. Changes in incidence, underlying diseases, and pathology. Am J Clin Pathol 1977; 68:29–38

26. Oels HC, Harrison EG Jr, Carr DT, Bernatz PE. Diffuse malignant mesothelioma of the pleura: a review of 37 cases. Chest 1971; 60:564–570

27. Press GA, Glazer HS, Wasserman TH, Aronberg DJ, Lee JK, Sagel SS. Thoracic wall involvement by Hodgkin disease and non-Hodgkin lymphoma: CT evaluation. Radiology 1985; 157:195–198

28. Rabinowitz JG, Efremidis SC, Cohen B, et al. A comparative study of mesothelioma and asbestosis using computed tomography and conventional chest radiography. Radiology 1982; 144:453–460

29. Ring NP, Addis BJ. Thymoma: an integrated clinicopathological and immunohistochemical study. J Pathol 1986; 149:327–337

30. Roberts GH. Distant visceral metastases in pleural mesothelioma. Br J Dis Chest 1976; 70:246–250

31. Salyer WR, Eggleston JC. Thymoma: a clinical and pathological study of 65 cases. Cancer 1976; 37:229–249

32. Sarosi GA, Davies SF. Blastomycosis. Am Rev Respir Dis 1979; 120:911–938

33. Schlienger M, Eschwege F, Blache R, Depierre R. [Malignant pleural mesothelioma. Study of 39 cases, 25 by autopsy.] Bull Cancer 1969; 56:265–308

34. Schwarz J, Baum GL. Actinomycosis. Semin Roentgenol 1970; 5:58–63

35. Schwarz J, Salfelder K. Blastomycosis. A review of 152 cases. Curr Top Pathol 1977; 65:165–200

36. Shin MS, Bailey WC. Computed tomography of invasive pleural mesothelioma. J Comput Tomogr 1983; 7:389–394
37. Shirkhoda A, Lopez-Berestein G, Holbert JM, Luna MA. Hepatosplenic fungal infection: CT and pathologic evaluation after treatment with liposomal amphotericin B. Radiology 1986; 159:349–353
38. Solomon A. Radiological features of diffuse mesothelioma. Environ Res 1970; 3:330–338
39. Stark P. Invasion of the sternum by lymphoma—role of CT. Radiology 1984; 24:130–132
40. Taryle DA, Lakshminarayan S, Sahn SA. Pleural mesotheliomas—an analysis of 18 cases and review of the literature. Medicine 1976; 55:153–162
41. Young JL Jr, Percy CL, Asire AJ (eds). Surveillance, epidemiology, and end results: incidence and mortality data, 1973–77. National Cancer Institute Monograph 57. US Dept of Health and Human Services, Public Health Service, NIH Publication no. 81–2330. Bethesda, MD: National Cancer Institute; 1981:15
42. Zerhouni EA, Scott WW Jr, Baker RR, Wharam MD, Siegelman SS. Invasive thymomas: diagnosis and evaluation by computed tomography. J Comput Assist Tomogr 1982; 6:92–100

Notes

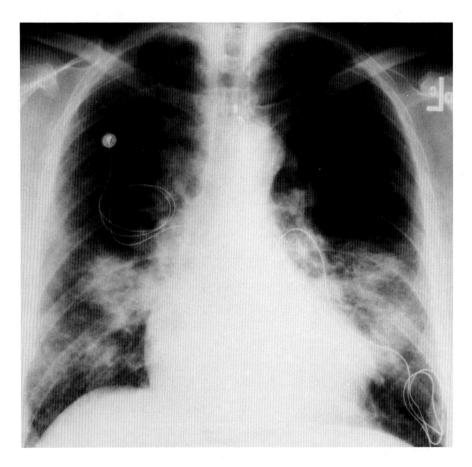

Figure 12-1. This 56-year-old man had a long history of ventricular arrhythmia and moderate rheumatoid arthritis. He had a 48-hour history of progressive dyspnea on exertion, mucoid sputum production, and mild chills. There was no hemoptysis, paroxysmal nocturnal dyspnea, or orthopnea. Medications included digitalis, amiodarone, and nonsteroidal anti-inflammatory drugs. The pulmonary capillary wedge pressure was 8 cm of water. A radiograph obtained 1 month earlier (not shown) demonstrated clear lungs and moderate cardiomegaly. You are shown the admission frontal radiograph.

Case 12: Amiodarone Toxicity

Question 61

Considering the history and radiographic findings, which *one* of the following is the MOST likely diagnosis?

(A) Congestive heart failure
(B) Rheumatoid lung
(C) Digitalis toxicity
(D) Amiodarone toxicity
(E) Aspiration pneumonia

The diagnosis of congestive heart failure (Option (A)) is excluded by the clinical information and the radiographic appearance. The history of arrhythmia and exertional dyspnea suggests the possibility of congestive heart failure. However, the patient experienced chills and had neither paroxysmal nocturnal dyspnea nor orthopnea. The pulmonary capillary wedge pressure (PCWP) of 8 cm of water militates further against a diagnosis of congestive heart failure. On the admission radiograph (Figure 12-1), the heart is borderline enlarged, and there are bilateral alveolar opacities located centrally and inferiorly. The opacities are rather focal, and the upper lobe vessels are of normal size with sharp margins. Central vessels are not enlarged, and both peribronchial cuffing and pleural effusion are absent. Congestive heart failure is, therefore, unlikely.

Given the history of rheumatoid arthritis, the possibility of rheumatoid lung (Option (B)) must be considered. The history of rather rapid onset of symptoms, coupled with the radiographic appearance, makes rheumatoid lung unlikely. When rheumatoid disease affects the lung, the pattern is usually one of interstitial pneumonitis or fibrosis or discrete pulmonary nodules.

Whenever there are unexplained parenchymal opacities in a patient receiving medication, the possibility of a drug reaction must be considered. The history indicated that this patient was receiving digitalis, amiodarone, and nonsteroidal anti-inflammatory drugs. Digitalis has both cardiovascular and systemic side effects. The major cardiovascular side effect is that of rhythm disturbance (such as ventricular premature beats, atrial arrhythmia, ventricular arrhythmia, and atrioventricular conduction disturbance). These could conceivably lead to congestive heart failure. Systemic side effects include anorexia, nausea, vomiting, diarrhea, gynecomastia, and visual disturbances. Direct pulmonary toxicity from digitalis (Option (C)) has not been reported, except for a rare case of digitalis-induced lupus erythematosus that affected the lung.[8] Digitalis toxicity is, therefore, unlikely.

The bilateral alveolar opacities, especially inferiorly, are consistent with aspiration pneumonia (Option (E)). The vast majority of episodes of aspiration are associated with a depressed state of consciousness. Other causes include neuromuscular disorders of the swallowing mechanism, head and neck surgery, and nighttime regurgitation. The history does not suggest any of the foregoing. Aspiration pneumonia is thus unlikely.

Amiodarone, a drug recently released in the United States, has proven to be effective in the treatment of both supraventricular and ventricular arrhythmias refractory to other forms of drug therapy. Unfortunately, side effects appear to be relatively common. Frequently reported side effects include skin discoloration, alteration of thyroid function, corneal deposits, neural toxicity, and myocardial depression. The side effects of specific interest to the radiologist are pneumonitis and hepatic dysfunction due to accumulation of the drug in the liver.

Pulmonary toxicity is a major clinical problem affecting 5 to 10% of patients receiving the drug.[2,7,14,15,24] Toxicity is rare in the first few weeks of treatment. Although pneumonitis may first appear 1 to 4 months after the initiation of treatment, it usually occurs later. The majority of patients with lung toxicity receive more than 400 mg per day. In a small percentage, the radiographic abnormalities precede the clinical symptoms. Exertional dyspnea, often severe, is the most frequent symptom. Fever, dry cough, and anorexia are also common. The onset of symptoms may be gradual or rapid. There is frequently evidence of amiodarone toxicity involving other organ systems at the time the pulmonary problem surfaces. The erythrocyte sedimentation rate is usually elevated, and the diffusing capacity is often depressed.

A review of 22 cases revealed that dense focal alveolar opacities are the most frequent radiographic finding.[2,7,14,15,24] Ten patients had only airspace consolidation, while six had airspace consolidation along with diffuse interstitial disease (Figures 12-2 and 12-3). Six patients had only interstitial disease. Pleural disease is present in 25% of patients, usually

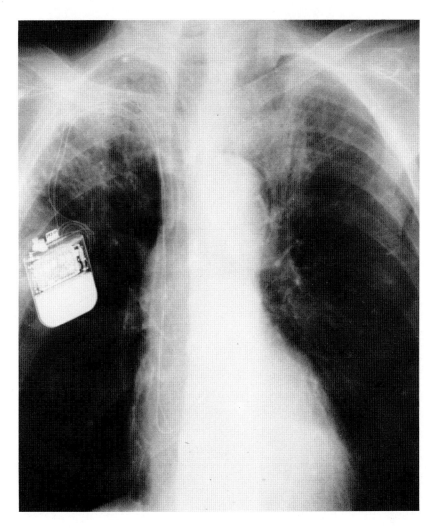

Figure 12-2

Figures 12-2 and 12-3. Amiodarone toxicity. This 70-year-old man with ventricular fibrillation had been receiving high doses of amiodarone for 5 months when he developed weakness, fatigue, dyspnea, weight loss, and low-grade fever. His chest radiograph (Figure 12-2) shows biapical opacities suggestive of tuberculosis. A CT scan (Figure 12-3) shows the process predominantly in the posterior segment of each upper lobe. Bronchoscopy recovered foamy macrophages compatible with drug toxicity. Stains and cultures for tuberculosis were negative. The amiodarone dose was decreased to 100 mg twice a week. The symptoms gradually subsided, and a follow-up radiograph 4 months later was normal.

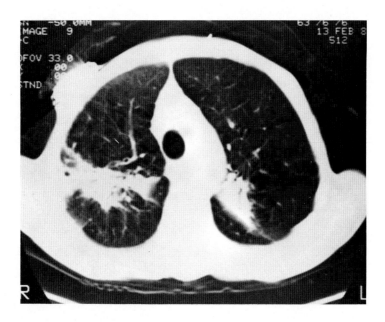

Figure 12-3

in consort with the lung disease. When the pulmonary involvement is diffuse, differentiation from congestive heart failure may be difficult. Gallium scintigraphy is usually positive in amiodarone lung disease but negative in congestive heart failure. **Option (D) is, therefore, the most likely diagnosis.**

The microscopic appearance of amiodarone lung is nonspecific (Figure 12-4). There are diffuse alveolar damage, thickening of the alveolar septa, and foamy intra-alveolar macrophages. With time, the exudate organizes and fibrosis appears. Electron microscopy shows granular and lamellar membranous bodies in the lung and elsewhere. This appearance is nonspecific and is found in cases of drug toxicity due to other amphiphilic drugs as well (Figure 12-5).

The response to the cessation of medication varies. In most patients, symptoms diminish over several weeks. Resolution of radiographic findings often requires several months, and scars may remain. A review of several series indicates that approximately 25% of those patients with documented amiodarone pulmonary opacities die.[2,7,14,15,24] Death may be due to rapidly progressing pulmonary insufficiency or slowly progressing pulmonary inflammation and fibrosis.

Of additional interest is the accumulation of amiodarone in the liver. This drug, an amphiphilic iodinated amine, is stored in the lysosomes of

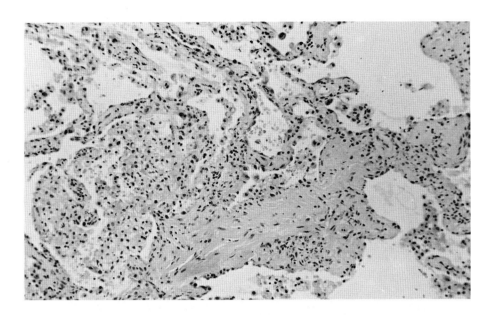

Figure 12-4

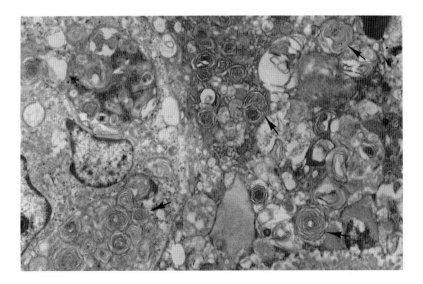

Figure 12-5
Figures 12-4 and 12-5. Amiodarone toxicity (biopsy from the patient in Figure 12-1). Figure 12-4 shows marked interstitial thickening with cellular infiltrate and fibrosis. Alveolar spaces are filled with established, and organizing fibrous connective tissue and foamy macrophages. An electron micrograph (Figure 12-5) demonstrates numerous lamellar whirls (arrows) in lysomes, a finding typical of many drug reactions.

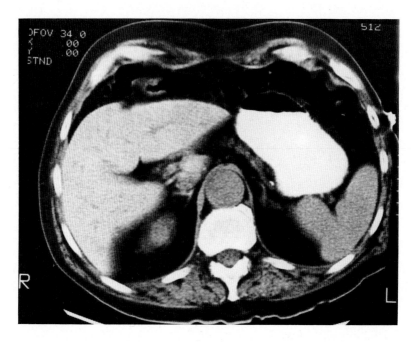

Figure 12-6. Amiodarone in liver. A non-contrast-enhanced CT scan through the liver and spleen in a patient on long-term therapy shows the liver at 90 to 98 HU and the spleen at 63 to 68 HU, both above normal. Because of greater hepatic than splenic concentration, the difference in density between the two organs is accentuated as well.

the liver; thus, a high hepatic concentration may result. The extra iodine will cause the liver to appear dense on computed tomography (CT). In a study of seven patients, Goldman et al.[9] found that the unenhanced liver measured 95 to 145 Hounsfield units (HU) in contrast to normal values of 30 to 70 HU (Figure 12-6). The spleen may be slightly denser than normal as well. These findings are associated with mild alterations in liver function, such as increased alkaline phosphatase and lactic dehydrogenase levels. In most cases, the change in liver function does not appear to have major clinical significance, although the long-term consequences are not clear.[9]

The dense liver from amiodarone accumulation must be differentiated from that due to other causes, such as that due to iron and glycogen storage.

Question 62

Concerning collagen vascular diseases that affect the lung,

- (A) the most frequent intrathoracic manifestation of rheumatoid arthritis is rheumatoid nodules
- (B) pulmonary opacities in systemic lupus erythematosus are most often due to diseases other than lupus pneumonitis
- (C) drug toxicity is responsible for approximately 10% of cases of systemic lupus erythematosus
- (D) radiographically, pulmonary fibrosis in scleroderma is characteristically perihilar
- (E) patients with polymyositis/dermatomyositis commonly develop diaphragmatic weakness

It has long been recognized that various arthritic conditions are, in fact, systemic disorders affecting many organs. Each of the collagen vascular diseases has characteristic, but sometimes overlapping, systemic manifestations. Although the intrathoracic manifestations are quite variable, they also frequently overlap.[11]

Pulmonary and pleural disease in rheumatoid arthritis has a predilection for male patients, although the arthritis itself is twice as frequent in female patients. The overall frequency of pulmonary and pleural disease has been estimated at 10 to 50%, depending on the patient population studies and the criteria for disease.[11] In general, there is a correlation between exacerbation of the arthritis, subcutaneous nodules, and the presence of intrathoracic disease. However, in a small percentage of patients, pulmonary and pleural disease typical of rheumatoid arthritis may present before other symptoms. When such is the case, serologic markers for rheumatoid arthritis are usually positive.

Most investigators divide the intrathoracic manifestations of rheumatoid disease into distinct categories, although more than one may appear in a given patient at any given time or in serial fashion.[11,13] Serositis, in the form of pleurisy, pleural effusion, or pericardial effusion, is the most frequent intrathoracic manifestation of rheumatoid arthritis (**Option (A) is false**). At autopsy, approximately 50% of patients have evidence of active or healed disease of the serosal membranes. Pleural effusions may be symptomatic or asymptomatic and tend to be unilateral. Although they may resolve spontaneously, they characteristically persist for months or years. Concomitant pulmonary changes are present in fewer than one-third of patients. The fluid is an exudate and has a glucose concentration usually below 25 mg/dL, despite a normal blood glucose level, and a lactic dehydrogenase level that is usually elevated. The fluid may contain polymorphonuclear cells that have dense black granules (the "RA" cells).

Interstitial lung disease is found in as many as 20% of patients with long-standing rheumatoid arthritis. Approximately one-half of the patients with pulmonary function abnormalities suggesting pulmonary fibrosis have negative chest radiographs initially. An early radiographic finding is a parenchymal pattern that may mimic miliary tuberculosis. With time, a linear fibrotic pattern may be visible in a predominantly basilar location. The pattern is similar to idiopathic pulmonary fibrosis, but the clinical and radiographic progression is usually less rapid and less severe (Figure 12-7).

Rheumatoid necrobiotic nodules are relatively rare and usually associated with advanced rheumatoid disease, the presence of subcutaneous nodules, and other evidence of intrathoracic rheumatoid disease. Rheumatoid nodules may be single or multiple and range in diameter from several millimeters to several centimeters. Cavitation and bronchopleural fistula are not uncommon. The nodules tend to subside when the arthritis is in remission. Caplan's syndrome refers to the presence of rheumatoid nodules in the lung in patients with rheumatoid arthritis and pneumoconiosis. These nodules generally appear when the arthritis flares and when subcutaneous nodules are present, and they are radiographically similar to the conventional rheumatoid nodules.

Pulmonary arteritis may complicate any of the above lesions or may be the sole manifestation of rheumatoid arthritis. The radiographic appearance is similar to that of idiopathic pulmonary hypertension with pruning of peripheral vessels, dilatation of the central vessels, and eventual right-sided cardiac enlargement.

Pleural and pericardial diseases are more common in systemic lupus erythematosus (SLE) than in any of the other collagen vascular diseases; they are eventually seen in 50 to 70% of patients.[11] Regarding the pleura, patients usually present clinically with unilateral pleurisy. Most, but not all, have concomitant small to moderate-sized effusions that usually respond well to steroids or cytotoxic drugs such as azathioprine. Another frequent cause of pleural effusions is hypoproteinemia secondary to lupus nephrosis. These effusions are transudates, are not associated with pain, are often large, and do not respond to the aforementioned treatment. They regress with treatment of the renal disease.

Although statistics vary from study to study, most agree that the majority of pulmonary parenchymal abnormalities found in patients with SLE are due to causes other than lupus involvement of the lung itself (lupus pneumonitis) **(Option (B) is, therefore, true).**[1,10-12,21] Diminished

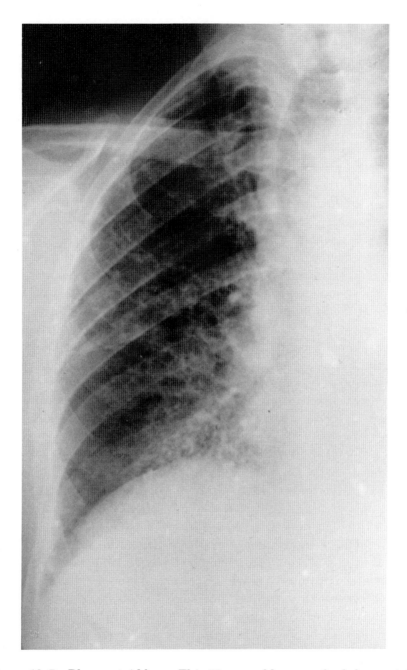

Figure 12-7. Rheumatoid lung. This 52-year-old woman had rheumatoid arthritis for over 20 years, and lung disease had been present for several years. This detailed view of the right lung was taken during the quiescent phase of her arthritis and respiratory symptoms. Note the elevated diaphragm, the diffuse interstitial pattern with some areas suggesting honeycombing, and the predominant basilar location of the parenchymal abnormality.

diaphragmatic excursion is common in SLE and is due to either splinting from pleurisy or diaphragmatic dysfunction. Therefore, the most frequent parenchymal abnormalities are basilar atelectasis and diminished lung volumes. Pulmonary infection (bacterial, fungal, and mycobacterial) is the next most frequent parenchymal finding. Both the SLE itself and many of the drugs used to treat the disease alter host immunity, promoting a situation conducive to the development of infection. *Nocardia* is the organism most often responsible for opportunistic infection. In lupus patients with cavitary lung lesions, infection and pulmonary infarction are the most likely etiologies. Local vasculitis leading to nodule and cavity formation is much less common.[26] Pulmonary edema, another abnormality in SLE, is most often attributable to congestive heart failure, renal failure, or aspiration pneumonitis. Additionally, most cases of acute pulmonary hemorrhage are attributable to infection, heart failure, uremia, or aspiration.[5]

It is estimated that between 2 and 18% of pulmonary lesions are not easily explainable on the basis of concomitant disease. The diagnosis of any of the lesions discussed below requires, at a minimum, the exclusion of the secondary diseases discussed above. Lupus pneumonitis, seen in a small percentage of patients, is usually a severe, acute illness with major systemic and respiratory symptoms.[5] The radiograph usually shows unilateral or bilateral acute alveolar opacities with or without pleural effusion. Histologically, there is a combination of vasculitis, hemorrhage, and edema. Pulmonary nodules, acute hemorrhage, and progressive pulmonary hypertension are only occasionally due to vasculitis. Basilar interstitial fibrosis, as a primary manifestation of SLE, is a controversial entity. If it in fact does occur, it is definitely much less common than the interstitial fibrosis associated with other collagen vascular diseases.

It has been estimated that approximately 10% of all cases of SLE are drug induced **(Option (C) is true).**[8] The drug-induced disease is similar, but not necessarily identical, to disease that is unrelated to drugs. Arthralgia and arthritis are present in 90% of patients, and pleuropulmonary disease is present in approximately 30%. As with non-drug-induced SLE, serositis and atelectasis are the most common radiographic manifestations. Pneumonitis and interstitial lung disease are less common. Radiographic findings in drug-induced SLE are indistinguishable from those in the non-drug-induced disease (Figure 12-8). In the drug-induced disease, however, renal and central nervous system involvement are much less common. Moreover, affected patients are older and almost exclusively Caucasian.

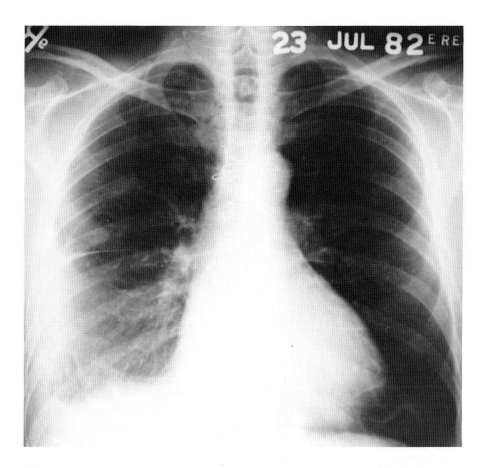

Figure 12-8. Drug-induced systemic lupus erythematosus. This 52-year-old man had a previous coronary artery bypass and aneurysmectomy. The patient was being treated with procainamide (Pronestyl) for persistent ventricular arrhythmias. After 6 months of treatment, he developed dyspnea, malaise, pleuritic chest pain, and anorexia over a 2-to 3-week period. Arthralgias were also present without arthritis. His chest radiograph shows cardiomegaly (unchanged from prior radiographs), a large right effusion, and blunting of the left costophrenic angle (not shown on this study). The pleural effusion was a clear nonbloody exudate with 1,800 leukocytes per μL (88% of which were polymorphonuclear cells) and a markedly elevated antinuclear antibody level. Serum tests for lupus were likewise positive. A diagnosis of drug-induced lupus was made. After the drug was discontinued, the patient's symptoms gradually improved. Amiodarone was substituted for Pronestyl, and the patient developed amiodarone pneumonitis several months later (not shown).

Table 12-1 lists the drugs that may induce SLE.[8] Hydralazine, procainamide, diphenylhydantoin, chlorpromazine, and isoniazid are unique because a large percentage of patients taking these drugs develop antinuclear antibodies, but only a small percentage develop SLE. The other drugs listed rarely induce antinuclear antibodies, and SLE is an uncommon sequela as well. Almost all patients with drug-induced SLE have antinuclear antibodies demonstrated by immunofluorescence, and 75% have positive lupus preparations. A smaller percentage have a positive Coombs test, positive rheumatoid factor, positive Wasserman test, and cryoglobulinemia. Antibodies to double-stranded DNA are rare in cases of drug-induced lupus and common in cases of non-drug-induced lupus. Cessation of the drug and treatment with aspirin or nonsteroidal anti-inflammatory agents are usually associated with resolution of symptoms and radiographic findings within several weeks. Steroids are rarely required. However, serum markers for SLE often persist for years after withdrawal of the drug.

In contrast to SLE, in cases of scleroderma primary pulmonary lung involvement is very common and of major clinical importance. In its late stages, the interstitial fibrosis of scleroderma is histologically indistinguishable from Hamman-Rich pulmonary fibrosis. In addition to, or instead of, the interstitial fibrosis there may be a primary vasculitis in the lungs.

Although basilar fibrosis is almost universally present at autopsy and the majority of patients show evidence of restrictive lung disease in pulmonary function tests, the clinical and radiographic evidence of disease often lags behind the functional abnormality. The chest radiograph, when positive, usually demonstrates a fine reticular pattern in the lower lung zones **(Option (D) is false)**, a pattern that often becomes progressively coarser with time. Progressive volume loss may develop, and small cysts may appear (Figures 12-9 to 12-12). A dilated esophagus may also be seen. Pleural disease is uncommon. In patients with predominant vasculitis, there may be evidence of progressive pulmonary arterial hypertension with or without other radiographic evidence of lung disease. Additional problems include the increased incidence of aspiration pneumonia and malignancy (adenocarcinoma and bronchioloalveolar cell carcinoma) associated with long-standing pulmonary fibrosis (Figures 12-10 through 12-12).

Polymyositis is a diffuse muscle disease affecting mainly the striated muscles of the limbs, the limb girdles, the neck, and the pharynx.[3,4,20] When characteristic skin lesions (dusky, red patches) are present, the disease is termed dermatomyositis. The respiratory complications for

Table 12-1. Drugs that may induce systemic lupus erythematosus*

1. Antiarrhythmic drugs	5. Antituberculous drugs
Practotol	Isoniazid†
Procainamide†	Para-aminosalicylic acid
Quinidine	Streptomycin
2. Antibiotics	6. Phenothiazines
Griseofulvin	Chlorpromazine†
Nitrofurantoin	Levomepromazine
Penicillin	Perazine
Sulfonamides	Perphenazine
Tetracycline	Promethazine
	Thioridazine
3. Anticonvulsant drugs	
Carbamazepine	7. Miscellaneous
Diphenylhydantoin†	Amoproxan
Ethosuximide	Anthiomaline
Mephenytoin	D-Penicillamine
Phenylethylacetylurea	Methysergide
Primidone	Methylthiouracil
Trimethadione	Oral contraceptives
Phenylbutazone	Oxyphenisatin
	Propylthiouracil
4. Antihypertensive drugs	Tolazamide
Guanoxan	
Hydralazine†	
L-Dopa	
Methyldopa	

*Reprinted with permission from Ginsburg WW [8].
†Drugs that elicit antinuclear antibodies in a large percentage of individuals using the drug.

both are similar. Frank respiratory failure due to diaphragmatic weakness is present in only 4 to 8% of patients **(Option (E) is false).** Such failure is usually found with well-established disease and usually associated with severe generalized muscle weakness and pharyngeal dysfunction. Since the striated muscles of the soft palate, pharynx, and the upper esophagus are often involved, the symptoms of dysphagia, nasal regurgitation, and aspiration occur frequently. Patchy opacities in gravity-dependent pulmonary segments are most often due to aspiration. Diffuse interstitial lung disease similar to that described for scleroderma is present in approximately 5% of patients (Figure 12-9). Clinically, patients may follow a rapidly progressive fatal course or be asymptomatic. Pleural disease and pulmonary arterial hypertension are rare, and infection is uncommon unless the patient is being treated with steroids

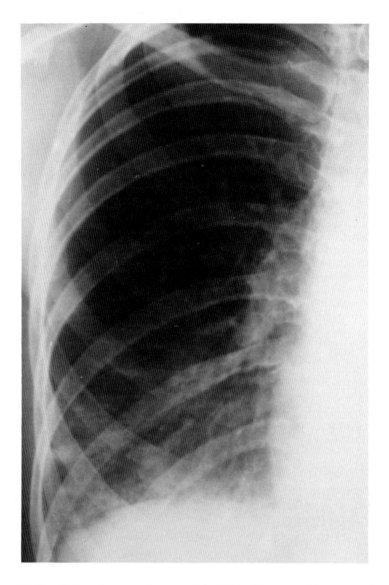

Figure 12-9. Scleroderma-polymyositis. This 34-year-old woman had a 1-month history of cough, fever, and hemoptysis initially thought to be due to infection. She did not respond to antibiotics. A view of the right lung shows basilar atelectasis. Interstitial disease was also suspected. The process progressed, and an open-lung biopsy, followed by muscle and skin biopsies, showed characteristics of both scleroderma and polymyositis. The patient was treated with steroids. Six weeks later, the symptoms completely resolved, and the radiograph appeared to be essentially normal.

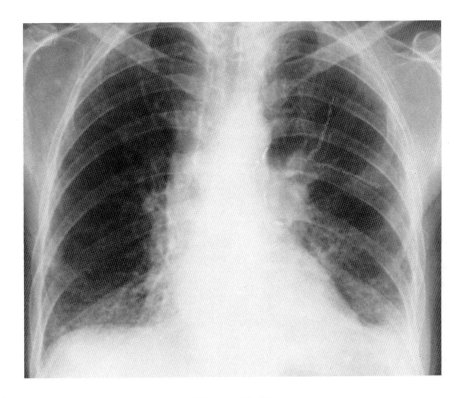

Figure 12-10
Figures 12-10 through 12-12. Scleroderma and lung cancer. This 59-year-old woman had a long history of arthritis and a history of mild dyspnea for several years. A prior chest radiograph showed bibasilar fibrosis and a left hilar mass. Thoracotomy revealed an unresectable adenocarcinoma. The radiograph shown in Figure 12-10 was obtained 2 weeks after surgery. The left hilar mass is still visible, along with a fine bibasilar pattern suggesting fibrosis. A CT scan (Figure 12-11) slightly below the carina shows a large mass behind the left pulmonary artery. A CT scan (Figure 12-12) at a lower level shows the bibasilar pattern consistent with fibrosis.

or cytotoxic drugs. Lung cancer due to pulmonary fibrosis does not appear to be a major problem.

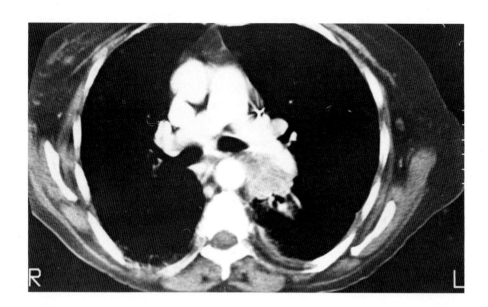

Figure 12-11

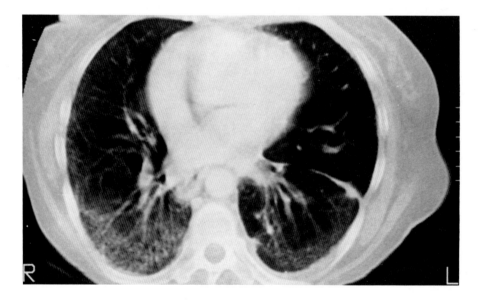

Figure 12-12

Questions 63 through 67

For each of the drugs listed below (Questions 63 through 67), select the *one* lettered side effect (A, B, C, D, or E) MOST closely associated with it. Each side effect may be used once, more than once, or not at all.

63. Nitrofurantoin (Furadantin)
64. Methysergide
65. Sulfonamides
66. Methadone
67. Adriamycin

    (A) Acute pneumonitis or chronic fibrosis
    (B) Pleural fibrosis
    (C) Cardiac toxicity
    (D) Noncardiac edema
    (E) Loeffler-type pneumonitis

Intrathoracic side effects associated with drug therapy are numerous. However, a working knowledge of certain frequently prescribed drugs or drugs with unique toxicities is useful. Some of these drugs are discussed below.[17-19,22,27]

Nitrofurantoin (Furadantin) is a bacteriostatic drug used most often for acute or chronic urinary tract infections. Maintenance therapy may be given for months or years. The most serious side effects are hypersensitivity reactions involving the skin, blood vessels, liver, and lung. Although pulmonary toxicity is not common, this drug is so widely used that it is one of the most frequent causes of drug-induced pulmonary disease.[16,17] It is somewhat unique in that it may either produce an acute hypersensitivity pneumonitis within hours or days of initiation of therapy or cause slowly progressive chronic pulmonary fibrosis with prolonged medication use **(Option (A) is the correct answer to Question 63).** With the acute disease, there is rapid onset of fever, chills, dyspnea, and chest pain. Peripheral eosinophilia is present in approximately 20 to 30% of cases. The radiograph usually shows a diffuse interstitial pattern, more severe at the bases. Pleural effusions are rare. Severe involvement may result in patchy, alveolar opacities as well (Figure 12-13). Cessation of the drug usually leads to rapid clinical and radiographic resolution. Residual lung damage from the acute pneumonitis is unusual. A lupus-like reaction is rarely seen with Furadantin administration.

A less frequent but potentially more serious side effect of Furadantin is chronic interstitial fibrosis complicating long-term use of the drug. This does not appear to be the end-stage of the acute disease but rather

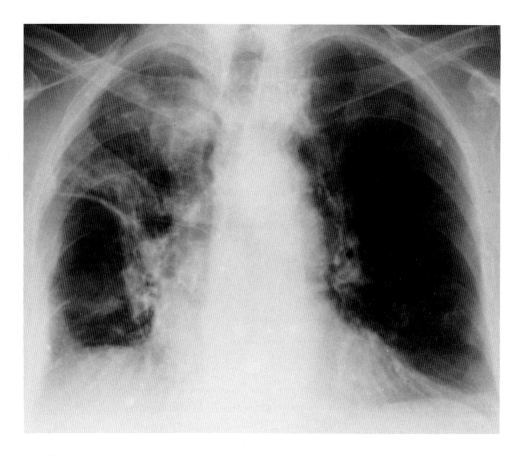

Figure 12-13. Nitrofurantoin pneumonitis. This 78-year-old woman had been using Furadantin for 2 years for recurrent urinary tract infections. She had experienced mild fatigue, mild anterior chest pain, and a nonproductive cough over the last month. The chest radiograph shows an elevated right hemidiaphragm (unchanged since her right nephrectomy 2 years earlier). Several areas of patchy alveolar opacities with mild volume loss are present in the right upper lobe. Similar but smaller patchy areas are present in the right lung base, with a few in the left lung. Her work-up resulted in a diagnosis of Furadantin pneumonitis. The drug was discontinued, with gradual partial regression of the patient's symptoms and radiographic abnormalities.

appears to be a separate entity. There is an insidious onset of exertional dyspnea and nonproductive cough 6 months to several years after initiation of therapy. The erythrocyte sedimentation rate is often elevated, but the eosinophil count is usually normal. The radiographic pattern is one of interstitial disease and volume loss, predominantly at the bases. Cessation of the drug will lead to a diminution of symptoms and radiographic findings in the majority of patients.

Methysergide (Sansert) is an ergot derivative used for the control of migraine headaches. The most serious side effect is retroperitoneal fibrosis. A less common side effect is pleural fibrosis with or without evidence of retroperitoneal fibrosis **(Option (B) is the correct answer to Question 64).**[6] The pleural fibrosis may follow long-term drug-induced effusions or may be seen without prior effusions. Cough, fever, and dyspnea are usually insidious in onset. The radiograph shows free or loculated pleural effusions. Diffuse bilateral or unilateral pleural thickening may be present. Biopsy usually demonstrates fibrosis and inflammation. Cessation of the drug often leads to regression even when "fibrosis" is present. This drug may rarely produce fibrosis elsewhere (mediastinum, pericardium, cardiac valves, and lungs).

With the development of other antibiotics, the use of sulfonamides has diminished. However, the recent combination of trimethoprim and sulfamethoxazole (e.g., Bactrim and Septra) has resulted in a resurgence of sulfonamide therapy. Adverse reactions occur approximately 5% of the time and may involve the hematopoietic tissues, the urinary tract, or the liver. A hypersensitivity vasculitis may involve the lungs and the skin (e.g., Stevens-Johnson syndrome and Behcet's disease). A lupus-like reaction has also been reported. The majority of pulmonary reactions are acute or subacute and are characterized by coughing and shortness of breath. Fever, skin rash, and peripheral eosinophilia also occur. Radiographs usually show fleeting patchy alveolar opacities that are often peripherally located (Figure 12-14) **(Option (E) is the correct answer to Question 65).** Pleural effusions are uncommon. Many other drug reactions present with similar clinical and radiographic findings, with or without peripheral eosinophilia (penicillin, chlorpropamide, cromolyn sulfate, and methotrexate). The close temporal relationship between the initiation of drug therapy and lung involvement usually makes the diagnosis fairly straightforward.

Methadone hydrochloride, a synthetic narcotic, has pharmacologic properties similar to those of morphine.[23,28] Given orally, methadone hydrochloride will suppress symptoms associated with heroin withdrawal. Intravenous or oral overdose may lead to acute noncardiac pulmonary edema **(Option (D) is the correct answer to Question 66).** Clinically, patients present with depressed consciousness, constricted pupils, and respiratory distress with rales. Most are hypoxic and acidotic. Pulmonary edema is the predominant radiographic pattern, although symmetrical bilateral involvement is the exception. Rather, the most

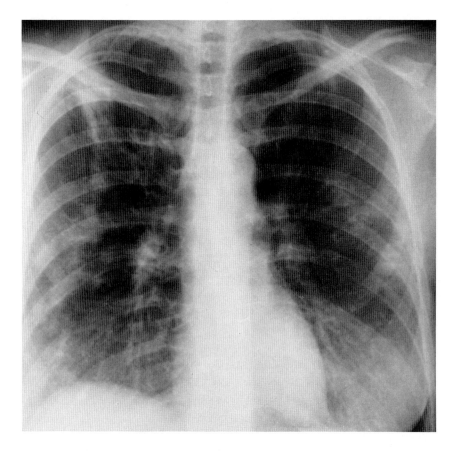

Figure 12-14. Sulfonamide pneumonitis. This 30-year-old asthmatic woman developed wheezing and dyspnea while receiving Bactrim (trimethoprim-sulfamethoxazole) for postoperative pelvic infection. The eosinophil counts ranged from 15 to 30%. The chest radiograph shows multiple ill-defined pulmonary opacities located predominantly peripherally. Symptoms, radiographic findings, and the eosinophil count returned to normal within 2 weeks after the discontinuance of the drug and the administration of steroids.

frequent appearance is that of patchy, asymmetrical, bilateral opacities. Unilateral or lobar disease is uncommon. In a small number of cases, the initial radiograph appears to be normal, with edema developing later. Narcotic antagonists will acutely diminish the symptoms, and radiographic resolution is usually visible within 24 to 72 hours.

Adriamycin (Doxorubicin) is a tumoricidal agent used to treat leukemia, lymphoma, and many solid tumors (such as breast carcinoma, small cell cancer of the lung, and sarcomas).[25] Cardiac toxicity, however, limits the total cumulative dose and thus the usefulness of this drug **(Option (C) is the correct answer to Question 67).** During the first few weeks of therapy, 10 to 25% of patients develop electrocardiographic abnormalities. A small percentage develop acute pericardial or myocardial inflammation, the latter at times causing severe myocardial dysfunction. However, it is the chronic myocardial damage that presents the major challenge to clinical management. The tumoricidal effects of the drug must be titrated against the potential damage to the heart. As a general rule, severe myocardial damage is rarely seen before a cumulative dose of 500 mg/m^2. It is estimated that less than 1% of patients receiving 500 mg/m^2 or less develop myocardial damage, whereas more than 30% of patients receiving greater than 600 mg/m^2 develop significant cardiac toxicity. Various tests have been proposed as indicators of cardiac damage before it becomes irreversible and permanently disabling. Radionuclide ventriculography and myocardial biopsy appear to be the two most definitive tests. When adriamycin cardiomyopathy is present, the clinical and radiographic presentation is one of increasing congestive heart failure and progressive cardiomegaly.

SUGGESTED READINGS

1. Carette S, Macher AM, Nussbaum A, Plotz PH. Severe, acute pulmonary disease in patients with systemic lupus erythematosus: ten years of experience at the National Institutes of Health. Semin Arthritis Rheum 1984; 14:52–59

2. Darmanata JI, van Zandwijk N, Düren DR, et al. Amiodarone pneumonitis: three further cases with a review of published reports. Thorax 1984; 39:57–64

3. Dickey BF, Myers AR. Pulmonary disease in polymyositis/dermatomyositis. Semin Arthritis Rheum 1984; 14:60–76

4. Frazier AR, Miller RD. Interstitial pneumonitis in association with polymyositis and dermatomyositis. Chest 1974; 65:403–407

5. Gamsu G, Webb WR. Pulmonary hemorrhage in systemic lupus erythematosus. J Can Assoc Radiol 1978; 29:66–68

6. Gefter WB, Epstein DM, Bonavita JA, Miller WT. Pleural thickening caused by Sansert and Ergotrate in the treatment of migraine. AJR 1980; 135:375–377

7. Gefter WB, Epstein DM, Pietra GG, Miller WT. Lung disease caused by amiodarone, a new antiarrhythmic agent. Radiology 1983; 147:339–344

8. Ginsburg WW. Drug-induced systemic lupus erythematosus. Semin Respir Med 1980; 2:51–58

9. Goldman IS, Winkler ML, Raper SE, et al. Increased hepatic density and phospholipidosis due to amiodarone. AJR 1985; 144:541–546
10. Haupt HM, Moore GW, Hutchins GM. The lung in systemic lupus erythematosus. Analysis of the pathologic changes in 120 patients. Am J Med 1981; 71:791–798
11. Hunninghake GW, Fauci AS. Pulmonary involvement in the collagen vascular diseases. Am Rev Respir Dis 1979; 119:471–503
12. Levin DC. Proper interpretation of pulmonary roentgen changes in systemic lupus erythematosus. AJR 1971; 111:510–517
13. Macfarlane JD, Dieppe PA, Rigden BG, Clark TJ. Pulmonary and pleural lesions in rheumatoid disease. Br J Dis Chest 1978; 72:288–300
14. Marchlinski FE, Gansler TS, Waxman HL, Josephson ME. Amiodarone pulmonary toxicity. Ann Intern Med 1982; 97:839–845
15. Olson LK, Forrest JV, Friedman PJ, Kiser PE, Henschke CI. Pneumonitis after amiodarone therapy. Radiology 1984; 150:327–330
16. Prakash UBS. Pulmonary reaction to nitrofurantoin. Semin Respir Med 1980; 2:70–75
17. Rosenow EC III. The spectrum of drug-induced pulmonary disease. Ann Intern Med 1972; 77:977–991
18. Rosenow EC III. Miscellaneous drug-induced pulmonary disease. Semin Respir Med 1980; 2:76–88
19. Rosenow EC III. Chemotherapeutic drug-induced pulmonary disease. Semin Respir Med 1980; 2:89–96
20. Schwarz MI, Matthay RA, Sahn SA, Stanford RE, Marmorstein BL, Scheinhorn DJ. Interstitial lung disease in polymyositis and dermatomyositis: analysis of six cases and review of the literature. Medicine 1976; 55:89–104
21. Segal AM, Calabrese LH, Ahmad M, Tubbs RR, White CS. The pulmonary manifestations of systemic lupus erythematosus. Semin Arthritis Rheum 1985; 14:202–224
22. Seltzer SE, Goldstein JD, Herman PJ. Iatrogenic thoracic complications induced by drugs. In: Herman PG (ed), Iatrogenic thoracic complications. Radiology of iatrogenic disorders. New York: Springer-Verlag; 1983
23. Stern WZ, Subbarao K. Pulmonary complications of drug addiction. Semin Roentgenol 1983; 18:183–197
24. Suárez LD, Poderoso JJ, Elsner B, Bunster AM, Esteva H, Bellotti M. Subacute pneumopathy during amiodarone therapy. Chest 1983; 83:566–568
25. Unverferth DV, Magorien RD, Leier CV, Balcerzak SP. Doxorubicin cardiotoxicity. Cancer Treat Rev 1982; 9:149–164
26. Webb WR, Gamsu G. Cavitary pulmonary nodules with systemic lupus erythematosus: differential diagnosis. AJR 1981; 136:27–31
27. Weiss RB, Muggia FM. Cytotoxic drug-induced pulmonary disease: update 1980. Am J Med 1980; 68:259–266
28. Wilen SB, Ulreich S, Rabinowitz JG. Roentgenographic manifestations of methadone-induced pulmonary edema. Radiology 1975; 114:51–55

Notes

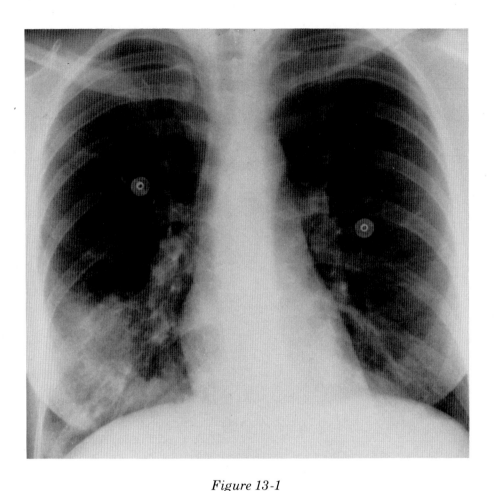

Figure 13-1

Figures 13-1 and 13-2. This otherwise healthy 38-year-old woman presented with a 10-day history of productive cough (watery sputum) and a 3-day history of chills, fever, nausea, vomiting, and diarrhea. Her temperature was 40.4°C, her respiratory rate was 20/minute, and her leukocyte count was 5,200/µL (84% segmented neutrophils, 2% bands, and 14% lymphocytes). There was no growth on routine sputum cultures or blood cultures. You are shown posteroanterior and lateral chest radiographs.

Case 13: Legionnaires' Disease

Question 68

Considering the history and radiographic findings, which *one* of the following is the MOST likely diagnosis?

    (A) Legionnaires' disease
    (B) *Pneumocystis carinii* pneumonia
    (C) Blastomycosis
    (D) Pneumococcal pneumonia
    (E) Primary tuberculosis

The history suggests an acute pneumonia in an otherwise healthy 38-year-old woman. The infection caused a mild lower respiratory illness for a few days followed by severe systemic symptoms (high fever and chills) and gastrointestinal symptoms (nausea, vomiting, and diarrhea). The leukocyte count was essentially normal except for an increased percentage of segmented neutrophils, and sputum and blood cultures were negative. The admission radiographic examination (Figures 13-1 and 13-2) demonstrated focal air-space disease in the right and left lower lobes, without associated pleural effusion. Although radiographic findings do not substitute for a culture-proven diagnosis, they often figure prominently, along with clinical clues, in the early decision process before culture results are available.

Pneumocystis carinii pneumonia (Option (B)), seen almost exclusively in debilitated newborns and in patients who are immunocompromised, is not likely in this patient, who is otherwise healthy. However, some of the clinical features of the acute respiratory illness seen in this case are similar to those seen with pneumocystis pneumonia in an immunocompromised patient. The majority of pneumocystis pneumonias are acute in onset, although mild symptoms may be present for weeks before the clinical "flare." The most frequent symptoms include fever, nonproductive cough, dyspnea, and chest pain. Gastrointestinal symptoms are infrequent, as are rales. The leukocyte count is often normal, and sputum cultures are usually negative. In the vast majority of patients, the chest

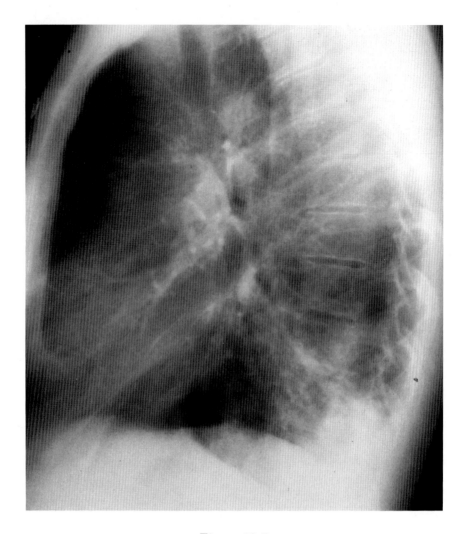

Figure 13-2

radiograph shows *diffuse* bilateral interstitial or air-space disease, unlike the pattern seen in this test case. The process often progresses rapidly and may spare the periphery of the lung. Uncommon appearances include patchy focal or lobar disease, cavitation, unilateral disease, pleural effusion, and extra-alveolar air.[17,28] Adenopathy is not a feature of pneumocystis pneumonia but may be present because of an underlying disease.[28]

The clinical presentation of an acute pneumonia with focal lower lobe air-space disease makes the diagnosis of blastomycosis (Option (C)) unlikely. Blastomycosis of the lung is usually a subacute or chronic illness, and the chest radiographic appearance, which is very variable, is most often that of a slowly progressive, nonsegmental, focal air-space process. The upper lobes are most often involved. Adenopathy and cavitation may occasionally be seen; however, in an older person, these findings more often suggest a malignant process.[6,20]

Blastomycosis is caused by *Blastomyces dermatitidis*, a dimorphic fungus seen most frequently in the central and southern United States, although it also occurs elsewhere (especially in Central America and South America as well as in Africa). It is an airborne infection from a soil reservoir. The vast majority of affected patients are men. Early symptoms of the disease include malaise, cough, and low-grade fever. Within weeks to months, the symptoms increase, as does the production of sputum, which may become blood-streaked. Dissemination is frequent and causes mucocutaneous abscesses, skin ulcerations, osteomyelitis, and urogenital disease (infection of the prostate, epididymis, and seminal vesicles).

Primary tuberculosis (Option (E)) may occur in an adult as a moderately acute pneumonia from which an organism is not recovered by routine staining or cultures. However, the onset is seldom so rapid with high fevers and abdominal symptoms as in the test patient. Although the leukocyte count may be normal, there is often mild leukocytosis, with elevation of the lymphocyte count. Bilateral lower lobe disease is uncommon. Primary tuberculosis is, therefore, unlikely.

The two best diagnostic choices among those offered are pneumococcal pneumonia (Option (D)) and Legionnaires' disease (Option (A)), but the distinction between them is difficult to make both clinically and radiographically. Both are acute pneumonias with overlapping clinical and radiographic findings. When the patient is first seen, clinical decisions must be made on incomplete evidence. In this case, however, the combination of clinical, laboratory, and radiographic findings is more suggestive of Legionnaires' disease than of pneumococcal pneumonia, as explained in the following paragraphs.

The test patient is an otherwise healthy 38-year-old woman with a mild 7-day prodrome. Although pneumococcal pneumonia is probably the most frequent community-acquired bacterial pneumonia, it is usually seen at the extremes of life (<5 years and >60 years of age) unless there is an underlying systemic problem (alcoholism, chronic heart disease, etc.).[13,24] Legionnaires' disease has a broader distribution in the community and probably accounts for a much larger percentage of pneumonias than previously believed.[4,16,18] Pneumococcal pneumonia is more likely to have a very explosive onset and follow a bout of coryza, whereas Legionnaires' disease is usually more gradual in onset, frequently with a prodrome of a nonproductive or watery cough (as in our test patient) and marked systemic symptoms (weakness, malaise, and anorexia) prior to the onset of the acute pneumonia. Pneumococcal pneumonia usually has a rapid onset of high fever, a *single* shaking chill, and pleurisy. Within hours, severe dyspnea and tachycardia are often present, as is purulent sputum (often bloody). With Legionnaires' disease, despite the high fever and *recurrent* chills, dyspnea and tachycardia are usually not as striking. In fact, many patients have a relative bradycardia (pulse of <100/minute, and fever of >40°C). Only a minority of patients develop purulent sputum or hemoptysis.

Upper abdominal symptoms are common with both infections, but watery diarrhea (as in our test patient) is a frequent finding in Legionnaires' disease. Disorientation, confusion, and other central nervous system symptoms are present in approximately one-third of patients hospitalized with Legionnaires' disease. With pneumococcal pneumonia, the leukocyte count is markedly elevated, with a shift to the left in all but the most debilitated or severely immunocompromised patients. In Legionnaires' disease, the leukocyte count is often normal; however, if leukocytosis is present, it is usually mild, with only one-half of the patients showing a shift to the left. In view of the foregoing, pneumococcal pneumonia is less likely than Legionnaires' disease; **thus Option (A) is the most likely diagnosis.**

Routine examination of the sputum may be helpful in documenting pneumococcal pneumonia, but less so for Legionnaires' disease. Interestingly, *Streptococcus pneumoniae* is frequently found in the sputum of normal patients but may be absent on smears and cultures in up to one-third of patients with proven pneumococcal disease. Approximately 25% of patients with pneumococcal pneumonia have positive blood cultures. Therefore, although the majority of patients have positive sputum or blood cultures, a significant minority have neither and must be treated on clinical grounds. With Legionnaires' disease, the Gram stain of the sputum may be a clue because of the paucity of leukocytes and lack of predominant organisms. *Legionella pneumophila* has staining properties similar to those of other gram-negative upper respiratory tract flora. The organism does not grow on routine cultures but may now be grown with special culture techniques. Rapid diagnosis is possible by direct immunofluorescence examination of the sputum and/or immunoassay of body fluids.

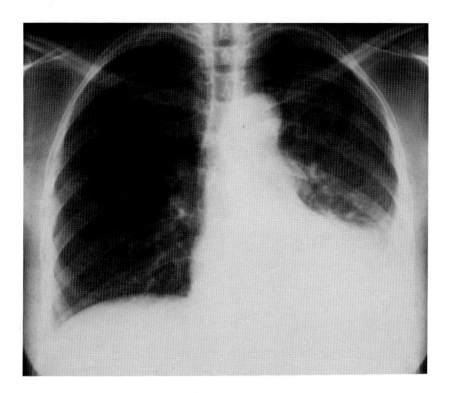

Figure 13-3. Pneumococcal pneumonia. This 54-year-old woman had a 2-day history of cough and malaise, followed by a shaking chill and rapidly rising temperature. Her radiograph, taken 24 hours after admission, shows dense consolidation of the left lower lobe, with little or no volume loss, and a moderate left pleural effusion that regressed as the pneumonia resolved. In the vast majority of pneumococcal pneumonias, the pleural effusion is a parapneumonic one that is not infected.

S. pneumoniae is usually aspirated into the lungs from the upper airway and often reaches gravity-dependent segments. The initial infection is peripheral and spreads to adjacent alveoli via the pores of Kohn. Thus, the chest radiograph shows dense air-space consolidation with air bronchograms and little or no volume loss. The process may spread from segment to segment but usually does not cross the fissures. In most instances, the disease is confined to a lobe, but the entire lobe is not consolidated (Figure 13-3). Multiple lobes are involved in one-third of patients.[6,8,12,13,29] A review of radiographs of hospitalized patients suggested that patchy bronchopneumonia or interstitial disease may be as likely as lobar consolidation with pneumococcal pneumonia.[13] It is probable that this changing pattern is due, at least in part, to earlier

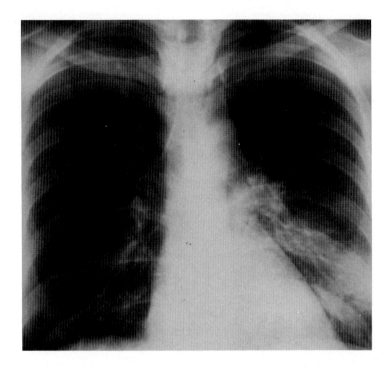

Figure 13-4. Legionnaires' disease. This is the husband of the test patient presented in Figures 13-1 and 13-2. He had a 3-day history of malaise, myalgias, and fever of 39.4°C, followed 2 days later by vomiting, cough productive of brownish sputum, pleuritic chest pain, chills, and headache. The leukocyte count was 7,000/μL, with 26% bands. His chest radiograph, taken on admission 5 days after the onset of symptoms, shows moderate air-space consolidation of the left lower lobe. Organisms were identified by the immunofluorescence technique.

diagnosis of the disease and the presence of emphysema or underlying cardiopulmonary disease in many of the patients.[29] In our test patient, large focal areas of lower lobe consolidation are certainly consistent with a diagnosis of pneumococcal pneumonia.

Radiographically, Legionnaires' disease usually shows progressive multilobar consolidation. Our test patient had *L. pneumophila* confirmed by a marked rise in serum antibody titers measured by the indirect immunofluorescence technique. Shortly after her hospitalization, her husband presented with similar signs and symptoms and the radiographic appearance shown in Figure 13-4. Both received and responded to erythromycin therapy.

Question 69

Concerning the radiographic appearance of Legionnaires' disease,

(A) at presentation, patchy or confluent lower lobe air-space disease is most frequent
(B) with time, the disease progresses to multilobar involvement in most patients
(C) progression to lobar consolidation occurs in under 10% of patients
(D) cavitation occurs in under 10% of nonimmunocompromised patients
(E) pleural effusion is present in one-third to one-half of the cases
(F) hilar or mediastinal adenopathy is present in about one-half of the cases

Although there is no radiographic appearance pathognomonic of Legionnaires' disease, certain features may help in suggesting the diagnosis. Numerous investigators describe slightly different radiographic patterns and slightly different frequencies of occurrence of these patterns. However, the general consensus is that of a predominantly patchy or confluent air-space process that usually begins in the lower lobes **(Option (A) is true)**. Typically, a portion of the lower lobe is initially involved, with subsequent progression to segmental or lobar consolidation **(Option (C) is false)**. With this progression, other lobes become involved, most often with patchy air-space disease **(Option (B) is true)**. At the peak of the disease, the typical patient has dense consolidation of the lower lobe initially involved, air bronchograms and volume loss in this lobe, and patchy air-space involvement of other lobes. Consolidation may involve lobes other than the lower lobes (Figures 13-5 through 13-7). Pleural effusion first appears during the height of the illness in 30 to 50% of cases **(Option (E) is true)**. Hilar or mediastinal adenopathy is seen in less than 5% of cases **(Option (F) is false)**.

Several investigators have noted that the disease often progresses to dense consolidation during the first week in spite of early initiation of erythromycin therapy. Despite the apparent radiographic worsening with treatment, continued erythromycin therapy usually results in clinical and radiographic resolution. Several series indicate that complete clearing may take several months. Most other bacterial pneumonias usually clear more rapidly.

The foregoing generalities are based on series of both community-acquired disease and disease in hospitalized and immunocompromised patients.[5,15,16,18] A study in renal transplant patients indicated that cavitation, which is uncommon in the normal host, may be more frequent in immunocompromised patients[22] **(Option (D) is true)**.

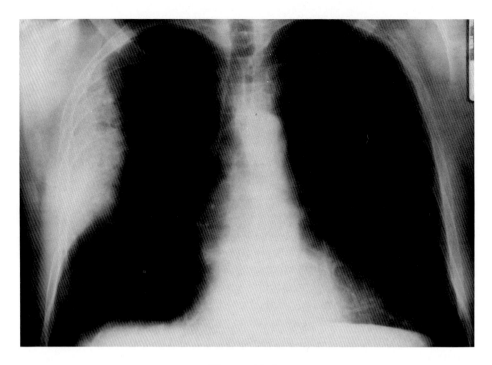

Figure 13-5

Figures 13-5 through 13-7. Legionnaires' disease. This 60-year-old man had a 2-day history of malaise, anorexia, fever, and chills and a 1-day history of dyspnea and diarrhea. His temperature was 40°C, and he had left lung basilar rales and a leukocyte count of 15,300/μL, with 22% bands. The admission chest radiograph (Figure 13-5) shows very dense peripheral consolidation in the right upper lobe. Three days later (Figure 13-6), the entire right upper lobe was consolidated. Five days later (Figure 13-7), the dense consolidation was located centrally, and there was mild volume loss. The central area required several weeks to clear completely.

Another recently described pneumonia is that caused by the Pittsburgh pneumonia agent (*Legionella micdadei*).[23] This pneumonia is also both a sporadic community-acquired infection and an opportunistic hospital-acquired infection. Again, the initial presentation is one of a unilobar disease most often in one of the lower lobes (Figure 13-8). Unlike Legionnaires' disease, Pittsburgh pneumonia usually remains confined to its initial site. Small effusions are seen in one-third of cases, and cavitation is rare. Complete clearing may take a few months. When patients are infected with both *L. pneumophila* and *L. micdadei*, the pneumonia is unusually severe.

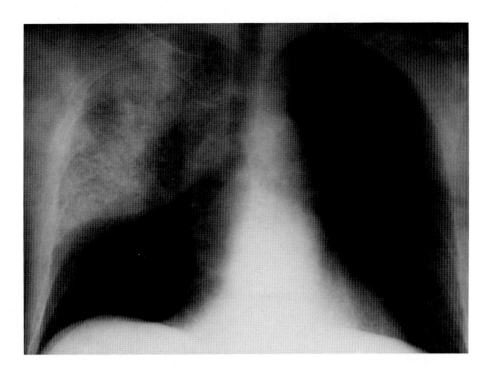

Figure 13-6

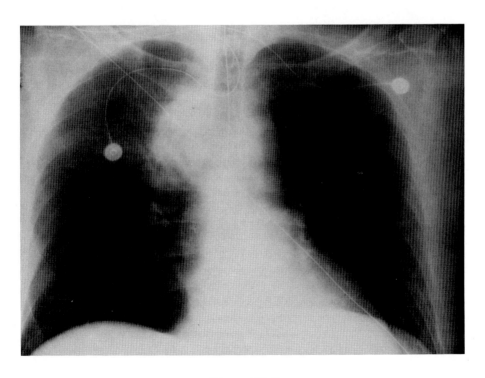

Figure 13-7

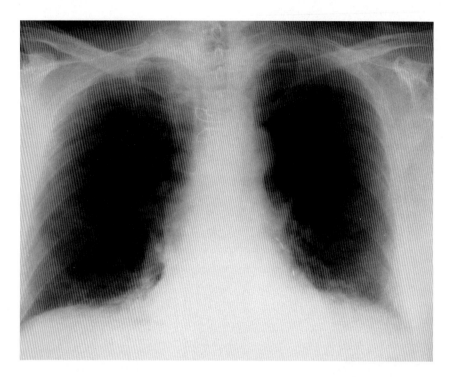

Figure 13-8. Pittsburgh pneumonia. This patient with poorly differentiated lymphocytic lymphoma and chronic obstructive pulmonary disease developed fever, cough, and hypoxia. Rales were heard at the lung bases. The chest radiograph shows patchy, ill-defined opacities in both lower lobes, with possible left pleural effusion. *L. micdadei* was isolated from the patient's sputum. Treatment with erythromycin led to a rapid recovery.

Question 70

Concerning primary tuberculosis,

    (A) adenopathy is more frequent than in postprimary tuberculosis
    (B) the predominant location is in the apical or apical posterior segments of the upper lobes
    (C) the majority of effusions are empyemas
    (D) the Ghon focus is a residuum
    (E) it is rarely seen after 15 years of age

Over the last three decades, there has been an 80% drop in the frequency of tuberculosis in the United States.[2,7,9,14,21,26] As a result of this dramatic decline, the number of people exposed to tuberculosis during childhood has also decreased. In Philadelphia in 1948, 16.4% of teenagers had a positive tuberculin skin test, whereas in 1968 only 1.4% did. The vast majority of the U.S. population, therefore, is now entering adulthood without prior sensitization.

A large proportion of new cases of tuberculosis in young and middle-aged adults are primary tuberculosis **(Option (E) is false)**. The diagnosis of primary tuberculosis is more difficult than that of postprimary (reinfection) tuberculosis because both the clinical and radiographic presentations are less characteristic for primary tuberculosis than for postprimary tuberculosis. Many of the "atypical" appearances seen in adults simply represent primary disease in the adult. The radiologist must be aware of this changing appearance.

In the majority of patients, the initial exposure to tuberculosis results in the rapid development of cell-mediated immunity, with little or no clinical disease. Within the first few weeks, the organisms are engulfed by phagocytosis. Caseous necrosis develops, and healing then begins. The only residua of that initial encounter are a positive skin test and a Ghon lesion (calcified or noncalcified parenchymal scar) **(Option (D) is true)**. The Ranke complex (Ghon lesion and calcified hilar or paratracheal node) is visible in approximately one-third of patients with a positive skin test.

When untreated, approximately 5 to 15% of people with converted skin tests develop active primary tuberculosis within 5 years. Another 5% develop active disease beyond 5 years. Active primary disease in the adult is similar in most respects to active primary disease in children, but the radiographic appearance may vary. In children, unilateral or asymmetrical hilar and mediastinal adenopathy are almost universally present. Hilar and mediastinal adenopathy are present in only 10 to 20% of adults with primary tuberculosis. As in children, the adenopathy is

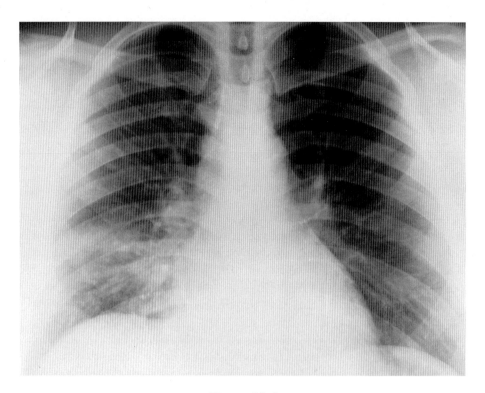

Figure 13-9
Figures 13-9 through 13-11. Primary tuberculosis. This 32-year-old woman presented with cough, hemoptysis, malaise, and weakness lasting for several weeks. The cough was minimally productive and nonpurulent. Figures 13-9 and 13-10 show middle-lobe consolidation. The hilum is slighly prominent, but no definite enlarged nodes are visible. A tomogram (Figure 13-11) shows hilar enlargement on the right and left, with an enlarged azygos node as well. At bronchoscopy the right middle-lobe bronchus was narrowed by extrinsic pressure and had a friable mucosa. Biopsy yielded tuberculosis on both smear and culture.

often asymmetrical or unilaterally located on the side of the parenchymal disease (Figures 13-9 to 13-12). In contrast, adenopathy is typically absent in postprimary tuberculosis, so that **Option (A) is true.**[3,11]

In primary tuberculosis, whether in children or adults, the parenchymal disease tends to appear as focal, homogeneous, air-space consolidation with ill-defined margins. Cavitation is uncommon. Unlike postprimary tuberculosis, there is no characteristic segmental or lobar distribution in primary tuberculosis, which may be multilobar and bilaterally located (Figure 13-13) **(Option (B) is false).** With postprimary tuberculosis, the majority of the parenchymal abnormality is found in

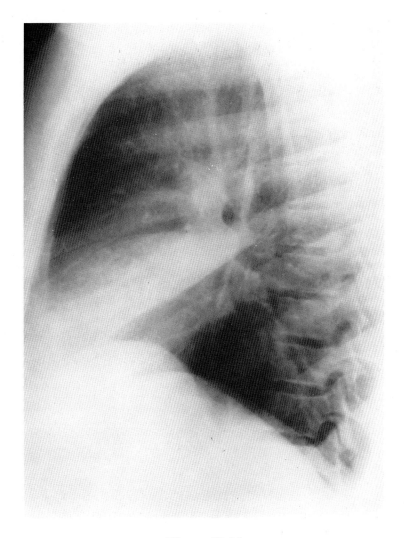

Figure 13-10

the apical or posterior segments of the upper lobe or the superior segment
of the lower lobe.

Another frequently encountered abnormality in primary tuberculosis
is pleural effusion, which is seen more often in adults than in children
(Figure 13-14). Ipsilateral parenchymal disease is visible in only
one-third of patients, and the skin test may be initially negative in as
many as one-third of patients. The pleural effusion, which may be
asymptomatic or associated with an acute febrile illness, is an exudate
high in polymorphonuclear leukocytes during the initial 2 weeks of its

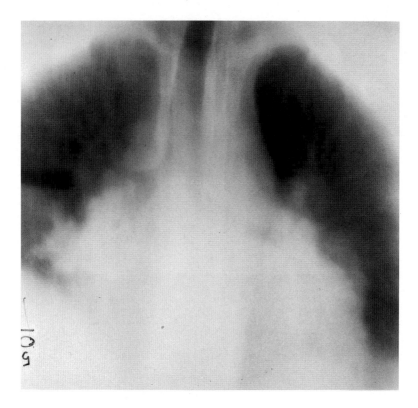

Figure 13-11

presence and high in small lymphocytes subsequently. Pleural fluid glucose concentration and pH have not proved to be reliable clues to the diagnosis. Stains of the pleural fluid seldom show organisms, and cultures are positive in less than 25% of patients **(Option (C) is false).** A needle biopsy of the pleura is often required for diagnosis. Great emphasis is placed on diagnosis and treatment at an early stage of pleural involvement, since two-thirds of untreated cases will develop active postprimary tuberculosis within the following year.[10,19,25]

Tuberculous empyemas or bronchopleural fistulas usually occur in older patients who have had prior tuberculous pleurisy. The majority have had stable pleural thickening or fibrothorax for many years and pneumothorax collapse therapy. Only a few have received appropriate chemotherapy. With advancing age, pleural infection recurs from a dormant focus in the pleura or adjacent lung. The pleural infection

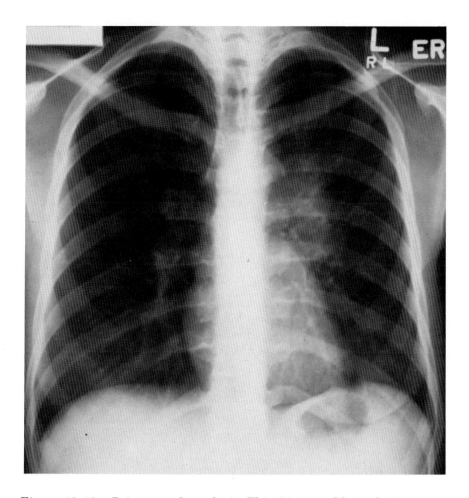

Figure 13-12. Primary tuberculosis. This 20-year-old psychotic woman presented with fever and cough lasting for several weeks. The chest radiograph shows a mass at the aortic pulmonary window and left hilum, along with a patchy opacity located laterally. The spleen was moderately enlarged clinically. Bronchoscopy showed severe extrinsic narrowing of the left upper lobe bronchus but did not reveal the cause of the patient's problem. At mediastinotomy, multiple enlarged nodes were biopsied, demonstrating tuberculosis.

eventually communicates with the lung (bronchopleural fistula) or the chest wall (empyema necessitans), causing air to appear in the pleural space (Figure 13-15). Schmitt et al.[25] have demonstrated that a persistent tuberculous empyema will prevent the visceral and parietal surfaces from apposing. Hulnick et al.[10] have found that computed tomography may be helpful in distinguishing an indolent empyema from severe tubercu-

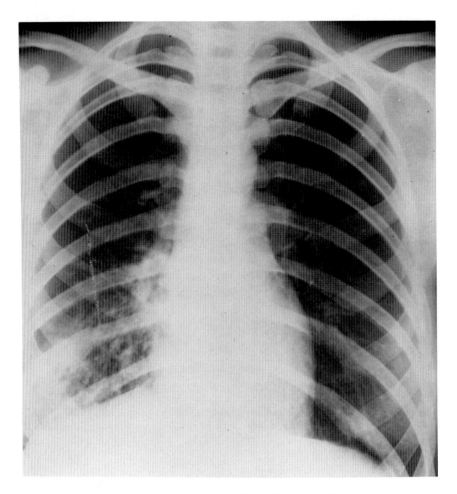

Figure 13-13. Primary tuberculosis. This 23-year-old pregnant woman presented with 2½ months of fever, cough, and chest pain. Sputum production was moderate. Her chest radiograph shows patchy, right lower lobe air-space disease. Sputum smear and culture were positive for tuberculosis.

lous scarring. In their study, all cases with fluid identified on computed tomography had active infection, whereas none with fibrothorax without a visible fluid collection had active disease.

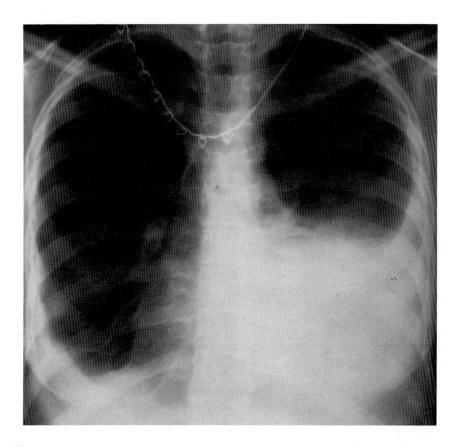

Figure 13-14. Primary tuberculosis. This 15-year-old girl was admitted with a low-grade fever, fatigue, dyspnea, and left pleuritic chest pain lasting for 2 weeks. One year earlier, her mother was diagnosed as having tuberculosis. At that time, the patient was found to have a positive skin test and a normal chest radiograph. She was treated but did not adhere to her treatment protocol. The current radiograph shows large left and moderate right pleural effusions. A small focus of parenchymal disease was seen in the left lung base after the exudative effusion was tapped. The sputum was heavily positive for tuberculosis. The effusions cleared over the next few months.

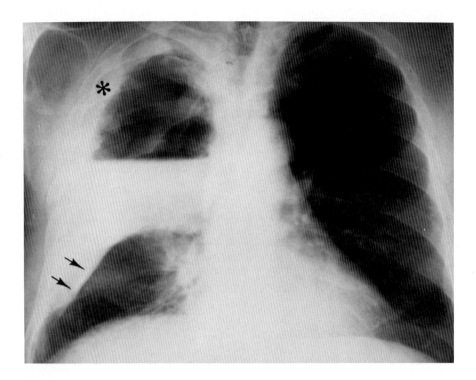

Figure 13-15. Bronchopleural fistula. At age 19, this elderly man began 5 years of pneumothorax therapy for tuberculous pleurisy. He never received drug treatment and continued to have a large homogeneous dense area in the upper two-thirds of his right hemithorax. The appearance remained stable for many years and was presumed to represent a fibrotic residuum. A few days after he coughed up a large amount of brownish material, his radiograph showed an air-fluid level, presumably in the pleural space. The parietal pleura (*) was remarkably thickened and nodular. Apart from the air-fluid level, the abnormality appeared identical to that seen 4 years earlier, when it was completely opaque. Faint calcification is suggested along the visceral pleural margin (arrows). Cultures of the expectorated material yielded mycobacteria.

Question 71

Concerning acute bacterial pneumonias,

- (A) adenopathy is more frequent in children than in adults
- (B) pneumatoceles secondary to staphylococcal pneumonia are more frequent in children than in adults
- (C) empyemas are more frequent with staphylococcal than with pneumococcal pneumonia
- (D) airborne pseudomonas pneumonia tends to be lobar

As discussed above, hilar and mediastinal adenopathy are present in the vast majority of children and in a small number of adults with primary tuberculosis. In adults, granulomatous infections such as histoplasmosis and coccidioidomycosis are most often associated with ipsilateral or asymmetrical hilar and mediastinal adenopathy. In histoplasmosis, severe nodal enlargement may be associated with mediastinal compression syndromes and may lead to fibrosing mediastinitis. In coccidioidomycosis, adenopathy often heralds diffuse dissemination and is an indication for antifungal therapy. As a general rule, however, most other fungal, bacterial, viral, and mycoplasmal infections are infrequently associated with adenopathy. Some of the less common bacterial infections (tularemia, pertussis, and anthrax) and certain viral infections (chicken pox, ornithosis, and mononucleosis) may be associated with adenopathy.[6] In contrast to adults, nodal enlargement is frequently present in children with air-space pneumonia (streptococcal, staphylococcal, etc.) and severe interstitial pneumonia (whooping cough, measles, influenza, etc.) **(Option (A) is true).** Moreover, mycoplasma pneumonia, the most frequently identified nonbacterial pneumonia, causes adenopathy rarely in adults but in 25% of children. Thus, for an adult presenting with adenopathy and parenchymal disease, the differential diagnosis includes granulomatous infection, one of the unusual bacterial or viral infections, or noninfectious causes (carcinoma, lymphoma, sarcoidosis, etc.) (Figure 13-16). For a child, this same presentation is most often due to infection.

Pneumonia caused by *Staphylococcus aureus* has been associated with mortality rates as high as 20 to 30%. In the majority of cases, it complicates a pre-existing viral respiratory infection or is due to seeding of the lung by a bacteremia. Young children and the elderly are most often affected, and the process behaves differently in the two groups. In children, a very acute severe pneumonia usually follows shortly after recovery from a viral respiratory illness. The clinical course is rapid, and

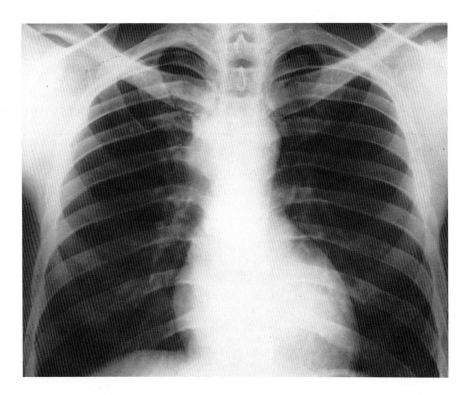

Figure 13-16. Coccidioidomycosis. This 38-year-old man presented with right paratracheal adenopathy and vague right apical disease. There was clinical evidence of a mild but persistent lower respiratory tract infection thought to represent tuberculosis. Transbronchial aspiration as well as lymph node biopsy were performed. The aspirate showed multinucleated giant cells that contained spherules of coccidioidal organisms and single spherules that were not intracellular. The lymph nodes contained areas of caseating necrosis and many multinucleated giant cells filled with coccidioidal organisms. Acid-fast stains were negative. As in this case, chronic fungal infections may mimic primary tuberculosis.

the radiograph shows very rapid progression from patchy bronchopneumonia to consolidation. Pleural effusions, which also develop rapidly and early, are frequently large and infected, occurring in up to 90% of cases. Pneumatoceles, a rather distinctive feature of childhood infection, occur in approximately one-half of the cases. They appear during the first week of infection as rapidly developing, thin-walled cystic lucencies that may occupy a large portion of the lung. They do not necessarily occur in the areas of maximal involvement and may simulate pneumothorax or lead to one. Regression is seen as the pneumonia clears.[1,6,8,19]

In adults, staphyloccocal infection may also follow influenza or another viral respiratory infection. The onset of symptoms is more variable in speed and severity, and the radiographic appearance is that of patchy bronchopneumonia involving several lobes (Figure 13-17). Widespread dense consolidation is uncommon. Abscesses, occurring in 25 to 75% of patients, have shaggy inner walls and indistinct outer margins. They often contain air-fluid levels, whereas pneumatoceles usually do not (Figure 13-18). For reasons unknown, abscesses are more frequent in adults, while pneumatoceles, effusions, and empyemas are more common in children **(Option (B) is true)**.

A pleural effusion is present in approximately 40% of patients with acute bacterial pneumonia. These parapneumonic effusions may be complicated or uncomplicated. In the latter, the Gram stain and cultures are negative, and the pleural fluid pH is typically greater than 7.20, with a lactic dehydrogenase level of <1,000 IU/L. Such an effusion usually resolves without the need for drainage. In contrast, the complicated effusion or empyema has a positive Gram stain and cultures, a pH typically lower than 7.00, and a glucose concentration of less than 40 mg/dL or a lactic dehydrogenase level of >1,000 IU/L. This type of effusion is associated with high morbidity and mortality unless drained early.

Currently, anaerobic pneumonias are the leading causes of empyemas, and most are hospital-acquired. Approximately 90% of effusions associated with such pneumonias are infected. The majority of effusions associated with gram-positive infections are community-acquired, empyemas being most common with staphylococcal infections. Approximately 80% of childhood and 20% of adult staphylococcal effusions are infected, whereas less than 5% of pneumococcal effusions are infected **(Option (C) is true)**. Of the aerobic gram-negative pneumonias, *Escherichia coli* and *Pseudomonas* species most often lead to empyemas.[6,8,19,27]

Pseudomonas aeruginosa is an infrequent cause of community-acquired bacterial pneumonia (<5%), whereas it is the most frequently identified bacterial organism in hospital-acquired lower respiratory tract infection. This is especially true in immunocompromised patients or those with cancer. There are three accepted routes of infection. The majority of cases are due to microaspiration of nasopharyngeal secretions that have become colonized with aerobic gram-negative bacilli during hospitalization. Hematogenous dissemination from the bladder, the skin, or the gastrointestinal tract is less common. Finally, respiratory

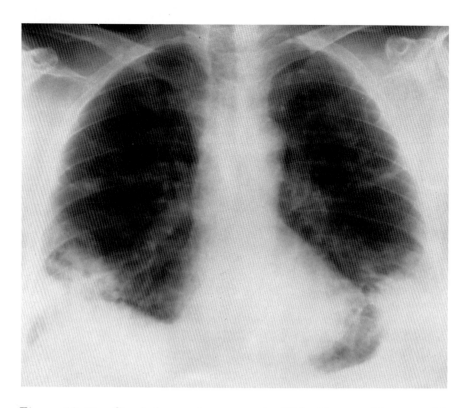

Figure 13-17. Staphylococcal pneumonia. This 52-year-old man with Hodgkin's disease had an influenza-like syndrome that was treated with erythromycin. He gradually improved but then experienced a rapid onset of fever and progressively increasing respiratory symptoms. A radiograph taken 2 days after his increase in symptoms showed a pattern typical of bronchopneumonia. No definite cavitation was present, but there was a left pleural effusion which later increased. Aspiration of the fluid yielded purulent material positive for staphylococci.

equipment may become contaminated with *Pseudomonas* species, resulting in an aerosolized spread of infection.

The majority of pneumonias caused by aspiration of pseudomonads have a diffuse patchy or somewhat nodular lower-lobe appearance. The pneumonia often spreads to involve the lung diffusely **(Option (D) is false)**. Small lucencies are often visible and may represent uninvolved areas of lung. Later in the course of the disease, microabscesses form with coalescence into larger abscesses (Figures 13-19 and 13-20). Complicated effusions are frequent. Infection caused by septicemia is more likely to present as diffuse ill-defined nodules throughout the

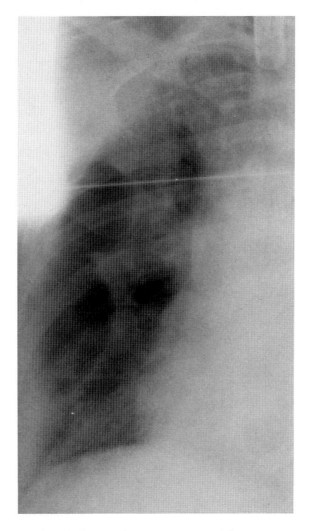

Figure 13-18. Staphylococcal pneumonia with pneumatoceles. This 64-year-old diabetic woman developed staphylococcal pneumonia after an infection at an amputation site. The initial radiograph showed diffuse disease throughout the entire right lung and minimal disease in the left lung. Several days after the onset of pneumonia, this radiograph was taken. Multiple thin-walled cystic lucencies (pneumatoceles) were visible on the right; they were not visible on a study film taken 48 hours earlier. A right pleural effusion was also seen. The rapid emergence of thin-walled cystic lucencies without air-fluid levels is most suggestive of pneumatoceles rather than abscesses. Her pneumatoceles enlarged and eventually resulted in a tension pneumothorax on the right.

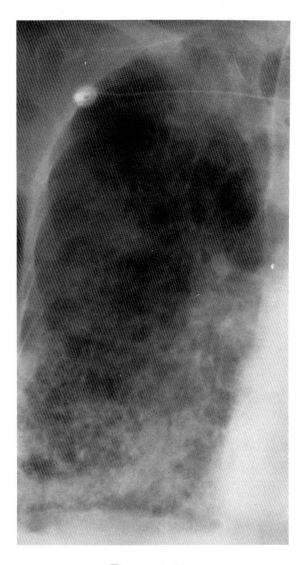

Figure 13-19

Figures 13-19 and 13-20. Pseudomonas pneumonia. This 58-year-old woman with severe chronic obstructive pulmonary disease was admitted to the hospital for respiratory failure. After several weeks of intermittent support on a ventilator, she rapidly developed signs and symptoms of acute pneumonia. A view of the right lung (Figure 13-19) showed a diffuse air-space pneumonia. Multiple small lucencies were seen within it and may represent pre-existing bullae, areas of lung not yet involved, or small abscesses. Four days later (Figure 13-20), many of the small lucencies seen at the right lung base had enlarged and become confluent. This pattern of progression is typical for pseudomonas pneumonia.

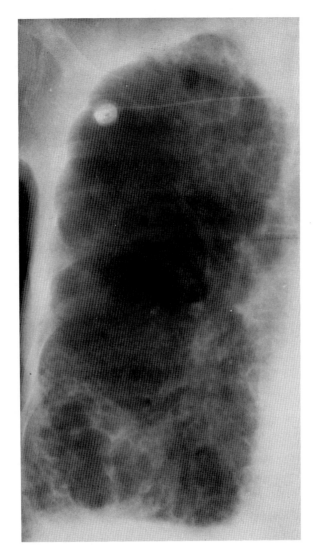

Figure 13-20

lung. The infection may progress rapidly and appear similar to one caused by aspiration.[6,27]

SUGGESTED READINGS

1. Caffey J. Pediatric x-ray diagnosis. Chicago: Year Book Medical Publishers; 1978:394–416
2. Choyke PL, Sostman HD, Curtis AM, et al. Adult-onset pulmonary tuberculosis. Radiology 1983; 148:357–362
3. Dhand S, Fisher M, Fewell JW. Intrathoracic tuberculous lymphadenopathy in adults. JAMA 1979; 241:505–507
4. Edelstein PH, Meyer RD. Legionnaires' disease. A review. Chest 1984; 85:114–120
5. Fairbank JT, Mamourian AC, Dietrich PA, Girod JC. The chest radiograph in Legionnaires' disease. Further observations. Radiology 1983; 147:33–34
6. Fraser RG, Paré JAP. Diagnosis of diseases of the chest, 2nd ed, vol II. Philadelphia: WB Saunders; 1978:787–791
7. Glassroth J, Robins AG, Snider DE Jr. Tuberculosis in the 1980s. N Engl J Med 1980; 302:1441–1450
8. Goodman LR, Goren RA, Teplick SK. The radiographic evaluation of pulmonary infection. Med Clin North Am 1980; 64:553–574
9. Hadlock FP, Park SK, Awe RJ, Rivera M. Unusual radiographic findings in adult pulmonary tuberculosis. AJR 1980; 134:1015–1018
10. Hulnick DH, Naidich DP, McCauley DI. Pleural tuberculosis evaluated by computed tomography. Radiology 1983; 149:759–765
11. Irving HC, Brown TS. Tuberculous mediastinal lymphadenopathy in Bradford. Clin Radiol 1980; 31:685–690
12. Jay SJ, Johanson WG Jr, Pierce AK. The radiographic resolution of *Streptococcus pneumoniae* pneumonia. N Engl J Med 1975; 16:798–801
13. Kantor HG. The many radiologic faces of pneumococcal pneumonia. AJR 1981; 137:1213–1220
14. Khan MA, Kovnat DM, Bachus B, Whitcomb ME, Brody JS, Snider GL. Clinical and roentgenographic spectrum of pulmonary tuberculosis in the adult. Am J Med 1977; 62:31–38
15. Kirby BD, Peck H, Meyer RD. Radiographic features of Legionnaires' disease. Chest 1979; 76:562–565
16. Kirby BD, Snyder KM, Meyer RD, Finegold SM. Legionnaires' disease: clinical features of 24 cases. Ann Intern Med 1978; 89:297–309
17. Kovacs JA, Hiemenz JW, Macher AM, et al. *Pneumocystis carinii* pneumonia: a comparison between patients with the acquired immunodeficiency syndrome and patients with other immunodeficiencies. Ann Intern Med 1984; 100:663–671
18. Kroboth FJ, Yu VL, Reddy SC, Yu AC. Clinicoradiographic correlation with the extent of Legionnaires' disease. AJR 1983; 141:263–268
19. Light RW. Pleural disease. Philadelphia: Lea & Febiger: 1983:101–125
20. Macher A. Histoplasmosis and blastomycosis. Med Clin North Am 1980; 64:447–459
21. Miller WT, MacGregor RR. Tuberculosis: frequency of unusual radiographic findings. AJR 1978; 130:867–875

22. Moore EH, Webb WR, Gamsu G, Golden JA. Legionnaires' disease in the renal transplant patient: clinical presentation and radiographic progression. Radiology 1984; 153:589–593
23. Muder RR, Reddy SC, Yu VL, Kroboth FJ. Pneumonia caused by Pittsburgh pneumonia agent: radiologic manifestations. Radiology 1984; 150:633–637
24. Mylotte JM, Beam TR Jr. Comparison of community-acquired and nosocomial pneumococcal bacteremia. Am Rev Respir Dis 1981; 123:265–268
25. Schmitt WG, Hübener KH, Rücker HC. Pleural calcification with persistent effusion. Radiology 1983; 149:633–638
26. Tead WW, Kerby GR, Schlueter DP, Jordahl CW. The clinical spectrum of primary tuberculosis in adults. Confusion with reinfection in the pathogenesis of chronic tuberculosis. Ann Intern Med 1968; 68:731–745
27. Unger JD, Rose HD, Unger GF. Gram-negative pneumonia. Radiology 1973; 107:283–291
28. Young LS. Clinical aspects of pneumocystis in man. In: Young LS (ed), *Pneumocystis carinii* pneumonia. New York: Marcel Dekker; 1984:139–174
29. Ziskind MM, Schwarz MI, George RB, et al. Incomplete consolidation in pneumococcal lobar pneumonia complicating pulmonary emphysema. Ann Intern Med 1970; 72:835–839

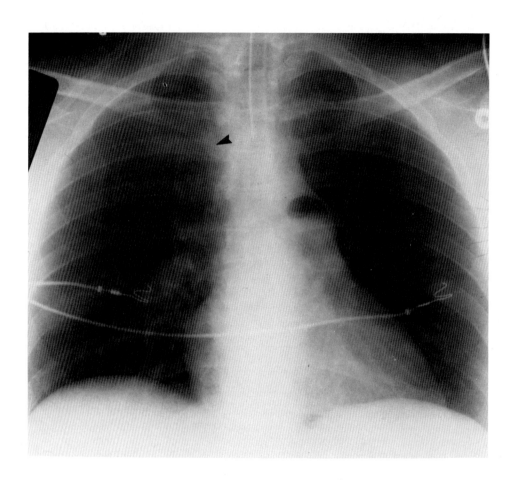

Figure 14-1. This erect portable radiograph was taken immediately after right internal jugular catheterization. An arrowhead indicates the tip of the internal jugular catheter.

Case 14: Air Embolism

Question 72

Which *one* of the following is the MOST likely diagnosis?

(A) Mediastinal air
(B) Paramediastinal bulla
(C) Pulmonary ligament air
(D) Pericardial air
(E) Pulmonary artery air

The portable radiograph (Figure 14-1), taken immediately after an apparently uncomplicated right internal jugular catheter insertion, demonstrates that the jugular venous catheter is positioned at the junction of the internal jugular and subclavian veins. The endotracheal tube is in satisfactory position in the mid trachea. The lungs are clear, and the heart is not enlarged. The only abnormality is a semicircular lucency just above the left main and upper lobe bronchi. There is no evidence of air elsewhere in the mediastinum, nor is there air in the subcutaneous tissues or pleural space. The patient was asymptomatic. Prior radiographs and a follow-up study 2 hours later were normal.

The semicircular lucency represents air in the upper main and left pulmonary arteries **(Option (E) is the most likely diagnosis).** This is the most frequent radiographic appearance of venous air embolism. Larger air infusions may cause visualization of the entire pulmonary artery and the right ventricle. Less specific signs of venous air embolism include pulmonary edema, focal oligemia, and atelectasis. If air crosses a patent foramen ovale or other septal defect, air may be seen in the left heart and systemic vessels as well.

It is likely that venous air embolism occurs considerably more often than is generally recognized clinically and radiographically. In many reported cases, radiographs are normal, with only a presumptive diagnosis being made. Nonetheless, venous air embolism is an unusual occurrence. In a patient with a new central venous pressure (CVP) catheter and an endotracheal tube for artificial ventilation, other causes of extrapulmonary air are more likely. A pneumomediastinum (Option (A)) is often the first radiographic sign of pulmonary barotrauma. The air collections are usually flat or oval and are usually vertical in orientation rather than horizontal, as in our test case. Moreover, the air is often seen at multiple levels in the mediastinum and is continuous with subcutaneous and deep cervical emphysema.

A paramediastinal bulla (Option (B)), even if located perfectly in front of or behind the left pulmonary artery, should not cause the pulmonary artery to appear as lucent as it does in Figure 14-1.

The inferior pulmonary ligament is composed of two pleural layers that cover the hilum anteriorly and posteriorly and contact one another below the inferior pulmonary vein. At this point, the ligament is formed and descends toward the diaphragm. The air collection seen in Figure 14-1 is located too high for the anatomic position of the inferior pulmonary ligament (Option (C) is unlikely). The ligament attaches the medial surface of the lower lobe to the adjacent mediastinum and may be attached to the diaphragmatic pleura or end in a free border without diaphragmatic attachment. The mediastinal attachment of the ligament relates to the inferior vena cava and ascending azygos vein on the right and to the esophagus and descending aorta on the left. On computed tomography (CT), the inferior pulmonary ligament is outlined by the lower lobe and is easily identified.[8,19] After trauma or esophageal rupture, air may enter the ligament. This has the appearance of an oval lucency parallel to the spine with extension downward from the inferior pulmonary vein to the diaphragm. Erect radiographs may show an air-fluid level in the ligament. CT scans may demonstrate that air thought to be in the pulmonary ligament is actually located elsewhere (Figures 14-2 and 14-3).[7,18]

The pericardium extends superiorly on the left to the main pulmonary artery, so that a small pneumopericardium (Option (D)) on an erect radiograph might be visible in the location shown in Figure 14-1. However, the air should sharply outline the main pulmonary artery, unlike the situation in this case.

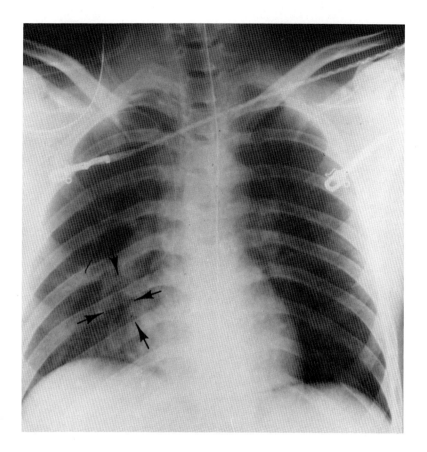

Figure 14-2
Figures 14-2 and 14-3. Post-traumatic pulmonary laceration simulating air in the inferior pulmonary ligament. The chest radiograph (Figure 14-2) and CT (Figure 14-3) were done within 6 hours of an automobile accident. On the radiograph, note the vague opacity in the lower half of the right lung and a lucency (arrows) lateral to the right heart border. The lucency was interpreted as air in the inferior pulmonary ligament. However, on CT two distinct pulmonary lacerations in the contused right lower lobe were seen. There was no air in the inferior pulmonary ligament.

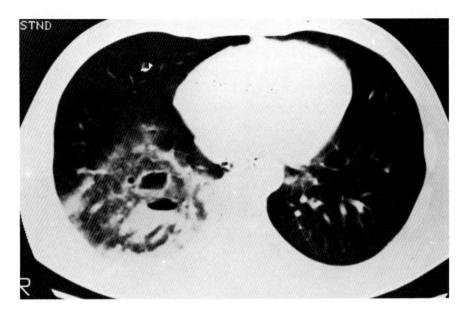

Figure 14-3

Question 73

Concerning ventilator-induced barotrauma,

(A) pneumothorax is usually due to rupture of a peripheral bulla or bleb through the pleura
(B) interstitial air, although usually present, is seldom visible radiographically in adults
(C) when pneumoperitoneum or pneumoretroperitoneum is a complication, pneumomediastinum is visible in only one-half of patients

The spontaneous pneumothorax seen in young adults is usually due to rupture of a peripheral bulla or bleb. Pneumothorax associated with blunt trauma, peripheral infection, or tumor is usually due to disruption of the visceral pleura. Pneumothorax seen with penetrating trauma may be due to an open wound of the chest wall or visceral pleural disruption. In contrast, patients developing air leaks from positive pressure therapy or asthma, coughing, Valsalva maneuver, etc., usually develop interstitial emphysema first. In such cases, the alveoli or peripheral airways rupture. Air may travel in the interstitial compartment toward the mediastinum centrally or toward the visceral pleura peripherally. The air travelling centrally may enter the mediastinum to result in pneumomediastinum.[13] Any subsequent rupture of the mediastinal or visceral pleura then allows the mediastinal air to enter the pleural space, resulting in pneumothorax **(Option (A) is false)**.

Although the mechanism described above would indicate that interstitial emphysema is generally present with ventilator-induced barotrauma, it is seldom visible in adults **(Option (B) is true)**. It is much more readily visible in newborns, since the interstitial connective tissue in children is supposedly looser and accommodates focal air collections more readily. Even in this age group, interstitial emphysema is best visualized when there is pulmonary consolidation. The air most often appears as an irregular branching or mottled pattern in the lower one-half to two-thirds of the lung. When linear and branching, the air may simulate an air bronchogram. Unlike the air in an air bronchogram, however, the air in interstitial emphysema is distributed irregularly and the branching lucencies do not taper (Figure 14-4).

When interstitial air surrounds a blood vessel that is tangential to the frontal x-ray beam, the vessel on end appears as a dense circle surrounded by a collar of lucency. A more frequent manifestation of interstitial emphysema in the adult, however, is the round or oval air cyst formed by air collecting in the loose connective tissue of the pleura. Such air cysts develop and increase in size rapidly.[1,26] When they occur at the lung base, they may mimic a subpulmonic pneumothorax. Differentiation from postinfectious pneumatoceles may be impossible.

The above-described signs of interstitial emphysema are important because they may be initial clues to barotrauma before symptoms, pneumomediastinum, or pneumothorax develops. Since pulmonary interstitial emphysema usually progresses to pneumothorax, treatment should be altered accordingly. Efforts should be made to diminish positive pressure ventilation or institute high-frequency high-volume ventilator assistance. Some have advocated the insertion of prophylactic chest tubes or, at least, a level of preparedness for an eventual pneumothorax.

The mediastinum may communicate with both the neck and the retroperitoneum.[15] In the neck, only one of three distinct fascial compartments communicates with the mediastinum. The previsceral space anteriorly extends from the mandible to the sternum and does not normally communicate with the mediastinum. The prevertebral space posteriorly extends from the base of the occiput to the upper thoracic spine and does not communicate with the mediastinum. The visceral compartment of the neck, located between the anterior and posterior

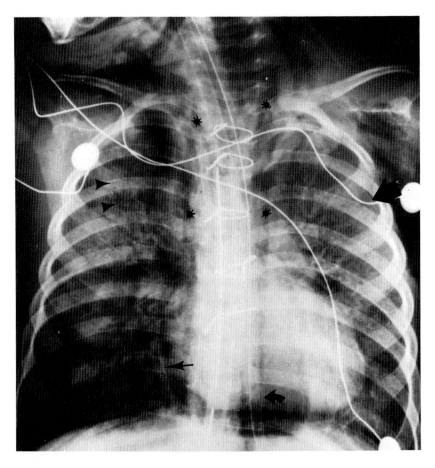

Figure 14-4. Barotrauma after cardiac surgery in a child. This radiograph shows multiple features of barotrauma. Interstitial air was found diffusely throughout both lungs, most readily appreciated on the right, where multiple branching irregular structures simulated disordered air bronchograms (arrowheads). Deep mediastinal emphysema and cervical emphysema were seen (*), with the mediastinal pleura noted behind the heart (curved arrow). Marked subcutaneous emphysema was present along the shoulders. It is difficult to be certain whether an air collection (horizontal arrow) lateral to the right heart border was a pneumomediastinum, a medial pneumothorax, or a local pneumopericardium. A left lung pneumothorax was diagnosable by virtue of the small amount of air collected in the left costophrenic angle and visualization of the visceral pleura (solid large arrow). Mediastinal air had dissected downward into the retroperitoneum. (Case courtesy of Barbara Rohlfing, M.D., San Francisco, Calif.)

compartments, communicates with the mediastinum and shares with it some common structures (trachea, esophagus, great vessels, and vagus nerves). Thus, if interstitial emphysema reaches the mediastinum, cervical emphysema may follow (Figure 14-4).

The mediastinum may communicate with the retroperitoneum via the esophageal hiatus and the aortic hiatus. In turn, the retroperitoneum is in continuity with the flanks. Thus, a ventilator-induced pneumomediastinum may result in pneumoretroperitoneum and air in the flanks (Figure 14-4). Pneumoperitoneum may follow pneumoretroperitoneum just as pneumothorax may follow pneumomediastinum. Retroperitoneal air is often crescentric and seen along the lateral and posterior aspects of the liver. It may outline the psoas muscles and kidneys and does not move with a change in patient position. Peritoneal air moves with patient positioning, tends to collect centrally under the diaphragm, and may produce visualization of the outer margin of the bowel wall (Figures 14-5, 14-6, and 14-7).

When pneumoretroperitoneum or pneumoperitoneum complicates ventilator-induced barotrauma, air is invariably seen in the mediastinum as well **(Option (C) is false).**[21] Therefore, in the artificially ventilated patient, pneumoperitoneum in association with pneumomediastinum and a clinically benign abdomen may very well be due to barotrauma. Pneumoperitoneum in the absence of visible mediastinal air should raise suspicion for a gastrointestinal perforation or other abdominal source of air.

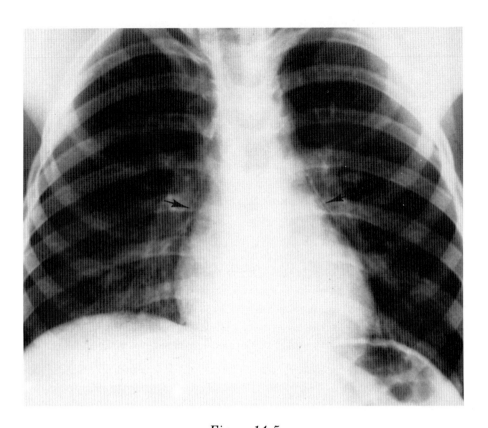

Figure 14-5

Figures 14-5 through 14-7. Mediastinal air due to a retrorectal abscess. This young patient experienced air dissection from the presacral area (retrorectal abscess) into the retroperitoneum and then into the mediastinum. Note the pneumomediastinum (arrows) on the frontal chest radiograph (Figure 14-5). The lateral chest radiograph (Figure 14-6) shows streaks of a pneumoretroperitoneum posteriorly (arrows). A view of the upper abdomen (Figure 14-7) shows air outlining the right kidney and in each flank (arrows), as well as the continuous diaphragm sign of pneumomediastinum (arrowheads).

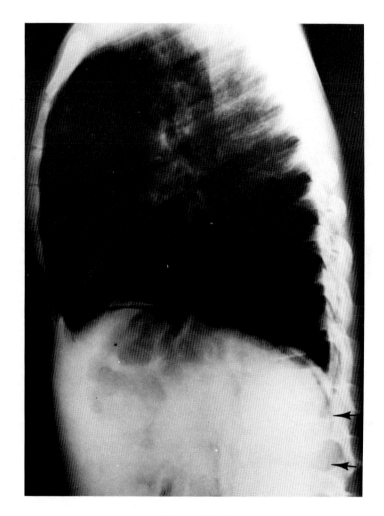

Figure 14-6

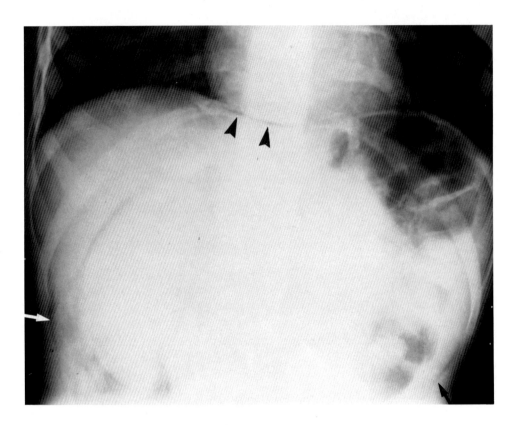

Figure 14-7

Question 74

Concerning the various substances that may embolize to the lung,

(A) death occurs with venous air embolization only if the air crosses a patent foramen ovale to enter the systemic circulation
(B) coagulopathy is a major cause of morbidity and mortality following amniotic fluid embolization
(C) the fat embolism syndrome more closely resembles the adult respiratory distress syndrome than it does venous thromboembolism
(D) intravenous metallic mercury injections usually cause minimal symptoms and dramatic radiographs
(E) oil embolism complicating lymphangiography causes a mild to moderate decrease in diffusing capacity in the majority of patients

Numerous substances other than venous thrombi may embolize to the lungs. The clinical effects of embolization and the underlying mechanisms vary greatly depending on the material that embolizes, the volume of material, and its source. Venous air embolization may be due to air entry during venous catheterization, surgery, childbirth, or fistula formation between an air-containing structure and an appropriate vessel.[2,9,10,11] Arterial air embolization results when air gains access to the pulmonary veins or the arterial circulation or when a venous air embolism crosses a patent foramen ovale or other septal defect due to elevated right-sided pressures. With venous air embolization, the air and blood are whipped into a foam within the right atrium and ventricle. Small foam bubbles embolize to the pulmonary arteries. In addition, fibrin plugs are formed and embolize as well. These events may cause transient vasoconstriction, capillary-permeability edema, pulmonary hypertension, cor pulmonale, and eventually death **(Option (A) is false).** In patients with arterial air embolization, symptoms are present with much smaller volumes of air and are usually due to vascular occlusion, most notably in the brain and heart (Figures 14-8 and 14-9).

Although venous air embolization may be rapidly fatal, it is not necessarily so. In the test case, the patient was asymptomatic, received no treatment, and had a follow-up radiograph that showed resolution. It is possible that many cases are asymptomatic, and many symptomatic cases are confused with other acute cardiopulmonary events. Symptomatic patients usually experience dyspnea, cough, and chest pain and demonstrate tachypnea, tachycardia, hypotension, wheezing, and a transient "mill wheel" murmur. As soon as the diagnosis is suspected, the patient should be placed in the left lateral decubitus position to "collect" the air in the right heart. Oxygen should be administered, both

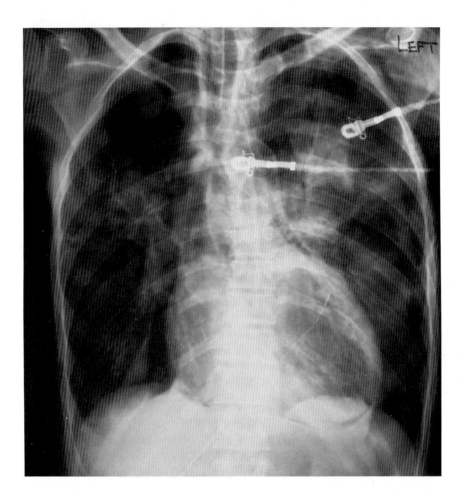

Figure 14-8

Figures 14-8 and 14-9. Arterial air embolization. This 51-year-old man was intubated after cardiac arrest and was difficult to ventilate. Bilateral pleural taps were performed for possible pneumothoraces, but there was no attempt to insert a CVP catheter. Resuscitation was unsuccessful, and these radiographs were taken immediately after the patient's demise. The chest radiograph (Figure 14-8) shows a right upper lobe fungus ball, left upper lobe air-space disease, and bilateral pneumothoraces. The left ventricle, ascending aorta, and aortic knob were filled with air. Note the difference between this appearance and that shown in Figure 14-1. Air was clearly present in the right axillary artery, and there was a pneumomediastinum as well. A view of the upper abdomen (Figure 14-9) shows air in the abdominal aorta (+) and air in the splenic and hepatic arteries. It is postulated that the positive pressure ventilation forced air into a right upper lobe pulmonary vein in the region of the cavity containing the fungus ball. The air may have been disseminated peripherally by cardiac massage at the time of attempted resuscitation. (Case courtesy of Heber McMahon, M.D., Chicago, Ill.)

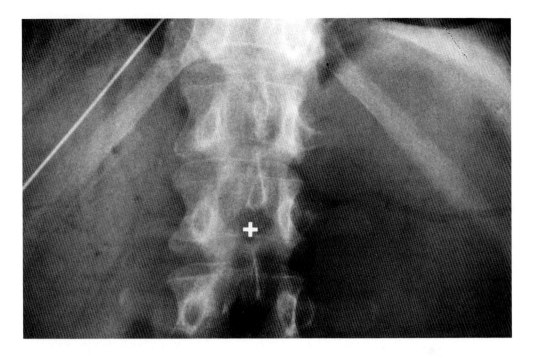

Figure 14-9

to improve arterial hypoxemia (if present) and to speed resolution of the air embolus; the intravascular N_2 gas will dissolve more quickly in blood when the partial pressure of N_2 in blood is lowered by raising the f_iO_2. Cardiopulmonary resuscitation may be necessary.

Although amniotic fluid embolization is uncommon, it may account for approximately 5% of maternal deaths and is the most common cause of death during and immediately following labor. Predisposing factors include a tumultuous labor, uterine stimulants, intrauterine fetal death, premature rupture of the membranes, and multiparity. Amniotic fluid may enter the circulation through the endocervical veins or at the placental site when there is premature separation, placenta previa, or uterine rupture. Several factors contribute to the profound dyspnea, cyanosis, shock, and bleeding that usually lead to death. With large infusions of amniotic fluid, particulate matter obstructs the pulmonary arteries, causing pulmonary arterial hypertension, diminished systemic blood flow, and peripheral vascular collapse. In those who survive the immediate embolic insult, bleeding due to a consumption coagulopathy may lead to a hemorrhagic death. A major cause of death with amniotic fluid embolization relates to its potent thromboplastic activity, which causes a consumption coagulopathy and disseminated intravascular coagulation **(Option (B) is true)**. The differential diagnosis of severe intra- and postpartum cardiopulmonary insufficiency also includes hemorrhagic shock, venous thromboembolism, venous air embolization, massive aspiration, gram-negative sepsis, and pulmonary edema. In most instances of amniotic fluid embolization, the radiograph is negative or shows evidence of noncardiac pulmonary edema.[14]

Although bone marrow embolizes to the lung in almost every patient with long bone fractures, pelvic fractures, and major orthopedic procedures, it is estimated that only 5% of patients develop the fat embolism syndrome.[3,4] This syndrome is characterized by dyspnea and hypoxia developing 1 to 2 days after the insult. Nonspecific neurologic abnormalities are frequently present as well. The chest radiograph may be normal or reveal diffuse patchy areas of consolidation or signs of interstitial or alveolar edema. Most patients require ventilator support and clear within a few days. A smaller number of patients develop progressive respiratory compromise and many of the features of the adult respiratory distress syndrome, such as high alveolar-arterial oxygen gradients, markedly decreased compliance, and pulmonary opacities (Figure 14-10) **(Option (C) is true)**. The neutral triglycerides carried to the lung undergo lipolysis, with the release of fatty acids. These free fatty acids increase capillary permeability, leading to edema and hemorrhage. In many of these cases progressing to the adult respiratory distress syndrome, there is also evidence of diffuse intravascular coagulation and a consumption coagulopathy.

Metallic mercury may be injected intravenously as a suicide gesture, as an attempt to enhance one's muscular prowess, or as a complication of using mercury as an anaerobic seal for blood gas determination. In the vast majority of cases, patients experience either mild transient respiratory distress or no clinical symptoms **(Option (D) is true)**. The radiographic appearance is very striking because of the extremely dense mercury droplets seen in the peripheral pulmonary arterial system (Figure 14-11). In the dependent portions of the lung, branching vessels may be opacified by the mercury. Mercury droplets may be found in the antecubital fossa (the usual injection site) and in the right ventricle. Paradoxical embolization distributes tiny droplets throughout the systemic circulation. Injection of large amounts may cause severe respiratory distress. However, complications are more frequently due to chronic mercurialism from absorption of the mercury as it is oxidized in the body. Signs and symptoms include hypersalivation, gingivitis,

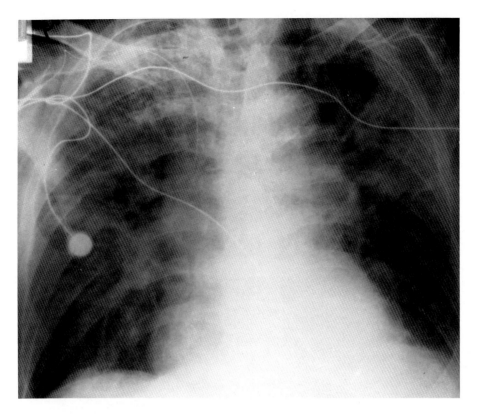

Figure 14-10. Fat embolism syndrome. This elderly patient suffered multiple lower extremity fractures in an automobile accident, never became hypotensive, and never lost consciousness. His radiograph, taken 2.5 days after the accident, shows diffuse interstitial and some patchy alveolar opacities which worsened during the next 48 hours. The clinical course closely resembled the adult respiratory distress syndrome.

metallic taste, diarrhea, renal disease, tremors, and personality changes.[16,17,24]

Mercury may be aspirated when the mercury bag of a small bowel tube ruptures or when mercury is ingested as a suicide gesture. The mercury pattern in the small airways may be similar to that in the arterial system, but the mercury may not be located as far peripherally (Figure 14-12). There may also be evidence of mercury elsewhere in the tracheobronchial tree or gastrointestinal tract.

Following lymphangiography, the oil-based contrast medium travels via the thoracic duct into the venous system and eventually to the lungs. Although embolization occurs in 100% of patients, acute respiratory

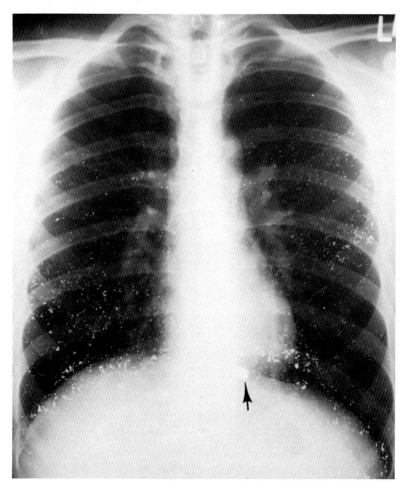

Figure 14-11. Intravenous self-administration of metallic mercury. This 43-year-old man was anorexic and had moderate dyspnea and mild ataxia after an accidental 0.5-mL injection of metallic mercury. His physical examination was unremarkable, and laboratory values indicated a pO_2 of 74 mm Hg, a pCO_2 of 33 mm Hg, and a pH of 7.4. The radiograph shows numerous tiny metallic droplets widely and peripherally distributed throughout the lungs. Note also the presence of mercury within the heart (arrow). He was asymptomatic at the time of discharge. (Reprinted with permission from Vas et al. [25].)

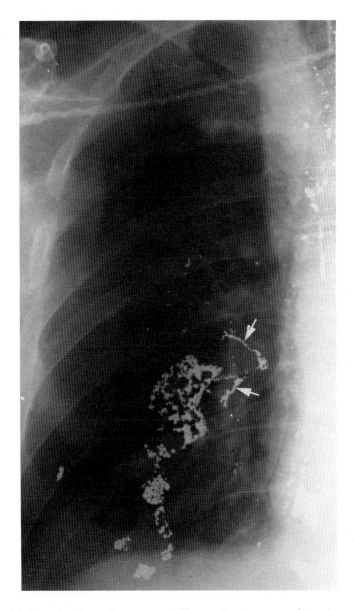

Figure 14-12. Aspirated mercury. The patient was undergoing esophageal resection and gastric pullthrough when the mercury balloon in the
esophagus was accidentally punctured, allowing mercury to escape into
the mediastinal and pleural spaces and the esophagus. The radiograph
shows mercury in the mediastinum, esophagus, and dependent posterior
pleural space. Branching mercury (arrows) was noted within bronchi
confirmed on a lateral view (not shown) as belonging to the superior
segment of the right lower lobe. It is presumed that some of the mercury
in the esophagus must have been aspirated to produce this appearance.

symptoms occur in less than 2%.[22] Symptoms are most frequent in those who have had embolization of large amounts of oil because of injection of excessive amounts (e.g., over 8 mL per leg) directly into a vein or when lymphatic obstruction causes lymphaticovenous connections. A group of patients at high risk are those with decreased cardiopulmonary reserve because of emphysema, heart failure, etc. Symptoms usually include mild cough, dyspnea, fever, and chills and are self-limited. Severe cases may lead to respiratory insufficiency and death. Although only a small number of patients develop symptoms, most suffer a decrease in diffusing capacity **(Option (E) is true).** The decrease usually varies from 10 to 30% but has been reported to be as great as 60%. It occurs during the first 48 hours and correlates directly with the amount of oil reaching the lungs. A delayed second fall in diffusing capacity may occur as the oil is lipolyzed into free fatty acids, which increase capillary permeability. In approximately one-half of patients, the chest radiograph shows evidence of the embolization as a very fine reticular or nodular (almost miliary) pattern throughout the lungs. The pattern is so fine that unless a preprocedure chest radiograph is available for comparison, subtle changes are often difficult to detect (Figure 14-13). Diffuse pulmonary uptake of Ga-67 is another finding associated with embolization of lymphangiographic contrast medium and is reported to occur in about 50% of patients.

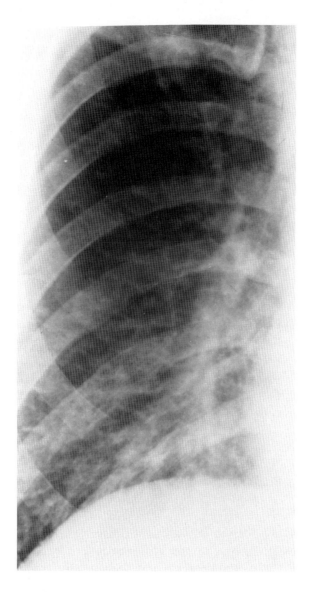

Figure 14-13. Oil embolization following lymphangiogram. This patient with lymphomatoid granulomatosis had a lymphangiogram as part of his initial work-up. A radiograph taken several days earlier was normal. The lymphangiogram was without incident, but it was noted on sequential abdominal studies that little or no contrast material was being absorbed by the para-aortic lymph nodes. A recheck of the lower extremities confirmed that the injection was indeed intralymphatic rather than intravenous. Within a few hours after completion of the study, the patient became progressively dyspneic, febrile, and extremely hypoxic, requiring ventilator support for several days. This radiograph, taken the day after the lymphangiogram, shows a diffuse interstitial pattern. The majority of patients with radiographically visible evidence of oil embolization have a finer (almost miliary) appearance and few or no symptoms.

Question 75

Concerning support and monitoring devices,

(A) to ensure accurate central venous pressure readings, a central venous pressure catheter is ideally positioned in the right atrium

(B) on the radiograph, a Swan-Ganz catheter is ideally positioned in a segmental pulmonary artery

(C) pulmonary capillary wedge pressures are affected by positive pressure ventilation

(D) aortic counter-pulsation catheters are ideally positioned with the tip in the aortic knob

(E) flexion of the neck advances an endotracheal tube toward the carina

A CVP catheter in the superior vena cava provides an indirect measurement of right atrial pressure and also provides access to a large vein for hemodialysis and infusion of various substances. The ideal location for a CVP catheter is beyond the last valve in the subclavian vein, which is approximately at the level of the first anterior rib. Catheters proximal to this valve do not truly reflect right atrial pressure. If the catheter is beyond the valve, there is no advantage to having the catheter tip in the right atrium **(Option (A) is false)**. A right atrial location has been associated with perforation of the atrial wall, which may result in cardiac tamponade due to either hemorrhage or infusion of intravenous fluid into the pericardial space. Tricuspid valve injury is another, albeit infrequent, complication of right atrial positioning. A catheter in the right atrium may also pass across the tricuspid valve, irritate the right ventricular wall, and cause ventricular arrhythmias. With the increasing use of larger, stiffer catheters for hemodialysis and chemotherapy, these complications may become more frequent.[5,25]

The Swan-Ganz catheter is a useful guide to circulatory resuscitation and fluid balance monitoring. After the catheter has been inserted into a major vein, its balloon is inflated, allowing the catheter to float into the main pulmonary artery. When measurements are not being taken, the tip of the catheter is optimally positioned within a few centimeters of the main pulmonary artery bifurcation. To measure the pulmonary capillary wedge pressure (PCWP), the balloon is inflated and floated farther distally into a wedged position. When the balloon is deflated, it should return to its original position, where it sits until it is reinflated for additional measurements. On the chest radiograph, the catheter should not be positioned in a segmental pulmonary artery because of the danger of wedging which, if prolonged, may cause pulmonary arterial obstruction, thrombosis, and infarction in as many as 7% of patients **(Option (B) is false).**[6]

Although the PCWP is the "gold standard" by which many clinical decisions are made, several interacting factors may alter the reading. An accurate wedge pressure reading is dependent upon continuity of pressure between the wedged catheter tip and the left atrium. If the alveolar pressure exceeds the pulmonary capillary pressure, as with high levels of positive pressure ventilation, the microvasculature collapses, and the PCWP determination is inaccurately elevated **(Option (C) is true).** Several factors are important in the relationship between the catheter and the left atrium. These factors are outlined in Figure 14-14.[20,23,24]

When the catheter tip is at or above the left atrium but the left atrial pressure is low, large differences develop between PCWP and left atrial readings. As the left atrial pressure increases, this effect diminishes. As positive end-expiratory pressure (PEEP) is increased, the external pressure on the vessels increases, and differences between these readings also increase. In as many as 40% of patients, the final wedged position of the catheter is at or above the left atrium. Portable lateral chest radiographs taken at the same time as the postcatheterization anteroposterior radiograph may help to confirm the correct position of the catheter tip.[20,23]

In addition to the changes outlined above, the use of PEEP causes many other cardiovascular effects. It usually decreases right and left ventricular preload, increases right ventricular afterload (resistance), decreases left ventricular afterload (resistance), and diminishes the heart rate response to decreased stroke volume. In sum, cardiac output frequently falls at high levels of PEEP.[12]

The intra-aortic counter-pulsation balloon provides support for patients who are hemodynamically compromised. Major indications for counter-pulsation include cardiogenic shock, low output states, pre- and postinfarction angina, and intractable congestive heart failure. The balloon is inflated during diastole and forcibly deflated during systole, a sequence that increases diastolic pressure in the aorta proximal to the balloon, thereby increasing perfusion to the coronary arteries. As the balloon deflates, it helps to propel the blood distally. By decreasing the afterload, the balloon diminishes left ventricular work and myocardial oxygen demand.

The balloon is inserted through a Dacron graft or percutaneously into the femoral artery and advanced retrogradely up the aorta. In most instances, fluoroscopic monitoring is not used. The tip is ideally placed

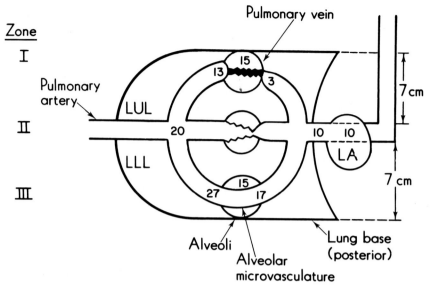

Zone

I

II

III

Pulmonary vein

Pulmonary artery

LUL

LLL

15
13
3
20
10   10
LA
15
27   17

Alveoli

Alveolar microvasculature

Lung base (posterior)

7 cm

7 cm

Figure 14-14. The three-zone model, adapted from Tooker et al. [24], helps explain the interrelationship between catheter position, left atrial pressure, and PEEP. In the diagram of a supine patient, the mean pulmonary artery pressure is 20 cm of H_2O, the alveolar pressure is 15 cm H_2O, and the left atrial pressure is 10 cm of H_2O. In upper zone I, the alveolar pressure exceeds the arterial pressure (15 > 13 cm of H_2O) and will affect the continuity of pressure between the wedged catheter tip and the left atrium (pulmonary venous pressure). In middle zone II, the alveolar pressure exceeds the venous pressure (15 > 10 cm of H_2O) and will also affect the continuity. In lower zone III, the arterial and venous pressures both exceed the alveolar pressure (27 > 17 > 15 cm of H_2O), so that continuity between the wedged arterial catheter tip and the left atrium is present. LUL = left upper lobe; LLL = left lower lobe; LA = left atrium.

distal to the left subclavian artery and appears to be sitting in the aortic knob on portable radiographs **(Option (D) is true).** When the balloon is inflated, the sausage-shaped lucency is visible on the radiograph. If the catheter is advanced too far, it may enter or obstruct the left subclavian artery or other vessels branching from the arch. In the case of a tortuous aorta, the surgeon may underestimate the length of the aorta so that the balloon is positioned more distally than desired in the descending aorta. This position decreases the effectiveness of the counter-pulsation mechanism. When the tip of the catheter is in the mid descending aorta, for example, the fusiform balloon, measuring approximately 26 cm long, may obstruct abdominal aortic vessels. Major complications, such as ischemia distal to the femoral insertion site, aortic injury or dissection, and local wound infection and hemorrhage occur in 7 to 10% of patients.

Flexion of the head and neck causes the endotracheal tube to advance toward the carina, while extension causes the tube to move away from the carina **(Option (E) is true).** The average excursion from flexion to extension is approximately 4 cm. Therefore, a tube tip 3 cm from the carina when the neck is extended may enter the right main bronchus when the neck is flexed. Likewise, a tube tip 3 cm beyond the vocal cords when the neck is flexed may be pulled out of the trachea when the neck is extended.

SUGGESTED READINGS

1. Albelda SM, Gefter WB, Kelley MA, Epstein DM, Miller WT. Ventilator-induced subpleural air cysts: clinical, radiographic, and pathologic significance. Am Rev Respir Dis 1983; 127:360–365
2. Cholankeril JV, Joshi RR, Cenizal JS, Ketyer S, O'Connor WT. Massive air embolism from the pulmonary artery. Radiology 1982; 142:33–34
3. Curtis AM, Knowles GD, Putman CE, McLoud TC, Ravin CE, Smith GJW. The three syndromes of fat embolism: pulmonary manifestations. Yale J Biol Med 1979; 52:149–157
4. Dines DE, Burgher LW, Okazaki H. The clinical and pathologic correlation of fat embolism syndrome. Mayo Clin Proc 1975; 50:407–411
5. Ducatman BS, McMichan JC, Edwards WD. Catheter-induced lesions of the right side of the heart. A one-year prospective study of 141 autopsies. JAMA 1985; 253:791–795
6. Foote GA, Schabel SI, Hodges M. Pulmonary complications of the flow-directed balloon-tipped catheter. N Engl J Med 1974; 290:927–931
7. Friedman PJ. Adult pulmonary ligament pneumatocele: a loculated pneumothorax. Radiology 1985; 155:575–576
8. Godwin JD, Vock P, Osborne DR. CT of the pulmonary ligament. AJR 1983; 141:231–236
9. Kashuk JL, Penn I. Air embolism after central venous catheterization. Surg Gynecol Obstet 1984; 159:249–252
10. Kizer KW, Goodman PC. Radiographic manifestations of venous air embolism. Radiology 1982; 144:35–39
11. Lambert MJ III. Air embolism in central venous catheterization; diagnosis, treatment and prevention. South Med J 1982; 75:1189–1191
12. Lentle BC, Castor WR, Khaliq A, Dierich H. The effect of contrast lymphangiography on localization of ^{67}Ga-citrate. J Nucl Med 1975; 16:374–376
13. Luce JM. The cardiovascular effects of mechanical ventilation and positive end-expiratory pressure. JAMA 1984; 252:807–811

14. Macklin CC. Transport of air along sheaths of pulmonic blood vessels from alveoli to mediastinum. Arch Intern Med 1939; 64:913-926

15. Masson RG, Ruggieri J, Siddiqui MM. Amniotic fluid embolism: definitive diagnosis in a survivor. Am Rev Respir Dis 1979; 120:187–192

16. Maunder RJ, Pierson DJ, Hudson LD. Subcutaneous and mediastinal emphysema. Pathophysiology. Arch Intern Med 1984; 144:1447–1453

17. Naidich TP, Bartelt D, Wheeler PS, Stern WZ. Metallic mercury emboli. AJR 1973; 117:886–891

18. O'Quin RJ, Lakshminarayan S. Venous air embolism. Arch Intern Med 1982; 142:2173–2176

19. Ravin CE, Smith GW, Lester PD, McLoud TC, Putman CE. Post-traumatic pneumatocele in the inferior pulmonary ligament. Radiology 1976; 121:39–41

20. Rohlfing BM, Webb WR, Schlobohm RM. Ventilator-related extra-alveolar air in adults. Radiology 1976; 121:25–31

21. Rost RC Jr, Proto AV. Inferior pulmonary ligament: computed tomographic appearance. Radiology 1983; 148:479–483

22. Shasby DM, Dauber IM, Pfister S, et al. Swan-Ganz catheter location and left atrial pressure determine the accuracy of the wedge pressure when positive end-expiratory pressure is used. Chest 1981; 80:666–670

23. Silvestri RC, Huseby JS, Rughani I, Thorning D, Culver BH. Respiratory distress syndrome from lymphangiography contrast medium. Am Rev Respir Dis 1980; 122:543–945

24. Tooker J, Huseby J, Butler J. The effect of Swan-Ganz catheter height on the wedge pressure—left atrial pressure relationships in edema during positive-pressure ventilation. Am Rev Respir Dis 1978; 117:721–725

25. Vas W, Tuttle RJ, Zylak CJ. Intravenous self-administration of metallic mercury. Radiology 1980; 137:313–315

26. Von Hugo R, Graeff H. Thrombohemorrhagic complications in the obstetric patient. In: Colman RW, Hirsh J, Marder VJ, Salzman EW (eds), Hemostasis and thrombosis. Basic principles and clinical practice. Philadelphia: JB Lippincott; 1987:926–941

27. Wechsler RJ, Byrne KJ, Steiner RM. The misplaced thoracic venous catheter: detailed anatomical consideration. CRC Crit Rev Diagn Imaging 1984; 21:289–305

28. Westcott JL, Cole SR. Interstitial pulmonary emphysema in children and adults: roentgenographic features. Radiology 1974; 111:367–378

Notes

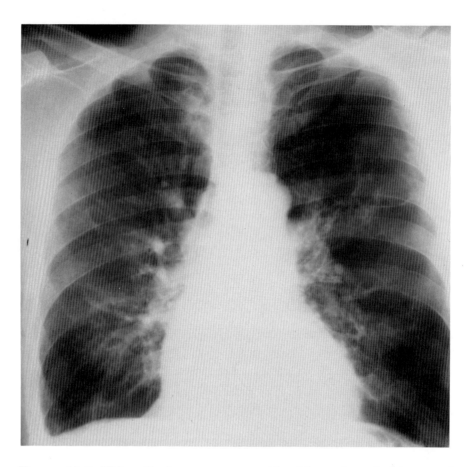

Figure 15-1. This elderly man presented with a 1-week history of shortness of breath. You are shown a posteroanterior chest radiograph taken at the time of admission.

Case 15: Emphysema with Pulmonary Edema

Question 76

Which *one* of the following is the MOST likely diagnosis?

(A) Emphysema with pulmonary edema
(B) Adult respiratory distress syndrome
(C) Emphysema with pneumonia
(D) Swyer-James syndrome
(E) Alpha-1-antitrypsin deficiency

Figure 15-1 shows evidence of severe emphysema with upper lobe bullae on the left, oligemic areas, and low hemidiaphragms. Additional findings include markedly distended right upper lobe vessels, enlarged and somewhat indistinct hila, peribronchial cuffing (Figure 15-2), end-on vessels larger than adjacent bronchi, and effusion at the right costophrenic angle. The heart appears somewhat larger than expected for the severe emphysema present (the heart is usually smaller). All in all, the radiographic appearance suggests pulmonary edema (asymmetrical) in a patient with emphysema **(Option (A) is the most likely diagnosis).**

The diagnosis of congestive heart failure with pulmonary edema in the presence of emphysema may be difficult both clinically and radiographically. Frequently, patients do not have a history of cardiac disease but experience an insidious onset of mild cough, dyspnea, and fatigue, all of which may be incorrectly attributed to worsening emphysema or emphysema with infection. When the edema is interstitial, rales are not heard. When the edema is alveolar, rales may be falsely attributed to bronchitis, retained secretions, or pneumonia. The chest radiograph may be equally misleading, since features such as a thickened interstitium, peribronchial cuffing, and redistribution of blood flow to upper lobe vessels may be seen in emphysema uncomplicated by congestive heart failure and pulmonary edema.

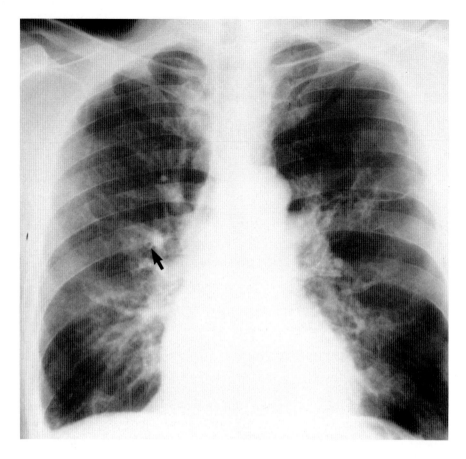

Figure 15-2 (Same as Figure 15-1). Emphysema with pulmonary edema. Note the peribronchial cuffing (arrow).

Careful comparison with prior radiographs is essential in diagnosing mild edema complicating emphysema. Clues to congestive failure and edema in a patient with emphysema include a mild increase in heart size, an increased size of vessels, and increased peribronchial cuffing. The interstitial edema may cause focal areas of haziness with blurring of the hilar vessels. In some patients, the decreased lung compliance with edema causes a decreased level of inflation. Thus, congestive heart failure and edema may change some of the radiographic findings of severe emphysema to more normal appearances: less hyperinflation and less of a decrease in heart size. Bed rest, treatment for congestive heart failure, and serial chest radiographs may help in proving the diagnosis (Figure 15-3).[12,17]

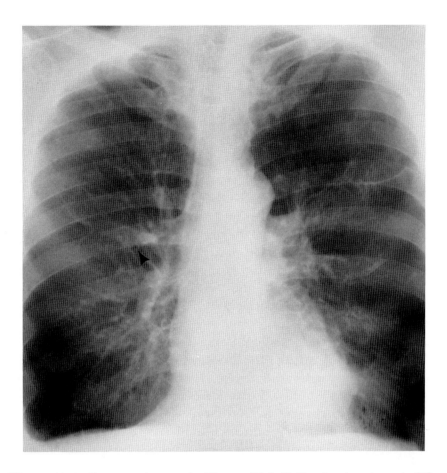

Figure 15-3. Same patient as in Figure 15-1. Following treatment of the patient, the chest radiograph improved considerably. Note that the upper lobe vessels on the right and both hila are smaller and better defined, and that the peribronchial cuffing has improved (arrowhead). Moreover, the heart is now slightly smaller.

Emphysema with pneumonia (Option (C)) is a reasonable consideration. However, considering the constellation of radiographic findings described and the absence of fever, emphysema with pulmonary edema is a better choice.

The Swyer-James syndrome (Option (D)) classically shows a unilateral hyperlucent lung (sometimes the entire lung is not involved) with contralateral hyperperfusion.[4] In this syndrome, the involved hemithorax is normal or slightly diminished in volume and has smaller-than-usual peripheral and central vessels. These features are not seen in the test case.

Alpha-1-antitrypsin deficiency (Option (E)) is an inherited disorder leading to emphysema in adulthood. The genetics are complex, but for practical purposes the clinical syndrome is only present in homozygotes. Unlike the more common forms of emphysema, there is no sex predilection. The disease is usually apparent by 40 years of age, and progression is usually rapid. Bronchitis, with cough and sputum production, is an infrequent problem.

The radiographic appearance of alpha-1-antitryspin deficiency is distinctive. There is severe panacinar emphysema predominantly in the lower zone of each lung (unlike the predominant upper zone changes in the test case). Accordingly, the lower zones show hyperlucency and diminished vascularity, while the upper zones show increased vascularity (Figures 15-4 and 15-5). In the more common form of panacinar emphysema, the lung disease is more evenly distributed, although basilar predominance may be seen.[4]

Although the edema of the adult respiratory distress syndrome (Option (B)) usually appears patchy with a widespread symmetrical distribution, it may be an asymmetrical process. However, the adult respiratory distress syndrome, which is due to increased capillary permeability, is preceded by a major event (shock, trauma, sepsis, etc.). Symptoms of the adult respiratory distress syndrome usually surface 24 hours after the insult. The patient presented in the test case had neither the precipitating event nor the characteristic progression of symptoms of the adult respiratory distress syndrome.

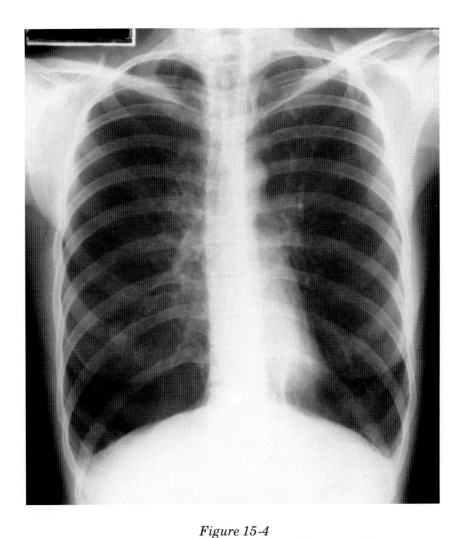

Figure 15-4

Figures 15-4 and 15-5. Alpha-1-antitrypsin deficiency. The posteroanterior radiograph (Figure 15-4) of this 39-year-old woman shows severe flattening of the hemidiaphragms, diminished vascularity in the lower zones of both lungs, and increased vascularity in the upper zones of the lungs. The heart appears small. The supine tomogram (Figure 15-5) demonstrates similar findings.

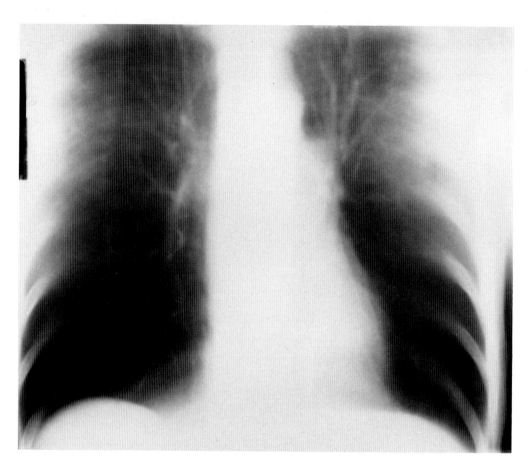

Figure 15-5

Question 77

Concerning the adult respiratory distress syndrome,

- (A) shock is a prerequisite for its development
- (B) the radiographic opacities usually lag behind the patient's symptoms for the first 24 to 36 hours
- (C) pulmonary opacities usually start peripherally and progress centrally
- (D) increased pulmonary capillary permeability is a prominent feature
- (E) its diagnosis requires lung biopsy

The adult respiratory distress syndrome is the final common pathway for numerous severe bodily insults that may involve the lungs directly or indirectly. The hallmarks of the adult respiratory distress syndrome are impaired lung mechanics, disordered gas exchange, intrapulmonary shunting, and opacities on the chest radiograph. These all combine to produce a hypoxia that is difficult to reverse with conventional support.

This syndrome first drew attention as a battlefield problem in Vietnam. The usual sequence of events included a battlefield injury leading to considerable blood loss, shock, and treatment with massive transfusions. The patient often appeared to be improving but then took a sudden turn for the worse on the following day. The terms "shock lung," "Da Nang lung," and "traumatic wet lung" were used to describe these patients. In the years that followed, it became apparent that similiar clinical, physiologic, and radiologic abnormalities may appear in civilian life for reasons other than shock (Tables 15-1 and 15-2) **(Option (A) is false)**.[1,3,5,16,19]

The evolution of the adult respiratory distress syndrome is traditionally described in terms of four discrete phases. However, these may not be clearly identifiable, and their speed of progression is variable. It may take hours to days to develop the full-blown syndrome, depending on the nature of the initial injury. In the first phase, immediately after the initial injury, there may be no clinical evidence of respiratory difficulty, or there may be early evidence of hyperventilation, tachypnea, dyspnea, and hypocarbia without auscultatory evidence of pulmonary disease. This may be followed by a brief period (second phase) of clinical stability, although hyperventilation and hypocarbia may persist, with evidence of shunting and decreased compliance. Also, in the second phase (24 to 36 hours after the injury), good-quality radiographs may appear normal or show the first signs of interstitial edema rapidly progressing to alveolar edema (Figure 15-6) **(Option (B) is true)**. The patient's low lung volumes may be reflected on the radiograph as an appearance of "poor inspiration."

Table 15-1. Diseases Associated with the Adult Respiratory Distress Syndrome

Amniotic fluid embolism	High-altitude pulmonary edema
Arterial emboli	Major surgery
Aspiration	Malaria
Bowel infarction	Multiple transfusions
Burns and smoke inhalation	Oxygen toxicity
Carcinomatosis	Pancreatitis
Cardiopulmonary bypass	Peripheral vascular disease
Clostridial sepsis	Pulmonary contusion
Disseminated intravascular coagulation	Radiation pneumonitis
Drug abuse	Ruptured aneurysm
Eclampsia	Shock (hypovolemic or endotoxic)
Fat embolism	Transfusion reaction
Fractures	Transplantation
Gram-negative sepsis	Trauma
Heat stroke	Viral pneumonia (influenza)

*From: Goodman LR, Putman CE (eds), Intensive care radiology: imaging of the critically ill. Philadelphia: WB Saunders, 1983:114–123

Table 15-2. Synonyms for the Adult Respiratory Distress Syndrome

Adult hyaline membrane disease	Progressive respiratory distress
Adult respiratory insufficiency syndrome	Pulmonary edema
Bronchopulmonary dysplasia	Pulmonary hyaline membrane disease
Congestive atelectasis	Pulmonary microembolism
Da Nang lung	Pump lung
Fat embolism	Respirator lung
Hemorrhagic lung syndrome	Shock lung
Oxygen toxicity	Solid lung syndrome
Postperfusion lung syndrome	Stiff lung syndrome
Post-transfusion lung	Transplant lung
Post-traumatic atelectasis	Traumatic wet lung
Post-traumatic pulmonary insufficiency	Wet lung
Progressive pulmonary consolidation	White lung syndrome

*From: Goodman LR, Putman CE (eds), Intensive care radiology: imaging of the critically ill. Philadelphia: WB Saunders; 1983:114–123

During the third phase, respiratory insufficiency progresses to the point where mechanical ventilation and supplemental oxygen are required. The lungs become stiffer, with evidence of increased intrapulmonary shunting and increased physiologic dead space. Interstitial edema rapidly gives way to diffuse alveolar edema (Figure 15-7). The radiographic appearance then stabilizes and, depending on the severity

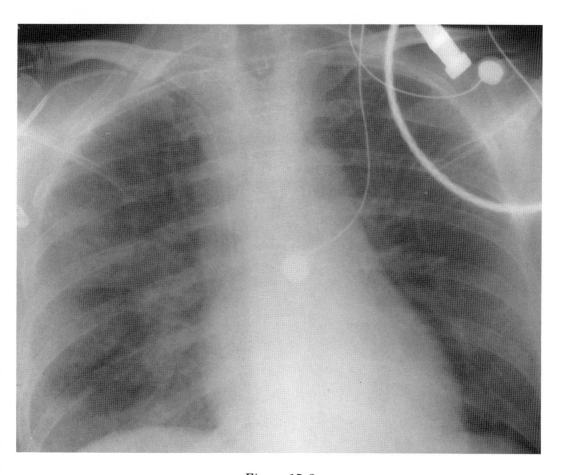

Figure 15-6

Figures 15-6 and 15-7. Adult respiratory distress syndrome. Two days after a colectomy for Crohn's disease, this 40-year-old woman developed increasing respiratory difficulty. Her preoperative chest radiograph and first postoperative one were negative. A view taken approximately 48 hours after surgery (Figure 15-6) shows some patchy areas of consolidation bilaterally along with a mild interstitial edema pattern. The heart is not enlarged. A Swan-Ganz catheter inserted shortly thereafter showed a normal wedge pressure. The patient's condition deteriorated. A radiograph obtained several hours after intubation (Figure 15-7) showed a marked progression in bilateral edema. The heart is not enlarged, and there is no evidence of pleural effusion. A radiograph obtained on the following day showed a slight further increase in edema.

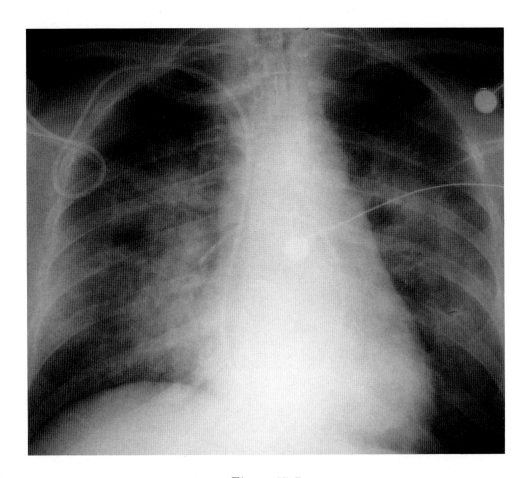

Figure 15-7

of the injury, may vary from patchy areas of consolidation to almost complete parenchymal opacification. Pre-existing pulmonary disease (e.g., emphysema, pulmonary embolism) or acute pulmonary disease (e.g., aspiration, contusion) may cause an asymmetrical edema pattern. In most instances, the diffuse capillary injury produces diffuse lung disease without a predilection for specific areas (**Option (C) is false).**

During the fourth phase, the intrapulmonary shunting increases further, and carbon dioxide and lactic acid levels both increase to result in metabolic and respiratory acidosis. Secondary infection and secondary organ failure may be present at this time. The radiographic appearance is often stable, despite the patient's worsening condition. The initiation of positive end-expiratory pressure during the third or fourth phase may cause an artificial hyperinflation of the lungs, so that they appear less opaque and falsely improved.[20]

Increased pulmonary capillary permeability is the major event evident early in the adult respiratory distress syndrome, regardless of the etiologic event **(Option (D) is true).** Numerous mechanisms appear to combine to make the capillaries more permeable. Complement activation causes leukocyte aggregation in the lungs, and aggregated neutrophils liberate toxic oxygen radicals and proteases that injure the endothelial cells. Many other factors, such as coagulopathy, platelet abnormalities, and microemboli, have been implicated.

In addition to edema, atelectasis is another major feature of the adult respiratory distress syndrome and occurs for several reasons. Interstitial edema decreases pulmonary compliance and leads to shallow breathing. Edema and secretions may plug peripheral airways. Surfactant, which normally lines the pulmonary alveolar surfaces and acts as an anti-atelectasis factor, is diminished. Type II pneumocytes responsible for surfactant production are injured, and with diminished surfactant, surface tension increases during expiration and atelectasis results.

As the name implies, the adult respiratory distress syndrome is a syndrome consisting of progressive respiratory distress with severe hypoxia, rigid lungs, and characteristic radiographic findings. Although there are certain histologic features that occur in each of its four phases, lung biopsy is not required to make the diagnosis **(Option (E) is false).** During the first phase, the lungs may be normal, or there may be evidence of interstitial edema or fibrin platelet emboli, with minimal hemorrhage. This is followed by vascular congestion, increased edema, and atelectasis. As these abnormalities increase, there are intra-alveolar hemorrhage and formation of hyaline membranes. In the final phase, there is a proliferation of reparative cells, and, if the process does not reverse itself, severe fibrosis results.

Although the term "adult respiratory distress syndrome" is helpful both in conceptualizing the final common pathway for various etiologies of lung injury and in formulating a plan for support and therapy of the patient, some have suggested abandoning it. Many consider that lumping a diverse collection of diseases into a single entity neglects the underlying initiating mechanism and compromises further thought. One misses the opportunity to understand the pathogenesis, natural history, prevention, treatment, and prognosis of these diseases. "Gradually, most clinics have adopted an intermediate position which takes the etiology into account; not only is the distinctive picture of respiratory insufficiency identified, but its etiology is also indicated, e.g., 'adult respiratory distress syndrome secondary to pancreatitis.' "[2,3]

Question 78

Conditions associated with unilateral or asymmetrical pulmonary edema include:

(A) rapid re-expansion of the lung after a pneumothorax or hydrothorax
(B) pulmonary embolism
(C) left atrial myxoma
(D) gravitational shift in a patient with congestive heart failure

Many conditions have been associated with unilateral or asymmetrical pulmonary edema. The atypical distribution of fluid may be due to asymmetrical edema formation or asymmetrical edema resorption. Factors that influence edema formation include pulmonary perfusion, pulmonary hydrostatic pressure, and capillary permeability. Factors that limit edema resorption include obstruction of lymphatic drainage and interference with the bellows function of the lungs.

A well-known, but somewhat uncommon, cause of unilateral pulmonary edema is rapid re-expansion of the lung after a pneumothorax or hydrothorax **(Option (A) is true).** Although the majority of cases have occurred after the lung has been collapsed for many days or when excessive negative pressure has been applied to the chest tube, such is not always the case. Edema has been reported with less than 48 hours of collapse and with relatively gentle suction. The edema is usually diffusely distributed in the re-expanded lung (Figure 15-8). Although it is usually present immediately, it may increase for 24 hours. In a patient with a normal cardiopulmonary reserve, the edema is of minor clinical significance. In compromised patients, however, it may be a potentially fatal problem. The edema usually subsides over several days without specific therapy. The pathophysiology of the injury has not been thoroughly elucidated. However, increased capillary permeability secondary to endothelial damage appears to be a responsible mechanism.[8,10]

Pulmonary embolism may cause asymmetrical or local pulmonary edema by several mechanisms **(Option (B) is true).** In patients who survive a massive pulmonary embolism, edema may develop in the areas not occluded by the emboli. Since a large amount of blood flow is diverted to the relatively normal areas, there is a high precapillary hydrostatic pressure, along with a high flow. This causes an "overperfusion"

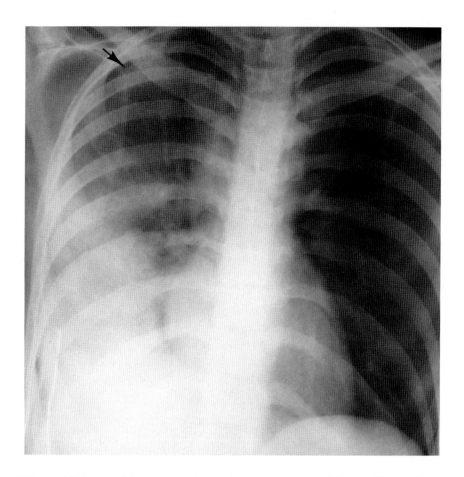

Figure 15-8. Rapid re-expansion pulmonary edema. This radiograph was taken several hours after a chest tube had been inserted for a hydropneumothorax of unknown duration. There is diffuse consolidation of the lower half of the right lung as well as more moderate consolidation of the upper half. A small pneumothorax persists (arrow). The left lung is clear and had normal vessels, and the heart is not enlarged. The right pulmonary edema cleared over the next 2 days.

pulmonary edema due to hydrostatic pressure forces. In other circumstances, patients with a pulmonary embolism may develop congestive heart failure or increased permeability edema unrelated to the embolic disease. Because the embolism prevents perfusion to the involved lung, edema does not form in this area. The edema forms elsewhere in the lung, where perfusion is normal, and does not, therefore, appear symmetrical (Figures 15-9 and 15-10). A variation on this theme is the development

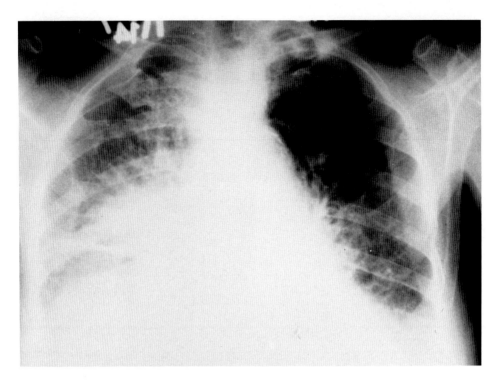

Figure 15-9

Figures 15-9 and 15-10. Asymmetrical pulmonary edema with pulmonary embolism. This middle-aged woman with long-standing mitral valve disease presented with signs of congestive heart failure. Her anteroposterior radiograph (Figure 15-9) shows an enlarged heart, bilateral pleural effusions, and pulmonary edema of the right lung and the lower half of the left lung; the upper half of the left lung is spared. Her pulmonary angiogram (Figure 15-10) demonstrates flow to the edematous areas and no flow to the upper half of the left lung.

of congestive heart failure and pulmonary edema in a patient with a pneumothorax. In such an instance, only the normal lung is adequately perfused and thus capable of developing edema. When the collapsed lung is re-expanded, it does not appear edematous. If the left ventricular problem is not corrected, edema should eventually appear in the re-expanded lung as well.[9,18]

Gravity has a major influence on the distribution of pulmonary blood flow and capillary hydrostatic pressure. Whether the patient is in the erect, supine, prone, or decubitus position, capillary hydrostatic pressure increases in the dependent areas and causes a balance of forces to favor escape of fluid from the capillaries to the interstitium. The shift of blood

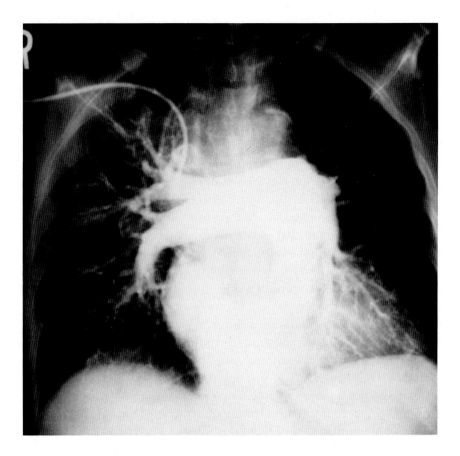

Figure 15-10

to the dependent areas is exaggerated further in patients on positive pressure ventilation. In the normal lung, these shifts have little effect on lung water, since pulmonary lymphatics are capable of increasing their capacity at least 10-fold to keep the lung relatively dry. In patients with pulmonary edema, the hydrostatic forces cause edema formation at a rate greater than that at which the already overtaxed lymphatics are able to function. Thus, edema forms predominantly in the dependent areas. In the upright patient, edema occurs predominantly in the lung bases, whereas in the supine patient, it occurs predominantly posteriorly. Likewise, patients lying in the decubitus position develop edema in the dependent lung **(Option (D) is true).**

This phenomenon of gravity dependence may be used to diagnostic advantage. In acutely ill patients it is sometimes difficult to distinguish pulmonary edema from other types of diffuse consolidation (pneumonia, etc.). If the patient is placed on his or her side with the least-diseased lung dependent for 2 hours, a repeat radiograph will show shifting of the edema toward the dependent side, whereas other diseases will not be altered by this maneuver. In a carefully controlled study of 33 patients, Zimmerman et al. found the positive predictive value of shift to be 84% (Figures 15-11 and 15-12).[21]

A frequent cause of asymmetrical pulmonary edema is congestive heart failure complicating emphysema. Emphysema destroys the capillary bed in a nonuniform fashion. In their classic article, Hublitz and Shapiro discussed the various patterns and speculated on the physiology of the same.[7] They basically identified two major patterns. The first, designated as a regional pattern, showed edema in some areas, while other areas remained relatively free of edema. The areas with edema corresponded to areas showing a relatively normal vascular bed on the chest radiograph or on the pulmonary angiogram. Conversely, the areas without edema corresponded to those showing a diminished vascular bed on the chest radiograph, pulmonary angiogram, or pulmonary perfusion scintigram. The second pattern identified was one of asymmetrically altered interstitial "markings." The interstitial markings varied from coarse interstitial lines (Kerley A and B lines) to a diffuse reticular pattern (Kerley C lines) to a fine miliary nodular pattern. These patterns were considered to be due to a decreased ability of the lymphatic system to clear the lung of edema. The authors postulated that emphysema altered the local lymphatics, decreased pulmonary compliance, and decreased elasticity. In addition, the decreased ventilation of the emphysematous lung was said to diminish the pumping action necessary to promote lymphatic drainage.[7,12,15]

Other, less frequently encountered causes of unilateral or asymmetrical edema include focal congenital or acquired pulmonary arterial disease (e.g., pulmonary artery hypoplasia, arterial invasion by tumor), other causes of lung disease (e.g., the Swyer-James syndrome), and unilateral veno-occlusive disease or unilateral obstruction of lymphatics (e.g., by tumor or radiation). The cause of asymmetrical edema may not be apparent from clinical and radiographic examinations. However, recurrent bouts of edema tend to appear in the same areas. A left atrial myxoma, which may obstruct the mitral valve, would not be expected to cause a focal increase in venous pressure and thus should not produce asymmetrical edema **(Option (C) is false).**

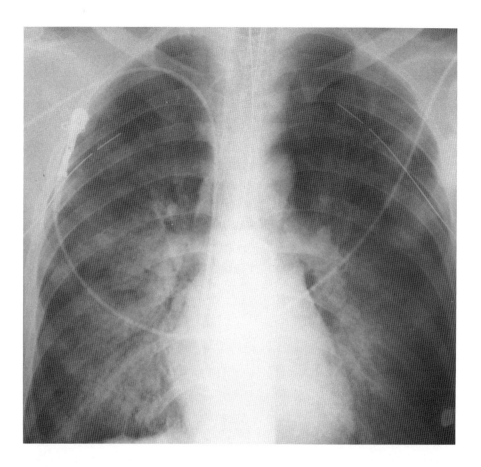

Figure 15-11

Figures 15-11 and 15-12. Gravitational shift of pulmonary edema. The patient had the adult respiratory distress syndrome due to venous air embolism and severe fluid overload (14.5 L net positive balance and a pulmonary wedge pressure of 20 mm Hg). The supine radiograph (Figure 15-11) shows bilateral pulmonary edema, more severe on the right than the left. A repeat radiograph (Figure 15-12) obtained after the patient had been in the left lateral decubitus position for 2 hours shows increased edema in the dependent left lung and decreased edema in the nondependent right lung. This positive gravitational shift test indicated that there was mobilizable lung water. Diuretics were administered, and the patient's urine output was 8.5 L over the next 48 hours. This led to partial clearing of the edema bilaterally. A repeat shift test (not shown) again was positive on the dependent side. Additional diuresis resulted in further clearing. (Reprinted with permission from Zimmerman et al. [21].)

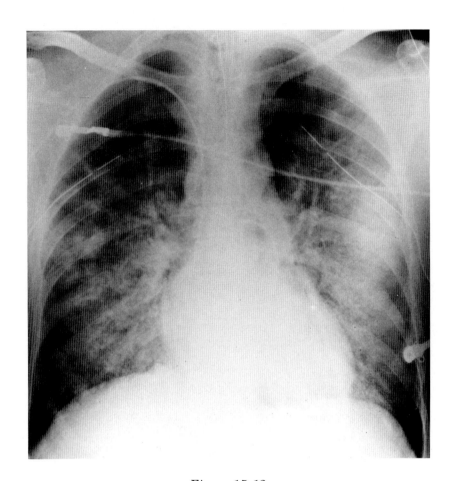

Figure 15-12

Question 79

Regarding obstructive pulmonary disease,

(A) the chest radiograph is a sensitive indicator of mild emphysema
(B) redistribution of blood flow to the upper lobes in a patient with emphysema indicates concomitant left heart failure
(C) hyperinflation is a more prominent feature of centrilobular than of panacinar emphysema
(D) a unilateral hyperinflated lung with a large hemithorax strongly suggests the Swyer-James syndrome

The radiographic diagnosis of emphysema is difficult. Emphysema, as defined by various international congresses, is a diagnosis based on anatomic examination of the lung rather than on clinical, functional, or radiologic features. Some define emphysema as enlargement of air spaces beyond the terminal bronchioles. Some definitions require lung destruction, while others do not.[4,6,14] Further difficulty arises with regard to the subgroups into which emphysema has been categorized. These subgroups, which are helpful for didactic purposes, are not often present in pure form. They are panacinar (panlobular), centriacinar (centrilobular), paraseptal, focal dust, and compensatory emphysema.

Panacinar emphysema destroys lung tissue distal to the terminal bronchioles, resulting in generalized hyperinflation and symptoms associated with the "pink puffer." In its pure form, it corresponds to "arterial deficiency" emphysema, in which overinflated and oligemic areas of pulmonary destruction are seen.[4]

Centriacinar emphysema causes destruction at the center of the acinus, altering the respiratory bronchioles but sparing the more distal alveolar ducts and alveoli. Ongoing proximal destruction is often associated with inflammation and mucous plugging. Marked hyperinflation is not a major component **(Option (C) is false),** and the patient's symptoms are most often those of the "blue bloater." This type of emphysema is often associated with chronic bronchitis, which is a disease defined on clinical rather than pathologic grounds. Chronic bronchitis refers to chronic or recurrent sputum production occurring for at least 3 consecutive months and for at least 2 successive years without another identifiable cause. The radiographic appearance of centriacinar emphysema corresponds to "increased markings" emphysema, in which the pulmonary markings are often prominent, irregular, and indistinct rather than attenuated.[4] The lung has the appearance of the so-called "dirty chest." Signs of pulmonary artery hypertension, with or without cardiac enlargement, are usually present.

Paraseptal emphysema is a mild form of peripheral bulla formation along septa, and it is seldom of clinical significance. This type of emphysema is more easily seen on axial computed tomography sections than on conventional chest radiographs. Focal dust emphysema resembles centriacinar emphysema and is seen in patients with occupational exposure to carbon dust. Compensatory emphysema is basically overinflation of the lung without evidence of pulmonary destruction. It is a response of the normal lung to volume loss elsewhere in the thorax.

Asthma, like chronic bronchitis, has a clinical definition: reversible bronchial obstruction elicited by various stimuli. Although its clinical hallmark is wheezing, wheezing may be seen in many other conditions, such as chronic bronchitis, congestive heart failure, pulmonary embolism, foreign body aspiration, etc.

With this wide overlapping spectrum of diseases defined in various ways, it is very difficult to judge the sensitivity of the chest radiograph in diagnosing them. The majority of studies based on radiologic correlation with clinical, functional, or autopsy findings indicate that the chest radiograph will diagnose most cases of severe emphysema and miss most cases of mild emphysema **(Option (A) is false)**. Fraser and Paré emphasize that moderate success may be achieved only by recognizing the two distinct patterns, arterial deficiency as generally seen in panacinar emphysema and increased markings as seen in centriacinar emphysema with or without chronic bronchitis.

Milne and Bass[11] present a dissenting point of view regarding radiologic recognition of emphysema. Pathologic grading, which is the gold standard, is strictly a morphologic measure of the amount of visible disease. The pathologic severity may not correlate with the amount of disability experienced by the patient during life. The authors developed a clinical severity index based on smoking history, clinical signs and symptoms, and pulmonary function tests. Using the clinical/functional index as the gold standard and a specific set of criteria for grading radiographs, they found a good correlation between the radiologic diagnosis of emphysema and the clinical/functional assessment of disease.

Although panacinar emphysema tends to involve the lungs diffusely, it usually is more severe in the lower zones. When this is the case, the capillary bed is destroyed at the lung bases, with resultant shunting of blood to the upper zones. Therefore, prominent upper zone vessels may be seen without evidence of left heart failure **(Option (B) is false)**. Similarly, if the capillary bed is destroyed predominantly in one hemithorax, hyperperfusion may be evident on the opposite side. In patients with prominent upper zone vessels resulting from congestive heart failure, interstitial edema often produces basilar haziness or indistinct margins of the lower zone vessels. In patients with basilar emphysema who do not have edema, basilar vessels may be sparse, but they should be sharply marginated.

Although the Swyer-James syndrome is a form of lobar or unilateral obstructive airways disease, ipsilateral hyperinflation is not a common feature. The obliterative bronchiolitis that occurs during childhood causes obstruction, but the injury to the growing lung probably retards its growth. Therefore, the involved hemithorax is usually normal or small in size **(Option (D) is false)**.

SUGGESTED READINGS

1. Divertie MB. The adult respiratory distress syndrome. Mayo Clin Proc 1982; 57:371–378
2. Effros RM, Mason GR. An end to "ARDS" (editorial). Chest 1986; 89:162–163
3. Fishman AP. Adult respiratory distress syndrome. In: Fishman AP (ed), Pulmonary diseases and disorders, vol II. New York: McGraw-Hill; 1980:1667–1681
4. Fraser RG, Paré JAP. Diagnosis of diseases of the chest. Philadelphia: WB Saunders; 1979:1297–1473
5. Greene R, Jantsch H, Boggis C, Strauss HW, Lowenstein E. Respiratory distress syndrome with new considerations. Radiol Clin North Am 1983; 21:699–708
6. Heitzman ER, Markarian B, Solomon J. Chronic obstructive pulmonary disease: a review, emphasizing roentgen pathologic correlation. Radiol Clin North Am 1973; 11:49–75
7. Hublitz UF, Shapiro JH. Atypical pulmonary patterns of congestive failure in chronic lung disease. The influence of pre-existing disease on the appearance and distribution of pulmonary edema. Radiology 1969; 93:995–1006
8. Humphreys RL, Berne AS. Rapid re-expansion of pneumothorax. A cause of unilateral pulmonary edema. Radiology 1970; 96:509–512
9. Hyers TM, Fowler AA, Wicks AB. Focal pulmonary edema after massive pulmonary embolism. Am Rev Respir Dis 1981; 123:232–233
10. Mahajan VK. Re-expansion pulmonary edema (editorial). Chest 1983; 83:4
11. Milne ENC, Bass H. The roentgenologic diagnosis of early chronic obstructive pulmonary disease. J Can Assoc Radiol 1969; 20:3–15
12. Milne ENC, Bass H. Roentgenologic and functional analysis of combined chronic obstructive pulmonary disease and congestive cardiac failure. Invest Radiol 1969; 4:129–147

13. Putman CE, Ravin CE. Adult respiratory distress syndrome. In: Goodman LR, Putman CE (eds), Intensive care radiology: imaging of the critically ill. Philadelphia: WB Saunders; 1983:114–122

14. Reich SB, Weinshelbaum A, Yee J. Correlation of radiographic measurements and pulmonary function tests in chronic obstructive pulmonary disease. AJR 1985; 144:695–699

15. Rigler LG, Surprenant EL. Pulmonary edema. Semin Roentgenol 1967; 2:33–48

16. Rinaldo JE, Rogers RM. Adult respiratory-distress syndrome: changing concepts of lung injury and repair. N Engl J Med 1982; 306:900–909

17. Rosenow EC III, Harrison CE Jr. Congestive heart failure masquerading as primary pulmonary disease. Chest 1970; 58:28–36

18. Steckel RJ. Unilateral pulmonary edema after pneumothorax. N Engl J Med 1973; 289:621–622

19. Unger KM, Shibel EM, Moser KM. Detection of left ventricular failure in patients with adult respiratory distress syndrome. Chest 1975; 67:8–13

20. Zimmerman JE, Goodman LR, Shahvari MBG. Effect of mechanical ventilation and positive end-expiratory pressure (PEEP) on chest radiograph. AJR 1979; 133:811–815

21. Zimmerman JE, Goodman LR, St. Andre AC, Wyman AC. Radiographic detection of mobilizable lung water: the gravitational shift test. AJR 1982; 138:59–64

Notes

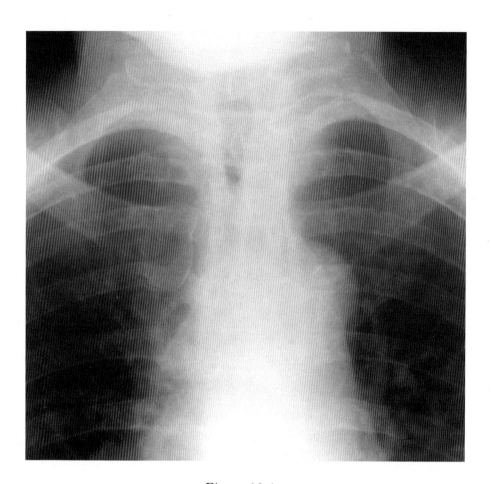

Figure 16-1
Figures 16-1 and 16-2. This 56-year-old woman presented with insidious onset of shortness of breath over the last 6 to 12 months. You are shown anteroposterior (Figure 16-1) and oblique (Figure 16-2) radiographs of the upper thorax.

Case 16: Postintubation Tracheal Stenosis

Question 80

Which *one* of the following is the MOST likely diagnosis?

(A) Saber-sheath trachea
(B) Laryngotracheal papillomatosis
(C) Mounier-Kuhn syndrome
(D) Postintubation tracheal stenosis
(E) Tracheoesophageal fistula

The anteroposterior radiograph (Figure 16-1) shows that the trachea is narrowed just above the thoracic inlet. Its left-to-right dimension at the level of the clavicles is approximately 45% of that in the upper cervical trachea. There is neither tracheal deviation nor a mass in the neck or upper mediastinum. The oblique radiograph (Figure 16-2) shows the trachea to better advantage, demonstrating that the narrowing is concentric and that the intrathoracic trachea appears spared. Whether studying the trachea with conventional radiographs, xeroradiographs, or tomograms, right-angle views are essential to fully appreciate any abnormality of this cylindrical structure, since a mass may compress the trachea in one plane and completely spare it in another. For the low cervical trachea and upper thoracic trachea, the lateral view is often inadequate because of the shoulders. Oblique views or lateral tomograms are often required (Figure 16-3).

Of the five choices offered, postintubation tracheal stenosis is the most likely diagnosis **(Option (D) is correct).** A focal narrowing for several centimeters above the thoracic inlet is typical in location for postintubation tracheal stenosis due to cuff injury. The narrowing is often concentric but not necessarily uniform. Symptoms of postintubation stenosis are usually gradual in onset and start several weeks after extubation. However, in this case, the onset of shortness of breath was extremely

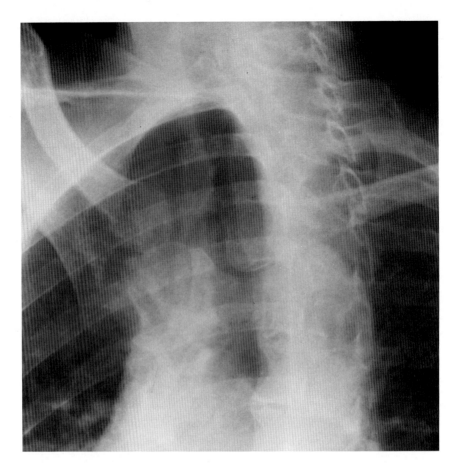

Figure 16-2

gradual; both the patient and her physician had attributed the dyspnea to her underlying cardiopulmonary disease.

The occurrence of postintubation tracheal injuries has diminished since the high-volume, low-pressure cuff has replaced the low-volume, high-pressure cuff. The new cuff seals the trachea with less pressure on the mucosa. Following extubation, there is bronchoscopic evidence of mucosal injury in the majority of patients. In most cases, however, either the trachea heals completely or the patient is left with some minimal tracheal narrowing of no clinical significance. Symptomatic obstruction is usually first noticed when there is a 50 to 75% narrowing of the trachea or when its diameter is reduced to 5 to 6 mm. While long-term complications of endotracheal intubation result from injury to the glottis,

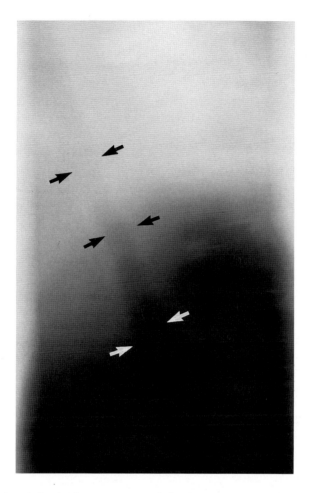

Figure 16-3. A lateral tomogram of the patient shown in Figures 16-1 and 16-2 demonstrates a long segment of tracheal narrowing (black arrows). The white arrows delineate the lower extent of the lesion.

subglottis, and the trachea at the level of the cuff and tube tip, major sites of injury following tracheostomy include the anterior tracheal wall just above the stoma, the level of the stoma itself, and the level of the cuff and tube tip (Figure 16-4).

Evaluation of the trachea should include its entire length from the vocal cords to the carina (Figures 16-5, 16-6, and 16-7). Multiple stenotic lesions are not infrequent. Anteroposterior and lateral tomograms are usually adequate to demonstrate areas of fixed stenosis and to approximate lengths of lesions (Figures 16-8, 16-9, and 16-10). Such static

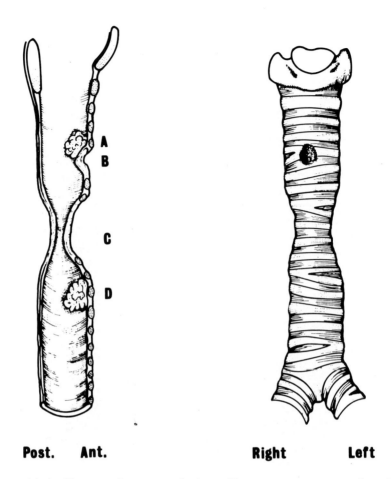

Post.   Ant.   **Right   Left**

Figure 16-4.   Post-tracheostomy lesions. Four common types of tracheal injury are: (A) polypoid granuloma above the stoma; (B) posterior depression of the anterior tracheal wall at the stoma; (C) circumferential narrowing of the trachea at the cuff site; and (D) polypoid granuloma along the anterior wall of the tube tip. (Reprinted with permission from Goodman and Putman [10].)

images, however, are inadequate for evaluating dynamic changes. Fluoroscopy, with videotaping if available, is required to evaluate cord motion and areas of tracheomalacia. Positive-contrast tracheography is the most definitive study for evaluating the length and dynamic character of a stenotic lesion prior to corrective surgery (Figure 16-11). Computed tomography (CT) does not adequately evaluate the length of the narrowed segment or its dynamic character.[6,7,9,10,12-14,20,21]

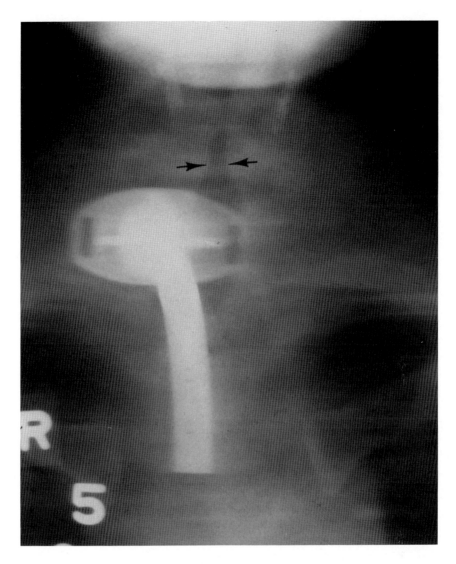

Figure 16-5
Figures 16-5 through 16-7. Severe subglottic stenosis after prolonged endotracheal intubation. The anteroposterior tomogram (Figure 16-5) shows concave margins at the subglottic trachea (arrows). On the lateral tomogram (Figure 16-6), the subglottic airway is not well demonstrated. Whenever possible, the trachea should be evaluated without the tracheostomy tube in place so as to avoid overlooking other major lesions. A portable radiograph taken several months earlier (Figure 16-7), while the patient was intubated, demonstrates the overdistended tracheal cuff in the subglottic airway (arrows). Compare the size of the balloon with the normal width of the trachea (arrowheads). (Case courtesy of Barbara Rohlfing, M.D., San Francisco, Calif.)

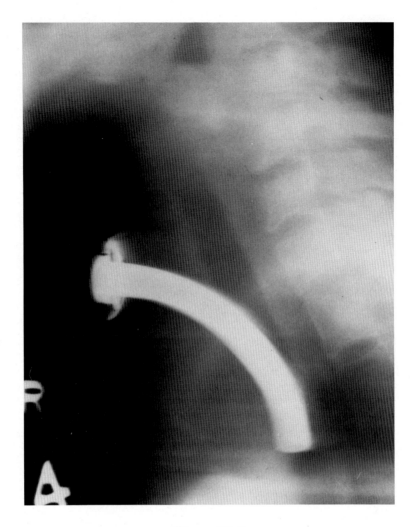

Figure 16-6

The other choices offered in the test question have different radiographic appearances than postintubation tracheal stenosis. The saber-sheath trachea (Option (A)) is usually seen in patients with chronic obstructive pulmonary disease. The frontal radiograph (Figure 16-12) demonstrates right-to-left narrowing of the trachea from the thoracic inlet to the carina, while the cervical trachea is normal.[11]

Laryngotracheal papillomatosis (Option (B)), usually seen in childhood, presents as multiple recurrent wart-like papillomas of the vocal cords and upper trachea. Following removal, they frequently recur. With

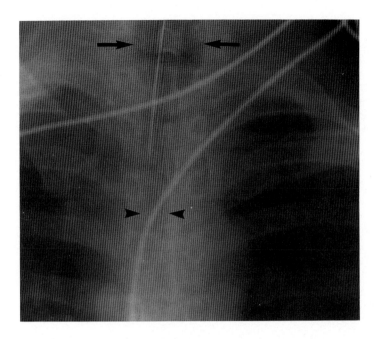

Figure 16-7

increasing age, they migrate down the tracheobronchial tree. As the child approaches adulthood, there is usually a slowing or cessation of the process. The radiographic appearance is one of irregularity of the internal tracheal wall caused by numerous small nodules (usually less than 1 cm). Initially, the lesions are more severe in the cervical trachea. When the papillomas involve the bronchi as well, there may be areas of obstruction, pneumonitis, or air-trapping. Occasionally, pulmonary nodules occur and may cavitate, leaving multiple moderately thin-walled cavities. Since such findings are absent in our test case, laryngotracheal papillomatosis is unlikely.

Mounier-Kuhn syndrome (tracheobronchomegaly) (Option (C)) causes tracheal widening rather than narrowing (Figures 16-13 and 16-14). This is the most common cause of tracheal enlargement; other causes include Ehler-Danlos syndrome, cutis laxa, and an occasional case of relapsing polychondritis which widens rather than narrows the trachea.

Tracheoesophageal fistula (Option (E)) is not an appropriate diagnosis based on the radiographs presented. Most tracheoesophageal fistulas are due to trauma, tumor, or infection. There is no supporting radiographic or historical evidence for this diagnosis in our test case. The majority of tracheoesophageal fistulas are intrathoracic rather than cervical.

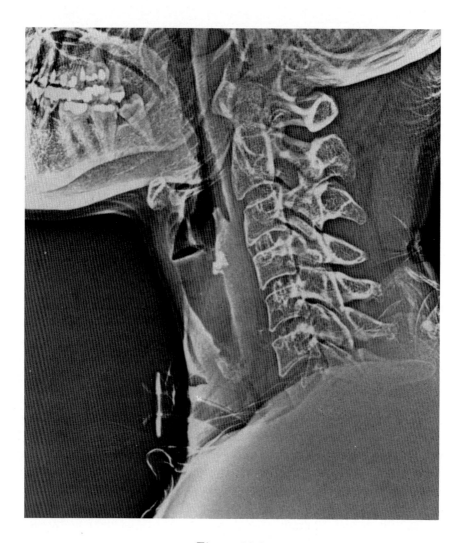

Figure 16-8

Figures 16-8 through 16-10. Post-tracheostomy stenosis. A lateral xeroradiograph (Figure 16-8) shows severe narrowing of the cervical trachea above the tracheostomy. A radiograph taken after the tracheostomy tube had been removed (Figure 16-9) demonstrates the tracheal stoma (asterisk). Note the stenosis above (upper two arrows) and below (lower four arrows) the stoma. An anteroposterior tomogram (Figure 16-10) shows normal glottic and subglottic areas, but there is almost complete stenosis (arrows) just above the level of the tracheal stoma (asterisk). This corresponds to the area of narrowing seen on the prior images. The trachea below the stoma is also narrowed.

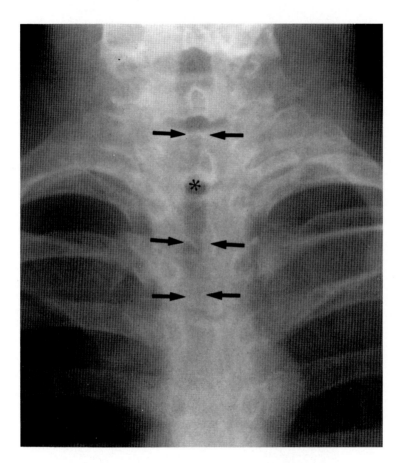

Figure 16-9

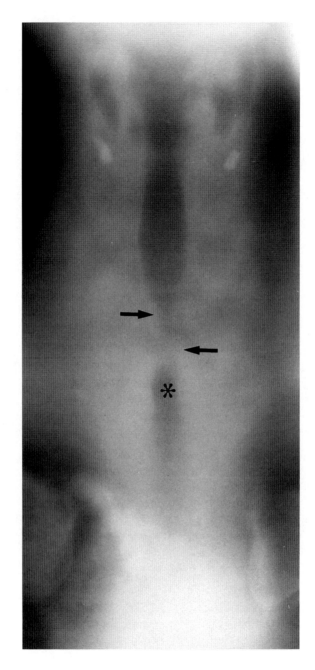

Figure 16-10

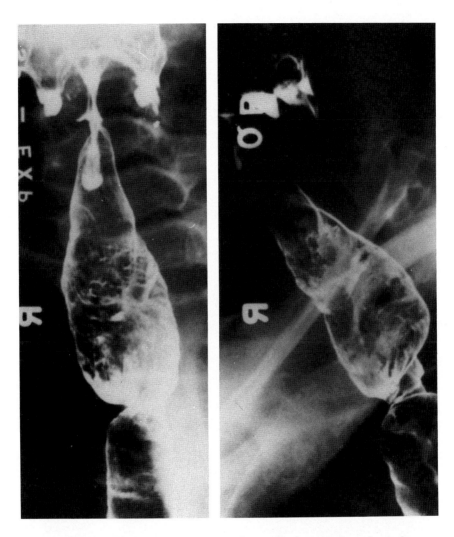

Figure 16-11. Tracheal stenosis at the cuff. A tantalum bronchogram in two projections demonstrates circumferential narrowing of the trachea at the thoracic inlet. (Reprinted with permission from Goodman and Gamsu [9].)

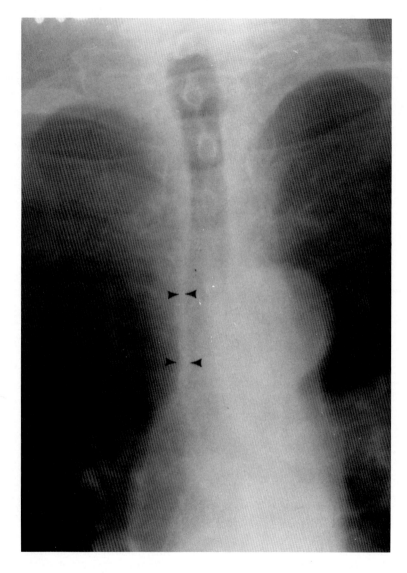

Figure 16-12. Saber-sheath trachea. This elderly patient, known to have severe chronic obstructive pulmonary disease, has a narrowed intrathoracic trachea. The tracheal wall is also shown (arrowheads).

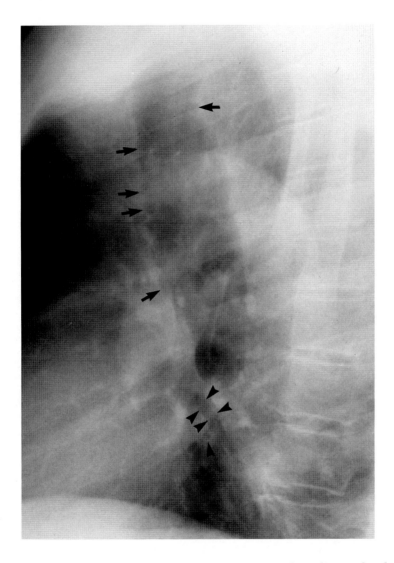

Figure 16-13. Tracheobronchomegaly. A lateral radiograph shows marked enlargement of the trachea and main bronchi. Multiple diverticula (arrows) are easily seen, especially along the anterior tracheal wall. Note other bronchi (arrowheads) as well.

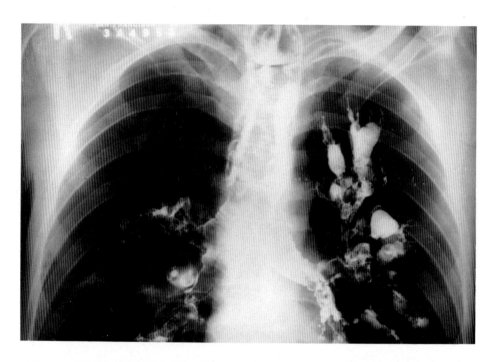

Figure 16-14. Tracheobronchomegaly. A bronchogram demonstrates marked enlargement of the entire trachea and the main bronchi. The lobar and segmental bronchi are also dilated. In this case, the bronchial dilatation is central, similar to that seen in allergic bronchopulmonary aspergillosis, except that the trachea and main bronchi are not characteristically enlarged in the latter.

Question 81

Concerning tracheal narrowing,

    (A) computed tomography is the most definitive imaging study for tracheal stenosis secondary to trauma or intubation

    (B) when viewed fluoroscopically, areas of tracheomalacia in the thorax collapse upon inspiration

    (C) dyspnea seldom occurs until the tracheal diameter is narrowed at least 50%

    (D) on spirometry, the forced expiratory volume in 1 second (FEV$_1$) is sufficient to evaluate tracheal function

    CT offers an excellent cross-sectional view of the trachea. The trachea may be round, oval, pear-shaped, or slightly concave posteriorly. The wall is thin, sharply defined internally, and may contain calcifications. CT also defines the relationship between the trachea and surrounding structures. A distinct fat plane between the trachea and the esophagus is present in less than half of patients.

    The unique cross-sectional view of the trachea with CT is ideally suited to the evaluation of intratracheal masses, the thickness of the tracheal wall, and the relationship of tracheal lesions to the mediastinum (and vice versa). Extrinsic causes of tracheal narrowing are well seen on CT. However, for tracheal injuries, tracheal stenosis, and tracheal webs, more conventional images (radiographs, xeroradiographs, tomograms, and tracheograms) are superior to CT. For short segments of stenosis or webs, CT may fail to define the lesion. For longer stenotic segments, CT measurements tend to overestimate the degree of stenosis and underestimate the length of the lesion **(Option (A) is false)**. It is uncertain whether coronal and sagittal reconstructions overcome some of these deficiencies.[7-10,17]

    In addition to stenosis, severe tracheal damage may destroy the cartilage rings and lead to focal collapse of the tracheal skeleton (tracheomalacia). Tracheomalacia usually, but not always, appears in conjunction with stenosis. The fluoroscopic appearance of tracheomalacia varies because different physiologic forces act on the cervical trachea and the intrathoracic trachea. In the thorax, expiration causes an increase in intrathoracic pressure, resulting in subsequent collapse of the malacic segment. Conversely, as the intrathoracic pressure decreases with inspiration, the trachea dilates to its maximal width **(Option (B) is false)**. The reverse is true in the cervical trachea. On inspiration, the diminished intratracheal pressure draws the malacic segment in. On expiration, the increased intratracheal pressure dilates the trachea.

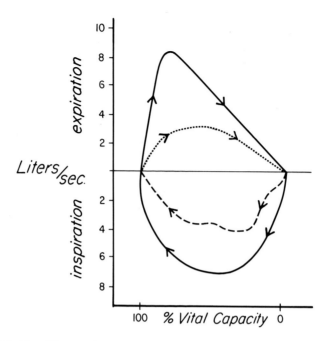

Figure 16-15. Flow-volume loop. The solid line represents a normal curve. In expiration, the peak air flow is reached in the early phase, whereas in inspiration, the peak air flow is reached in the midphase. The dotted line represents expiratory obstruction with a markedly diminished peak air flow. Similarly, the dashed line represents inflow obstruction with diminished inspiratory air flow.

Fixed areas of stenosis (no malacia) do not change with respiratory maneuvers. Stenotic lesions may be both intra- and extrathoracic, with or without malacia. In addition, paralysis of the vocal cords also may be present.[7,14,21]

The forced expiratory volume in 1 second (FEV_1), which is a basic physiologic measurement for obstructive lung disease, is not sufficient for evaluating upper airway disease. Recording the forced expiratory capacity and the forced inspiratory capacity as a flow-volume loop provides a more accurate assesssment of dynamic changes in the diameter of the trachea **(Option (D) is false)**. In normal patients, during the forced expiratory capacity maneuver, normal expiratory maximal flow reaches 6 to 12 L/second within the first 25% of the expiration. It then trails off during the remainder of the expiration. Normally, the forced inspiratory capacity maneuver produces a more gradual curve and peak flow toward the middle of inspiration (Figure 16-15). Fixed obstructions in the airway, such as stenosis or tumor, reduce peak flow in both inspiration and expiration. In patients with variable intrathoracic lesions (tracheomalacia), the trachea narrows on expiration and the expiratory flow-volume loop plateaus. The inspiratory loop is normal or close to normal. In cervical tracheomalacia, forced inspiration causes inward motion of the walls and a plateau of the inspiratory loop. The expiratory loop is close to normal. These flow-volume loops are more difficult to interpret in patients with compound lesions.[6,12,16]

As previously mentioned, the clinical diagnosis of a postintubation tracheal lesion is frequently missed because the patient's slowly increasing symptoms are attributed to underlying cardiopulmonary disease or because the patient's wheezing is mistakenly attributed to a new onset of "asthma." The vast majority of patients with normal hearts and lungs tolerate mild to moderate tracheal narrowing with little or no symptomatology. Symptomatic obstruction is usually noticed when there is a 50 to 75% narrowing of the tracheal diameter or when the tracheal diameter is reduced to 5 to 6 mm **(Option (C) is true).** Often an acute respiratory infection, with associated increased secretions, precipitates acute deterioration. A high degree of suspicion and careful attention to the appearance of the trachea are required in every patient developing any "cardiopulmonary" symptoms in the weeks and months following extubation.

Questions 82 through 85

For each of the tracheal abnormalities listed below (Questions 82 through 85), select the *one* lettered statement (A, B, C, D, or E) MOST closely associated with it. Each statement may be used once, more than once, or not at all.

82. Mounier-Kuhn syndrome
83. Laryngotracheal papillomatosis
84. Saber-sheath trachea
85. Rhinoscleroma

    (A) is believed to be viral in origin
    (B) is characterized by tracheobronchial diverticula
    (C) is associated with pneumothorax
    (D) may involve nasal sinuses, nose, and pharynx
    (E) is strongly correlated with chronic obstructive pulmonary disease

Tracheobronchomegaly, or Mounier-Kuhn syndrome, is one of the few recognized causes of diffuse enlargement of the entire trachea and main bronchi. It is predominantly a disease of men 30 to 50 years old. Symptoms of chronic bronchitis or bronchiectasis are usually present early, and there is usually evidence of increased pulmonary dead space. Radiographically, the trachea is 3 cm or more in diameter and usually has a scalloped appearance. The scalloping is due to outpouching of the tracheal mucosa and connective tissue between the cartilaginous rings so that broad diverticula are formed (Figures 16-13 and 16-14) **(Option (B) is most closely associated with Question 82)**. Fluoroscopically, there is evidence of increased flaccidity of the tracheal wall, with excessive tracheal collapse during forced expiration or coughing. In addition to the tracheal and proximal bronchial abnormalities described, recurrent infections result in radiographic evidence of pneumonia, bronchiectasis, and chronic fibrosis.[2,4]

The exact etiology of laryngotracheal papillomatosis is uncertain. Many consider it to be of viral etiology and analogous to cutaneous warts **(Option (A) is most closely associated with Question 83)**. A dissenting view maintains that the papillomas are benign mucosal overgrowths. The process often appears in young children, requires frequent excision, and may necessitate tracheostomy. However, when confined to the larynx and trachea the papillomas are usually self-limited and may diminish by young adulthood. With bronchial extension into the lung, mortality and morbidity increase.

Microscopically, the papillomas consist of a connective tissue stroma with diffuse lymphocytic infiltration, covered by well-differentiated squamous epithelium. These papillomas of childhood must be distinguished from the isolated bronchial papilloma seen in adults. Malignant transformation is infrequent in the childhood form, whereas such transformation is not uncommon in the adult (isolated) form.[1,5,18]

The radiographic appearance of saber-sheath trachea has already been discussed. In this condition, the internal coronal tracheal diameter at 1 cm above the aortic arch is less than two-thirds of the sagittal diameter. Of the 60 patients studied by Greene,[11] 57 (95%) had clinical evidence of chronic obstructive pulmonary disease **(Option (E) is most closely associated with Question 84).** Of 60 control patients, only two had evidence of saber-sheath trachea. Both were eventually found to have chronic obstructive pulmonary disease. In the group of patients with saber-sheath trachea, only 55% had other radiographic evidence of chronic obstructive pulmonary disease. Thus, saber-sheath trachea, even in the absence of other radiographic evidence, strongly suggests the diagnosis. The converse, however, is not true. Many patients with severe chronic obstructive pulmonary disease do not have a saber-sheath tracheal configuration.

Rhinoscleroma, a progressive infectious disease of the nasopharynx and upper airway, is caused by *Klebsiella rhinoscleromatis*. In the United States, it is mainly seen in immigrants from Central America, South America, North Africa, Central Europe, and Eastern Europe. The majority of patients are young adults, and the history often extends over many years. Initial symptoms are those of the common cold, at which time the diagnosis is usually not made. This is followed by a proliferative stage in which there is progressive infiltration by granulation tissue of the nasal mucosa, paranasal sinuses, pharynx, glottis, and proximal trachea **(Option (D) is most closely associated with Question 85).** In the narrowing stage, airway scarring may lead to dyspnea.

Radiographically, the vast majority of patients with rhinoscleroma show either diffuse sinus opacification or mucosal thickening. Bone destruction is rare. The usual clinical and radiologic diagnosis is that of chronic sinusitis. A study of the nose by conventional radiography or tomography often demonstrates either normal anatomy or atrophy of the inferior and middle turbinates. Glottic and tracheal involvement is not invariably present. When present, there is usually evidence of laryngeal and subglottic tracheal deformity and rigidity. Transglottic stenosis is not uncommon, and nodules may be present as well. Appropriate antibiotic treatment may arrest the disease, but surgery may be necessary to relieve obstructed areas.[3,4]

Question 86

Concerning an acquired tracheoesophageal fistula,

(A) respiratory symptoms usually exceed esophageal symptoms
(B) when due to prolonged intubation, it usually presents with mediastinal emphysema
(C) the most frequent etiology is infection
(D) it frequently follows intubation with a Sengstaken-Blakemore tube

Acquired tracheoesophageal fistulas are most often due to trauma, intubation, or tumor. Infection as a primary cause of fistulas is uncommon **(Option (C) is false).**

Although symptoms are due at least in part to the underlying disorder, the dominant symptoms are respiratory **(Option (A) is true).** Food and secretions pass from the esophagus to the trachea and lungs. Thus, coughing and dyspnea at mealtime and evidence of aspiration in the gravity-dependent lung segments are most frequent.[12,15,19,22]

Fistulas due to prolonged intubation usually do not cause signs of mediastinitis or mediastinal emphysema. The majority of such fistulas result from prolonged damage to the mucosa of the posterior tracheal membrane. Chronic inflammation of the connective tissue between the trachea and the esophagus usually results. Thus, when the final erosion occurs, the two structures have been welded together and material passes between them without contaminating the mediastinum. Mediastinitis and mediastinal emphysema are more likely to occur in an acute post-traumatic tracheoesophageal fistula, in which there is no inflammatory welding **(Option (B) is false).**

In patients with cancer in the mediastinum, a tracheoesophageal fistula frequently complicates radiation or chemotherapy. If the tumor has invaded the walls of both the esophagus and the trachea, the fistula opens as the tumor undergoes necrosis. On occasion, such fistualization may occur even without any therapy.

The radiographic appearance of a tracheoesophageal fistula is variable. Frequently, basilar pneumonitis is present due to aspiration of gastric contents. In patients on ventilators, air may distend the esophagus and stomach (Figures 16-16 and 16-17). If a tracheoesophageal fistula is suspected, care should be exercised when giving water-soluble oral contrast material, since such contrast medium, unlike barium, is irritating to the lung (Figure 16-18).

An infrequent but potentially fatal complication of Sengstaken-Blakemore tubes is esophageal rupture. This may occur from overdisten-

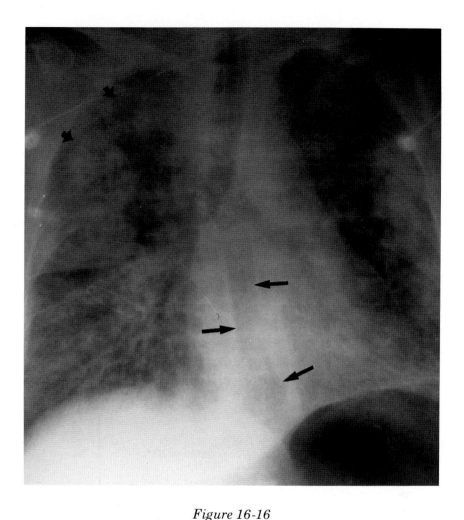

Figure 16-16

Figures 16-16 and 16-17. Tracheoesophageal fistula secondary to lymphoma. The patient presented with a large mediastinal mass and compression of the distal trachea due to Hodgkin's disease. Several days after radiotherapy, he developed dyspnea and severe pneumonitis necessitating intubation. His chest radiograph (Figure 16-16) shows bilateral pulmonary opacities, air filling the lower esophagus (long arrows), and marked gastric dilatation. A pneumothorax also developed at this time (short arrows). The patient died shortly thereafter. The pathologic specimen of the trachea (Figure 16-17), viewed frontally, shows a tumor at the carina (T). A fistula was present in this mass connecting the trachea and the esophagus.

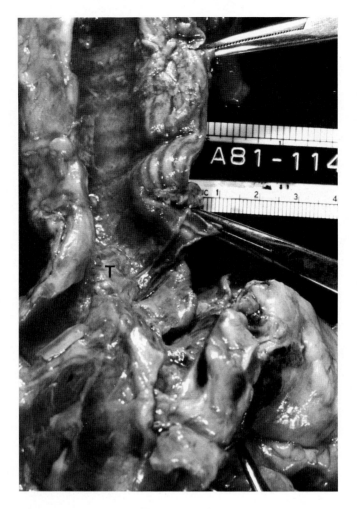

Figure 16-17

tion of the sausage-shaped esophageal balloon but is more frequently due to inflation of the gastric balloon in the distal esophagus. The gastric balloon may lodge in the distal esophagus during the initial placement or may be pulled from the stomach to the esophagus when tension is applied to the tube. This often results in a tear of the left wall of the esophagus, with direct communication between the esophagus and the pleural space. Mediastinitis and mediastinal emphysema are uncommon, perhaps because the mediastinum is decompressed directly into the pleural space. Since the esophageal injury usually occurs at the distal esophagus, far removed from the trachea, a tracheoesophageal fistula does not result **(Option (D) is false).**[22]

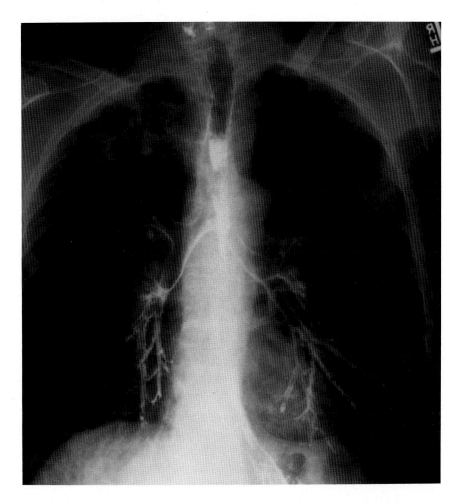

Figure 16-18. Tracheoesophageal fistula secondary to esophageal tumor. This 55-year-old man presented with bibasilar pneumonia and a history of dysphagia. A barium swallow showed a mass at the mid esophagus, with no barium entering the trachea during the first few swallows. Suddenly, barium flooded the trachea. A subsequent chest radiograph (Figure 16-18) shows barium outlining the tracheobronchial tree.

SUGGESTED READINGS

1. Al-Saleem T, Peale AR, Norris CM. Multiple papillomatosis of the lower respiratory tract. Clinical and pathologic study of eleven cases. Cancer 1968; 22:1173–1184
2. Bateson EM, Woo-Ming M. Tracheobronchomegaly. Clin Radiol 1973; 24:354–358
3. Becker TS, Shum TK, Waller TS, et al. Radiological aspects of rhinoscleroma. Radiology 1981; 141:433–438

4. Choplin RH, Wehunt WD, Theros EG. Diffuse lesions of the trachea. Semin Roentgenol 1983; 18:38–50

5. Felson B. Neoplasms of the trachea and main stem bronchi. Semin Roentgenol 1983; 18:23–37

6. Gamsu G, Borson DB, Webb WR, Cunningham JH. Structure and function in tracheal stenosis. Am Rev Respir Dis 1980; 121:519–531

7. Gamsu G, Webb WR. Computed tomography of the trachea: normal and abnormal. AJR 1982; 139:321–326

8. Godwin JD. The thoracic airway, trauma. In: Godwin JD (ed), Computed tomography of the chest. Philadelphia: JB Lippincott; 1984:474–481

9. Goodman LR, Gamsu G. Tracheostomy. In: Teplick JG, Haskin ME (eds), Surgical radiology. Philadelphia: WB Saunders; 1981:1090–1105

10. Goodman LR, Putman CE (eds). Intensive care radiology: imaging of the critically ill. Philadelphia: WB Saunders; 1983:31–33

11. Greene R. "Saber-sheath" trachea: relation to chronic obstructive pulmonary disease. AJR 1978; 130:441–445

12. Grillo HC. The trachea—tumors, strictures, and tracheal collapse. In: Glen WWL (ed), Thoracic and cardiovascular surgery, 4th ed. Norwalk: Appleton-Century-Crofts; 1983:308–325

13. Hemmingsson A, Lindgren PG. Roentgenologic examination of tracheal stenosis. Acta Radiol (Diagn) 1978; 19:753–765

14. James AE Jr, MacMillan AS Jr, Eaton SB, Janower ML, Grillo HC. Radiological considerations of granuloma and stenosis at the site of tracheostomy. Radiology 1970; 96:513–520

15. Obrecht WF Jr, Richter JE, Olympio GA, Gelfand DW. Tracheoesophageal fistula: a serious complication of infectious esophagitis. Gastroenterology 1984; 87:1174–1179

16. Payne WS, Leonard PF, Miller RD, Rosenow EC III, DeSanto LW. Physiologically based assessment and management of tracheal strictures. Surg Clin North Am 1973; 53:875–884

17. Pearlberg JL, Sandler MA, Kvale P, Beute GH, Madrazo BL. Computed-tomographic and conventional linear-tomographic evaluation of tracheobronchial lesions for laser photoresection. Radiology 1985; 154:759–762

18. Rosenbaum HD, Alavi SM, Bryant LR. Pulmonary parenchymal spread of juvenile laryngeal papillomatosis. Radiology 1968; 90:654–660

19. Schmitz GL. Acquired tracheoesophageal fistula. Otolaryngol Clin North Am 1979; 12:823–827

20. Stauffer JL, Olson DE, Petty TL. Complications and consequences of endotracheal intubation and tracheotomy. A prospective study of 150 critically ill adult patients. Am J Med 1981; 70:65–76

21. Stitik FP, Bartelt D, James AE Jr, Proctor DF. Tantalum tracheography in upper airway obstruction: 100 experiences in adults. AJR 1978; 130:35–41

22. Wechsler RJ, Steiner RM, Goodman LR, Teplick SK, Mapp E, Laufer I. Iatrogenic esophageal-pleural fistula: subtlety of diagnosis in the absence of mediastinitis. Radiology 1982; 144:239–243

Case 17: Post-thoracotomy Fluid Collections

Question 87

Concerning this patient's images,

    (A) there is fluid in the anterior mediastinum
    (B) there is fluid in the major fissure
    (C) there is dense consolidation of the left upper lobe
    (D) the chest tube does not communicate with the pleural collections

The portable radiograph (Figure 17-1) shows, parallel to the upper lateral left ribs, a homogeneous opacity, most likely due to a loculated pleural effusion or an extrapleural fluid collection. The location of the large homogeneous opacity situated more medially is considerably less certain. Lateral and decubitus radiographs (not shown) did not help to elucidate its location. A chest tube (arrowheads) seen along the left hemidiaphragm had ceased draining well approximately 3 days earlier. A computed tomographic (CT) examination (Figures 17-2, 17-3, and 17-4) was performed for clarification and to help determine the appropriate diagnostic and therapeutic approaches.

The CT images document fluid, varying from 4 to 12 Hounsfield units (HU), in several locations. The fluid in the anterior mediastinum (Figure 17-5) has a triangular configuration similar to what one might expect from a thymic abnormality in a man of this age **(Option (A) is true).** The oval density in the left mid hemithorax represents fluid in the major fissure (Figure 17-6) **(Option (B) is true).** On the lung windows (not shown) this fissural fluid minimally displaced pulmonary markings and had a sharp interface with the pulmonary parenchyma.

In Figure 17-5, note that two focal fluid collections are present on the left. Both bulge toward the lung, do not contain air bronchograms, and do not conform to the anatomic distribution of the upper lobe **(Option (C) is false).** Although small or patchy areas of parenchymal disease are

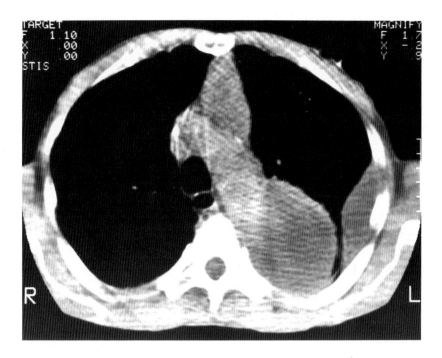

Figure 17-2

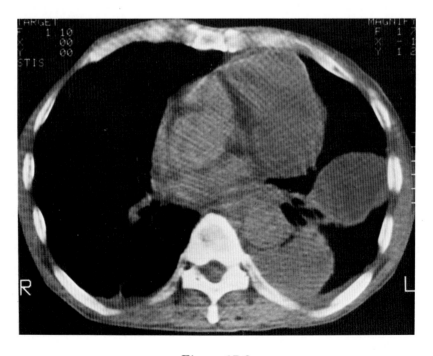

Figure 17-3

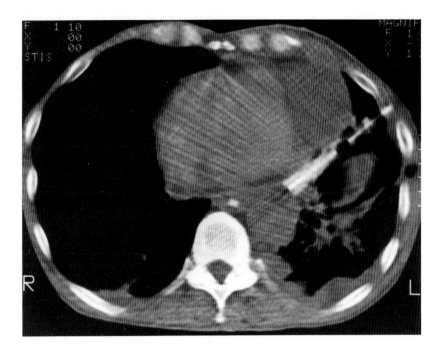

Figure 17-4

not always visible at mediastinal windows, consolidation of the left upper lobe should be.

Examination of the entire CT study indicated that continuity was present between some of the pleural collections, while others appeared isolated. The lateral collection shown in Figure 17-5 did not appear continuous with others, so that one might consider it as possibly extrapleural. However, it is also likely to be in the pleural space, since adjacent extrapleural fat was not obliterated (as might be expected with an extrapleural collection). The anterior collection seen in Figure 17-6 was lateral to mediastinal fat and, therefore, probably in the pleural space as well.

Although the chest tube is seen on the CT scan, it does not communicate with the loculated fluid collections (Figure 17-7) **(Option (D) is true).** The tube had been draining fluid well for the first several days, but the output gradually diminished in the days preceding the studies shown. Lack of chest tube drainage in the presence of fluid collections indicates that the fluid has become loculated or that there is a mechanical problem with the tube (fibrin sheath, debris plugging the tube, or kink, etc.). In this patient, even if the chest tube had drained the pleural collections, the mediastinal collection would have persisted.

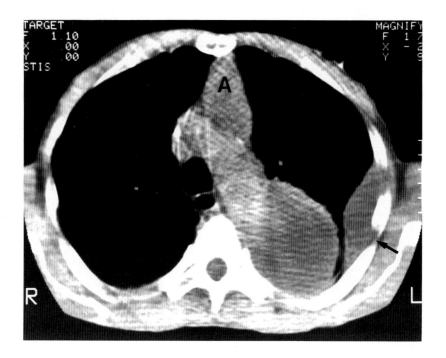

Figure 17-5

Figures 17-5 through 17-7 (Same as Figures 17-2 through 17-4, respectively). In Figure 17-5, note the anterior mediastinal collection (A) and the preservation of extrapleural fat (arrow) adjacent to the lateral pleural collection. An upper lobe distribution of disease is not seen. In Figure 17-6, note the fissural fluid (+) in the mid left hemithorax and the anterior collection (probably pleural) lateral to mediastinal fat (F). In Figure 17-7, the chest tube (white band) is seen. Also noted is loculated fluid (+) anteriorly on the left.

The majority of correctly placed chest tubes drain well and do not require sophisticated imaging evaluation. In problem cases, the antero-posterior radiograph may fail to identify the cause of suboptimal drainage. A lateral view may reveal that the tube is not in direct continuity with the fluid collection or that the tube is in the major fissure and, thus, probably isolated from the remaining fluid in the pleural space. When the frontal and lateral radiographs fail to reveal the cause for poor drainage, or when multiple loculations are suspected, CT is often extremely helpful (Figure 17-8).[18] For the test case shown, CT not only demonstrated the tube separate from the pleural collections but also demonstrated that reinsertion of a single tube would not successfully drain the various collections (they did not all communicate with each

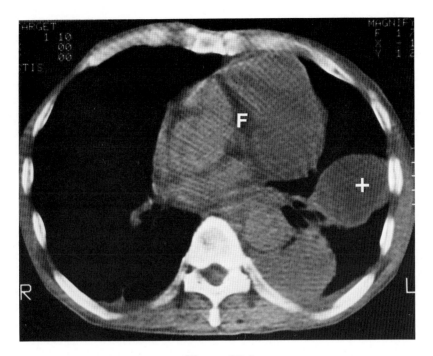

Figure 17-6

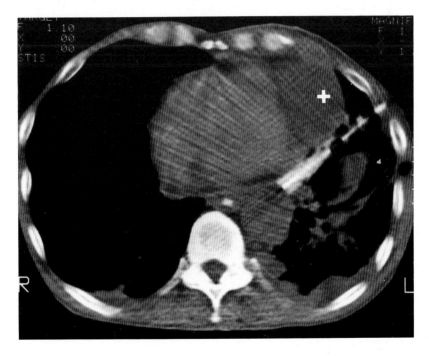

Figure 17-7

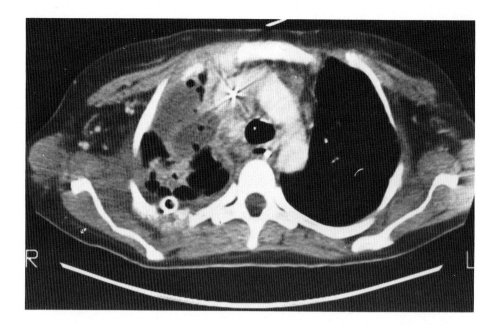

Figure 17-8. Chest tube isolated from pleural collection. The patient had had direct trauma to her right apex and a subsequent large hemothorax. Chest tube drainage was initially successful but eventually ceased. On posteroanterior and lateral radiographs (not shown) the chest tube appeared to be in an appropriate position. CT showed that the anterior collection did not communicate with the chest tube (white ring) located posteriorly.

other). With the CT scans indicating locations, each separate collection was drained under fluoroscopic guidance. The anterior mediastinal collection was slightly turbid as compared to the other, clear ones. A catheter was inserted into that collection. Subsequent cultures of all the fluid collections proved negative, however.

Question 88

Concerning the computed tomographic differentiation between lung abscesses and empyemas,

(A) a lung abscess characteristically has a thin wall
(B) a lung abscess characteristically displaces adjacent lung markings (vessels, bronchi)
(C) a lung abscess has a distinct interface with normal lung
(D) an empyema is usually elliptical rather than round

Making the distinction between a lung abscess and a collection in the pleural space (such as empyema, bronchopleural fistula, or loculated fluid) may be difficult. As a general rule, the air-fluid level of a bronchopleural fistula is longer on one radiographic view and shorter on the other view taken at 90 degrees to it.[7] Such an appearance reflects the nonspherical shape of most intrapleural collections. On one of the two views, the air-fluid level will often reach the chest wall. Conversely, an abscess cavity tends to be round, and its air-fluid level tends to be the same length on both views taken at 90 degrees to each other. The fluid level usually reaches neither the surrounding lung opacity nor the chest wall.

In the majority of patients with uncomplicated empyemas or abscesses, the above guidelines are adequate for most diagnostic or therapeutic purposes.[7] However, in patients with complex pleuroparenchymal disease, CT has proved to be extremely helpful. CT will frequently distinguish between parenchymal disease and pleural disease, indicate when both are present, and demonstrate their relationship to other intrathoracic structures. Such distinction is based on various criteria.[19,22] In most empyemas, the thickened visceral and parietal pleura are visible as distinct linear structures separated by fluid (split-pleura sign). Intravenous contrast material enhances the visibility of the thickened pleura (Figures 17-9, 17-10, and 17-11). A lung abscess tends to have a thicker wall of surrounding pneumonic process, whereas the wall of an empyema is usually thinner (only the thickened pleura itself) **(Option (A) is false)**. Pleural collections may displace adjacent lung markings (vessels, bronchi), whereas abscesses occur within the lung and usually do not **(Option (B) is false)**.[17] The interface with the normal lung is usually indistinct for an abscess, whereas an empyema has a relatively distinct interface where its pleural covering displaces the lung (Figure 17-12) **(Option (C) is false)**. As a general rule, pleural fluid collections tend to be oval or elliptical rather than round since they conform to the

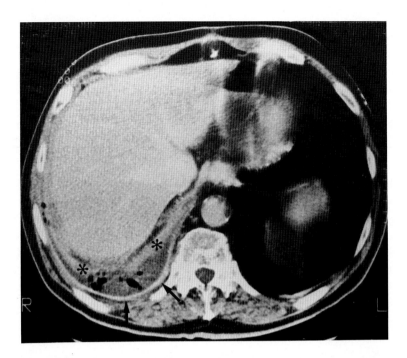

Figure 17-9. Empyema. The patient developed an empyema following coronary artery surgery. Initial drainage was considered successful. However, fever recurred several days after removal of the chest tube. A CT scan through the lower right hemithorax showed a thickened parietal pleura (arrows) enhanced by contrast material and fluid in the pleural space containing multiple small air collections. The anterior boundary of the fluid likely represents the inferior part of the lower lobe (asterisks) rather than the hemidiaphragm.

pleural space **(Option (D) is true).** However, a large pleural collection at the lower hemithorax may be round rather than oval and may form an acute angle with the chest wall, a feature usually expected with an abscess instead (Figure 17-13).

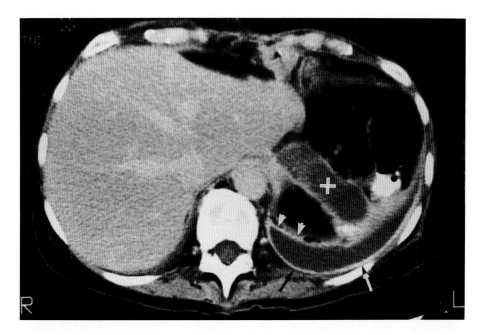

Figure 17-10
Figures 17-10 and 17-11. Pleural effusion and subphrenic abscess. The patient had several gastric surgical procedures and evacuation of several subphrenic abscesses. Fluid is seen in the left lower posterior pleural space (Figure 17-10) separating the parietal pleura (arrows) from the hemidiaphragm (arrowheads). Centrally, an upper abdominal loculated fluid collection (+) is present. Aspiration of the upper abdominal collection yielded pus which was successfully drained by a percutaneous catheter. At a higher level (Figure 17-11), loculated pleural fluid is seen medially (2). The parietal pleura is thickened when compared to that on the other side. The infected collection is oval and displaces the contrast-enhanced lung anterior to it. Incidentally noted are loculated fluid anterolaterally on the left and free fluid posteriorly on the right.

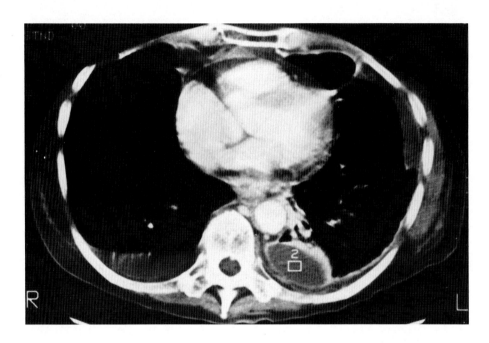

Figure 17-11

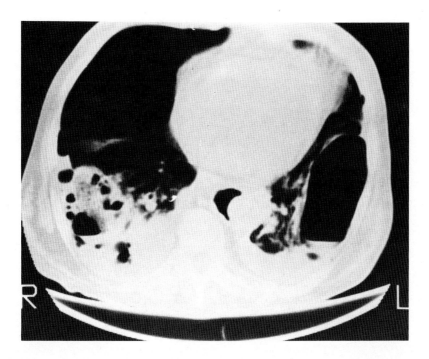

Figure 17-12. Abscess and bronchopleural fistula. On the right, an area of dense consolidation with ill-defined margins is seen. Multiple air pockets, as well as air-fluid levels and possible air bronchograms, are seen within it. Medially, the findings are characteristic of an abscess. Laterally, one cannot totally exclude a coexistent pleural collection. On the left, the oval lateral air collection has a thin wall, has a sharp anteromedial interface with the lung, and displaces some of the lung medially. The small air-fluid level within it contacts the lateral chest wall. These are all features of a pleural collection, in this case due to a bronchopleural fistula. The air medial to the descending aorta has an unusual shape but probably lies within the esophagus.

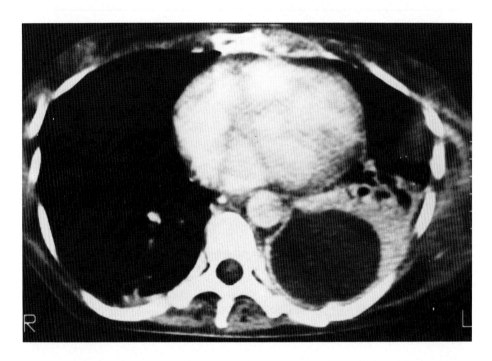

Figure 17-13. Round loculated pleural effusion. The patient had previous upper abdominal surgery. The conventional radiographs showed a left basilar opacity, and differentiation between a pleural or a parenchymal process was not possible. The CT examination shows a rounded homogeneous left fluid collection with a thick posterior parietal pleura and marked displacement of the adjacent lung. Due to the extent of opaque lung adjacent to the loculated fluid collection, associated basilar pneumonia cannot be completely excluded.

Question 89

Concerning potential complications following median sternotomy,

    (A) a 20% increase in mediastinal width in the first 48 hours after coronary bypass surgery implies the need for reoperation

    (B) pulmonary edema secondary to cardiopulmonary bypass is present radiographically in the majority of patients

    (C) after the first postoperative week, computed tomography is of little value in separating postoperative changes from pathologic processes

    (D) a thin midline lucency in the sternum is a reliable radiographic predictor of impending sternal dehiscence

    (E) left lower lobe atelectasis after coronary artery surgery is partially attributable to temporary paralysis of the left hemidiaphragm

In the first several days after cardiac or mediastinal surgery, many abnormalities are noted on the chest radiograph. Some are of no clinical significance and simply reflect expected alterations due to the surgery. Others portend potential complications or represent current complications requiring intervention.[3,8,12] For example, following coronary artery surgery, the mediastinum in almost every patient. This widening is undoubtedly due to a combination of hemorrhage and edema and is usually self-limited. At the time of surgery, tubes are usually placed in the anterior mediastinum and beneath the heart to permit adequate drainage of the mediastinum. Katzberg et al.[12] compared the width of the mediastinum on the preoperative posteroanterior radiograph with that on the postoperative anteroposterior radiograph. They found that stable patients, without clinical evidence of significant bleeding, exhibit mediastinal widening of approximately 35% **(Option (A) is false).** Patients with moderate clinical evidence of bleeding, who did not require reoperation, had increases in their mediastinal width of approximately 50%. Patients requiring reoperation had increases in width of approximately 60%. There was considerable overlap between groups, so that the radiographic appearance alone is not a reliable determinant of the need for reoperation. The decision is usually made based on the rate of drainage of blood from the chest tubes, the stability of the patient's blood pressure, and the patient's cardiac output. On occasion, the drainage tubes malfunction and fluid collects in the mediastinum, resulting in mediastinal widening and the appearance of "apical caps." The patient may develop hypotension due either to hypovolemia or to low cardiac output from tamponade of the superior vena cava or right atrium.

Pulmonary edema resulting from extracorporeal circulation was a frequent problem with early bypass equipment. Improved mechanics and filtering have diminshed this complication so that currently, less than one-fourth of patients develop postoperative pulmonary edema **(Option (B) is false)**. When edema occurs, it is usually seen in the first 72 hours after surgery. Approximately one-half of the patients have edema resulting from elevated left-sided pressures (heart failure), whereas the other half show normal wedge pressures. In this group, edema is believed to be due to a dilutional hypoproteinemia which occurs in almost all patients on cardiopulmonary bypass.[13]. Edema develops in approximately 75% of patients whose serum proteins fall to less than 4 g/dL, whereas it develops in only 15% of patients with serum protein values greater than 4 g/dL. In most patients, the edema is mild and responds to diuretics.

CT may be of great value, even in the early postoperative period.[9] In the vast majority of patients, CT shows a fairly constant pattern by the end of the first week. The tissues of the chest wall have returned to normal or are only mildly edematous. The sternum itself is either well approximated or may show minor step-offs, impactions, or gaps. The anterior mediastinum and mid mediastinum often appear normal or close to normal. In a majority of patients, mediastinal fat planes have returned to normal or are only slightly edematous. Small, well-circumscribed collections of fluid may persist beyond the first week. Many measure above 30 HU, as might be seen with resolving hematomas. Tiny bubbles of air may also be present in the anterior mediastinum for a few days after the removal of anterior drainage tubes. By the end of the second or third week, these abnormalities have resolved as well. Thus, due to the foregoing expected CT findings, CT is of great value in separating postoperative changes from pathologic processes **(Option (C) is false)**.

Although serious complications after coronary artery surgery are infrequent, they have a high mortality and morbidity if they are not diagnosed and treated early. With an understanding of the expected changes outlined above, one should be able to diagnose postoperative mediastinal infection earlier with CT than with more conventional methods (Figure 17-14). In other situations, there will be concern as to whether a fluid collection is infected or represents a resolving hematoma (Figure 17-8). CT mapping allows one to guide the aspiration of a fluid collection for diagnostic and, possibly, therapeutic purposes. Although CT is more sensitive than tomography or conventional radiography for detection of sternal osteomyelitis, it is not as sensitive as one might like for detection of early sternal changes.[9] The sternum may appear normal when osteomyelitis is first suspected clinically. This may be followed by marked, visible lysis of the sternum within 1 week. Scintigraphy with

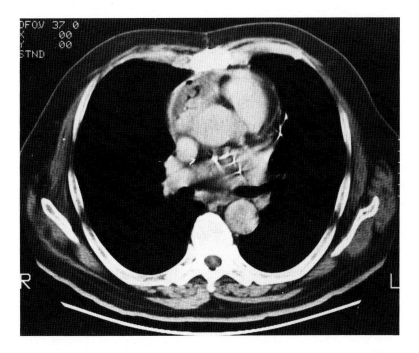

Figure 17-14. Pericardial abscess after coronary artery surgery. The patient returned 3 weeks after coronary artery surgery with fever and an elevated white blood cell count. His chest radiograph was normal and unchanged from the discharge radiograph. CT showed a right anterior pericardial collection containing gas bubbles. The abnormality was confined to this area only. CT localization permitted a local rib resection and drainage rather than a repeat sternotomy.

Tc-99m MDP or Ga-67 may be helpful for early diagnosis of sternal osteomyelitis prior to the development of radiographic changes.

Sternal dehiscence is associated with very high mortality and morbidity but fortunately is an infrequent complication of median sternotomy. It is frequently associated with deep wound infections and osteomyelitis. Both the infection and the unstable sternum are often apparent earlier clinically than radiographically. In most instances, radiographic evidence of mediastinal infection is lacking and conventional radiographic and tomographic evaluations of the sternum for osteomyelitis are insensitive and nonspecific. The thin (1 to 3 mm) midline sternal lucency seen in 30 to 60% of patients after sternotomy is not a reliable predictor of eventual dehiscence **(Option (D) is false).** Unless the lucency is extremely wide or shows progressive widening, it is of no diagnostic signficance.[2] As dehiscence progresses, the sternal wires tend to shift position. They cut through the diseased sternum, some migrating with the right half of the sternum, and some migrating with the left.

Several factors contribute to the frequent occurrence of left basilar atelectasis following coronary artery surgery, including manipulation of the lung during surgery, mechanical compression of the lower lobe by the enlarged heart, and splinting. Moreover, in patients requiring nasotracheal suction, the catheter enters the right bronchus in the majority of instances and, thus, mucous plugging on the left is more likely. An additional interesting etiologic factor is left diaphragmatic paresis or paralysis. During surgery, topical cardiac hypothermia is produced by chilling the pericardial sac with cold physiologic saline or applying an ice pack to the ventricular surface. This decreases the metabolic needs of the myocardium during surgery. However, the phrenic nerve found on the surface of the pericardium may be injured. Since the institution of topical hypothermia several years ago, the frequency of postoperative left lower lobe atelectasis has risen from approximately 30 to 80%, as shown in one study.[14] Fluoroscopy of such patients demonstrates markedly decreased or absent motion of the left hemidiaphragm during the immediate postoperative period up to 70% of the time **(Option (E) is true)**. Paresis may last for weeks or months.

Question 90

Concerning postoperative fluid collections,

- (A) after laparotomy, pleural effusions are present in approximately 50% of patients
- (B) the initial radiographic signs of subphrenic abscess, such as pleural effusion, atelectasis, or diaphragmatic elevation, are usually present by the fifth postoperative day
- (C) immediately following hemorrhage, a hemothorax is usually isodense with respect to unopacified soft tissue (muscle) on computed tomographic scans
- (D) a pleural effusion developing 2 to 6 weeks after cardiac surgery is more likely due to the postpericardiotomy syndrome than to infection

Postoperative pleural effusions are more common than generally believed, being found in as many as 60% of patients after upper abdominal surgery and 35% of patients after lower abdominal surgery **(Option (A) is true)**.[15] Even after vaginal or caesarean deliveries, small pleural effusions are common.[11] Patients with ascites may develop effusion by leakage through the diaphragm. Effusions occurring after upper quadrant surgery tend to be larger and ipsilaterally located. In the vast majority of patients, the effusions are self-limited and are not associated with major postoperative complications, prolonged mortality, or morbidity. If the clinical examination does not suggest an etiology for the postoperative effusion (such as pancreatitis, congestive heart failure, pulmonary embolism, etc.), a more extensive work-up may not be rewarding. In general, the effusions regress within a week or two without specific therapy.

The initial radiographic signs of subphrenic abscess, such as diaphragmatic elevation, pleural effusion, atelectasis, or subphrenic air collections, usually become apparent during the second week after abdominal surgery **(Option (B) is false)**.[5,7] These signs may appear somewhat earlier if the peritoneal space is soiled prior to surgery, as from a colonic or gastric perforation or penetrating abdominal trauma. Early diagnosis is often difficult because the signs and symptoms suggestive of subphrenic abscess are often present prior to the radiographic findings described. In patients on antibiotics or steroid therapy, the abscess may progress with only mild or nonspecific symptoms.

Prior to the advent of CT and modern ultrasonography, the conventional work-up for a subphrenic abscess included conventional radiographs of the chest and abdomen, fluoroscopy of the diaphragm, contrast-enhanced studies of the gastrointestinal and urinary tracts, and liver-lung scintigraphy. These latter studies were insensitive unless large fluid collections were present. CT and ultrasonography have dramatically altered the diagnostic approach to a subphrenic abscess.[1,10,16] These modalities are both noninvasive and highly sensitive and should be used whenever the diagnosis is being seriously considered clinically, even if chest radiographic findings are absent (Figures 17-15 and 17-16). The presence of air-fluid levels and multiple bubbles of gas within the collection, or extensive soft tissue edema adjacent to the collection, strongly suggests that the fluid collection is infected. However, in the majority of cases, differentiation between infected and sterile fluid collections is not possible, so that CT and sonography serve as guides for percutaneous diagnostic aspiration and drainage, as appropriate. In most studies comparing CT and sonography, CT has proven to be slightly more sensitive and to give a broader and more detailed display of the extent of disease and its relationship to adjacent abdominal structures.

Extravascular collections of blood, regardless of their location in the body, go through several stages of evolution. These stages are documented by CT. Immediately following hemorrhage, the blood collection approximates the density of the adjacent unenhanced soft tissue (muscle)

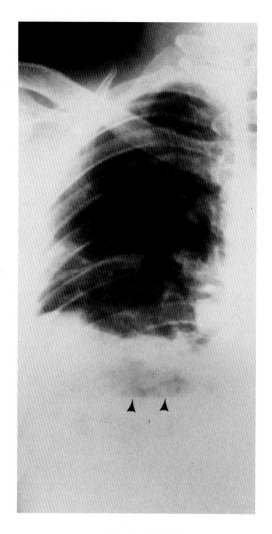

Figure 17-15
Figures 17-15 and 17-16. Subphrenic abscess. The patient had prior biliary surgery, drainage of a subphrenic abscess, and subsequent recurrence of symptoms. The chest radiograph (Figure 17-15) shows a relatively uniform opaque area in the lower third of the right hemithorax. An air-fluid level is visible (arrowheads). CT (Figure 17-16) shows a large right posterior pleural effusion bordered anteriorly by collapsed, contrast-enhanced lung (asterisk). Anterior to the lung is a large irregular collection of air and fluid within the abdomen. No air collections are identified within the lung or pleural space. The diagnosis of a large subphrenic abscess was confirmed surgically. A follow-up chest radiograph showed marked improvement. (Case courtesy of E. T. Stewart, M.D., Medical College of Wisconsin, Milwaukee.)

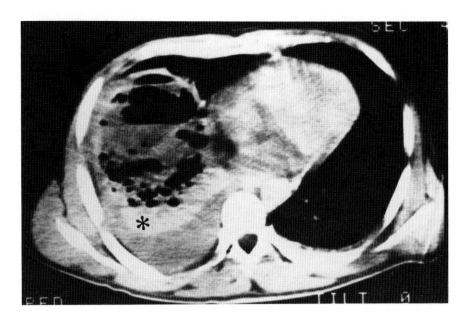

Figure 17-16

(Option (C) is true). During the first 48 hours, there may be clot retraction and some dehydration, causing increased concentration of hemoglobin and resultant focal hyperdensity (60 to 80 HU) (Figures 17-17, 17-18, and 17-19). A seroma may form around the clot, or the serum may layer above the clot (hematocrit effect seen in anticoagulated patients). This fluid is considerably less dense. As the clot lyses, the fluid again becomes isodense with respect to muscle and finally hypodense (20 HU or less) within a few weeks.

Over 90% of hematomas occurring in closed spaces, such as muscle, solid organs, brain, and retroperitoneum, behave in such a fashion. However, in the pleural and peritoneal spaces, the hyperdense phase occurs considerably less frequently and lasts for a shorter period of time. In these spaces, it is probable that respiratory motion alters clotting, either preventing it completely or speeding up the process of clot lysis.[6,20] It is also probable that the pleural and peritoneal surfaces exude fluid to dilute the deteriorating blood products. Nevertheless, within the first 2 weeks after hemorrhage into the pleural space, focal dense areas abutting the chest wall should not be confused with tumor or other significant pathology. With regard to the head, it should be noted that a fresh hemorrhage into the brain (approximately 50 HU) will appear hyperdense relative to the normal brain (approximately 40 HU).

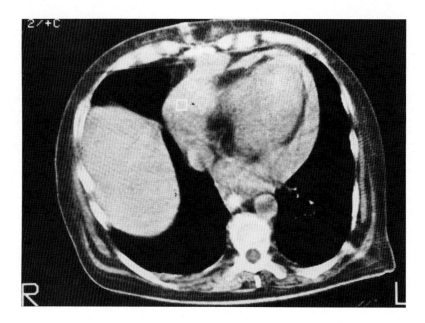

Figure 17-17. Hemopericardium after coronary artery surgery. Widening of the mediastinum approximately 8 days after surgery suggested mediastinal infection or hemorrhage. CT showed distention of the pericardial space on the left. A right anterolateral collection, mediastinal versus pericardial in location, had an attenuation value of 74 HU. These findings were considered more suggestive of hemorrhage than of infection, and fine-needle aspiration was not performed. The patient made an uneventful recovery. Had infection been considered more likely, needle aspiration of the right-sided lesion would have been helpful.

Several factors determine the density of a fluid collection. First, the protein content of many of these fluids overlap. Second, the CT number depends on many factors unrelated to the fluid itself: size of the collection, its relationship to adjacent structures, volume averaging, and variation from one scanner to another. Another factor is intrinsic body motion. Vock et al. have shown that the standard deviation of fluid measured in a dog thorax is 19 HU, but this drops to 9 HU when the heart is stopped.[21] The authors also performed experiments in vitro, with control of many of the above-mentioned factors, and found a correlation of 0.85 to 0.89 between fluid specific gravity and CT density. Unfortunately, the in vitro accuracy cannot be reproduced in the living patient.

The most common explanation for a pleural effusion 2 to 6 weeks after cardiac surgery is the postpericardiotomy syndrome **(Option (D) is true).** Infection in the pleural space after cardiac surgery is uncommon.

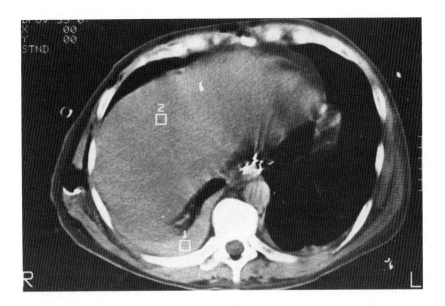

Figure 17-18. Hemothorax. A CT scan 2 days after an automobile accident demonstrates a hyperdense pleural fluid collection (1) measuring 77 HU. This compares with a poorly contrast-enhanced liver (2) that measures 57 HU. Subcutaneous emphysema is also present on the right.

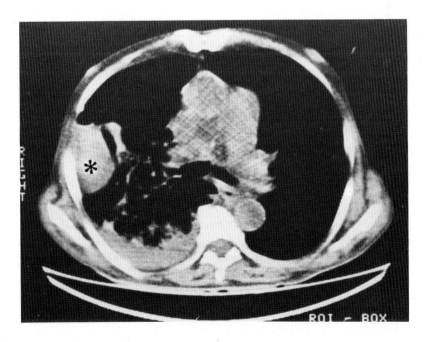

Figure 17-19. CT of the thorax 11 days after a large pleural hemorrhage reveals a lateral mass (*) measuring approximately 95 HU. Although an underlying pleural mass was considered, a chest radiograph obtained prior to the hemorrhage showed no pleural lesion. A follow-up radiograph several weeks later showed marked improvement.

Postpericardiotomy syndrome, however, develops in 10 to 30% of patients within a few weeks after surgery and may occur up to 1 year after surgery. Relapses have been reported. Patients usually experience fever, malaise, and dyspnea, similar to the findings with postmyocardial infarction syndrome (Dressler's syndrome). There may be clinical and radiographic evidence of pericardial effusion, pleural effusions, and pneumonitis. Radiographic findings appear within 48 hours preceding or following the onset of symptoms. There may be a mild leukocytosis, and the erythyrocyte sedimentation rate is usually elevated. Pericardial effusion may, on occasion, lead to cardiac tamponade. The usual differential diagnosis includes postoperative infection, myocardial infarction, pulmonary embolism, congestive heart failure, or pericardial hemorrhage from excessive anticoagulation. In general, the syndrome is self-limited, and patients respond to bed rest and anti-inflammatory agents. A patient's long-term prognosis is not affected by the occurrence of the syndrome.[4]

SUGGESTED READINGS

1. Alexander ES, Proto AV, Clark RA. CT differentiation of subphrenic abscess and pleural effusion. AJR 1983; 140:47–51
2. Berkow AE, Demos TC. The midsternal stripe and its relationship to postoperative sternal dehiscence. Radiology 1976; 121:525
3. Carter AR, Sostman HD, Curtis AM, Swett HA. Thoracic alterations after cardiac surgery. AJR 1983; 140:475–481
4. Engle MA, Klein AA, Hepner S, Ehlers KH. The postpericardiotomy and similar syndromes. Cardiovasc Clin 1976; 7:211–217
5. Fataar S, Schulman A. Subphrenic abscess: the radiological approach. Clin Radiol 1981; 32:147–156
6. Federle MP, Jeffrey RB Jr. Hemoperitoneum studied by computed tomography. Radiology 1983; 148:187–192
7. Friedman PJ, Hellekant CAG. Radiologic recognition of bronchopleural fistula. Radiology 1977; 124:289–295
8. Goodman LR. The post thoracotomy radiograph. In: Goodman LR, Putman CE (eds), Intensive care radiology: imaging of the critically ill. Philadelphia: WB Saunders; 1983:124–140
9. Goodman LR, Kay HR, Teplick SK, Mundth ED. Complications of median sternotomy: computed tomographic eveluation. AJR 1983; 141:225–230
10. Halber MD, Daffner RH, Morgan CL, et al. Intraabdominal abscess: current concepts in radiologic evaluation. AJR 1979; 133:9–13
11. Hughson WG, Friedman PJ, Feigin DS, Resnik R, Moser KM. Postpartum pleural effusion: a common radiologic finding. Ann Intern Med 1982; 97:856–858

12. Katzberg RW, Whitehouse GH, deWeese JA. The early radiologic findings in the adult chest after cardiopulmonary bypass surgery. Cardiovasc Radiol 1978; 1:205–215

13. Klancke KA, Assey ME, Kratz JM, Crawford FA. Postoperative pulmonary edema in postcoronary artery bypass graft patients. Chest 1983; 84:529–534

14. Kohorst WR, Schonfeld SA, Altman M. Bilateral diaphragmatic paralysis following topical cardiac hypothermia. Chest 1984; 85:65–68

15. Light RW, George RB. Incidence and significance of pleural effusion after abdominal surgery. Chest 1976; 69:621–625

16. Lundstedt C, Hederström E, Holmin T, Lunderquist A, Navne T, Owman T. Radiological diagnosis in proven intraabdominal abscess formation: a comparison between plain films of the abdomen, ultrasonography and computerized tomography. Gastrointest Radiol 1983; 8:261–266

17. Proto AV, Merhar GL. Central bronchial displacement with large posterior pleural collections. Findings on the lateral chest radiograph and CT scans. J Can Assoc Radiol 1984; 35:128–132

18. Stark DD, Federle MP, Goodman PC. CT and radiographic assessment of tube thoracostomy. AJR 1983; 141:253–258

19. Stark DD, Federle MP, Goodman PC, Podrasky AE, Webb WR. Differentiating lung abscess and empyema: radiography and computed tomography. AJR 1983; 141:163–167

20. Swensen SJ, McLeod RA, Stephens DH. CT of extracranial hemorrhage and hematomas. AJR 1984; 143:907–912

21. Vock P, Effmann EL, Hedlund LW, Lischko MM, Putman CE. Analysis of the density of pleural fluid analogs by computed tomography. Invest Radiol 1984; 19:10–15

22. Williford ME, Godwin JD. Computed tomography of lung abscess and empyema. Radiol Clin North Am 1983; 21:575–583

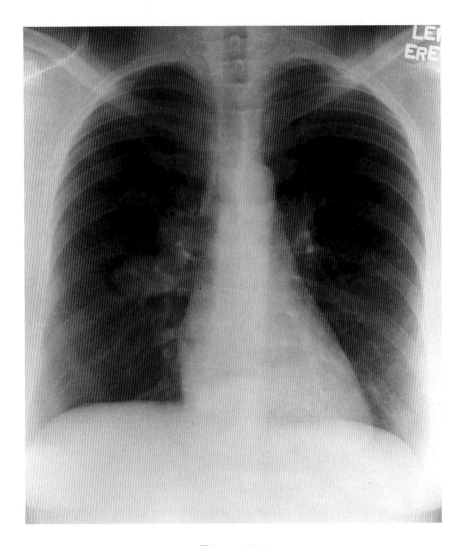

Figure 18-1
Figures 18-1 and 18-2. This 26-year-old woman presented with complaints of dyspnea and hemoptysis. You are shown posteroanterior and lateral chest radiographs.

Case 18: Arteriovenous Malformation

Question 91

Which *one* of the following is the MOST likely diagnosis?

(A) Carcinoid tumor
(B) Metastatic carcinoma
(C) Primary tuberculosis
(D) Hodgkin's lymphoma
(E) Arteriovenous malformation

There are several observations that must be made on the posteroanterior and lateral chest radiographs (Figures 18-1 and 18-2) in order to arrive at the correct diagnosis. First, the masses are multiple. Although on the posteroanterior view the right perihilar mass is most evident, an additional mass is projected over the right heart border (Figure 18-3). On the lateral view (Figure 18-4), this additional mass is clearly seen within the right middle lobe and is associated with two large vessels, one each presumably entering and exiting it.

The above findings suggest that arteriovenous malformation is the most likely diagnosis **(Option (E) is therefore correct).** This diagnosis was confirmed at subsequent pulmonary angiography, which clearly showed a large arteriovenous malformation in the right middle lobe with a single feeding and a single draining vessel (Figure 18-5). The frontal angiographic projection demonstrated the more central arteriovenous malformation, which resembled hilar adenopathy, as well as the one in the anteromedial right middle lobe (Figure 18-6). Angiographic evaluation of the left lung (Figure 18-7) revealed another arteriovenous malformation which was not seen on the posteroanterior and lateral views, illustrating the importance of complete angiographic evaluation. Occasionally, the larger arteriovenous malformations may be correctly diagnosed by computed tomography (Figures 18-8).

Failure to recognize the right middle lobe mass and associated vessels in Figures 18-1 and 18-2 leaves only the right perihilar mass, which

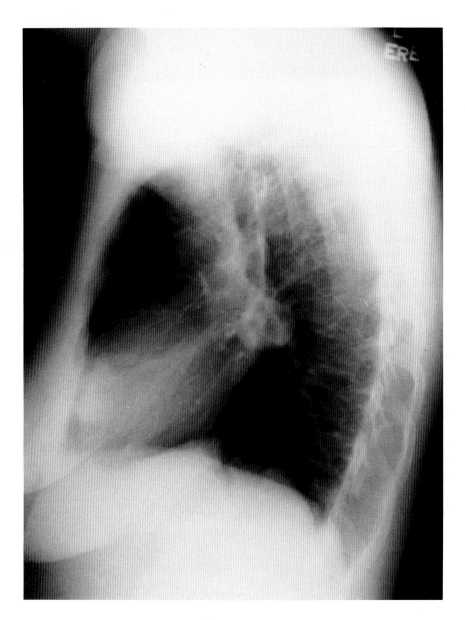

Figure 18-2

might be interpreted as lymphadenopathy, suggesting the possibility of Hodgkin's lymphoma (Option (D)) or primary tuberculosis (Option (C)). Recognition of multiple masses, with failure to identify the associated vessels for the mass in the right middle lobe, would raise the possibility of metastatic carcinoma (Option (B)). Finally, the complaint of hemopty-

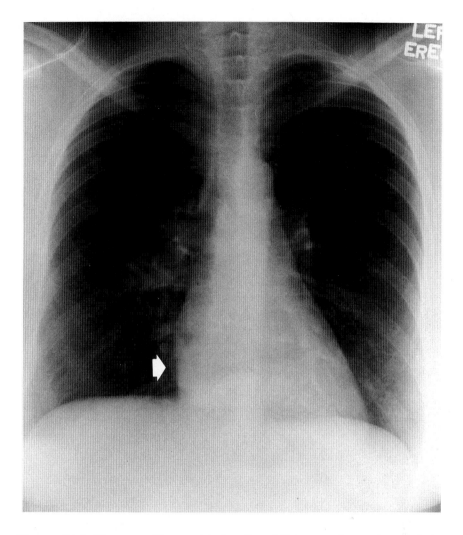

Figure 18-3 (Same as Figure 18-1). In addition to the right perihilar mass, note the mass (arrow) projected at the right heart border.

sis in a young woman might have led to a consideration of carcinoid tumor (Option (A)). However, when the appropriate radiographic observations are made (multiple intraparenchymal masses and associated vessels), the correct diagnosis of arteriovenous malformation is clear.

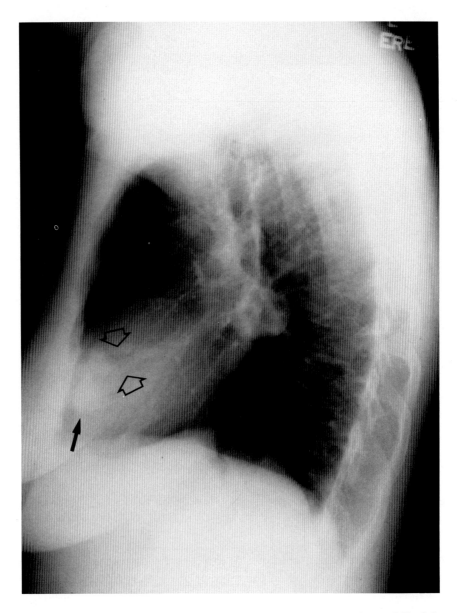

Figure 18-4 (Same as Figure 18-2).   The mass in the right middle lobe
(closed arrow), projected at the right heart border in Figure 18-3, has two
vessels (open arrows) associated with it.

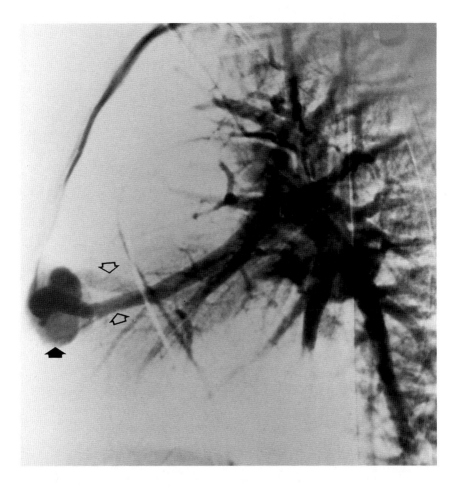

Figure 18-5. This lateral angiogram confirms the arteriovenous malformation (closed arrow) and associated vessels (open arrows). Compare with Figure 18-4.

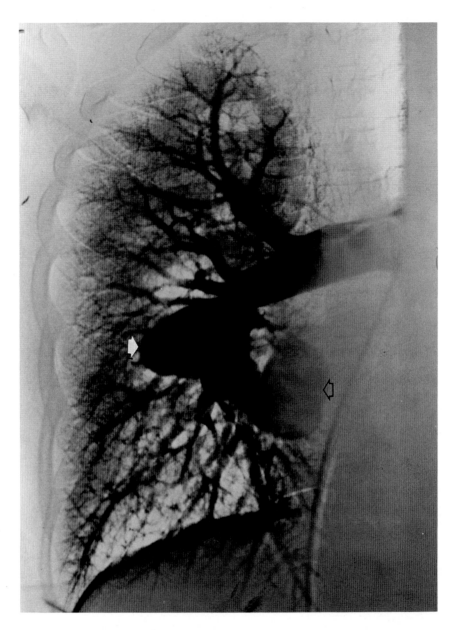

Figure 18-6. This frontal angiogram shows the central arteriovenous malformation (white arrow) and the arteriovenous malformation in the right middle lobe (open arrow). The closer approximation of the arteriovenous malformations on the angiogram is due to projectional differences when compared with the posteroanterior view (Figure 18-3).

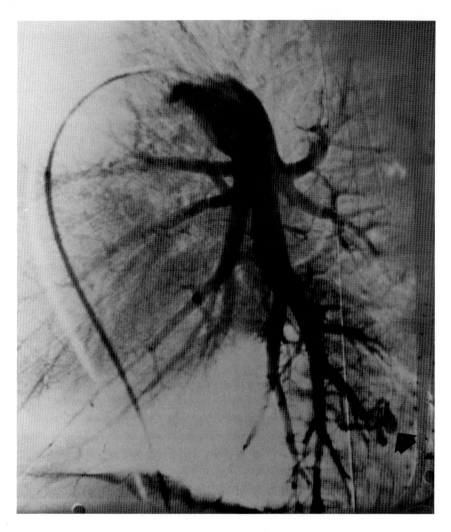

Figure 18-7. A lateral angiogram of the left lung shows another arteriovenous malformation (arrow) in the lower lobe.

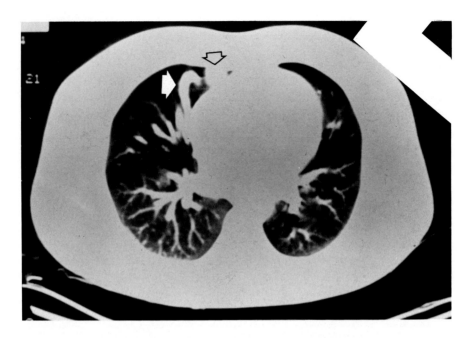

Figure 18-8. A computed tomogram of the patient shown in Figures 18-1 through 18-7 clearly demonstrates the right middle lobe arteriovenous malformation (open black arrow) and one of its associated vessels (solid white arrow).

Question 92

Concerning carcinoid tumors,

- (A) they are benign bronchial adenomas
- (B) they are most common in the sixth decade of life
- (C) hemoptysis is a common feature
- (D) the majority are located in the peripheral airways
- (E) calcification is commonly recognized on conventional chest radiographs

Carcinoid tumors account for less than 5% of all primary lung neoplasms.[1,8,10,14-16] Although they have been traditionally included under the category of bronchial adenomas, it should be noted that the term "adenoma" implies a benign epithelial lesion. Since carcinoid tumors are, in truth, of low-grade malignant potential, they are not true benign adenomas **(Option (A) is false).** Carcinoid tumors, which are now considered to be of Kultschitzky cell neural crest origin, metastasize to regional lymph nodes in 10 to 15% of cases.[1,16]

The tumors of malignant potential previously included under the category of bronchial adenomas, along with the true bronchial adenomas, are carcinoid tumor, cylindroma (adenoid cystic carinoma), and mucoepidermoid carcinoma. The carcinoid type is by far the most common, accounting for 85 to 90% of all four types previously termed bronchial adenomas. While the carcinoid type is said to metastasize to regional lymph nodes in 10 to 15% of cases, metastases are more frequent from cylindromas and less frequent from mucoepidermoid carcinomas.

In most series, carcinoid tumors are found more frequently in female patients. Approximately 90% of the patients are less than 50 years old when the tumor is noted **(Option (B) is false).** Approximately 80% of carcinoid tumors arise in the major bronchi and are thus located centrally **(Option (D) is false).** Because of their vascular nature and central location, hemoptysis is a common feature **(Option (C) is true).** Although calcification may be seen within the lesions pathologically, it is unusual to recognize such calcification on conventional radiographs **(Option (E) is false).**

The radiographic manifestations of carcinoid tumors are largely dependent upon the location of the mass. As noted, the vast majority of these lesions are located centrally and, thus, are manifested radiographically by evidence of bronchial obstruction. This obstruction may present as atelectasis, complete collapse, or air-trapping if collateral air drift is sufficient to maintain lung expansion.[14] In addition, infections may occur distal to the area of obstruction. For the 20% or so of carcinoid tumors arising peripherally and thus not causing bronchial obstruction, the radiographic appearance is most often that of a solitary pulmonary nodule. The appearance of such a nodule is indistinguishable from that of solitary pulmonary nodules of other etiologies.

Question 93

Concerning Hodgkin's lymphoma,

(A) at the time of presentation, it involves the lung parenchyma in approximately 30% of cases
(B) when pulmonary parenchymal involvement is present, associated mediastinal or hilar lymph node enlargement is seen in less than 60% of cases
(C) at the time of presentation, it involves the thorax more commonly than does non-Hodgkin's lymphoma
(D) involvement of the anterior mediastinal lymph nodes is infrequent
(E) at the time of presentation, pleural effusion is seen in approximately 50% of patients

Radiographic findings in Hodgkin's disease, a malignant lymphoma, relate to whether the patient is studied at time of presentation or following treatment. Once treatment is begun, the intrathoracic findings may be related to complications of therapy (including drug toxicity and/or radiation change), opportunistic superinfection, and recurrence or persistence of disease.[3-5,9,11,13]

A review of 300 consecutive untreated patients with Hodgkin's disease and non-Hodgkin's lymphoma seen at the Stanford University Medical Center indicated that intrathoracic disease was seen at the time of presentation in 67% of patients with Hodgkin's lymphoma, as compared with 43% of patients with non-Hodgkin's lymphoma **(Option (C) is true).**[5] This intrathoracic involvement was predominantly manifested as mediastinal and/or hilar adenopathy. Pulmonary parenchymal involvement, although more common overall in Hodgkin's lymphoma, was seen in less than 12% of patients, as compared with less than 5% of those with non-Hodgkin's lymphoma **(Option (A) is false).** Such parenchymal involvement in Hodgkin's disease occurs by direct extension from mediastinal and hilar nodes along bronchovascular pathways. It is almost always associated with radiographic evidence of hilar and/or mediastinal adenopathy, unless there has been previous irradiation of these nodes **(Option (B) is false).**

Involvement of the anterior mediastinal nodes in Hodgkin's lymphoma is very common and, indeed, may be helpful in differentiating the disease from sarcoidosis radiographically **(Option (D) is false).** Although Hodgkin's disease may resemble sarcoidosis, the latter far less commonly causes enlargement of anterior mediastinal lymph nodes visible on conventional radiographs.

Pleural effusions are seen in Hodgkin's lymphoma and have been reported in up to 30% of untreated cases **(Option (E) is false).** In general, however, other intrathoracic manifestations of the disease will be present when pleural effusions are seen. Hodgkin's disease does not commonly invade the pleura directly.

Question 94

Concerning pulmonary arteriovenous malformations,

    (A) they occur most often in the upper lobes
    (B) they are associated with hypertrophic osteoarthropathy
    (C) most are found in patients with hereditary hemorrhagic telangiectasia
    (D) bronchial artery embolotherapy is an accepted method of treatment
    (E) an associated complication is brain abscess

Pulmonary arteriovenous malformations may occur as either single or multiple lesions. The majority are associated with arteriovenous communications elsewhere in the body as part of a condition known as hereditary hemorrhagic telangiectasia or the Rendu-Osler-Weber syndrome **(Option (C) is true)**.[7] Radiographically, they present as round, oval, or lobulated masses. Correct diagnosis depends upon the recognition of associated feeding and draining vessels, as in the test case (Figures 18-1 and 18-2), or the fluoroscopic demonstration of a change in size with a change in intrathoracic pressure and/or blood flow. Pulmonary arteriovenous malformations are most commonly identified in the lower lobes; like any arteriovenous shunt, they may also be associated with hypertrophic osteoarthropathy **(Option (A) is false,** while **Option (B) is true)**.

Although systemic arteriovenous malformations are generally supplied by multiple communicating arteries, pulmonary arteriovenous malformations differ in that approximately 80% are supplied by a single feeder vessel arising from the pulmonary circulation and draining into a bulbous, nonseptated aneurysmal communication (the arteriovenous malformation) that empties into a single draining vein. The remaining 20% of pulmonary arteriovenous malformations are more complex and consist of two or more pulmonary artery branches communicating through the bulbous, septated aneurysmal portion of the lesion with two or more draining veins. Because the normal capillary bed of the lung is bypassed by the arteriovenous malformation, the arteriovenous malformation is in many ways similar to a right-to-left cardiac shunt. The normal filtering function of the pulmonary capillary bed is lost, so that embolization leading to stroke and/or brain abscess is a significant risk **(Option (E) is true)**. In fact, such embolization accounts for 10% mortality in such patients.

Until recently, surgical resection of pulmonary arteriovenous malformations was considered the therapy of choice. More recently, the technique of balloon embolotherapy has proven very effective.[2,6,17] In this technique, detachable silicone balloons are introduced into the feeding pulmonary artery and result in its occlusion **(Option (D) is false)**.

Prior to resecting or embolizing pulmonary arteriovenous malformations it is important to assess the patient for pulmonary arterial hypertension. Closing the malformation in patients with pulmonary artery hypertension results in the removal of a low-resistence shunt and may cause severe cor pulmonale and death.[12]

SUGGESTED READINGS

1. Attar S, Miller JE, Hankins J, McLaughlin JS. Bronchial adenoma—benign or malignant? South Med J 1978; 71:919–922
2. Barth KH, White RI Jr, Kaufman SL, Terry PB, Roland JM. Embolotherapy of pulmonary arteriovenous malformations with detachable balloons. Radiology 1982; 142:599–606
3. Blank N, Castellino RA. The intrathoracic manifestations of the malignant lymphomas and the leukemias. Semin Roentgenol 1980; 15:227–245
4. Desforges JF, Rutherford CJ, Piro A. Hodgkin's disease. New Engl J Med 1979; 301:1212–1222
5. Filly R, Bland N, Castellino RA. Radiographic distribution of intrathoracic disease in previously untreated patients with Hodgkin's disease and non-Hodgkin's lymphoma. Radiology 1976; 120:277–281
6. Gomes AS, Mali WP, Oppenheim WL. Embolization therapy in the management of congenital arteriovenous malformations. Radiology 1982; 144:41–49
7. Hodgson CH, Burchell HB, Good CA, Clagett OT. Hereditary hemorrhagic telangiectasia and pulmonary arteriovenous fistula: survey of a large family. New Engl J Med 1959; 261:625–636
8. Hurt R, Bates M. Carcinoid tumors of the bronchus: a 33 year experience. Thorax 1984; 39:617–623
9. Johnson DW, Hoppe RT, Cox RS, Rosenberg SA, Kaplan HS. Hodgkin's disease limited to intrathoracic sites. Cancer 1983; 52:8–13
10. Marks C, Marks M. Bronchial adenoma. A clinicopathologic study. Chest 1977; 71:376–380
11. North LB, Fuller LM, Hagemeister FB, Rodgers RW, Butler JJ, Shullenberger CC. Importance of initial mediastinal adenopathy in Hodgkin disease. AJR 1982; 138:229–235

12. Rodan BA, Goodwin JD, Chen JTT, Ravin CE. Worsening pulmonary hypertension after resection of arteriovenous fistula. AJR 1981; 137:864–866
13. Shuman LS, Libshitz HI: Solid pleural manifestations of lymphoma. AJR 1984; 142:269–273
14. Spitzer SA, Segal I, Lubin E, Nili M, Levy M. Unilateral increased transradiancy of the lung caused by bronchial carcinoid tumour. Thorax 1980; 35:739–744
15. Tolis GA, Fry WA, Head L, Shields TW. Bronchial adenomas. Surg Gynecol Obstet 1972; 134:605–610
16. Turnbull AD, Huvos AS, Goodner JT, Beattie EJ Jr. The malignant potential of bronchial adenoma. Ann Thorac Surg 1972; 14:453–464
17. White RI Jr, Mitchell SE, Barth KH, et al. Angioarchitecture of pulmonary arteriovenous malformations: an important consideration before embolotherapy. AJR 1983; 140:681–686

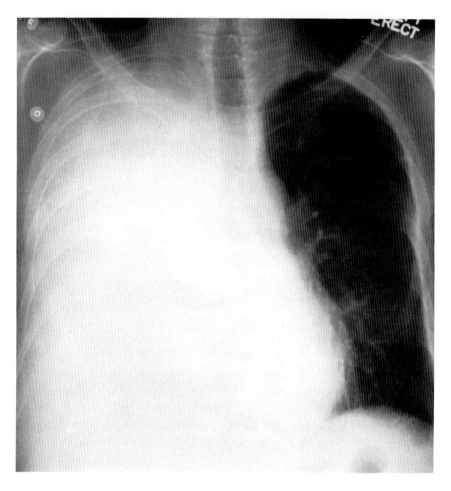

Figure 19-1. This 60-year-old alcoholic patient presented with shortness of breath. You are shown a posteroanterior chest radiograph.

Case 19: Hepatic Hydrothorax

Question 95

Which *one* of the following is the LEAST likely diagnosis?

(A) Malignant mesothelioma
(B) Atelectasis of the right lung
(C) Meigs' syndrome
(D) Hepatic hydrothorax
(E) *Klebsiella* pneumonia

The posteroanterior chest radiograph demonstrates complete opacification of the right hemithorax with associated contralateral mediastinal shift. This contralateral shift strongly suggests that right lung atelectasis alone would be very unlikely, since ipsilateral mediastinal shift would thus be expected **(Option (B) is the least likely diagnosis).**

A common cause of complete opacification of a hemithorax with contralateral mediastinal shift is pleural effusion. Thus, Meigs' syndrome (Option (C)) and hepatic hydrothorax (Option (D)), both associated with effusion, would be likely considerations. Malignant mesothelioma (Option (A)), also associated with effusion, is likely, although when extensive it may encircle the lung and show either ipsilateral shift or no shift of mediastinal structures. Finally, *Klebsiella* pneumonia (Option (E)), because of its necrotizing properties, may expand an involved lobe or lung and conceivably could produce the appearance shown in Figure 19-1.

Question 96

Concerning mesothelioma,

    (A) the benign form is associated with previous exposure to asbestos
    (B) the association of hypertrophic osteoarthropathy and a localized pleural mass suggests the benign form
    (C) pleural effusions are commonly seen in association with the benign form
    (D) when there is pleural effusion with the malignant form, the mediastinum is usually shifted contralaterally
    (E) the malignant form frequently has metastasized to distant sites at the time of initial detection

Mesothelioma may occur in a localized form, which is usually benign, or in a diffuse form, which is malignant. The latter form is frequently associated with previous exposure to asbestos, in particular to fibers of the crocidolite type.[2,8-10] The tumor spreads diffusely along the pleura and may encase the lung.[1,3,12] It is locally invasive but seldom metastasizes to distant sites **(Option (E) is false).** Although pleural effusion may be associated with malignant mesothelioma and may obscure it, the effusion uncommonly results in contralateral shift of the mediastinal structures **(Option (D) is false).** The exact explanation for this phenomenon is unclear. However, it is postulated that the tumor encases the lung to prevent normal lung inflation and, thus, decrease lung volume. Alternatively, invasion of the medial aspect of the lung by the neoplasm may occlude the bronchi and result in an element of atelectasis that decreases lung volume. Whatever the mechanism for the decreased volume, it may promote ipsilateral mediastinal shift or tend to counteract any contralateral shift from effusion.

The localized and usually benign form of mesothelioma arises from the visceral pleura much more frequently than from the parietal pleura and does not appear to be associated with asbestos exposure[7] **(Option (A) is false).** In general, the lesion uncommonly gives rise to clinical signs or symptoms, especially when small. However, clubbing of the fingers and hypertrophic osteoarthropathy may be seen **(Option (B) is true).** In contrast to the malignant form, pleural effusion is rarely associated with benign localized mesotheliomas **(Option (C) is false)** (See Case 33, Localized Fibrous Mesothelioma, for further discussion).

Question 97

Concerning Meigs' syndrome,

    (A) the original description included both benign and malignant ovarian tumors
    (B) pleural effusion indicates metastatic spread
    (C) ascitic fluid is generally absent
    (D) right-sided pleural effusions are more common than left-sided ones

In 1937, Meigs and Cass reported seven patients who each had benign ovarian fibroma associated with ascites and hydrothorax and who were cured by removal of the fibroma.[5] Benign ovarian fibroma associated with ascites and hydrothorax subsequently came to be known as Meigs' syndrome[4] **(Options (A) and (C) are false).** Attention was called to this constellation of findings because of the concern that patients with an ovarian mass, ascites, and hydrothorax might reasonably be assumed to have a malignant inoperable lesion that had metastasized rather than a benign operable one **(Option (B) is false).** The exact etiology of the ascites and explanation for the associated hydrothorax have not yet been elucidated. The pleural effusions may be small or large and are much more common on the right side than on the left **(Option (D) is true).** The term "Meigs' syndrome" is sometimes loosely applied to lesions of the ovary other than fibromas, contrary to Meigs' original description.

Question 98

Concerning hepatic hydrothorax,

    (A) the associated liver disease is cirrhosis
    (B) right-sided pleural effusions are more common than left-sided ones
    (C) ascites is uncommon
    (D) it is most likely secondary to pulmonary infection

Hepatic hydrothorax is a term that has been coined to call attention to the development of hydrothorax in cases of cirrhosis associated with ascites[11] **(Option (A) is true; Option (C) is false).** Generally, the condition is seen in fewer than 10% of patients with cirrhosis of the liver and ascites. Most commonly the effusions are right-sided, although less frequently they may be left-sided or bilateral **(Option (B) is true).** While the exact mechanism for development of pleural effusions is unclear, it is believed that ascitic fluid is most likely transported across the

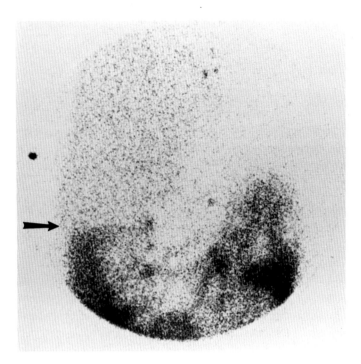

Figure 19-2. This anterior scintigram of the thorax and upper abdomen obtained after intraperitoneal injection of Tc-99m sulfur colloid shows activity in the right hemithorax. The position of the right hemidiaphragm is indicated by an arrow.

diaphragm either by the lymphatic system or through defects in the diaphragm **(Option (D) is false).** These defects are said to be more common on the right side, a situation which may explain the predominance of right-sided effusions.

The patient shown in Figure 19-1 suffers from hepatic hydrothorax. His hepatic cirrhosis was secondary to chronic alcohol abuse, and he had developed both ascites and a massive right-sided pleural effusion. To confirm the suspected diagnosis of hepatic hydrothorax, Tc-99m sulfur colloid was injected into the peritoneal cavity and sequential images were obtained. Over several hours the tracer was seen to move into the right hemithorax (Figure 19-2), confirming migration across the right hemidiaphragm either through diaphragmatic defects or via the lymphatics.

Patients undergoing peritoneal dialysis for renal failure may also develop hydrothorax.[6] The common denominator in the pathogenesis of these effusions and of hepatic hydrothorax seems to be a large amount of fluid in the peritoneal space (dialysate with renal failure, ascites with hepatic cirrhosis).

SUGGESTED READINGS

1. Alexander E, Clark RA, Colley DP, Mitchell SE. CT of malignant pleural mesothelioma. AJR 1981; 137:287–291
2. Becklake MR. Asbestos-related diseases of the lung and other organs: their epidemiology and implications for clinical practice. Am Rev Respir Dis 1976; 114:187–227
3. Lewis RJ, Sisler GE, Mackenzie JW. Diffuse, mixed malignant pleural mesothelioma. Ann Thorac Surg 1981; 31:53–60
4. Meigs JV. Fibroma of the ovary with ascites and hydrothorax—Meigs' syndrome. Am J Obstet Gynecol 1954; 67:952–984
5. Meigs JV, Cass JW. Fibroma of the ovary with ascites and hydrothorax. Am J Obstet Gynecol 1937; 33:249–267
6. Milutinovic J, Wu WS, Lindholm DD, Lapp NL. Acute massive unilateral hydrothorax: a rare complication of chronic peritoneal dialysis. South Med J 1980; 73:827–828
7. Okike N, Bernatz PE, Woolner LB. Localized mesothelioma of the pleura: benign and malignant variants. J Thorac Cardiovasc Surg 1978; 75:363–372
8. Rabinowitz JG, Efremidis SC, Cohen B, et al. A comparative study of mesothelioma and asbestosis using computed tomography and conventional chest radiography. Radiology 1982; 144:453–460
9. Selikoff IJ, Bader RA, Bader ME, Churg J, Hammond EC. Asbestosis and neoplasia. Am J Med 1967; 42:487–496
10. Selikoff IJ, Churg J, Hammond EC. Asbestos exposure and neoplasia. JAMA 1964; 188:142–146
11. Stanley NN, William AJ, Dewar CA, Blendis LM, Reid L. Hypoxia and hydrothoraces in a case of liver cirrhosis: correlation of physiological, radiographic, scintigraphic, and pathological findings. Thorax 1977; 32:457–471
12. Taryle DA, Lakshminarayan S, Sahn SA. Pleural mesotheliomas—an analysis of 18 cases and review of the literature. Medicine (Baltimore) 1976; 55:153–162

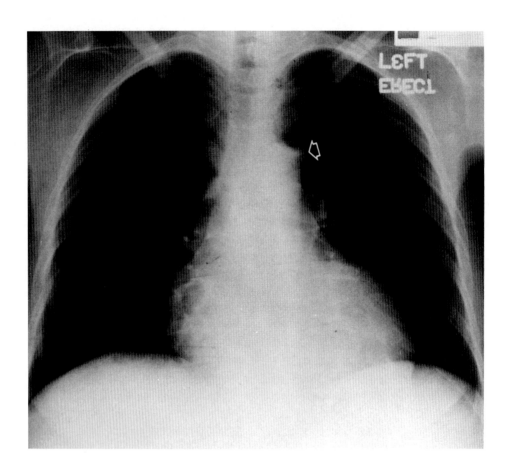

Figure 20-1. This 32-year-old woman has cardiac disease secondary to the carcinoid syndrome. You are shown a posteroanterior chest radiograph.

Case 20: Dilated Left Superior Intercostal Vein

Question 99

Which *one* of the following is indicated by the arrow in Figure 20-1?

(A) Aortic diverticulum
(B) Lymph node
(C) Ductus arteriosus
(D) Left superior intercostal vein
(E) Persistent left superior vena cava

The posteroanterior chest radiograph (Figure 20-1) demonstrates a "nipple-like" projection adjacent to the lateral margin of the aortic arch, cardiomegaly, some prominence of the right atrium, and mild distention of the azygos vein. The latter two findings are consistent with elevated systemic venous pressure secondary to the patient's tricuspid insufficiency associated with her carcinoid syndrome. In this clinical situation, the left superior intercostal vein is often distended. Of the options listed in Question 99, left superior intercostal vein is the best explanation for the radiographic finding **(Option (D) is the correct answer)**.

A number of normal systemic veins and arteries are routinely visualized on posteroanterior chest radiographs. The margins of the superior vena cava, azygos arch, and aortic arch are commonly seen and are only rarely confused with pathological findings. On the other hand, the left superior intercostal vein, seen less often, may occasionally be mistaken for neoplasm or lymphadenopathy (Option (B)). This vein, a single trunk that arises from the left second, third, and fourth posterior intercostal veins, courses anteriorly along the lateral wall of the aortic arch to drain into the left brachiocephalic vein. Communication with the accessory hemiazygos vein posteriorly is frequent.

End-on visualization of the left superior intercostal vein on the posteroanterior chest radiograph is responsible for the "nipple-like"

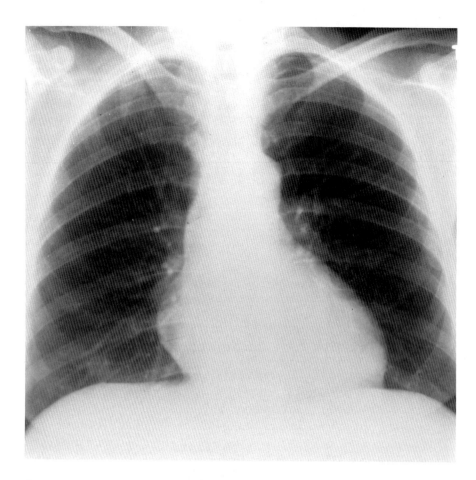

Figure 20-2. Posteroanterior radiograph of the patient shown in Figure
20-1, taken after placement of a tricuspid valvular prosthesis (not visible
on this view), shows decreased size of the left superior intercostal and
azygos veins (compare with Figure 20-1).

projection adjacent to the aortic arch.[1,5,6] In general, the appearance is
so characteristic as to allow easy identification, but if there is any
question, the vein may be examined fluoroscopically and advantage may
be taken of the fact that veins change in size with changes in patient
position or intrathoracic pressure. Dilatation of the vein occurs in
situations of increased blood flow, as when the vessel serves as a
collateral pathway, or in situations of increased pressure within the
systemic venous system, as occurred in the patient in this case.[2]
Following surgical correction of the patient's tricuspid insufficiency with
placement of a prosthetic valve, the left superior intercostal and azygos
veins both decreased in size (Figure 20-2).

Visualization of the ductus arteriosus (Option (C)) is not expected in an adult. Moreover, the position of the structure indicated by the arrow in Figure 20-1 is too high to represent a ductus arteriosus. A persistent left superior vena cava (Option (E)) produces a more vertically oriented soft tissue margin along the left upper mediastinum than that shown in Figure 20-1. Aortic diverticulum (Option (A)) is discussed below and also would not explain the findings in Figure 20-1.

Question 100

Concerning "carcinoid heart disease" secondary to an intra-abdominal primary carcinoid tumor,

    (A) metastatic spread of tumor to the liver is implied
    (B) it is generally secondary to metastatic involvement of the myocardium
    (C) the tricuspid and pulmonic valves are most commonly involved
    (D) echocardiography reveals metastasis to the valves

Cardiac disease associated with the carcinoid syndrome, so-called carcinoid heart disease, has been noted since the early 1930s.[8] The disease is characterized pathologically by fibrous lesions in the heart and great vessels; the histology of lesions is virtually pathognomonic in that the focal or diffuse collections of fibrous tissue are of a peculiar type free of elastic fibers and are deposited on the endocardium of the valvular cusps **(Options (B) and (D) are false).** The tricuspid and pulmonic valves are most commonly involved **(Option (C) is true).**

In the majority of patients, the site of the primary carcinoid tumor is the small intestine, and hepatic metastases are nearly always seen **(Option (A) is true).** The pathophysiology of the cardiac lesions is not well understood, but the serotonin secreted by the tumor is thought to play a major role in their formation. Such lesions are seen when carcinoid metastases to the liver are present or, less commonly, when there is drainage of the carcinoid tumor by routes other than the portal vein. Thus, it appears that serotonin-producing metastases in the liver or in a location bypassing the liver, where serotonin would normally be detoxified, are a requirement. The relative scarcity of left-sided cardiac lesions is attributed to inactivation of serotonin by monoamine oxidase during passage through the lungs.

Question 101

Concerning an aortic diverticulum,

(A) when visible, that found in adults at the aortoductal junction is generally seen better on the lateral than on the posteroanterior chest radiograph

(B) that seen with an aberrant right subclavian artery and a left aortic arch is thought to represent incomplete regression of the primitive distal right aortic arch

(C) that associated with a right aortic arch and an aberrant left subclavian artery is seen on the posteroanterior chest radiograph as a soft tissue opacity in the left paratracheal region

(D) that associated with a left aortic arch and an aberrant right subclavian artery is termed the "diverticulum of Kommerell"

Aortic diverticula, sac-like outpouchings of the aortic arch, may be confused with aneurysms or mediastinal masses of other etiology. In an excellent review of the subject, Salomonowitz et al. described three basic types of aortic diverticula.[9] The first type, seen with a left aortic arch and an aberrant right subclavian artery, occurs at the origin of the aberrant artery and has been termed the Kommerell diverticulum **(Option (D) is true)**.[10] The diverticulum (Figure 20-3) is considered to represent an incomplete regression of the primitive distal right aortic arch and is said to be present in the majority of cases of aberrant right subclavian artery **(Option (B) is true)**. Uncommonly, an aberrant right subclavian artery may be responsible for dysphagia and necessitate surgical intervention.[4,7] In such instances, it is important to recognize the nature of the Kommerell diverticulum so that it is not mistaken for an aneurysm and unnecessarily resected.

The second type of aortic diverticulum is seen in association with a right aortic arch and an aberrant left subclavian artery.[3] In this case, the diverticulum represents the remnant of the primitive distal left aortic arch and gives rise to the aberrant vessel. If identified on the posteroanterior chest radiograph, the diverticulum is seen as a soft tissue opacity in the left paratracheal region (Figure 20-4) **(Option (C) is true)**. A lateral esophagram will show a large horizontal indentation on the posterior wall of the esophagus. Aortography (Figure 20-5) nicely demonstrates the aortic diverticulum, although a less invasive study, such as computed tomography, may do the same.[12]

The third type of aortic diverticulum is seen at the aortoductal junction along the inner aspect of the aorta just distal to the left subclavian artery. This has sometimes been termed the ductus diverticulum or ductus bulge. It represents a remnant of the infundibular portion of the ductus

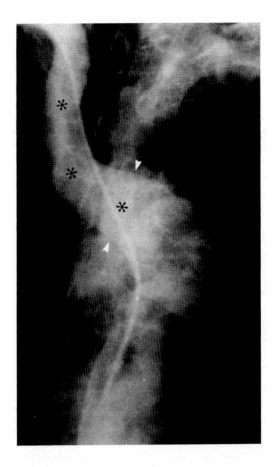

Figure 20-3. Anteroposterior angiogram shows the aberrant right subclavian artery (*) originating from the aortic arch. Note the wide origin of the vessel (arrowheads), the diverticulum of Kommerell. (Reprinted with permission from Proto et al. [7].)

arteriosus and is not normally identified in adults on posteroanterior chest radiographs. However, if visible, it may be noted as a soft tissue mass in the aortic-pulmonic window on the lateral chest radiograph **(Option (A) is true).**

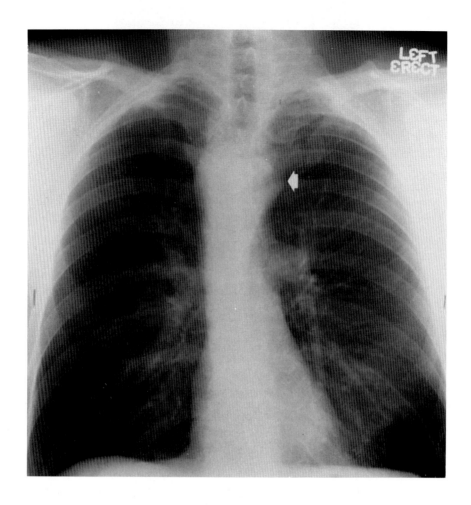

Figure 20-4
Figures 20-4 and 20-5. The posteroanterior view (Figure 20-4) of a patient with a right aortic arch and an aberrant left subclavian artery shows the associated diverticulum (arrow) in its typical location. An angiogram (Figure 20-5) further demonstrates the diverticulum (arrow).

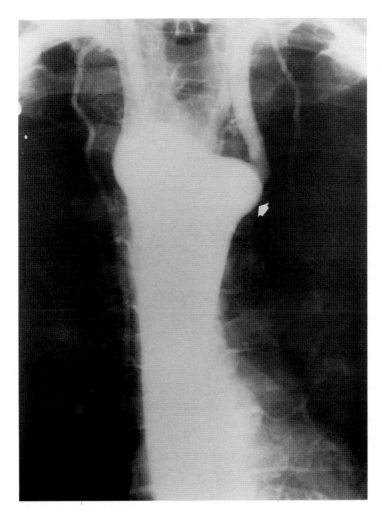

Figure 20-5

Discussion

Since the dilatation of the azygos vein was a key observation in the analysis of Question 99, some remarks should be made about it. The azygos vein begins at about the level of the first or second lumbar vertebral body, usually as a continuation of the right ascending lumbar vein. It enters the thorax through the aortic hiatus of the diaphragm and passes along the anterior portion of the thoracic vertebral column to the right of the midline up to the level of the fourth or fifth thoracic vertebra, at which point it arches forward to empty into the posterior wall of the superior vena cava.[11] The azygos vein receives drainage from the right superior intercostal vein and the hemiazygos venous system. Via its connection to the ascending lumbar vein, it also communicates with the inferior vena cava. Thus, the azygos vein provides a potential collateral pathway between the inferior vena cava below and the superior vena cava above. Like other veins throughout the body, it is quite distensible and may, therefore, dilate in response to increased flow through the vessel or increased pressure within the vessel. Changes in flow may be related to conditions that are either congenital (interruption of the inferior vena cava) or acquired (obstruction of the inferior vena cava from any cause). In addition, conditions that increase flow in the vessel, such as pregnancy, may also distend it. Moreover, any condition that increases the pressure in the systemic venous system, such as congestive heart failure or tricuspid insufficiency, may also dilate the vein.

It is the arch of the azygos vein that is seen end-on at the lower right paratracheal area on the posteroanterior chest radiograph. On radiographs obtained with the patient standing, the transverse diameter of the arch of the azygos vein should generally not exceed 1 cm. In fact, the transverse diameter in most patients is 7 mm or less. Increases in the transverse diameter of the vein beyond normal values should evoke considerations of increased pressure or flow through the azygos system.

SUGGESTED READINGS

1. Ball JB Jr, Proto AV. The variable appearance of the left superior intercostal vein. Radiology 1982; 144:445–452
2. Friedman AC, Chambers E, Sprayregen S. The normal and abnormal left superior intercostal vein. AJR 1978; 131:599–602
3. Jung JY, Almond CH, Saab SB, Lababidi Z. Surgical repair of right aortic

arch with aberrant left subclavian artery and left ligamentum arteriosum. J Thorac Cardiovasc Surg 1978; 75:237–243

4. Klinkhamer AC. Aberrant right subclavian artery. Clinical and roentgenologic aspects. AJR 1966; 97:438–446

5. Lane EJ, Heitzman ER, Dinn WM. The radiology of the superior intercostal veins. Radiology 1976; 120:263–267

6. McDonald CJ, Castellino RA, Blank N. The aortic "nipple." The left superior intercostal vein. Radiology 1970; 96:533–536

7. Proto AV, Cuthbert NW, Raider L. Aberrant right subclavian artery: further observations. AJR 1987; 148:253–257

8. Roberts WC, Sjoerdsma A. The cardiac disease associated with the carcinoid syndrome (carcinoid heart disease). Am J Med 1964; 36:5–26

9. Salomonowitz E, Edwards JE, Hunter DW, et al. The three types of aortic diverticula. AJR 1984; 142:673–679

10. Shannon JM. Aberrant right subclavian artery with Kommerell's diverticulum. J Thorac Cardiovasc Surg 1961; 41:408–411

11. Smathers RL, Buschi AJ, Pope TL Jr, Brenbridge AN, Williamson BR. The azygous arch: normal and pathologic CT appearance. AJR 1982; 139:477–483

12. Webb WR, Gamsu G, Speckman JM, Kaiser JA, Federle MP, Lipton MJ. CT demonstration of mediastinal aortic arch anomalies. J Comput Assist Tomogr 1982; 6:445–451

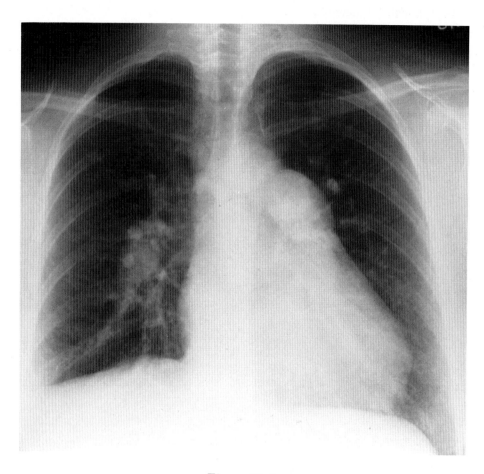

Figure 21-1
Figures 21-1 and 21-2. History withheld. You are shown posteroanterior
(Figure 21-1) and lateral (Figure 21-2) chest radiographs of a 32-year-old
woman.

Case 21: Pulmonary Arterial Hypertension

Question 102

Which *one* of the following is the MOST likely diagnosis?

(A) Lymphoma
(B) The Hughes-Stovin syndrome
(C) Pulmonic valvular stenosis
(D) Pulmonary arterial hypertension
(E) Sarcoidosis

Based on the patient's age and sex, each of the diagnostic considerations presented would be a reasonable consideration, with the exception of the Hughes-Stovin syndrome (Option (B)), which is far more common in men than in women. From a radiographic standpoint it is first necessary to determine whether the hilar enlargement is due to lymphadenopathy, in which case sarcoidosis and lymphoma would be the more likely considerations, or whether the enlargement is secondary to enlargement of the central pulmonary arteries, in which case pulmonary arterial hypertension or pulmonic valvular stenosis would be more likely. While lobulation of an enlarged hilum or the presence of obvious lymphadenopathy elsewhere in the mediastinum may be a clue on the posteroanterior view that the hilar enlargement is also due to adenopathy, the differentiation between enlarged hilar arteries and enlarged hilar lymph nodes is often greatly aided by the lateral view of the chest.[17] On the lateral view, enlarged hilar arteries will conform to the position and course of nonenlarged ones. The normal "clear space" seen below the left upper lobe bronchus is typically preserved. On the other hand, with hilar and, particularly, subcarinal adenopathy, this space is often filled with soft tissue opacity.

In the case presented here (Figures 21-1 and 21-2), the radiographic appearance on the lateral view favors enlarged hilar arteries, not nodes.

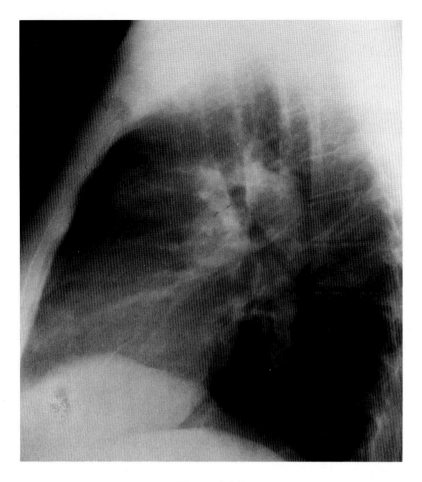

Figure 21-2

Hence, lymphoma (Option (A)) and sarcoidosis (Option (E)) are not likely. Additionally, both the posteroanterior and lateral views indicate enlargement of the main pulmonary artery. In view of the foregoing findings of centralized uniform pulmonary artery enlargement, along with apparent tapering of the peripheral vessels, the diagnosis of pulmonary arterial hypertension is strongly suggested **(Option (D) is most likely)**. Pulmonic valvular stenosis (Option (C)), when it results in pulmonary arterial enlargement, affects the main and left hilar pulmonary arteries but generally not the right. Thus, pulmonic stenosis is not likely. The Hughes-Stovin syndrome, which has as one of its components aneurysms of large and small pulmonary arteries, would not be a likely cause of the uniform arterial enlargement seen in Figures 21-1 and 21-2. Moreover, the syndrome is far more common in men than in women, as already mentioned.

Question 103

Concerning the Hughes-Stovin syndrome,

    (A) findings include aneurysms of large and small pulmonary arteries
    (B) most cases are associated with congenital cardiovascular defects
    (C) it occurs more commonly in women than in men
    (D) peripheral venous thrombosis is a feature
    (E) hemoptysis is uncommon

The Hughes-Stovin syndrome is characterized by aneurysms of both large and small pulmonary arteries associated with thrombosis of both peripheral veins and dural sinuses **(Options (A) and (D) are true)**. The syndrome was originally reported in 1959 by Hughes and Stovin, who described a disease process which they divided into three general stages.[12,14,22] In the early stage, the prominent feature was that of raised intracranial pressure due to thrombosis of the jugular veins and/or the dural sinuses. The next phase of the illness was one of recurrent thromboses of both superficial and deep systemic veins. This stage was also characterized by recurrent febrile episodes without evidence of septicemia. Such episodes responded to neither antibiotics nor steroid administration. In the third stage of the illness attention was drawn to the chest because of hemoptysis associated with aneurysms of both large and small pulmonary arteries **(Option (E) is false)**. Indeed, the demise of many of these patients was due to massive hemoptysis secondary to rupture of these aneurysms.

Most of the afflicted patients are men or boys, many of whom have had associated congenital cardiovascular defects, most often septal defects and patent ductus arteriosus **(Option (B) is true; Option (C) is false)**. Pulmonary thromboembolism has been a common associated finding.

Question 104

Concerning pulmonic valvular stenosis,

(A) radiographically, dilatation more commonly involves the main and left pulmonary arteries than the right pulmonary artery

(B) the associated dilatation of the main pulmonary artery is readily distinguished on chest radiographs from idiopathic dilatation of that artery

(C) there is poor correlation between the prominence of the pulmonary artery and the severity of valvular stenosis

(D) when complicated by both right ventricular hypertrophy and a right-to-left shunt at the atrial level, it is termed the "trilogy of Fallot"

Stenosis of the pulmonary valve is the most common form of right ventricular outflow tract obstruction and is said to account for approximately 6% of all congenital cardiac lesions.[4,5,21] There are various types of valvular stenoses, although the most common is that in which the valve has three fused commissures resulting in restriction of the central orifice. The size of the residual orifice is directly related to the degree of fusion of the commissures. While the valve may be minimally thickened, its mobility is preserved. Thus, during diastole there is inversion of the valve, followed during systole by the characteristic dome-shaped valve, which may be seen at angiography.

Blood passing through the stenotic valve creates a jet effect, which is thought to account, at least in part, for poststenotic dilatation of the main pulmonary artery. However, the degree of dilatation is not related to the severity of valvular stenosis **(Option (C) is true)**. In addition, because of the jet effect and the more direct continuation of the left than the right pulmonary artery with the main pulmonary artery, dilatation frequently involves the left pulmonary artery. The right pulmonary artery tends to be spared, as its orientation is for the most part perpendicular to that of the jet of blood. Accordingly, the main and left pulmonary arteries tend to dilate with pulmonic valvular stenosis, and there is selective flow of blood toward the left lung, which may be dramatically demonstrated by pulmonary perfusion scintigraphy **(Option (A) is true)**. With infundibular pulmonic stenosis there is no significant inequity of vascular distribution, a differentiating point that may help to distinguish this type of stenosis from valvular stenosis.

Poststenotic dilatation of the main pulmonary artery, due to pulmonic valvular stenosis, may be closely mimicked by idiopathic dilatation of that artery. This latter condition is a benign one in which the main pulmonary artery dilates without impairment of cardiac function, as opposed to pulmonic valvular stenosis in which right ventricular pressure is elevated.[1] Idiopathic dilatation of the main pulmonary artery is rarely encountered prior to the age of 4 years, and its etiology has not been established. On conventional chest radiographs such dilatation is difficult, if not impossible, to distinguish from that seen with pulmonic valvular stenosis **(Option (B) is false)**. A potential differentiating point relates to the dilatation of the left pulmonary artery that may be seen with valvular stenosis.

Pulmonic valvular stenosis may be associated with a variety of other congenital abnormalities. Perhaps one of the best known of these is tetralogy of Fallot, which consists of pulmonic valvular stenosis, interventricular septal defect, an ascending aorta that overrides the interventricular septum to receive blood from both ventricles, and right ventricular hypertrophy. This is contrasted with the less well known trilogy of Fallot, which consists of pulmonic valvular stenosis, right-to-left shunting at the atrial level through either a true atrial septal defect or a patent foramen ovale, and right ventricular hypertrophy **(Option (D) is true)**. In these patients, the ventricular septum is intact, and shunting occurs at the atrial level. Resultant cyanosis distinguishes patients with this entity from those with pulmonic valvular stenosis alone.

Question 105

Concerning primary pulmonary arterial hypertension,

    (A) the diagnosis is essentially one of exclusion
    (B) the disease most commonly affects young women
    (C) dyspnea on exertion is a common presenting complaint

Primary pulmonary hypertension is a term currently used to describe a disease state in which pulmonary arterial hypertension of unexplained etiology is present.[9] The diagnosis is established when other causes of pulmonary hypertension have been excluded **(Option (A) is true)**. These other causes include entities such as: pulmonary thromboembolism, which may be evaluated by ventilation-perfusion scintigraphy or by selective pulmonary angiography if the scintigraphic findings are indeterminate; chronic obstructive pulmonary disease, which may be evaluated by pulmonary function tests; elevated left ventricular filling pressures, which may be evaluated by pulmonary wedge pressure determination or by cardiac catheterization, if necessary; left-to-right shunts with Eisenmenger's physiology, which may be evaluated by cardiac catheterization; pulmonary arteritides, which may be evaluated with such studies as sedimentation rates and antinuclear antibodies; and parasitic diseases, particularly schistosomiasis. The importance of making an accurate diagnosis cannot be overstated, as the therapies for the other forms of pulmonary hypertension differ significantly from those currently utilized in primary pulmonary hypertension.

Primary pulmonary hypertension is relatively uncommon and has been characterized as an illness that predominantly affects young women **(Option (B) is true).** As recognition of the disease has improved, more male patients and older individuals of both sexes are being identified, and occasional familial cases have also been described.[11,19] Of interest, a group of patients developed pulmonary hypertension in Europe in the late 1960s following introduction of an appetite suppressant, aminorex fumarate. Pathologically, the lesions in these patients were indistinguishable from those noted in patients with true primary pulmonary hypertension, namely hypertrophy of the media in small pulmonary arterioles in a pattern reminiscent of that seen in response to chronic hypoxia.

Radiographically, the appearance is that of significant pulmonary arterial hypertension—dilatation of the main and central pulmonary arteries with tapering of the more peripheral arterial vessels. This results in apparent oligemia of the pulmonary periphery, an appearance which is particularly striking when viewed in association with dilated central pulmonary arteries. The pulmonary blood flow appears equalized and centralized, without evidence of cephalization.[18]

Symptoms are nonspecific and most commonly include complaints of dyspnea on exertion **(Option (C) is true),** easy fatigability, and a sensation of tiredness. The prognosis in most patients is relatively poor, and death occurs (usually as a result of cor pulmonale) within 2 to 10 years after initial symptoms appear. Treatment of the disease thus far with a variety of drug regimens has proven disappointing. The process is usually well advanced at the time of the initial diagnosis, and the course seems unaffected by most drugs that have been tried.

Question 106

Concerning sarcoidosis,

(A) pleural effusion is rarely, if ever, associated with it
(B) "eggshell" calcifications are an uncommon residuum
(C) enlargement of anterior mediastinal nodes occurs in approximately 15% of patients
(D) enlargement of subcarinal nodes is rare

Sarcoidosis is a systemic granulomatous disease of unknown etiology. The classical histologic appearance of noncaseating granulomas is relatively nonspecific, as similar findings may be seen in association with other diseases such as tuberculosis, mycotic infections, and lymphoma. The term "noncaseating" is somewhat misleading, as an element of granular necrosis may be present. In truth, the distinction between caseating and noncaseating granulomas is not absolute, so that the diagnosis may at times be in question. The term "sarcoidosis" encompasses clinical, radiographic, and pathologic findings, which, when taken in the aggregate, suggest the appropriate diagnosis. Nonetheless, the usage of the term to indicate an actual disease entity has become engrained in the medical literature and is generally accepted.

Due to the multisystem involvement and the wide variety of radiographic and clinical manifestations, it is not possible to review the entire spectrum of sarcoidosis.[8,16] However, several points of interest are worthy of note.

The most common radiographic abnormality noted in thoracic sarcoidosis is lymphadenopathy.[7,13,15] Initial reviews of multiple cases stressed involvement of the hilar and right paratracheal nodes. Subsequent reviews also pointed out that left paratracheal nodes are generally involved, although, unless specifically sought, such involvement was frequently less apparent radiographically. Strengthened by evidence gained from computed tomography, more recent reports have stressed that, in addition to hilar and paratracheal adenopathy, other intrathoracic lymph nodes are often involved.[3] A review of 87 patients with documented sarcoidosis demonstrated that 21% had involvement of the subcarinal nodes, 16% had involvement of the anterior mediastinal nodes, and 2% had involvement of the posterior mediastinal nodes **(Option (C) is true; Option (D) is false).**[2] Involvement of hilar nodes was present in 97% of the patients, while involvement of paratracheal nodes was present approximately 75% of the time. Thus, although involvement of hilar and paratracheal nodes is clearly the most common radiographic pattern of adenopathy, the disease process may also involve anterior, subcarinal, and, rarely, posterior mediastinal nodes.

It is often stressed that anterior mediastinal adenopathy as evidenced radiographically is far more common in lymphoma than in sarcoidosis; it occurs only rarely in sarcoidosis. It is now clear that anterior mediastinal adenopathy in sarcoidosis is not as rare as had once been thought. On the other hand, it would be highly unusual with sarcoidosis to encounter anterior mediastinal adenopathy without hilar adenopathy, whereas isolated involvement of anterior mediastinal lymph nodes would not be unusual with lymphoma.

One interesting feature of lymphadenopathy in sarcoidosis is eggshell calcification of hilar and mediastinal nodes.[14] Eggshell calcification, long considered as nearly pathognomonic of silicosis, does occur, although uncommonly with sarcoidosis (Figure 21-3) **(Option (B) is true)**. In the reported cases, patients have had systemic disease and steroid therapy had been initiated prior to the development of the calcification. The lymph node calcification was not associated with systemic hypercalcemia. Patients had demonstrated evidence of both lymphadenopathy and parenchymal disease, and eggshell calcification developed with regression of the parenchymal disease being treated with steroids.

A misconception concerning sarcoidosis is that pleural disease is not seen in uncomplicated cases. A review of 227 patients identified pleural reaction (pleural effusion and/or pleural thickening) in 23 (approximately 10%) **(Option (A) is false)**.[23] Of these 23 patients, 15 had pleural effusions, which were unilateral in 13 of the 15. Pleural effusion was encountered only when the disease showed signs of progression, such as involvement of the pulmonary parenchyma. Pleural effusion was not seen in patients whose only manifestation of the disease was mediastinal lymphadenopathy. Pleural thickening was seen in 8 of the 23 patients and was always associated with advanced sarcoidosis.

With regard to radiographic staging of sarcoidosis, several different systems have been proposed, although most are similar to the following: Stage I—mediastinal and hilar adenopathy; Stage II—mediastinal and hilar adenopathy plus parenchymal disease; Stage III—parenchymal disease without associated adenopathy; and Stage IV—parenchymal fibrosis.[6]

Histologically, it appears that the extent of parenchymal granulomatous involvement in Stage I disease (mediastinal adenopathy without parenchymal disease radiographically) is less than that in Stage II or Stage III (radiographic parenchymal involvement for both). In these latter two stages, characteristic granulomas are often demonstrated on

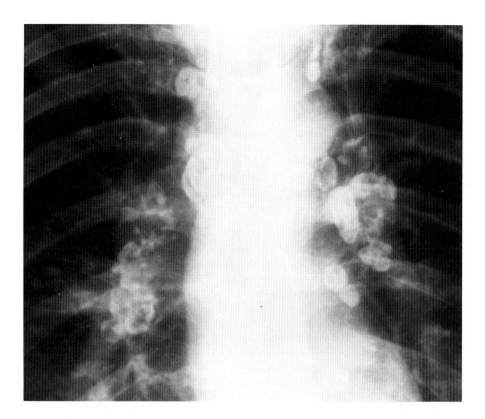

Figure 21-3. In this patient with a history of sarcoidosis, note the eggshell calcifications of mediastinal and hilar nodes, particularly evident at the right hilum. (Reprinted with permission from Gross et al. [10].)

transbronchial biopsy, so that open lung biopsy may not be required. For Stage I disease, open lung biopsy may be necessary to uncover parenchymal granulomas.[19]

SUGGESTED READINGS

1. Befeler B, MacLeod CA, Baum GL, Schwartz H. Idiopathic dilatation of the pulmonary artery. Am J Med Sci 1967; 254:667–674
2. Bein ME, Putman CE, McLoud TC, Mink JH. A reevaluation of intrathoracic lymphadenopathy in sarcoidosis. AJR 1978; 131:409–415
3. Berkmen YM, Javors BR. Anterior mediastinal lymphadenopathy in sarcoidosis. AJR 1976; 127:983–987

4. Castaneda-Zuniga WR, Formanek A, Amplatz K. Radiologic diagnosis of different types of pulmonary stenoses. Cardiovasc Radiol 1977–1978; 1:45–57

5. Chen JT, Robinson AE, Goodrich JK, Lester RG. Uneven distribution of pulmonary blood flow between left and right lungs in isolated valvular pulmonary stenosis. AJR 1969; 107:343–350

6. DeRemee RA. The roentgenographic staging of sarcoidosis. Historic and contemporary perspectives. Chest 1983; 83:128–133

7. Dunbar RD. Sarcoidosis and its radiologic manifestations. CRC Crit Rev Diagn Imaging 1978; 11:185–221

8. Espinosa GA. Sarcoidosis: multiple chest manifestations. Natl J Med Assoc 1978; 70:191–194

9. Fishman AP, Pietra GG. Primary pulmonary hypertension. Annu Rev Med 1980; 31:421–431

10. Gross BH, Schneider HJ, Proto AV. Eggshell calcification of lymph nodes. AJR 1980; 135:1265–1268

11. Gupta BD, Moodie DS, Hodgman JR. Primary pulmonary hypertension in adults: clinical features, catheterization findings and long-term follow-up. Cleve Clin Q 1980; 47:275–284

12. Hughes JP, Stovin PGI. Segmental pulmonary artery aneurysms with peripheral venous thrombosis. Br J Dis Chest 1959; 53:19–27

13. Kirks DR, McCormick VD, Greenspan RH. Pulmonary sarcoidosis. Roentgenologic analysis of 150 patients. AJR 1973; 117:777–786

14. Kopp WL, Green RA. Pulmonary artery aneurysms with recurrent thrombophlebitis. The "Hughes-Stovin syndrome." Ann Intern Med 1962; 56:105–113

15. McLoud TC, Putman CE, Pascual R. Eggshell calcification with systemic sarcoidosis. Chest 1974; 66:515–517

16. Mitchell DN, Scadding JG. Sarcoidosis. Am Rev Respir Dis 1974; 110:774–802

17. Proto AV, Speckman JM. The left lateral radiograph of the chest. Part 1. Med Radiogr Photogr 1979; 55:29–74

18. Ravin CE, Greenspan RH, McLoud TC, Lange RC, Langou RA, Putman CE. Redistribution of pulmonary blood flow secondary to pulmonary arterial hypertension. Invest Radiol 1980; 15:29–33

19. Rich S, Brundage PH. Primary pulmonary hypertension. Current update. JAMA 1984; 251:2252–2254

20. Rosen Y, Amorosa JK, Moon S, Cohen J, Lyons HA. Occurrence of lung granulomas in patients with stage I sarcoidosis. AJR 1977; 129:1083–1085

21. Singleton EB, Leachman RD, Rosenberg HS. Congenital abnormalities of the pulmonary arteries. AJR 1964; 91:487–499

22. Teplick JG, Haskin ME, Nedwich A. The Hughes-Stovin syndrome. Case report. Radiology 1974; 113:607–608

23. Wilen SB, Rabinowitz JG, Ulreich S, Lyons HA. Pleural involvement in sarcoidosis. Am J Med 1974; 57:200–209

Notes

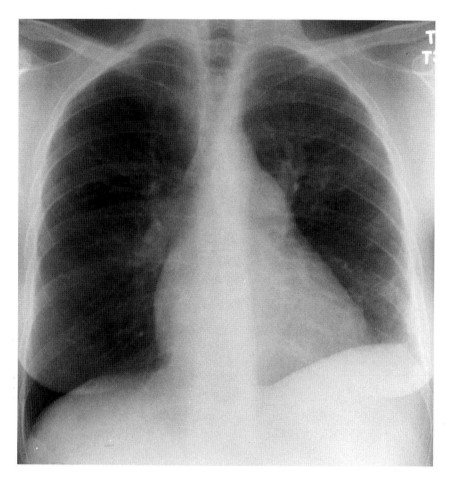

Figure 22-1. This 43-year-old woman suffered from progressive exertional dyspnea. You are shown a posteroanterior chest radiograph.

Case 22: Pulmonary Thromboembolism

Question 107

Which *one* of the following is the MOST likely diagnosis?

(A) Atrial septal defect
(B) Ventricular septal defect
(C) Pulmonary thromboembolism
(D) Acute myocardial infarction
(E) Chronic congestive heart failure

The posteroanterior chest radiograph (Figure 22-1) demonstrates enlargement of the hilar and main pulmonary arteries, mild cardiomegaly, increased size and number of vessels in the upper lung zones, and areas of diminished or absent perfusion in the right and left lower lung and left mid-lung zones. The foregoing findings are also associated with a blunted left costophrenic angle, apparent elevation of the left hemidiaphragm, and pleural thickening/effusion along the left lower chest wall. Overall, the radiographic features are most consistent with pulmonary thromboembolism **(Option (C) is most likely).** Pulmonary arterial hypertension was also present in this patient.

The other options offered are less likely in view of the radiographic appearance. A left-to-right shunt, such as atrial septal defect (Option (A)) or ventricular septal defect (Option (B)), would be expected to increase the size of pulmonary vessels diffusely and symmetrically throughout the lungs without areas of pulmonary oligemia. Additionally, a left-to-right shunt would not explain the left hemidiaphragmatic elevation and blunting of the left costophrenic angle. Redistribution of pulmonary blood flow, classically associated with elevated pulmonary venous pressure, may be seen with chronic congestive heart failure (Option (E)) or, less commonly, with acute myocardial infarction (Option (D)). In these situations, however, one would expect to see indistinct vessels due to edema rather than absent vessels at the lung bases.

Moreover, with congestive heart failure, right-sided or bilateral pleural effusion would be more common than an isolated left pleural effusion.

Question 108

Concerning atrial septal defect,

(A) the ostium primum type is often part of a complex malformation known as an endocardial cushion defect
(B) the left atrium is generally enlarged
(C) fixed splitting of the second heart sound is noted on physical examination
(D) it is more common in male patients
(E) it is a common cause of heart failure in infancy
(F) it is the only left-to-right shunt in which the pulmonary flow can be massive and the murmur not apparent

Left-to-right shunt lesions are characterized by passage of blood from a zone of higher pressure (the left side of the heart and systemic arteries) to a zone of lesser pressure (the right side of the heart and pulmonary arteries). Shunting occurs most commonly at the atria, ventricles, and great vessels.

The generic term atrial septal defect is used to describe several different cardiac defects: ostium secundum, ostium primum, and atrioventricularis communis.[2]

Ostium secundum defects include all defects of the atrial septum except those at the inferior margin of the septum. The lower edge of an ostium secundum defect is separated from the atrioventricular valves by atrial septal tissue. Occasionally, the entire atrial septum may be absent; however, if the atrioventricular valves are intact, the defect is still considered to be of the ostium secundum type.

Ostium primum defects involve the inferior margin of the atrial septum. Such a defect is invariably associated with a cleft of the anterior leaflet of the mitral valve, resulting in mitral insufficiency. Occasionally, the septal leaflet of the tricuspid valve is also affected. Ostium primum defects are generally large, and often the entire septum is absent, the defect then being recognized chiefly by the mitral cleft. Such a complex malformation is often referred to as an endocardial cushion defect **(Option (A) is true).**

Atrioventricularis communis represents a more extensive variety of the ostium primum defect. In this situation, the inferior margin of the atrial septum and the superior margin of the ventricular septum are absent. The mitral and tricuspid valves lose their separate identities, and there is generally a common atrioventricular valve, which is insufficient, resulting in communication of all four cardiac chambers.

The presence of a defect in the atrial septum results in passage of blood from the left to the right atrium. Shunted blood courses through the right side of the heart into the pulmonary vascular bed, resulting in enlargement of the right atrium, right ventricle, main and hilar pulmonary arteries, and pulmonary vascular bed. Of importance is the fact that the left atrium, although it carries extra blood, does not enlarge, since the septal defect allows the left atrium to decompress **(Option (B) is false).**

The murmurs that result from an atrial septal defect are related to increased blood flow through the right side of the heart. A systolic murmur is generated by increased flow across the pulmonic valve, while a diastolic murmur results from increased flow across the tricuspid valve. As the increased volume of blood in the right heart is relatively uninfluenced by respiration, right heart mechanical events are delayed at a constant interval from left heart events in all phases of the respiratory cycle. Thus, the time between the closing of the aortic and pulmonic valves remains wide and fixed, often referred to as "fixed splitting" of the second heart sound **(Option (C) is true).** This finding is an important clinical clue to the correct diagnosis on physical examination.

Atrial septal defects are not associated with cyanosis and only rarely cause heart failure in infancy **(Option (E) is false).** Typical right heart flow murmurs and fixed splitting of the second heart sound are often detectable within the first few weeks of life. Atrial septal defects are notable in that pulmonary blood flow may be massive and murmurs may not be apparent **(Option (F) is true).** Moreover, heart size may not be a good indicator of shunt volume, except insofar as small shunts do not generally cause substantial cardiac enlargement.

An atrial septal defect is the most common congenital cardiac abnormality detected initially during adult life. Women are twice as commonly afflicted as men **(Option (D) is false).** Interestingly, atrial septal defect and patent ductus arteriosus are the only two common congenital heart lesions that afflict women more often than men.

Radiographically, the pulmonary vascularity in patients with atrial septal defects is increased along with enlargement of the main pulmonary artery.[4,5,13] Vessels throughout the lungs are enlarged, consistent with shunt vascularity. The heart itself is usually of normal size or only mildly enlarged. With marked cardiac enlargement, one must consider additional complications such as associated mitral valve disease or right ventricular failure. The left atrium is normal in size as it is decompressed into the right atrium, a clue to distinguishing an atrial septal defect from a patent ductus arteriosus or ventricular septal defect. The aortic knob is of normal size, although it may appear small in comparison to the enlarged main pulmonary artery.

Question 109

Concerning ventricular septal defect,

    (A) in newborns, a murmur is immediately apparent
    (B) it is the most common left-to-right shunt present in adults
    (C) spontaneous closure occurs in 15 to 30% of patients
    (D) left atrial enlargement is the rule in adult patients

Ventricular septal defect is a common congenital cardiac malformation. The most common type of ventricular septal defect involves the membranous septum and adjacent muscle lying just below the aortic valve. Less commonly seen is the ventricular septal defect involving the muscular septum.

Ventricular septal defects allow the passage of blood from the left to the right ventricle. This is particularly true in systole when, with left ventricular contraction, blood is pushed through the septal defect into the right ventricle, causing a systolic murmur. With small defects and relatively little shunting (pulmonary-to-systemic flow ratio <1.5:1.0), pressures and resistances in the right heart generally remain normal, as does the chest radiograph. With larger defects, more blood crosses into the right ventricle, causing dilation of those structures carrying this extra volume. Importantly, the left atrium does not decompress and is enlarged, unlike the situation in an atrial septal defect.

A ventricular septal defect may occur as an isolated anomaly at least 20% of the time. It is the most common left-to-right shunt in newborns and is a common cause of congestive heart failure during infancy, although murmurs are generally not apparent immediately **(Option (A) is false)**. The reason for this initial absence of murmurs is that the two ventricles have similar systolic pressures early in life. However, after 4 to 6 weeks the right ventricular systolic pressure generally has decreased so that blood begins to move across the ventricular septal defect to generate a murmur. The intensity of the murmur may not reflect the size of the shunt, in that small ventricular septal defects may be associated with very loud murmurs. This is explained by the high velocity of the blood moving through the defect, rather than the actual amount of blood. While ventricular septal defect is the most common left-to-right shunt present in newborns, atrial septal defect is the most common one present in adults **(Option (B) is false).**

Interestingly, and importantly from a clinical standpoint, spontaneous closure of ventricular septal defects occurs in 15 to 30% of cases **(Option (C) is true).**[1] This generally happens within the first 2 years of life and is usually associated with defects of relatively small size. With larger septal defects, pressure rises in the right ventricle and pulmonary arterial system. Eventually, pulmonary resistance may approach systemic resistance, resulting in a decrease in left-to-right shunting across the ventricular septal defect. Individuals at this stage are often asymptomatic. Ultimately, the right ventricle tends to fail, resulting in either chronic congestive heart failure or syncopal attacks.

Radiographically, the pulmonary vascularity shows a generalized increase throughout the lungs along with expected enlargement of the main and central pulmonary arteries.[4,5,13] The heart may also be mildly enlarged, but the important specific observation in adults is that the left atrium is enlarged, unlike the situation in an atrial septal defect **(Option (D) is true).** The aortic knob is of normal size but often appears small in comparison to the enlarged main pulmonary artery.

From a radiographic standpoint, it is the size of the left atrium that is critical in determining the level of the intracardiac shunt. Shunt vascularity associated with a left atrium of normal size suggests an atrial septal defect, while the same vascularity associated with a large left atrium suggests a ventricular septal defect or a patent ductus arteriosus. If the aortic knob is large, a patent ductus arteriosus becomes more likely, whereas if the aortic knob is of normal size a ventricular septal defect is more likely. Unfortunately in adult patients the left atrium may indent the barium-filled esophagus to a similar degree in both atrial and ventricular septal defects. It is presumed that, in the setting of an atrial septal defect, the esophageal indentation is secondary to the enlarged right ventricle displacing the normal-sized left atrium posteriorly. In such situations, the configuration of the sternum has been suggested as a means of differentiating atrial septal defects from ventricular septal defects (lower sternal bulge with ventricular septal defect versus upper sternal bulge with atrial septal defect).

Question 110

Concerning pulmonary thromboembolism,

(A) pulmonary angiography is unsafe in patients suspected of having the chronic form
(B) the presence of stenoses or webs in pulmonary arteries suggests the acute form
(C) surgery has no role in the management of the chronic form
(D) pulmonary arterial hypertension is an absolute contraindication to pulmonary angiography
(E) when right ventricular end-diastolic pressures exceed 20 mm Hg there is increased risk of death during pulmonary angiography

The clinical, radiographic, and therapeutic considerations involved in acute pulmonary thromboembolism have been widely discussed and reviewed throughout the medical literature.[3,6-12] While pulmonary angiography remains the gold standard for diagnosis, it has been accepted that a completely normal pulmonary perfusion scintigram excludes the diagnosis of acute pulmonary thromboembolism. Abnormal ventilation/perfusion patterns are associated with varying degrees of likelihood of acute pulmonary thromboembolism.

In order to establish whether a particular patient with abnormal ventilation/perfusion scintigraphic findings actually has acute pulmonary thromboembolism, a pulmonary angiogram is required. However, only a small percentage of these patients actually undergo angiography in most institutions, which may in part be related to concerns over the morbidity and mortality of the procedure. Clearly, the potential risks will vary depending upon the experience of the angiographer. Recent publications suggest, however, that the frequency of complications is very low in experienced hands.[6-9,11,12] For example, a review of more than 1,300 pulmonary angiograms from the Duke University Medical Center showed that there were three deaths, a mortality rate of approximately 0.2%.[8] Such a rate seems low, given the potential severity of the disease process itself and the complications associated with anticoagulation. The three patients who died had severe pulmonary hypertension and, more importantly, elevation of the right ventricular end-diastolic pressure to a level equal to or greater than 20 mm Hg **(Option (E) is true)**. One of the three had a main pulmonary artery injection. The other two had selective injection of 25 to 30 ml of contrast material into the right pulmonary artery. It should be noted, however, that angiography was successfully performed in other patients with right ventricular end-diastolic pressures greater than 20 mm Hg.

The exact mechanism of death in patients undergoing pulmonary angiography is not clear. However the high osmolality of conventional radiographic contrast agents seems to result in an increase in pulmonary vascular resistance. This increased resistance further raises pulmonary arterial pressures and imposes increased afterload on the right ventricle. In those patients with a marginally compensated right ventricle, as evidenced by right ventricular end-diastolic pressures equal to or greater than 20 mm Hg, this additional stress of increased afterload may be sufficient to cause complete ventricular failure and death. Such a sequence of events may occur even with selective arterial injections, a technique previously recommended in the setting of pulmonary arterial hypertension. Thus, it is recommended that pressures be measured in the main pulmonary artery and right ventricle for all patients undergoing pulmonary angiography. If the right ventricular end-diastolic pressure is equal to or greater than 20 mm Hg, serious consideration should be given to terminating the procedure to avoid the injection of contrast material. In the setting of pulmonary hypertension with right ventricular end-diastolic pressures of less than 20 mm Hg, selective injections are recommended so that reduced amounts of contrast material are used **(Option (D) is false)**. Since the high osmolality of conventional contrast agents has been implicated in the increased pulmonary artery pressures often observed following injection, it is possible that the newer low-osmolality contrast agents may prove to be safer in the setting of pulmonary arterial hypertension.

Most acute emboli undergo resolution. The time for such resolution varies from individual to individual. It is apparently related to the underlying status of the cardiovascular system and is generally longer in those with cardiovascular compromise. In some cases, acute pulmonary emboli may fail to resolve and lead to chronic emboli. If a large enough portion of the pulmonary vascular bed is obstructed by such chronic emboli, signs and symptoms of cor pulmonale may result.

More experience is being gained with surgical removal of chronic emboli **(Option (C) is false)**.[9] Preoperative radiographic assessment includes pulmonary angiography to demonstrate the size and location of the central chronic emboli, since those emboli more central in location are more amenable to surgical removal **(Option (A) is false)**. Moreover, it has been noted at the time of surgery that "back-bleeding" from the cleared pulmonary artery is a good sign of both subsequent clinical improvement and maintained patency of the pulmonary artery. This back-bleeding is apparently from bronchial arterial collateral circulation to the pulmonary arteries distal to the obstructing embolus. Thus, the radiographic workup of a patient suspected of having chronic pulmonary emboli and considered a candidate for embolectomy is aided by bronchial arteriography.

Angiographic signs are different for acute and chronic emboli. The sign of an acute embolus is specific—direct visualization of an intraluminal filling defect. So-called secondary signs (abrupt vessel occlusion, perfusion defects) are nonspecific. The signs associated with a chronic embolus include stenoses and webs (Figure 22-2) **(Option (B) is false).** Additionally, those patients in whom bronchial arteriography shows enlarged bronchial arteries with collateral filling of the pulmonary arteries distal to the obstructing chronic embolus will have brisk back-bleeding at surgery (Figure 22-3).

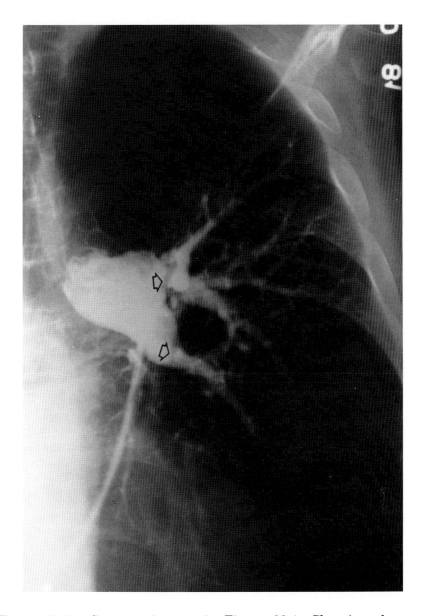

Figure 22-2. Same patient as in Figure 22-1. Chronic pulmonary thromboembolism. On the pulmonary angiogram, note the webs (arrows) associated with chronic emboli.

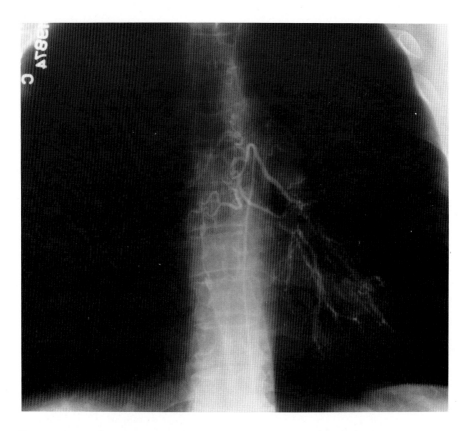

Figure 22-3. Same patient as in Figures 22-1 and 22-2. The bronchial arteriogram shows enlarged bronchial arteries with collateral filling of pulmonary arteries distal to the obstructing chronic emboli.

SUGGESTED READINGS

1. Alpert BS, Cook DH, Varghese PJ, Rowe RD. Spontaneous closure of small ventricular septal defects: ten-year follow-up. Pediatrics 1979; 63:204–206
2. Bedford DE. The anatomical types of atrial septal defect. Their incidence and clinical diagnosis. Am J Cardiol 1960; 6:568–574
3. Bell WR, Simon TL. Current status of pulmonary thromboembolic disease: pathophysiology, diagnosis, prevention, and treatment. Am Heart J 1982; 103:239–262
4. Dunne EG. Cardiac radiology. Philadelphia: Lea & Febiger; 1967:95–178
5. Elliott LP, Schiebler GL, et al. X-ray diagnosis of congenital cardiac disease, 2nd ed. Springfield, Illinois: Charles C Thomas; 1979:115–161

6. Frankel N, Coleman RE, Pryor DB, Sostman HD, Ravin CE. Utilization of lung scans by clinicians. J Nucl Med 1986; 27:366–369

7. Fulkerson WJ, Coleman RE, Ravin CE, Saltzman HA. Diagnosis of pulmonary embolism. Arch Intern Med 1986; 146:961–967

8. Mills SR, Jackson DC, Older RA, Heaston DK, Moore AV. The incidence, etiologies, and avoidance of complications of pulmonary angiography in a large series. Radiology 1980; 136:295–299

9. Mills SR, Jackson DC, Sullivan DC, et al. Angiographic evaluation of chronic pulmonary embolism. Radiology 1980; 136:301–308

10. Rosenow EC III, Osmundson PJ, Brown ML. Pulmonary embolism. Mayo Clin Proc 1981; 56:161–178

11. Sabiston DC Jr. Pathophysiology, diagnosis, and management of pulmonary embolism. Am J Surg 1979; 138:384–391

12. Sostman HD, Ravin CE, Sullivan DC, Mills SR, Glickman MG, Dorfman GS. Use of pulmonary angiography for suspected pulmonary embolism: influence of scintigraphic diagnosis. AJR 1982; 139:673–677

13. Swischuk LE. Plain film interpretation in congenital heart disease, 2nd ed. Philadelphia: Lea & Febiger; 1970:47–74

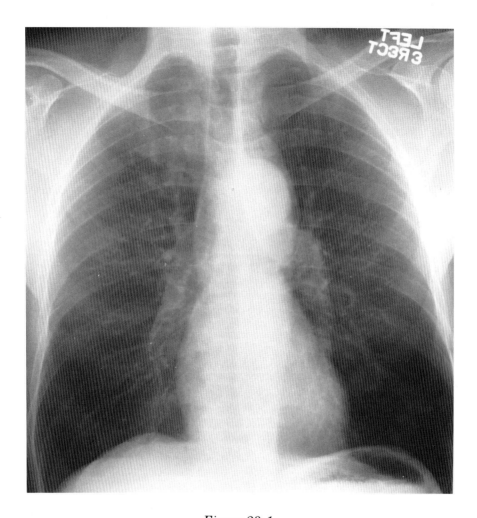

Figure 23-1
Figures 23-1 through 23-5. This 35-year-old woman with myasthenia gravis is being evaluated for thymoma. You are shown posteroanterior and lateral chest radiographs (Figures 23-1 and 23-2) and computed tomographic scans (Figures 23-3 through 23-5).

Case 23: Thymoma

Question 111

Which *one* of the following is the MOST likely diagnosis?

(A) Thymic hyperplasia
(B) Thymolipoma
(C) Substernal thyroid
(D) Thymoma
(E) Normal thymus

Posteroanterior (Figure 23-1) and lateral (Figure 23-2) chest radiographs demonstrate an anterior mediastinal mass. On the posteroanterior view (Figure 23-6), note that the mass projects to the left of the aortic knob, obliterates neither the lateral margin of the knob nor the proximal descending aorta, and terminates at the level of the anterior thoracic inlet (just below the clavicle). On the lateral view (Figure 23-7), the mass is clearly identified in the upper retrosternal area. No calcification or cavitation is identified within the lesion, and the trachea is not deviated.

The computed tomographic scans (Figures 23-3 through 23-5), obtained with intravenous contrast material, show the mass anterior to the aortic arch and great vessels (Figure 23-8 and 23-9). Note that the mass does not extend into the neck (Figure 23-5).

Given the radiographic findings of an anterior mediastinal mass in a patient with myasthenia gravis, the most likely diagnosis among those offered is thymoma **(Option (D) is most likely).** One would not expect thymic hyperplasia (Option (A)) or normal thymus (Option (E)) in an adult to produce a mass effect. Thymolipoma (Option (B)) would be expected to show significant fatty content on computed tomography (not demonstrated in this case). Substernal thyroid (Option (C)) is unlikely since there is no evidence of continuity of the mass with cervical thyroid tissue and since the trachea is not displaced.

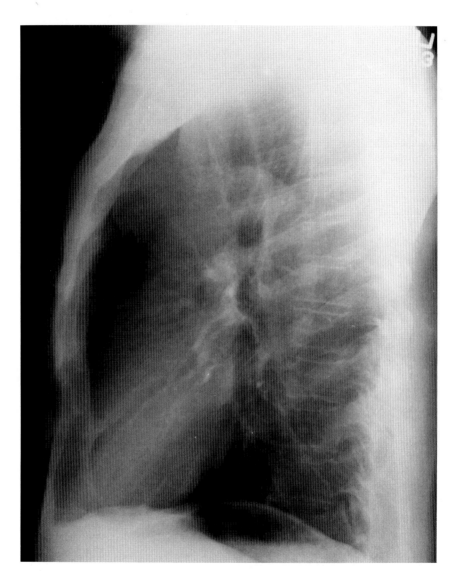

Figure 23-2

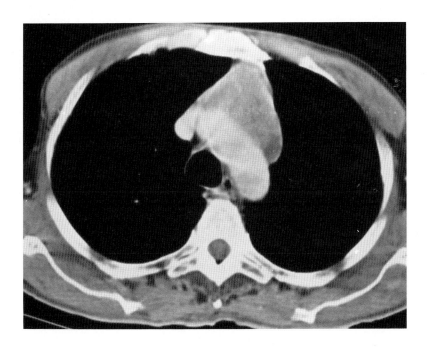

Figure 23-3

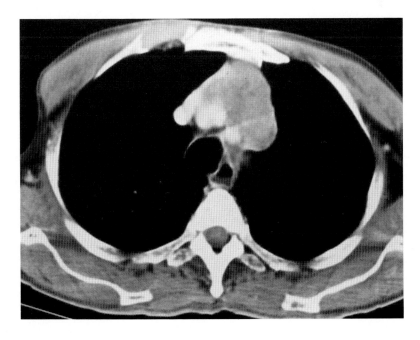

Figure 23-4

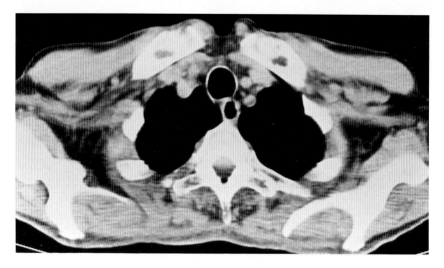

Figure 23-5

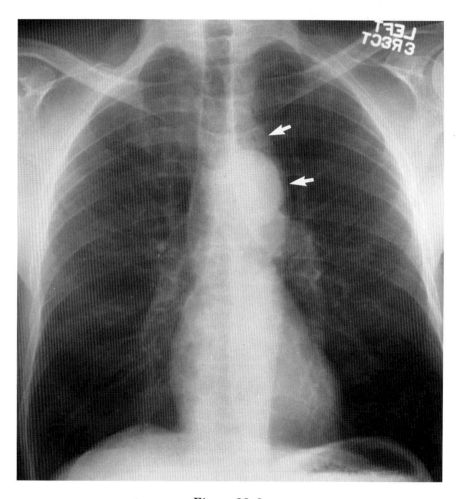

Figure 23-6
Figures 23-6 and 23-7 (Same as Figures 23-1 and 23-2, respectively).
Note the mass (arrows) as described in the text on the posteroanterior
(Figure 23-6) and lateral (Figure 23-7) views.

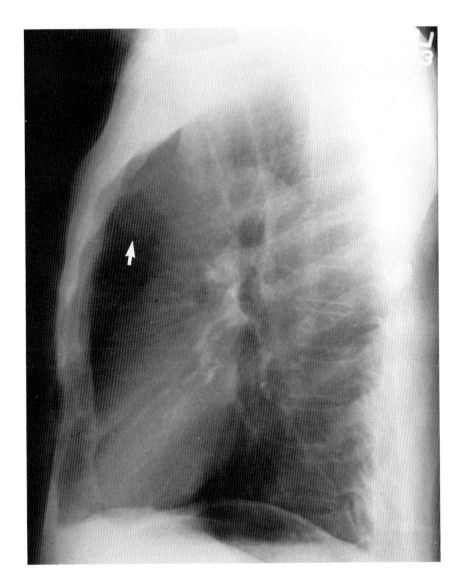

Figure 23-7

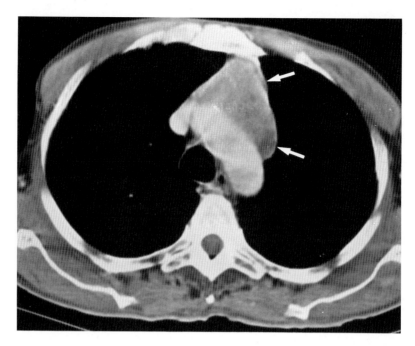

Figure 23-8

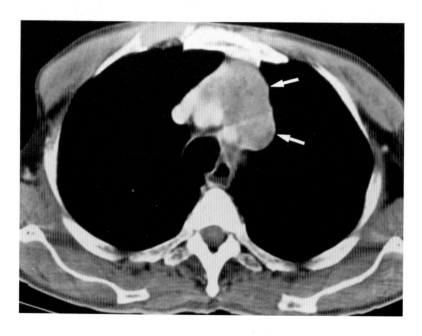

Figure 23-9
Figures 23-8 and 23-9 (Same as Figures 23-3 and 23-4, respectively). On computed tomography the mass (arrows) lies anterior to the aortic arch (Figure 23-8) and great vessels (Figure 23-9).

Question 112

Concerning patients with myasthenia gravis,

- (A) posteroanterior and lateral chest radiographs will demonstrate fewer than 10% of associated thymomas
- (B) approximately 10 to 15% have thymomas
- (C) 25 to 50% of patients with thymomas have the disease
- (D) distant metastases from malignant thymomas are common

Myasthenia gravis is a neuromuscular disorder clinically manifested by weakness and easy fatigability of voluntary muscles.[2,8] The basic defect is failure of transmission at the neuromuscular junction reflecting a reduction in the number of acetylcholine receptors on the postjunctional muscle membrane. In myasthenia gravis, there are specific autoantibodies directed against one or more of the subunits of the acetylcholine receptor. These appear to cause degradation of the receptors via a complement-mediated injury. The etiology of the autoimmune response in myasthenia gravis is unknown.[9]

Two-thirds of myasthenic patients are women; symptoms in women most often first appear during the third decade of life. Afflicted men tend to be older. In fact, most patients presenting over the age of 50 years are men.

The relationship between myasthenia gravis and abnormalities of the thymus gland remains poorly understood. However, there clearly is an association, as indicated by both the large number of pathologic changes in the thymus glands of patients with myasthenia and the favorable results of thymectomy. Approximately 75% of myasthenic patients have thymic abnormalities. By far, the most common abnormality is hyperplasia of the gland, while gross or microscopic thymomas are found in approximately 15% of myasthenic patients (**Option (B) is true**). Overall, approximately 10 to 15% of patients with myasthenia gravis will have a thymoma, while 25 to 50% of patients with thymomas will have myasthenia gravis (**Option (C) is true**).

Although the majority of thymic tumors are encapsulated, about 25% are reported to be locally invasive. Metastases, when they occur, are generally located on adjacent pleural surfaces. Distant metastases with malignant thymomas are distinctly uncommon (**Option (D) is false**).

Therapy for myasthenia gravis has markedly improved the prognosis of the disease. Anticholinesterase agents are the first line of treatment, and most patients will benefit to some degree. For patients in whom return to full activity is not achieved, further therapeutic measures, such as thymectomy and steroid therapy, are required. A number of studies have suggested that removal of the thymus gland leads to clinical improvement or remission in patients with myasthenia gravis. Improvement has been reported in 60 to 85% of such patients, and complete remission has been reported in 20 to 36%. Thymectomy in the absence of a demonstrated thymoma is controversial. Some argue that the potential advantage of permanent remission or improvement favors thymectomy despite the short-term risks of surgical morbidity and mortality. Others argue that surgery should only be used for those who do not respond to appropriate medical therapy, including corticosteroids.

The most widely accepted indication for thymectomy is the presence of a thymoma. Thus, demonstration of a thymoma is of great significance in patients with myasthenia gravis. Posteroanterior and lateral chest radiographs will detect the majority of thymomas, although computed tomographic scanning has proven extremely useful in cases in which the tumor is not evident **(Option (A) is false).**[3]

Question 113

Concerning thymolipomas,

(A) they contain both fat and epithelial elements of the thymus gland
(B) they characteristically cause symptoms early in their course
(C) when large they mold to the cardiac and diaphragmatic contours
(D) they constitute approximately 50% of thymic tumors

Thymolipomas, benign thymic neoplasms containing fatty tissue, make up less than 10% of all thymic tumors, only 50 cases having been reported through 1973 **(Option (D) is false).**[10] Histologically, the tumor consists of adult adipose tissue interspersed with areas of hyperplastic or atrophic thymic tissue **(Option (A) is true).** The tumor can grow to a huge size but, due to its benign and pliable nature, generally causes few symptoms **(Option (B) is false).** Indeed, in the majority of patients, the tumors are asymptomatic and are incidentally discovered at the time of chest radiographic examinations.

Radiographically, the fatty, pliable tumor often falls toward the diaphragm as it enlarges, adapting itself to the cardiac and diaphragmatic contours **(Option (C) is true).** Calcification has not been identified within these tumors, nor has associated pleural effusion been seen. Although some clues to the diagnosis of thymolipoma may be gained from the conventional chest radiograph, the diagnosis is more likely to be established by computed tomography, which more readily identifies fatty tissue.

Question 114

Concerning thymomas,

(A) they are common in children
(B) benign and malignant lesions are distinguished readily by histologic examination
(C) approximately 50% are predominantly cystic
(D) they are present in 50% of patients with aregenerative erythrocytic anemia
(E) on computed tomography, fat plane obliteration indicates mediastinal invasion

Thymomas constitute the most common "surgical" tumor of the anterior mediastinum.[11] Although they can occur at any age, they are extremely rare in children; almost all patients are older than 20 years **(Option (A) is false)**. Pathologically, the tumors arise from components of the normal thymus and are generally divided into four types based on the predominant cell present: lymphocytic, epithelial, lymphoepithelial, or spindle cell. Importantly, in individual cases it may be difficult to establish whether the lesion is benign or malignant by histologic examination alone **(Option (B) is false)**. Rather, gross characteristics at surgery of local invasion versus complete encapsulation have been more reliably associated with determining the ultimate prognosis. The majority of thymomas are solid, although multiple small cysts may be present. Approximately 5 to 10% of the time, the tumor is predominantly cystic **(Option (C) is false)**.

Radiographically, most thymomas are visualized at the base of the heart, near its junction with the great vessels. The tumors are round or oval with smooth or slightly lobulated margins. Calcification has been reported occasionally in thymoma, either at the periphery of or throughout the lesion.

As discussed above, 10 to 15% of patients with myasthenia gravis will have a thymoma, while 25 to 50% of patients with thymomas will have myasthenia gravis. Thymoma is also associated with various anemias and immunologic deficiencies. One example is aregenerative erythrocytic anemia (pure red cell aplasia). In this rare anemia, 50% of patients prove to have thymomas **(Option (D) is true)**. The patients are generally women and almost always over 50 years of age. Another example is acquired hypogammaglobulinemia, in which 5 to 15% of patients prove to have thymomas. Carcinoid of the thymus gland has been associated with Cushing's syndrome.

Although most thymomas will be detected on routine chest radiography, computed tomography plays an important role in recognition of smaller masses.[1,3,7] In order to make the appropriate diagnosis, one must distinguish a thymoma from normal thymic tissue.[4-6] Several reviews have suggested that the normal thymus has a bilobate, arrowhead appearance at all ages, with gradual focal or diffuse fatty replacement of the parenchyma occurring between the ages of 20 and 40 years. Residual islands of thymic tissue in patients with fatty replacement are generally small and appear linear, round, or oval. These islands of tissue do not produce a focal alteration of the lateral mediastinal border. On the other hand, a thymoma is spherical or oval and, if large enough, does produce a distinct focal bulge of the lateral mediastinal border. Several reports have noted that fat obliteration adjacent to a thymoma does not reliably indicate mediastinal invasion by the tumor **(Option (E) is false).** Whether such obliteration will be reliable when seen on more recent scanners with better resolution is not yet known.

The computed tomographic appearance of the normal gland is clearly age-related. In patients under the age of 10 years, the thymus exhibits extreme variability in appearance and is difficult to characterize. Throughout the first decade of life and until puberty, the gland enlarges as a function of age and tends to assume a more triangular cross-sectional appearance (Figure 23-10). After puberty, the gland has a characteristic triangular or arrowhead shape and begins to develop areas of inhomogeneity due to fatty replacement (Figure 23-11). As the patient ages, the thymus involutes and often shows increasing fatty replacement. By the time patients are 40 years or older, most will have total fatty replacement, although some still show residual thymic tissue (Figure 23-12). Importantly, however, the tissue does not produce any alteration in the lateral mediastinal border, unlike a thymoma (Figure 23-13).

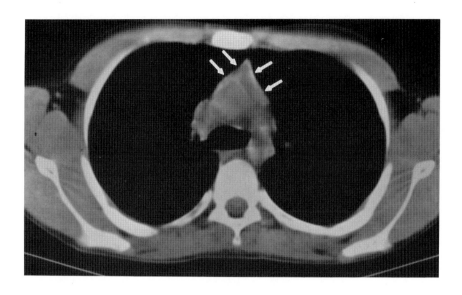

Figure 23-10. A normal thymus in a 15-year-old boy. Note the arrowhead configuration (arrows).

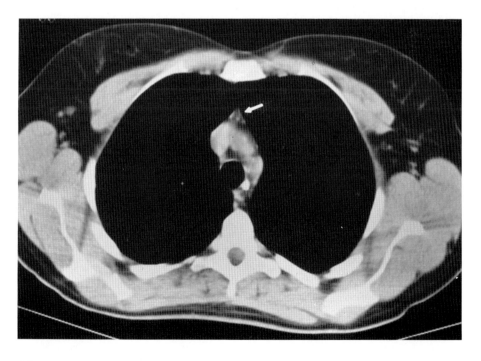

Figure 23-11. A normal thymus in a 30-year-old woman. Note the small size (arrow), some fatty replacement, residual islands of tissue, and flat lateral margins.

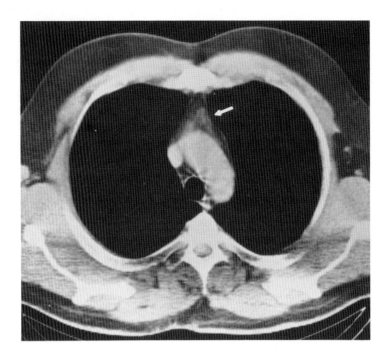

Figure 23-12. A normal thymus in a 40-year-old man. Note the flat or concave lateral margin (arrow) and inhomogeneous nature of the gland secondary to fatty replacement. Residual tissue does not alter the normal mediastinal border. (Compare with Figure 23-13.)

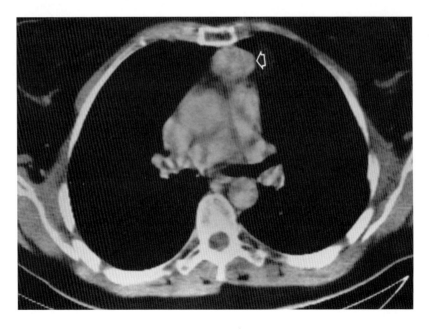

Figure 23-13. A thymoma in a 46-year-old woman with myasthenia gravis. Note the convex lateral margin (arrow) of the soft tissue mass.

SUGGESTED READINGS

1. Brown LR, Muhm JR, Sheedy PF II, Unni KK, Bernatz PE, Herman RC Jr. The value of computed tomography in myasthenia gravis. AJR 1983; 140:31–35

2. Drachman DB. Myasthenia gravis. N Engl J Med 1978; 298:136–142, 186–193

3. Ellis K, Gregg HG. Thymomas—roentgen considerations. AJR 1964; 91:105–119

4. Francis IR, Glazer GM, Bookstein FL, Gross BH. The thymus: reexamination of age-related changes in size and shape. AJR 1985; 145:249–254

5. Heiberg E, Wolverson MK, Sundaram M, Nouri S. Normal thymus: CT characteristics in subjects under age 20. AJR 1982; 138:491–494

6. Moore AV, Korobkin M, Olanow W, et al. Age-related changes in the thymus gland: CT-pathologic correlation. AJR 1983; 141:241–246

7. Moore AV, Korobkin M, Powers B, et al. Thymoma detection by mediastinal CT: patients with myasthenia gravis. AJR 1982; 138:217–222

8. Scadding GK, Havard CW. Pathogenesis and treatment of myasthenia gravis. Br Med J 1981; 283:1008–1012

9. Seybold ME. Myasthenia gravis. A clinical and basic science review. JAMA 1983; 250:2516–2521

10. Teplick JG, Nedwich A, Haskin ME. Roentgenographic features of thymolipoma. AJR 1973; 117:873–877

11. Wilkins EW Jr, Edmunds LH Jr, Castleman B. Cases of thymoma at the Massachusetts General Hospital. J Thorac Cardiovasc Surg 1966; 52:322–330

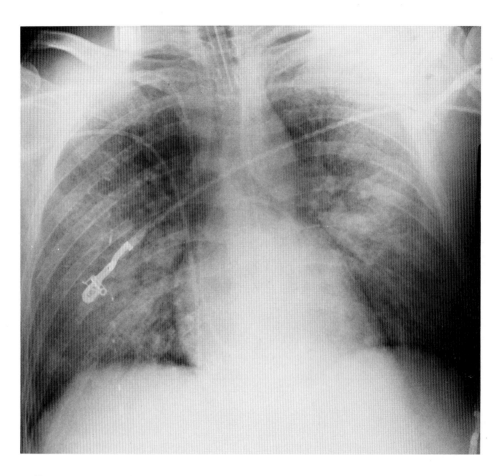

Figure 24-1. This 30-year-old man presented with a cough. You are shown a portable chest radiograph.

Case 24: *Pneumocystis carinii* Pneumonia

Question 115

Conditions that should be considered in the differential diagnosis include:

(A) *Pneumocystis carinii* pneumonia in a patient with acquired immunodeficiency syndrome (AIDS)
(B) chronic eosinophilic pneumonia
(C) atypical mycobacterial infection
(D) pulmonary edema due to heroin abuse
(E) pulmonary alveolar proteinosis

The portable chest radiograph (Figure 24-1) demonstrates bilateral perihilar opacification of the pulmonary parenchyma extending to the periphery of the lung with relative sparing of the costophrenic sulci. An air-bronchogram is faintly visible in the left upper lobe. The patient, a homosexual male with acquired immunodeficiency syndrome (AIDS) and *Pneumocystis carinii* pneumonia **(Option (A) is true),** also had brain abscesses due to *Toxoplasma gondii.*

A number of diffuse lung diseases, including pulmonary edema, pneumonia, ARDS (adult respiratory distress syndrome), fat embolism syndrome, pulmonary hemorrhage, pulmonary alveolar proteinosis, and eosinophilic lung disease, could produce such a radiographic appearance. Chronic eosinophilic pneumonia (Option (B)) should not be considered, however, since characteristically, the periphery of the lung is involved, especially the upper zones, with sparing of the perihilar regions (Figure 24-2) **(Option (B) is false).**[12] Chronic eosinophilic pneumonia is part of the spectrum of eosinophilic lung disease (Table 24-1). It affects middle-aged and elderly women in 83% of cases. A history of atopy or asthma can be elicited in up to 30% of patients. Signs and symptoms include fever, chronic eosinophilic pneumonia (90%), weight loss (79%), cough (75%), dyspnea (69%), and night sweats (69%). Steroid therapy can

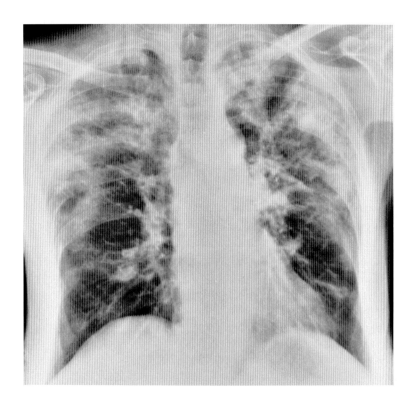

Figure 24-2. Chronic eosinophilic pneumonia. Note the peripheral distribution with predilection for the upper lung zones and sparing of the perihilar regions.

Table 24-1. Eosinophilic Lung Disease

Idiopathic
  Loeffler's syndrome
  Chronic eosinophilic pneumonia
  Hypereosinophilic syndrome
	Parasite-Induced
	  Ascariasis
	  Schistosomiasis
	  Toxocariasis
	  Tropical pulmonary eosinophilia

Drug-Induced
  Aminosalicylic acid
  Chlorpropamide
  Hydralazine
  Nitrofurantoin
  Penicillin
  Sulfonamides
	Fungus-Induced
	  Allergic bronchopulmonary aspergillosis
	
	Connective Tissue Disease/Vasculitis
	  Polyarteritis nodosa
	  Churg-Strauss disease
	  Wegener's granulomatosis

Chemical-Induced Nickel carbonyl	

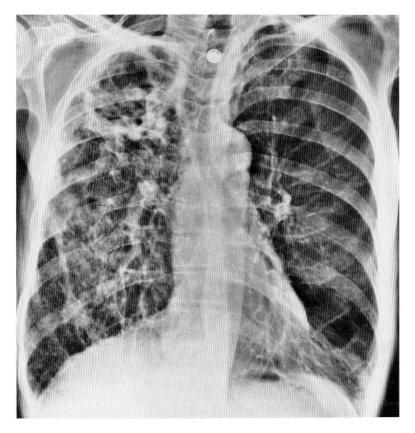

Figure 24-3. *Mycobacterium avium-intracellulare* (MAI) infection in a patient with emphysema. Note multiple cavities throughout the right lung. Loss of volume and a dominant cavity are visible in the right upper lobe.

produce remarkable results—symptoms may disappear within 24 to 48 hours, and the radiographic abnormalities may clear within a week.

Atypical mycobacterial disease of the lung should not be considered since bilateral symmetrical perihilar disease as in Figure 24-1 would be unusual **(Option (C) is false).** It more likely produces an appearance indistinguishable from that of tuberculosis. In the vast majority of patients (98%), the disease is located in the apical or posterior segments of the upper lobes. Although the distribution of disease is often bilateral (41 to 66% of cases), when unilateral it is found twice as often on the right as on the left. Cavitation is exceedingly common (88 to 96% of cases). The cavities usually measure over 4 cm in diameter, are multiple, and may be thin-walled (Figure 24-3). Cicatrization atelectasis occurs in 66% of patients, and bronchogenic spread of the disease can occur in 63 to 81% of patients. Pleural effusions, lymph node enlargement, and miliary disease are uncommon with atypical mycobacterial infection of the lung, except in patients with AIDS, in whom they may occur.[16,21]

Pulmonary edema due to heroin abuse is a distinct possibility for the radiographic appearance seen in Figure 24-1, since the pulmonary edema incited by intravenous drug abuse usually produces bilateral perihilar opacification **(Option (D) is true).** Since pulmonary alveolar proteinosis in its classical form may be radiographically indistinguishable from pulmonary edema, the former condition should be considered **(Option (E) is also true).**

Question 116

Concerning *Pneumocystis carinii* pneumonia,

(A) it is diagnosable by transbronchial biopsy
(B) the organism is rarely obtained with bronchial washings
(C) the typical radiograph shows multifocal patchy pneumonia
(D) a normal chest radiograph virtually excludes it in a patient with AIDS

AIDS is characterized by the occurrence of life-threatening opportunistic infections, Kaposi's sarcoma, or both, in previously healthy patients without obvious explanation for their profound deficiency of cell-mediated immunity.[2,11,13,18,22] The disease is induced by a retrovirus termed the human immunodeficiency virus (HIV), previously known as HTLV III.[2,18] Since the initial report of AIDS in 1981, more than 70,000 cases have been reported to the CDC. It is predicted that AIDS will develop in 30% of infected persons within 5 years of infection and that an estimated 270,000 cases of AIDS will have occurred in the United States by 1991.[18] Four population groups account for the vast majority of AIDS cases in the United States: (1) homosexual or bisexual men (73%); (2) intravenous drug users (17%); (3) hemophiliacs (1%) and recipients of blood transfusions before 1983, when testing of blood became possible (2%); and (4) cases of heterosexual transmission (4%) and perinatal transmission to children. Transmission of the HIV by routes other than intimate contact, blood products, or intravenous drug abuse is virtually unknown.[18] The HIV induces a profound immune defect, with both a decrease in the absolute numbers of T cells and a reversal of the normal T-cell helper-to-suppressor ratio (normal ratio, 2; ratio in AIDS patients, 0.2 to 0.4). The clinical manifestations of AIDS can be divided into those caused by the direct effects of the HIV, those related to the opportunistic infections, and those caused by Kaposi's sarcoma and other malignancies.

The direct effects of the HIV include an acute infectious mononucleosis-like illness 3 weeks to 3 months after exposure, with fevers, sweats, malaise, myalgias, arthralgias, headache, diarrhea, generalized lymph node enlargement, and a macular erythematous rash. More common than this acute illness is AIDS-related complex (ARC), a persistent generalized lymph node enlargement affecting 10 to 30% of persons who will ultimately develop AIDS within 1 year. However, radiographic intrathoracic lymph node enlargement should not be ascribed to ARC but rather to infection or tumor.[23] Another direct effect of HIV infection is that on the brain; it leads to AIDS encephalopathy and AIDS dementia, which can be found in two-thirds of patients.[18,25]

Pneumocystis carinii pneumonia (PCP) is the most common symptomatic pulmonary infection in patients with AIDS. It occurs in 62% of all such patients[7,13,18,24], followed by cytomegalovirus pneumonia and *Mycobacterium avium-intracellulare* (MAI) infection, which occur in up to 17 and 20% of patients, respectively. In 27% of patients, PCP coexists with some other infection. Tuberculosis can also be seen in 2 to 10% of patients,[4] and there is an increased susceptibility to developing cryptococcosis, aspergillosis, coccidioidomycosis, histoplasmosis (Figure 24-4), nocardiosis, and gram-negative bacterial pneumonias.

The typical radiographic pattern of PCP consists of early reticulonodular perihilar opacification that soon becomes coalescent, having an appearance of diffuse parenchymal homogeneous consolidation (Figure 24-5) **(Option (C) is false)**. The lung in the costophrenic sulci and the apices may be spared initially but becomes involved in more advanced cases (Figure 24-6). ARDS may ensue. In 30 to 50% of patients, atypical features of PCP can be encountered; they include asymmetric distribution, lobar consolidation, nodular lesions, abscesses, cavities, pneumatoceles, pneumothorax, and pleural effusions.[11] In 4% of patients, hilar or mediastinal lymph node enlargement can be seen.[11]

A significant minority of AIDS patients (6%) will have clinical symptoms of PCP in the face of a normal chest radiograph **(Option (D) is false)**.[15,18] In this setting, gallium-67 scintigraphy can be positive and prompt further investigation. The scintigraphic pattern can be either homogeneously or heterogeneously diffuse and has a positive predictive value approaching 90%.

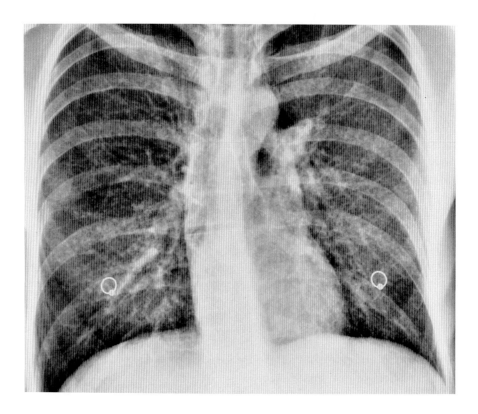

Figure 24-4. Miliary histoplasmosis in AIDS. Note diffuse miliary nodules throughout both lungs in a patient with bilateral nipple rings.

PCP is acquired by the aerogenous route and is characterized by an alveolitis. The alveolar spaces are filled with cysts and trophozoites associated with active infiltration and phagocytosis by alveolar macrophages. Foamy eosinophilic proteinaceous material fills the alveolar sacs as seen with hematoxylin and eosin staining.[14] Alveolar septa are secondarily thickened.

A definitive diagnosis of PCP requires the demonstration of the organism in lung tissue. The most dependable method of obtaining such tissue is open lung biopsy. Transbronchial biopsy is certainly an alternative procedure for diagnosis, with a reported sensitivity of 66 to 98% **(Option (A) is true)**. Bronchial washings may also yield the organism **(Option (B) is false)**. Sputum examination using immunofluorescence techniques with monoclonal antibodies will yield a diagnosis of PCP in a high percentage of patients, thus obviating the need for bronchoscopy and transbronchial biopsy. This ease of diagnosis is due to

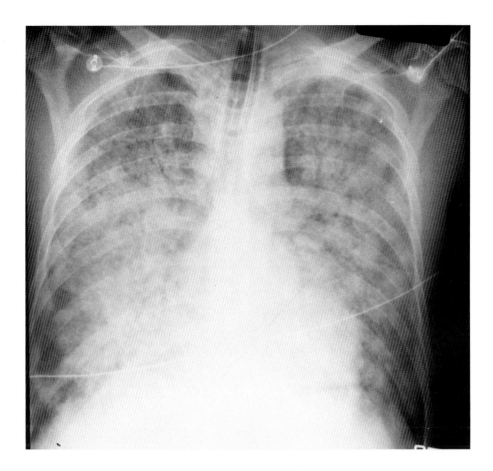

Figure 24-5. In this patient with AIDS and PCP the supine chest radiograph reveals diffuse consolidation of both lungs with resultant air-bronchograms.

the extremely large number of proliferating organisms in AIDS patients as compared with that in other immunocompromised hosts.[18]

As already mentioned, cytomegalovirus pneumonia occurs in up to 17% of patients with AIDS, either alone or in combination with other opportunistic infections. Cytomegalovirus is the most frequently found organism at autopsy, but it only infrequently produces symptoms. Its radiographic features of infection are virtually indistinguishable from those seen in PCP.

Nontuberculous mycobacterial infection can lead to patchy or nodular consolidation and hilar and mediastinal lymph node enlargement (Figure 24-7). As already noted, up to 20% of patients with AIDS are diagnosed

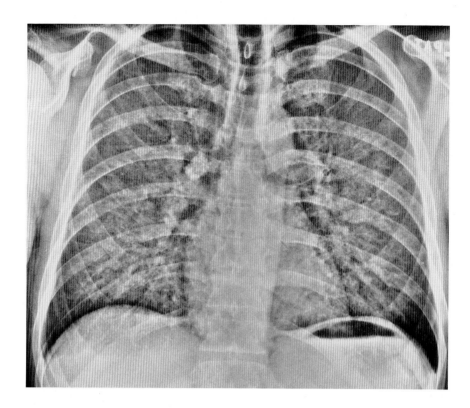

Figure 24-6. Early PCP. Note the sparing of apices and costophrenic sulci.

as having MAI infection during life. It is frequently a disseminated disease and produces thin-walled cavities in AIDS patients less frequently than in non-AIDS patients.

Kaposi's sarcoma develops in about 35% of patients with AIDS, primarily in the subgroup of homosexual men. The tumor is an aggressive multicentric lesion that usually involves the skin, lymph nodes, and, in 50% of cases, the abdominal viscera. Intrathoracic disease occurs in 14% of patients with AIDS. Typically, a multinodular or reticular parenchymal pattern is seen (Figure 24-8). Hilar and mediastinal lymph node enlargement are present in 92% of cases, and pleural effusions are present in 89%.[9,20]

Intrathoracic non-Hodgkin lymphoma can be seen in 2 to 4% of AIDS patients. It is usually a high-grade B-cell lymphoma. Lymph node enlargement predominates over lung involvement, which is found in only 1% of patients.[18,23]

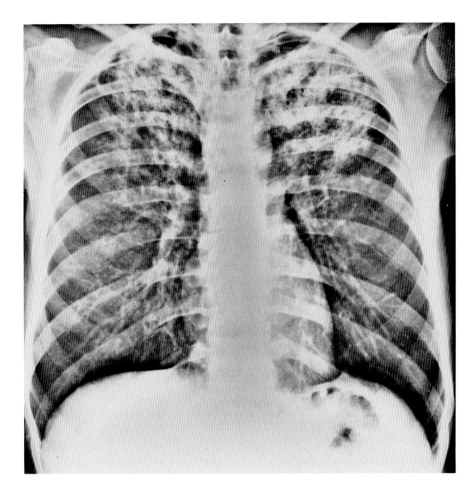

Figure 24-7. MAI in an AIDS patient. Bilateral upper lobe confluent opacities are demonstrated.

A nonspecific interstitial pneumonitis has also been described in up to 34% of AIDS patients—no organism could be identified at bronchoscopy or even open lung biopsy. It may be the result of HIV in the lung parenchyma.[19] A rapid increase in the number of AIDS patients diagnosed with lymphocytic interstitial pneumonia (LIP) has also been recorded. LIP can simulate infectious pulmonary processes, and lung biopsy is necessary for the diagnosis.[17] Radiographically, reticular, reticulonodular, and patchy opacification has been observed. LIP in children under 13 years of age indicates a high likelihood of infection

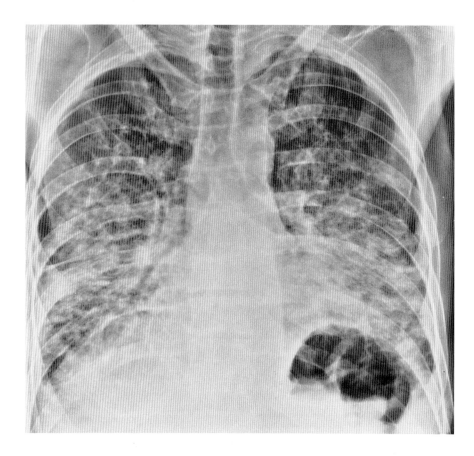

Figure 24-8. Kaposi's sarcoma in an AIDS patient. Reticular opacities involve both lungs. Small bilateral pleural effusions are also present.

with the AIDS virus. The course of LIP is slow and indolent compared with the course of untreated infections or neoplasms.

Congestive cardiomyopathy associated with AIDS has also been reported and has led to premature congestive heart failure in young males.[8]

Question 117

Concerning atypical mycobacterial infections,

    (A) they are rare in patients with AIDS
    (B) they are difficult to differentiate radiographically from tuberculosis
    (C) they do not destroy lung parenchyma
    (D) treatment regimens are similar to those used for typical tuberculosis
    (E) they are transmitted by person-to-person contact

Atypical mycobacterial infections are not rare in AIDS patients **(Option (A) is false)**. In a series of 52 patients with AIDS-related pneumonia, 6 cases were due to atypical mycobacteria.[13] Five patients had *Mycobacterium avium-intracellulare* infection, and one had *Mycobacterium kansasii* infection.

No definite feature allows easy radiographic differentiation from tuberculosis **(Option (B) is true)**. Atypical mycobacteria tend to produce infection in people with emphysema, resulting in thin-walled cavities with rare exudative pulmonary consolidation or pleural effusion.[1,5,26] Compared with classical tuberculosis, there is less scarring and loss of volume. However, irreversible destructive changes with formation of bullae may result if the infection is not recognized and treated promptly **(Option (C) is false)**.

Atypical mycobacteria are notorious for their drug resistance. The chemotherapeutic regimen frequently has to be expanded to include five or six drugs; thus, it is not similar to that used for typical tuberculosis **(Option (D) is false)**. Occasionally, if the disease is limited to a lobe, surgical therapy has to be considered. Unlike tuberculosis, pulmonary infections due to atypical mycobacteria are not considered contagious. The epidemiology of the infection is not entirely known, but as a rule person-to-person transmission is not said to occur **(Option (E) is false)**.

Question 118

Concerning pulmonary alveolar proteinosis,

    (A) initially it involves the interstitial compartment of the lung
    (B) it classically produces the "photographic-negative" image of pulmonary edema
    (C) it is associated with *Nocardia asteroides* infections
    (D) asbestos workers develop a similar radiographic appearance when massively exposed to asbestos fibers
    (E) the alveoli are filled with a surfactant-like material

Pulmonary alveolar proteinosis, also called phospholipidosis, is a diffuse lung disease, the hallmark of which is a dense accumulation of periodic acid–Schiff-positive phospholipid material in the alveoli. Initially, there is preservation of the architecture of the pulmonary interstitium, without involvement of this compartment **(Option (A) is false).**

The chest radiograph in patients with pulmonary alveolar proteinosis has classically been described as showing a "bat wing" pattern, with mainly perihilar parenchymal opacity (Figure 24-9). Although a variety of patterns are associated with this disease, the "photographic-negative" image of pulmonary edema is not the classical appearance **(Option (B) is false),** as is found with chronic eosinophilic pneumonia.

Superimposed infection often complicates the course of pulmonary alveolar proteinosis.[3] Bacterial infections are most common, but the number of infections by other organisms is striking. Foremost among the latter is *Nocardia asteroides,* although *Cryptococcus, Mucor*, and *Aspergillus* infections may also occur **(Option (C) is true).** An association of pulmonary alveolar proteinosis with hematologic malignancy and lymphoma has also been reported.[3]

Massive exposure to silica, not asbestos, over a short period of time may lead to a radiographic appearance similar to that of pulmonary alveolar proteinosis **(Option (D) is false).** This entity, termed silicoproteinosis, has been described primarily in sandblasters.

The alveoli of patients with pulmonary alveolar proteinosis are filled with a surfactant-like material **(Option (E) is true).** A phospholipid-rich substance may be recovered during bronchoalveolar lavage. It is considered that a derangement of normal surfactant reprocessing is the cause of the disease. Possible underutilization of released surfactant from lamellar bodies of Type II pneumocytes and secondary exhaustion of macrophage transport capacity may also contribute to the disease process.[6]

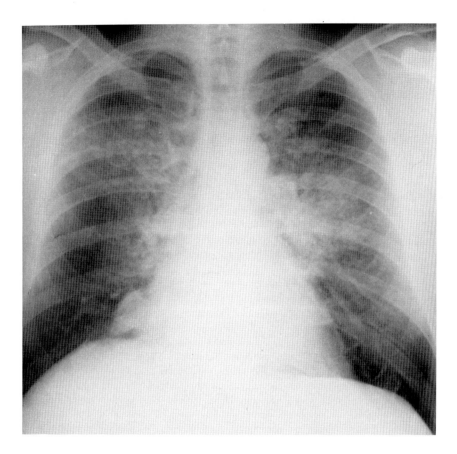

Figure 24-9. Bilateral perihilar parenchymal opacity is the classical appearance of pulmonary alveolar proteinosis.

SUGGESTED READINGS

1. Albelda SM, Kern JA, Marinelli DL, Miller WT. Expanding spectrum of pulmonary disease caused by nontuberculous mycobacteria. Radiology 1985; 157:289–296
2. Broder S, Gallo RC. A pathogenic retrovirus (HTLV-III) linked to AIDS. N Engl J Med 1984; 311:1292–1297
3. Carnovale R, Zornoza J, Goldman AM, Luna M. Pulmonary alveolar proteinosis: its association with hematologic malignancy and lymphoma. Radiology 1977; 122:303–306
4. Chaisson RE, Schechter GF, Theuer CP, Rutherford GW, Echenberg DF, Hopewell PC. Tuberculosis in patients with the acquired immunodeficiency syndrome. Am Rev Respir Dis 1987; 136:570–574
5. Christensen EE, Dietz GW, Ahn CH, et al. Pulmonary manifestations of *Mycobacterium intracellulare.* AJR 1979; 133:59–66

6. Claypool WD, Rogers RM, Matuschak GM. Update on the clinical diagnosis, management, and pathogenesis of pulmonary alveolar proteinosis (phospholipidosis). Chest 1984; 85:550–558

7. Cohen BA, Pomeranz S, Rabinowitz JG, et al. Pulmonary complications of AIDS: radiologic features. AJR 1984; 143:115–122

8. Corboy JR, Fink L, Miller WT. Congestive cardiomyopathy in association with AIDS. Radiology 1987; 165:139–141

9. Davis SD, Henschke CI, Chamides BK, Westcott JL. Intrathoracic Kaposi sarcoma in AIDS patients. Radiographic-pathologic correlation. Radiology 1987; 163:495–500

10. Doppman JL, Geelhoed GW, De Vita VT. Atypical radiographic features in *Pneumocystis carinii* pneumonia. Radiology 1975; 114:39–44

11. Epstein DM, Gefter WB, Conard K, Kelley MA, Miller WT. Lung disease in homosexual men. Radiology 1982; 143:7–10

12. Gaensler EA, Carrington CB. Peripheral opacities in chronic eosinophilic pneumonia: the photographic negative of pulmonary edema. AJR 1977; 128:1–13

13. Hopewell PC, Luce JM. Pulmonary involvement in the acquired immunodeficiency syndrome. Chest 1985; 87:104–112

14. Hughes WT. Pneumocystis carinii pneumonitis. Chest 1984; 85:810–813

15. Kramer EL, Sanger JH, Garay SM, Grossman RJ, Tiu S, Banner H. Diagnostic implications of Ga-67 chest-scan patterns in human immunodeficiency virus-seropositive patients. Radiology 1989; 170:671–676

16. Marinelli DL, Albelda SM, Williams TM, Kern JA, Iozzo RV, Miller WT. Nontuberculous mycobacterial infection in AIDS: clinical, pathologic, and radiographic features. Radiology 1986; 160:77–82

17. Oldham SA, Castillo M, Jacobson FL, Mones JM, Saldana MJ. HIV-associated lymphocytic interstitial pneumonia: radiologic manifestations and pathologic correlation. Radiology 1989; 170:83–87

18. Rubin RH. Acquired immunodeficiency syndrome. In: Rubenstein E, Federman DD (eds), Scientific American medicine. New York: Scientific American; 1988; 7; 11:1–19

19. Simmons JT, Suffredini AF, Lack EE, et al. Nonspecific interstitial pneumonitis in patients with AIDS: radiologic features. AJR 1987; 149:265–268

20. Sivit CJ, Schwartz AM, Rockoff SD. Kaposi's sarcoma of the lung in AIDS: radiologic-pathologic analysis. AJR 1987; 148:25–28

21. Snider DE Jr, Hopewell PC, Mills J, Reichman LB. Mycobacterioses and the acquired immunodeficiency syndrome. Am Rev Respir Dis 1987; 136:492–496

22. Stark P, Nguyen MC. *Pneumocystis* pneumonia caused by acquired immune deficiency (AIDS) syndrome in homosexual men. Prax Klin Pneumol 1984; 38:26–28

23. Stern RG, Gamsu G, Golden JA, Hirji M, Webb WR, Abrams DJ. Intrathoracic adenopathy: differential feature of AIDS and diffuse lymphadenopathy syndrome. AJR 1984; 142:689–692

24. Suster B, Akerman M, Orenstein M, Wax MR. Pulmonary manifestations of AIDS: review of 106 episodes. Radiology 1986; 161:87–93

25. Whelan MA, Kricheff II, Handler M, et al. Acquired immunodeficiency syndrome: cerebral computed tomographic manifestations. Radiology 1983; 477–484
26. Zvetina JR, Demos TC, Maliwan N, et al. Pulmonary cavitation in *Mycobacterium kansasii:* distinctions from *M. tuberculosis.* AJR 1984; 143:127–130

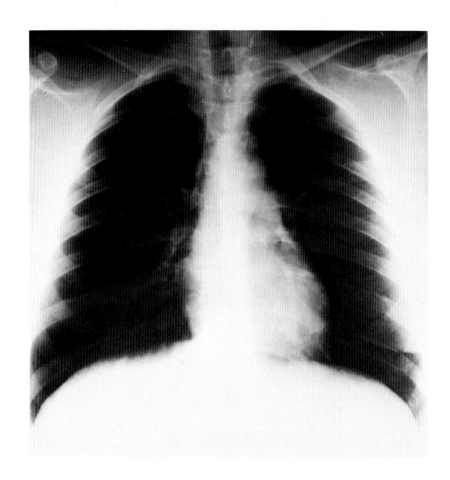

Figure 25-1
Figures 25-1 to 25-3. This 27-year-old woman presented with progressive wheezing. You are shown a posteroanterior view (Figure 25-1), a cone-down view (Figure 25-2), and a lateral view with barium in the esophagus (Figure 25-3).

Case 25: Adenoid Cystic Carcinoma of the Trachea

Question 119

Which *one* of the following is the MOST likely diagnosis?

(A) Pulmonary sling
(B) Leiomyoma of the esophagus
(C) Tracheal neoplasm
(D) Bronchogenic cyst
(E) Double aortic arch

Figures 25-1 and 25-2 show a mass protruding into the distal trachea from its left lateral wall (arrows, Figure 25-4). An extratracheal mass component separates the trachea from the esophagus, as evidenced by displacement of the barium column posteriorly (Figure 25-3). The findings are highly suggestive of a tracheal neoplasm **(Option (C) is correct).** In this young patient, an adenoid cystic carcinoma is most likely.

Leiomyoma of the esophagus (Option (B)) is an intramural tumor that might have an extraluminal component, as in Figure 25-3, but it would not likely protrude into the tracheal lumen, as in Figures 25-2 and 25-4.

A double aortic arch (Option (E)) would probably produce bilateral imprints on the tracheal wall. Also, the right arch would usually be larger and higher than the left and tracheal narrowing would be expected in a higher position than that seen in the test patient.

A bronchogenic cyst (Option (D)) classically occurs in a subcarinal location, and when large it may cause splaying of the carina. In rare instances, it may be found in a paratracheal or retrotracheal location; however, an intraluminal component would be distinctly unusual.

Pulmonary sling (Option (A)) refers to origination of the left pulmonary artery from the right. The anomalous vessel courses between the trachea and the esophagus. Although it may indent the posterior tracheal wall, it would not be expected to produce an intraluminal tracheal mass.

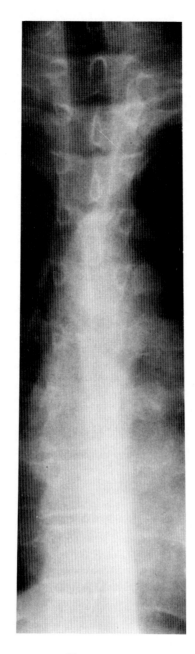

Figure 25-2

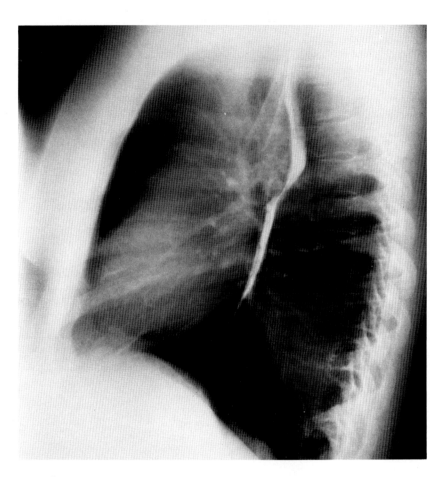

Figure 25-3

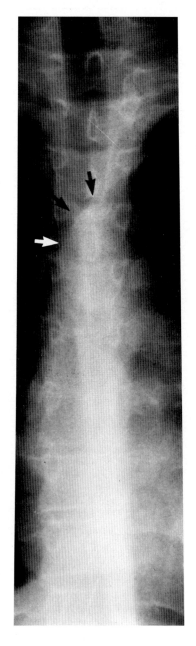

Figure 25-4 (Same as Figure 25-2).   The arrows outline the intraluminal mass.

Question 120

Concerning a pulmonary sling,

(A) it is usually detected in adulthood
(B) the left pulmonary artery originates from the right pulmonary artery
(C) the anomalous vessel produces an anterior imprint on the trachea
(D) the right main bronchus is not affected
(E) the left hilus is larger and higher than the right one

Pulmonary sling, more correctly termed anomalous left pulmonary artery, is usually detected in infancy because it causes progressive respiratory obstruction, particularly during the expiratory phase of respiration **(Option (A) is false)**. A mortality rate of up to 50% may be found, even after surgical treatment. An association of pulmonary sling with complete cartilage ring-tracheal stenosis has relatively recently been described and named the ring-sling complex.[1,5,9]

In patients with pulmonary sling, the left pulmonary artery originates from the right due to failure of the main pulmonary artery to bifurcate into right and left main branches **(Option (B) is true)**. The main pulmonary artery trunk is elongated, following the course of the right pulmonary artery and giving rise to the left pulmonary artery from its extrapericardial segment.

The anomalous left pulmonary artery produces a posterior tracheal imprint **(Option (C) is false)**. As the vessel wraps around the junction of the trachea and right main bronchus, it passes posterior to the trachea and anterior to the esophagus on its way towards the hilus of the left lung.

The proximal segment of the vessel may compress the right main bronchus, leading to atelectasis or obstructive pneumonia or emphysema on the right **(Option (D) is false)**. In patients with pulmonary sling, the left hilus is smaller and lower than the right **(Option (E) is false)**. The lower trachea deviates slightly to the left, rather than to the right as is normally seen. An important finding on the esophagram is a mediastinal opacity (the anomalous vessel) separating the trachea from the esophagus.

Question 121

Concerning tracheal neoplasms in adults,

(A) they are usually benign
(B) adenoid cystic carcinomas (cylindromas) are more common than squamous cell carcinomas
(C) adenoid cystic carcinomas are more common in the sixth than in the third decade of life
(D) adenoid cystic carcinomas usually arise from the posterolateral tracheal wall
(E) carcinoid tumors are among the most common

Most tracheal neoplasms in adults are malignant **(Option (A) is false)**. On the other hand, in children the vast majority of tracheal neoplasms are benign.[6,10] Squamous cell carcinoma is considered to be the most common malignant tracheal tumor in adults **(Option (B) is false)**. However, some variance in the relative frequencies of tracheal neoplasms does exist.[4] Adenoid cystic carcinomas occur in the third through the fifth decades of life **(Option (C) is false)**, whereas squamous cell carcinomas are found in the fifth through the seventh decades. Since minor salivary glands are located in the tracheal mucosa at the posterolateral tracheal wall, adenoid cystic carcinomas (cylindromas) usually arise from that location **(Option (D) is true)**. Carcinoid tumors typically are found in the central bronchi. They may invade the trachea secondarily. Only rarely do they originate primarily in the trachea **(Option (E) is false)**.[2]

Question 122

Concerning double aortic arch,

(A) typically, the left arch is larger than the right
(B) usually, the right arch is lower than the left
(C) it is usually associated with a bicuspid aortic valve
(D) it is the most common vascular ring in adults

The aortic arch system develops embryologically from the primitive aortic arches that supply the six branchial clefts. The third pair of arches forms the carotid arteries, the left fourth arch forms the normal adult aortic arch, and the right fourth arch forms the right subclavian artery. The sixth primitive arches form the central pulmonary arteries and the left ductus arteriosus. Persistence of the proximal segment of the right fourth arch explains embryologically the formation of a double aortic arch.

Double aortic arch is characterized by a vascular ring that encircles the trachea and esophagus. The ascending aorta arises anterior to the trachea and divides into two arches, each of which courses posteriorly along either side of the trachea and esophagus. Each arch also gives rise to its common carotid and subclavian arteries. The left and right arches then join behind the esophagus to form the upper descending aorta, which descends in the thorax either to the right or to the left of the midline (Figure 25-5). The ductus arteriosus may be present on the left or the right, or it may be bilateral. On occasion, the left arch may be hypoplastic or atretic, as a result of an embryologic attempt at regression. The most common type of double aortic arch exhibits a right arch that is larger and higher in position than its left-sided counterpart **(Options (A) and (B) are false)**, a left ductus arteriosus, and a left-sided upper descending aorta.[8] However, variation from the usual situation does exist (Figure 25-6).

Most infants with double aortic arch are "poor eaters." Respiratory problems, such as dyspnea, stridor, and recurrent pneumonia, predominate over manifestations of esophageal obstruction. A double aortic arch can be difficult to recognize in young children since it may be obscured by a large thymus. Widening of the mediastinum at the level of the right aortic arch with a subtle indentation on the tracheal air column is present. The smaller left arch can be seen at a slightly lower level, where there can be found a second tracheal indentation. A frontal barium esophagram shows bilateral asymmetric indentation of the esophagus produced by each arch. A lateral esophagram shows a large posterior imprint on the esophagus formed by the junction of the two arches.

The aortic valve in patients with a double arch is usually tricuspid **(Option (C) is false)**. Bicuspid aortic valve is found in 2% of the population and is associated with aortic valvular stenosis, coarctation, or atrial septal defects. Double aortic arch is usually symptomatic and thus uncovered early in life. It may be an incidental finding in older children or adults. However, the most common vascular ring in adults is seen with a right aortic arch and an anomalous left subclavian artery **(Option (D) is false)**.[3,8] The ring is completed with the left pulmonary artery and the ligamentum arteriosum and occurs in 1 out of 600 otherwise normal individuals.

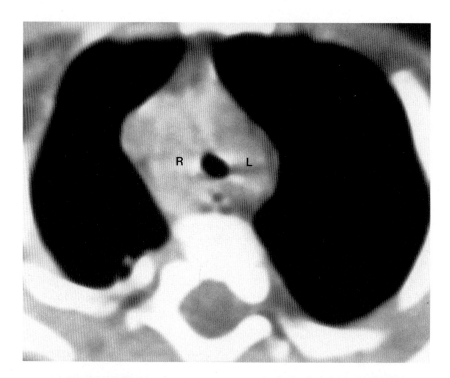

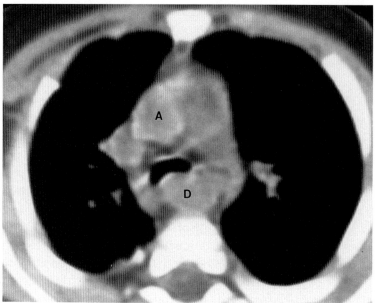

Figure 25-5. Infant with double aortic arch on CT. (Top) CT shows the right (R) and left (L) aortic arches encircling the trachea. The right arch is larger and higher than the left, which appears less dense due to its lower position and volume averaging. (Bottom) CT performed at a level 2 cm lower shows the common ascending (A) and descending (D) aorta.

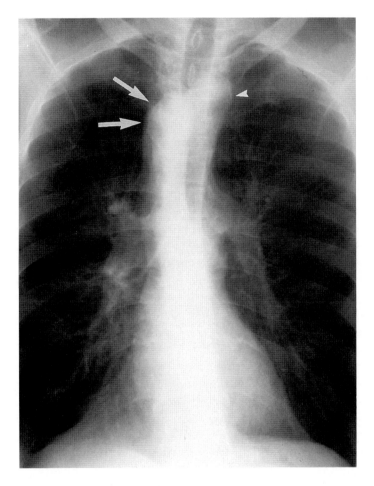

Figure 25-6. In this patient with double aortic arch, the left arch (one arrowhead) is positioned higher than the right (arrows), in variance with the typical appearance as explained in the text.

Discussion

Primary tracheal tumors are rare. They account for less than 0.1% of cancer deaths and are found in 1 of 2,000 autopsies. Tumors of the larynx and bronchi are 75 and 180 times more common, respectively, than tracheal tumors.

Adenoid cystic carcinoma of the trachea was previously classified along with carcinoid and mucoepidermoid carcinoma in the category of "bronchial adenoma." However, its biologic and topographic behavior differs from that of the more frequently encountered carcinoid tumor. Adenoid cystic carcinoma is predominantly a tracheal tumor that may secondarily involve the main bronchi. Carcinoid tumors only rarely occur *de novo* in the trachea; they are usually found in the central bronchi. Adenoid cystic carcinoma accounts for only 0.1 to 0.2% of all intrathoracic tumors, and for only 10% of the so-called "bronchial adenomas," but it accounts for 40% of all primary malignant tumors of the trachea. Only squamous cell carcinoma of the trachea is more common, although in a recent large series of tracheal tumors the adenoid cystic carcinoma predominated.[4] The peak age range of adenoid cystic carcinoma is 30 to 50 years, and it is slightly more common in women.

Overall, this neoplasm occurs more often in the salivary glands than in the trachea. The histology, however, is similar: a moderately well-differentiated, unencapsulated adenocarcinoma composed of small uniform cells forming small cystic spaces.[7] There is a tendency for perineural infiltration and spread along soft tissue planes.

Clinically, the tracheal tumor may cause only minor symptoms over months to years; initially, patients are misdiagnosed as having asthma. The most common symptoms at presentation are dyspnea, cough, inspiratory or expiratory stridor, hoarseness, hemoptysis, and recurrent pneumonias. A delay in diagnosis may be life-threatening since acute signs and symptoms of airway obstruction occur when the luminal diameter of the trachea decreases to about 5 mm. Consequently, a mucous plug or further tumor growth may lead to acute respiratory failure.

Adenoid cystic carcinoma arises in the middle and lower third of the trachea, with a predilection for its posterolateral aspect at the junction between the cartilaginous and the membranous wall. At this site there may be an agglomeration of glands from which the tumor originates. Chest radiographs may be interpreted as normal, especially if inadequately exposed for demonstration of mediastinal structures. High-kVp technique is necessary in such instances, although computed tomography (CT) usually elucidates the problem. The tumor presents usually as a

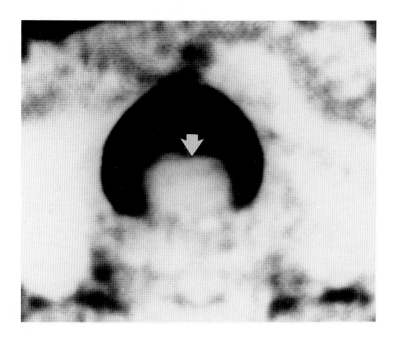

Figure 25-7
Figures 25-7 and 25-8. Axially (Figure 25-7) and coronally (Figure 25-8) reconstructed CT scans of a 29-year-old woman with stridor reveal a polypoid mass, adenoid-cystic carcinoma (arrow), that protrudes into the tracheal lumen.

broad-based lesion occupying the intraluminal space but occasionally also as a polypoid lesion (Figures 25-7 and 25-8). With entire circumferential involvement of the trachea, stenosis may result over a segment of 2 to 10 cm. Advanced tumors lead to an extraluminal mediastinal mass that is best demonstrated by CT. Involvement of the main bronchi may lead to atelectasis, obstructive pneumonia, or hyperexpansion of the distal lung.

The differential diagnosis for malignant tracheal tumor includes squamous cell carcinoma, adenoid cystic carcinoma, chondrosarcoma, mucoepidermoid carcinoma, and leiomyosarcoma. Invasion of the trachea may result from primary tumors of the thyroid gland, esophagus, lung, or larynx. Lymphoma, as well as hematogenous metastases from malignant melanoma and colon, renal, and breast carcinomas, may involve the tracheal wall. Granulomatous disease and amyloid deposits are additional causes of tracheal narrowing or masses.

The therapy of adenoid cystic carcinoma consists of primary sleeve resection of the tumor-bearing tracheal segment and end-to-end or

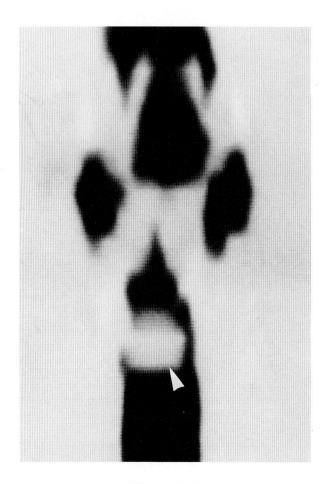

Figure 25-8

end-to-side anastomosis of the remaining large airways. Laryngeal release procedures allow the surgeon to resect up to one-half of the tracheal length. The limiting factor is the extension of tumor tissue into the neighboring mediastinal structures. Adjuvant and palliative radiotherapy have a role in treatment as well.

After surgical removal of the tumor, local recurrences or distant metastases to the lung, liver, brain, or bones occur in up to 50% of patients. The 5-year survival rate is 75%, but late recurrences can occur up to 30 years after removal of the primary tumor. Even with distant metastases, the patient may survive 10 to 15 years.

SUGGESTED READINGS

1. Berdon WE, Baker DH, Wung JT, et al. Complete cartilage-ring tracheal stenosis associated with anomalous left pulmonary artery: the ring-sling complex. Radiology 1984; 152:57–64
2. Briselli M, Mark GJ, Grillo HC. Tracheal carcinoids. Cancer 1978; 42:2870–2879
3. Garti IJ, Aygen MM, Levy MJ. Double aortic arch anomalies: diagnosis by countercurrent right brachial arteriography. AJR 1979; 133:251–256
4. Grillo HC. Tracheal tumors: surgical management. Ann Thorac Surg 1978; 26:112–125
5. Hatten HP Jr, Lorman JG, Rosenbaum HD. Pulmonary sling in the adult. AJR 1977; 128:919–921
6. Pearson FG, Todd TR, Cooper JD. Experience with primary neoplasms of the trachea and carina. J Thorac Cardiovasc Surg 1984; 88:511–518
7. Stark P. Adenoid-cystic carcinoma (cylindroma) of the trachea. An analysis of nine cases. ROFO 1982; 136:31–35
8. Stewart JR, Kincaid OW, Edwards JE. An atlas of vascular rings and related malformations of the aortic arch system. Springfield, IL: Charles C Thomas; 1964:1–37
9. Stone DN, Bein ME, Garris JB. Anomalous left pulmonary artery: two new adult cases. AJR 1980; 135:1259–1263
10. Weber AL, Grillo HC. Tracheal tumors. A radiological, clinical, and pathological evaluation of 84 cases. Radiol Clin North Am 1978; 16:227–246

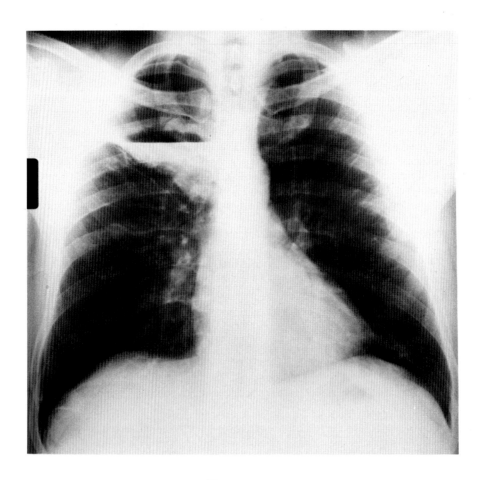

Figure 26-1
Figures 26-1 and 26-2. This 38-year-old man was examined because of
mild fever and cough. You are shown posteroanterior (Figure 26-1) and
lateral (Figure 26-2) chest radiographs.

Case 26: Infected Bulla

Question 123

Which *one* of the following is the MOST likely diagnosis?

(A) Anaerobic lung abscess
(B) Empyema
(C) Tuberculosis
(D) Wegener's granulomatosis
(E) Infected bulla

In the test patient, the most likely diagnosis is an infected bulla **(Option (E) is correct).** A spherical, smooth, thin-walled cavity with an air-fluid level occupies most of the right upper lobe (Figures 26-1 and 26-2). Although the cavity wall itself is not visible, one may infer that it is thin because of the absence of soft tissue separating the lung from the inner rib margins at the lung apex. A lung abscess (Option (A)) would be expected to exhibit a thicker wall and adjacent parenchymal reaction. An empyema (Option (B)), because of its nonspherical shape in most instances, usually exhibits unequal fluid level lengths on views taken at 90° to each other.[4]

Cavitation does occur with tuberculosis (Option (C)), both in primary disease (30% of patients) and in postprimary disease (over 50% of patients). Since between 75 and 90% of the cases of tuberculosis seen in the United States are of the postprimary variety, most cavities will be found in the apical and posterior segments of either upper lobe (90%) or in the superior segment of either lower lobe (10%). However, the cavities produced (Figure 26-3) are usually not as smooth and thin-walled as in the test case.

Wegener's granulomatosis (Option (D)) manifests with multiple pulmonary nodules that can cavitate in one-third to one-half of cases. Solitary cavities are less frequently described as the initial manifestation of the disease, and even if one were to occur, its wall would usually not be as smooth and thin as in the test case (Figure 26-4).

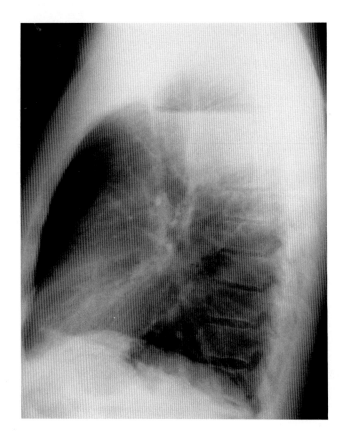

Figure 26-2

The thickness of the cavity wall has been used to differentiate benign from malignant disease. In a study by Woodring et al.,[13] all of the cavities with a wall 1 mm thick or thinner proved to be benign. Cavities with a wall thickness of between 1 and 4 mm were benign in 90% of instances, while those with a thickness of between 5 and 15 mm were benign just as often as malignant. A maximal wall thickness of more than 15 mm indicated malignancy in 90% of instances.

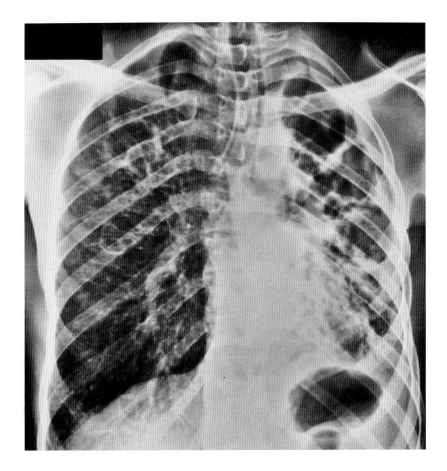

Figure 26-3. Tuberculosis. Note extensive destruction of the left upper lobe with a large cavity replacing the apex of the left lung. Smaller cavities are visible in the left midlung, the right upper lobe, and the right midlung.

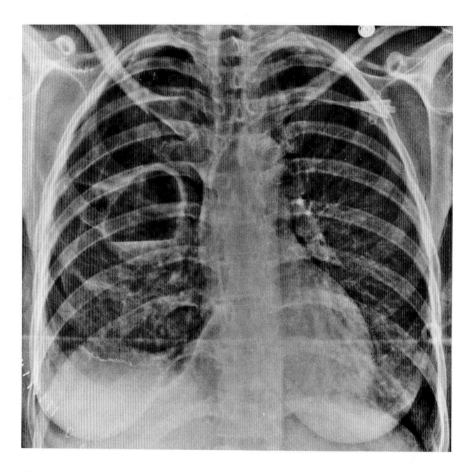

Figure 26-4. Patient with biopsy-proven Wegener's granulomatosis. Note the large cavity with a moderately thick wall, seen especially well along its superior margin.

Question 124

Concerning lung abscesses,

    (A) they usually result from aspiration
    (B) fewer than 1% occur as a result of hematogenous dissemination
    (C) CT is required to distinguish them from empyemas in most cases
    (D) the middle lobe is a common location
    (E) the treatments of abscesses and empyemas are similar

A lung abscess (Figure 26-5) may develop as the result of any bacterial pneumonia, but abscesses are particularly common after aspiration **(Option (A) is true).** They typically exhibit a mix of organisms, mainly anaerobic. In the course of hematogenous dissemination of an extrapulmonary infection or as a result of septic embolism, a lung abscess may result as well **(Option (B) is false).** However, this mechanism is less frequently responsible than aspiration. Computed tomography (CT) helps to differentiate an empyema from a lung abscess; however, in most cases conventional radiography will suffice **(Option (C) is false),** especially when a sequence of radiographs is available to show the development of the process (Table 26-1). Owing to the effect of gravity and the usually supine position of patients during aspiration, abscesses have a predisposition for the apical and posterior segments of the upper lobes, as well as the superior and basilar segments of the lower lobes.[1,3] In a series of 36 abscesses, the location of the cavity was as follows: posterior segment of the right upper lobe in 12 (33%), apicoposterior segment of the left upper lobe in 7 (19.5%), superior segment of either lower lobe in 7 (19.5%), and basilar segment of a lower lobe in 10 (28%).[2] The anterior aspects of the lungs, such as the middle lobe and lingula, are thus less likely to be involved **(Option (D) is false).**

The usual therapy for lung abscesses differs from that for empyemas **(Option (E) is false).** Empyemas necessitate drainage, whether through a large-bore chest tube inserted percutaneously, through a catheter placed by an interventional radiologist, or via thoracotomy. Abscesses, on the other hand, are usually treated medically with postural drainage and antibiotics.[3] Recent reports offer as an alternative the percutaneous drainage of abscesses, provided that the adjacent pleural space is obliterated to preclude causing pleural infection as a result of the needle puncture.[11]

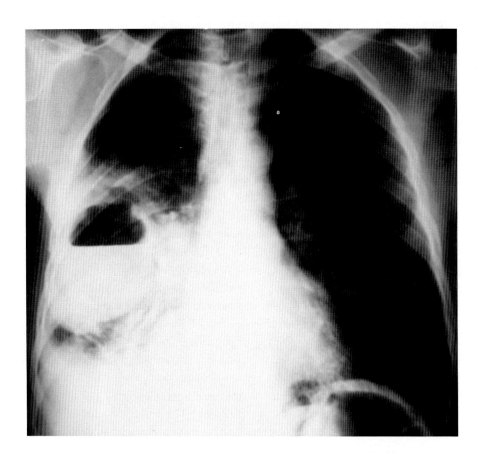

Figure 26-5. A large abscess cavity of the right lower lobe, with an air-fluid level and extensive surrounding pneumonia, is seen in this patient after difficult intubation for general anesthesia.

Table 26-1. Radiographic Differentiation of Empyema from Abscess*

Empyema	Abscess
Displaces vessels and bronchi	Obliterates or destroys vessels and bronchi
Does not conform to lobar boundaries	Has segmental or lobar boundaries
Forms obtuse angle with chest wall	Forms acute angle with chest wall
Is elliptical and forms unequal fluid levels on frontal and lateral radiographs	Is spherical and forms fluid levels of equal length on frontal and lateral radiographs
Fluid level extends up to chest wall	Fluid level not usually peripheral in location
Usually sharply defined by adjacent lung	Poorly defined due to adjacent pneumonia
On CT, visceral and parietal pleura separated by fluid ("split pleura sign")	On CT, intraparenchymal location away from enhancing, inflamed pleura

*Differentiating features apply to both conventional radiography and CT unless otherwise stipulated. Adapted from Stark DD, Federle MP, Goodman PC. Differentiating lung abscess and empyema: radiography and computed tomography. AJR 1983; 141:163–167

Question 125

Concerning Wegener's granulomatosis,

(A) it typically produces a solitary cavity in the lung
(B) it usually involves the upper airways and the kidneys
(C) the limited form involves the kidneys
(D) approximately 20% of patients develop lymphoma

Wegener's granulomatosis usually produces multiple parenchymal nonsharp nodules or areas of opacity, although up to 20% of patients may have solitary pulmonary lesions **(Option (A) is false)**. In the course of the disease, cavitation develops in one-third to one-half of patients.[5-7,9] The vast majority of patients present with symptoms referable to the paranasal sinuses or lungs. Pulmonary symptoms include cough, hemoptysis, and pleuritic pain. Renal involvement characterized by hematuria, pyuria, and azotemia occurs in most patients at some time during the course of the disease **(Option (B) is true)**. The frequency of organ involvement in one series was as follows: respiratory tract, 100%;

urinary tract, 83%; joints, 56%; skin and muscle, 44%; eyes or middle ear, 39%; heart or pericardium, 28%; and nervous system, 22%.[6]

Renal involvement is a major cause of mortality in Wegener's granulomatosis. The patient may initially be asymptomatic. Hematuria with progressive renal failure may eventually develop into the predominant feature of the disease. Only rarely does renal disease actually precede the onset of pulmonary disease.

The limited form of Wegener's granulomatosis involves the respiratory tract but spares the kidneys **(Option (C) is false).** This form of the disease occurs in up to 50% of patients afflicted with Wegener's granulomatosis, and it is associated with a better prognosis.[5]

Before the introduction of prednisone and cytoxan, the prognosis of Wegener's granulomatosis was poor; death occurred within 6 months of onset as a result of either renal or respiratory failure. In recent years, cytotoxic therapy has resulted in long-term remissions and even apparent cures. In contradistinction to lymphomatoid granulomatosis, Wegener's granulomatosis is not believed to evolve into malignant lymphoma **(Option (D) is false).**[8]

Question 126

Concerning bullae,

- (A) they are more common in emphysematous than in otherwise normal lungs
- (B) their walls usually are less than 3 mm thick
- (C) when infected, surgical intervention is the treatment of choice
- (D) they are usually found in the lower lobes
- (E) they are more likely to be infected by fungal than by bacterial pathogens

Parenchymal bullae exist either as solitary cystic spaces in otherwise normal lungs or, more frequently, as part of diffuse emphysema and chronic obstructive pulmonary disease **(Option (A) is true).** They are defined as cystic spaces larger than 1 cm in diameter with a thin wall that is less than 3 mm in thickness **(Option (B) is true).** Paraseptal emphysema is often responsible for the formation of these localized air cysts, which are usually found in the upper lobes **(Option (D) is false).**

In a recent series of 14 patients with infected bullae, the mean age at presentation was 47 years.[10] All patients in this group were smokers (mean, 38 pack-years). Two patients were asymptomatic, while the remaining twelve presented with cough, pleuritic pain, purulent or increasing sputum, fever, chills, or dyspnea. Chest radiographs showed one or more air-fluid levels, but only five patients had associated pulmonary consolidation. Most infections resulted from bacterial pathogens **(Option (E) is false).** Of 14 patients, 13 received oral antibiotics (penicillin or tetracycline). Their symptoms resolved, and there was a gradual radiographic clearing of fluid within 2 to 32 weeks (mean, 12 weeks). One patient was totally asymptomatic, and his fluid level cleared without any form of therapy.

Some authors consider an infected bulla an indication for surgery. However, experience indicates that surgery is often not necessary and that a conservative approach is appropriate **(Option (C) is false).**[12] In the course of healing, the involved bulla may significantly decrease in size or disappear altogether.[12] Disappearance is most likely due to the complete occlusion of the bronchial communication by the inflammatory process, with subsequent resorption of air from the bulla.

An infected bulla may be misinterpreted as either a lung abscess or an empyema with an air-fluid level. In contrast to an abscess, an infected bulla usually shows a very sharp inner outline and generally a lower air-fluid level. However, pneumonia around an infected bulla may reinforce the false impression of lung abscess.

An empyema tends to conform to the shape of the pleural space. As previously stated, the usually nonspherical shape of an empyema results in unequal fluid-level lengths on orthogonal views when air and fluid are present in the empyema.[1] Location of the process at the presumed site of a fissure or at the costophrenic sulcus may be another clue to a pleural, rather than parenchymal, abnormality.

SUGGESTED READINGS

1. Bartlett JG, Finegold SM. Anaerobic infections of the lung and pleural space. Am Rev Respir Dis 1974; 110:56–77
2. Bartlett JG, Finegold SM. In: Lung disease: state of the art. American Lung Association 1974–75 1975:207–228
3. Bartlett JG, Gorbach SL, Tally FP, Finegold SM. Bacteriology and treatment of primary lung abscess. Am Rev Respir Dis 1974; 109:510–518
4. Friedman PJ, Hellekant CA. Radiologic recognition of bronchopleural fistula. Radiology 1977; 124:289–295
5. Gohel VK, Dalinka MK, Israel HL, Libshitz HI. The radiological manifestations of Wegener's granulomatosis. Br J Radiol 1973; 46:427–432
6. Gonzalez L, Van Ordstrand HS. Wegener's granulomatosis. Review of 11 cases. Radiology 1973; 107:295–300

7. Landman S, Burgener F. Pulmonary manifestations in Wegener's granulomatosis. AJR 1974; 122:750–756

8. Liebow AA. The J. Burns Amberson lecture—pulmonary angiitis and granulomatosis. Am Rev Respir Dis 1973; 108:1–18

9. Maguire R, Fauci AS, Doppman JL, Wolff SM. Unusual radiographic features of Wegener's granulomatosis. AJR 1978; 130:233–238

10. Peters JI, Kubitschek KR, Gottlieb MS, Awe RJ. Lung bullae with air-fluid levels. Am J Med 1987; 82:759–763

11. Snow N, Lucas A, Horrigan TP. Utility of pneumonotomy in the treatment of cavitary lung disease. Chest 1984; 87:731–734

12. Stark P, Gadziala N, Greene R. Fluid accumulation in preexisting pulmonary air spaces. AJR 1980; 134:701–706

13. Woodring JH, Fried AM, Chuang VP. Solitary cavities of the lung: diagnostic implications of cavity wall thickness. AJR 1980; 135:1269–1271

Notes

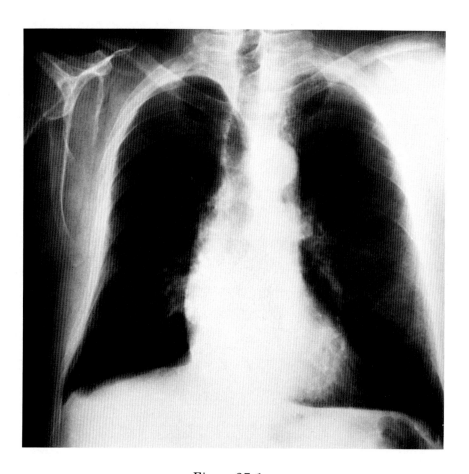

Figure 27-1

Figures 27-1 to 27-3. You are shown routine posteroanterior (Figure 27-1) and lateral (Figure 27-2) chest radiographs of a 53-year-old man. A computed tomographic (CT) scan was obtained subsequently (Figure 27-3).

Case 27: Rounded Atelectasis

Question 127

Which *one* of the following is the MOST likely diagnosis?

(A) Bronchogenic carcinoma
(B) Organized pulmonary infarct
(C) Cryptococcal granuloma
(D) Rounded atelectasis
(E) Plasma cell granuloma

Figures 27-1 and 27-2 show a parenchymal subpleural mass in the posterior aspect of the right lower lobe. Marked adjacent pleural thickening is also visible. Computed tomography (CT) of the chest (Figure 27-3) confirms the conventional radiographic findings and also illustrates curving vessels in association with the mass. This constellation of radiographic findings is highly suggestive of a rounded atelectasis **(Option (D) is correct).**

Bronchogenic carcinoma (Option (A)), organized pulmonary infarct (Option (B)), cryptococcal granuloma (Option (C)), and plasma cell granuloma (Option (E)) are all reasonable considerations for a solitary pulmonary mass. Pleural thickening could conceivably be seen with each of them, although the extent of thickening noted in Figure 27-2 would be unlikely except for bronchogenic carcinoma with spread along the pleural surface. None of these entities, however, would be expected to produce the curving vessels seen in Figure 27-3, a finding highly characteristic of rounded atelectasis in view of the mechanism by which rounded atelectasis is produced (see Discussion).

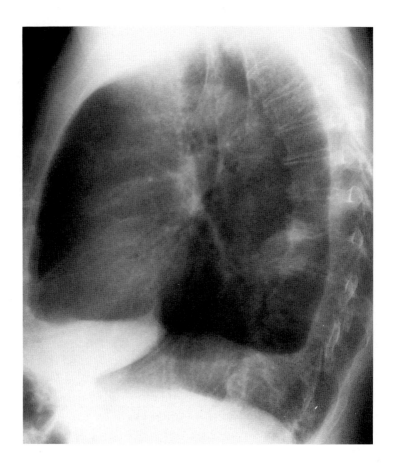

Figure 27-2

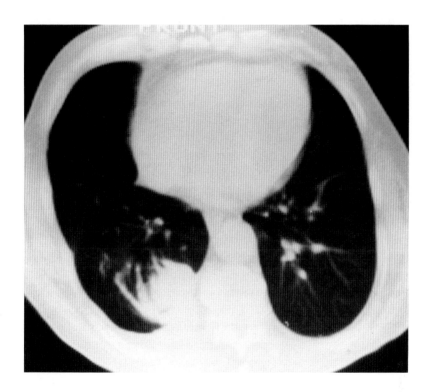

Figure 27-3

Question 128

Concerning bronchogenic carcinomas,

    (A) less than 50% of adenocarcinomas occur in the lung periphery
    (B) the "tail sign" is specific for the bronchioloalveolar cell type
    (C) visible calcification excludes the diagnosis
    (D) the most frequently cavitating type is small-cell carcinoma
    (E) a relationship to smoking is well established for all cell types

Approximately 75% of adenocarcinomas occur in the lung periphery, although recently an increased occurrence of hilar or mediastinal masses in poorly differentiated adenocarcinoma has been noted **(Option (A) is false)**.[14]

The "tail sign" has been described in patients with bronchioloalveolar cell carcinoma; a large percentage of these tumors exhibit a linear density that connects them to the pleura. The "tail" represents a desmoplastic reaction about the neoplasm leading to retraction of the visceral pleura with pleural puckering, wrinkling, or umbilication. However, two relatively recent studies could not convincingly demonstrate that the "tail sign" is specific for bronchioloalveolar cell carcinoma.[7,13] Pleural tails may also be found with other neoplastic processes and with granulomas and other inflammatory lesions. Thus, the "tail sign" is a nonspecific reflection of a desmoplastic reaction **(Option (B) is false)**.

The mere presence of visible calcification in a pulmonary mass does not exclude the diagnosis of bronchogenic carcinoma, especially when the calcium is eccentrically located **(Option (C) is false)**. Diffuse, central (target), concentric, or popcorn calcifications, on the other hand, are very good indicators that a lesion is benign. Calcium within a bronchogenic carcinoma is due either to calcification of necrotic areas (dystrophic calcification) or to engulfment of a granuloma by the malignancy. Radiographically visible calcification in peripheral pulmonary neoplasms is quite infrequent and occurs in less than 1% of lesions.[9]

Cavitation in bronchogenic carcinoma occurs in about 10% of cases. In a large series of 632 tumors, 16% cavitated; most of the cavitated tumors (82%) were squamous cell carcinomas **(Option (D) is false)**.[3] Large-cell carcinoma (11%) and adenocarcinoma (7%) accounted for the remaining ones. Cavitation usually results from central necrosis in the neoplasm.

The association of smoking with bronchogenic carcinoma is well known; 93% of patients with bronchogenic carcinoma are smokers. Many studies have shown that the risk of bronchogenic carcinoma increases in

Table 27-1. Bronchogenic Carcinoma Risk Factors

Cigarette smoking (93% of patients are smokers)	Arsenic
	Chromates
Marijuana smoking	Petrochemicals
Ionizing radiation	Concomitant emphysema
Bis-chloromethyl ether	Genetic predisposition
Asbestos	Deficiency in vitamins A and E, selenium,
Cadmium	β-carotene
Nickel	

Adapted from Skarin AT. Respiratory tract and head and neck cancer. In: Rubenstein E, Federman DD (eds), Scientific American medicine. New York: Scientific American, 1987; 12; 6:1–28

direct proportion to the number of cigarettes smoked. Compared with a nonsmoker, a smoker has a 16 to 30 times greater chance of developing a squamous or small-cell carcinoma and a 4 to 6 times greater chance of developing an adenocarcinoma or large-cell carcinoma.[5,8] Bronchioloalveolar cell carcinoma does not currently show a clear-cut positive association with smoking **(Option (E) is false).** Table 27-1 lists a number of risk factors for bronchogenic carcinoma. There is also a greater than expected frequency of bronchogenic carcinoma in patients with tuberculosis.

Early figures noting the frequency of squamous cell carcinoma (40 to 70%) and of adenocarcinoma (4 to 15%) are also changing. A significant increase in adenocarcinoma has been recorded within the last 15 years.[8] Currently, 35 to 40% of bronchogenic carcinomas are squamous cell carcinoma, 25 to 30% are adenocarcinoma, 20 to 25% are small-cell carcinoma, and 10 to 15% are large-cell undifferentiated carcinoma. In some series, adenocarcinoma is as common as squamous cell carcinoma.

Question 129

Concerning rounded atelectasis,

    (A) there is a correlation with asbestos exposure
    (B) the mass occurs at the site of maximum pleural thickening
    (C) the mass is composed of airless lung
    (D) calcification within the mass is common
    (E) it usually occurs at the lung apex

In a certain number of cases of rounded atelectasis, there is a correlation with previous asbestos exposure (**Option (A) is true**).[12] The mass, which is composed of airless lung (**Option (C) is true**), occurs at the site of maximum pleural thickening (**Option (B) is true**). As a rule, calcification does not occur within the mass of rounded atelectasis (**Option (D) is false**). Conceivably, however, the airless lung may contain a preexisting calcified granuloma. Rounded atelectasis is typically found in the posteroinferior or anteroinferior aspect of the lung (**Option (E) is false**). For further information, see the Discussion section.

Question 130

Concerning plasma cell granulomas,

    (A) there is usually a clinical history of pneumonia
    (B) they usually occur as multiple lesions
    (C) most are not calcified
    (D) transformation to multiple myeloma occurs in approximately 10% of cases
    (E) their diagnosis is readily established by percutaneous needle aspiration biopsy

Plasma cell granuloma, also known as inflammatory pseudotumor or histiocytoma of the lung, is characterized histologically by a mixture of fibroblasts, histiocytes, lymphocytes, and plasma cells. The pathogenesis of this lesion is uncertain. In only 20% of patients can an antecedent pneumonia be verified (**Option (A) is false**).[1,10] Although plasma cell granulomas may present as multiple lesions, they usually present as solitary nodular masses (**Option (B) is false**). Multiple nodules, cavitation, and calcification of these lesions are all unusual (**Option (C) is true**).

No known relationship exists between plasma cell granuloma and multiple myeloma (**Option (D) is false**). Plasma cell granuloma consists of a benign proliferation of plasma cells, granulation tissue, histiocytes, and lymphocytes, accompanied by deposits of hyaline material.[1] Occasionally, an aggressive local behavior may be exhibited, as evidenced by bronchial obstruction or infiltration of adjacent structures.[10]

The diagnosis of plasma cell granuloma is readily established by surgical resection of the nodule mass. The tissue sample obtained through percutaneous needle aspiration biopsy is often not sufficient for a specific diagnosis of a benign lesion **(Option (E) is false)**.

Discussion

Rounded atelectasis, a form of peripheral lung collapse, is also known as folded lung, atelectatic pseudotumor, and pleuroma.[11] The term "atelectatic pulmonary and pleural asbestotic pseudotumor" has been used, but it does not take into account the fact that rounded atelectasis may occur in people not exposed to asbestos.

Rounded atelectasis is invariably associated with extensive pleural thickening or a marked pleural peel.[6] Occasionally, a pleural effusion may be demonstrated. It is assumed that the following sequence of events leads to the formation of this peripheral pulmonary mass. Pleural fluid compresses a pulmonary lobe so that an atelectatic region of lung is formed. A cleft-like invagination of the visceral pleura surrounds this atelectatic region and separates it from the rest of the lung. Subsequent fibrinous deposits on the visceral pleura and in the cleft perpetuate the position and configuration of the atelectasis. In the wake of pleural fluid resorption, the normal lung expands and engulfs the atelectatic region to form the mass of rounded atelectasis.[6]

The causes of the initiating pleural effusion are numerous: tuberculosis, congestive heart failure, benign asbestos pleural effusion, pulmonary infarction, postmyocardial infarction (Dressler's) syndrome, and nonspecific pleurisy.[11] At the time of detection, little or no pleural effusion may be found. A pleural peel is a signpost of previous pleural activity, however. Biopsy of the pleura usually reveals nonspecific inflammation with fibrosis. At surgery, a sheet-like thickening of the visceral pleura may be discovered. In patients with asbestos exposure, pleural thickening is present.

Radiographically, rounded atelectasis presents as a subpleural, solitary mass, which may be oval, lobulated, or irregular and which can reach a diameter of 2.5 to 5 cm, sometimes even larger. It forms acute angles with the adjacent thickened pleura and thus appears intraparenchymal. Its margins may be sharp or poorly defined. Part of its circumference is blurred in one or more projections by bronchi and blood vessels connecting it to the central hilar area. The blood vessels curve and bundle together as they converge towards the mass along with the accompanying bronchi. This appearance has been termed the "comet tail" or "vacuum cleaner effect" and is well demonstrated on both conventional tomography and CT (Figure 27-3).[4,12] Such an appearance is crucial to the diagnosis of rounded atelectasis (Figures 27-4 to 27-7). A pleural peel is also essential to the diagnosis. Occasionally a pleural effusion is found. The pleural abnormality is more pronounced over the mass. The ipsilateral costophrenic sulcus is frequently blunted. This cancer-mimicking, atelectatic pseudotumor of the lung usually remains stable, although occasional spontaneous reduction or even disappearance of the mass over the course of several months to a year has been noted.

Once the typical radiographic findings are recognized and rounded atelectasis is diagnosed, a conservative approach is appropriate. A history of previous asbestos exposure or pleuritis may further help in making a decision. Periodic follow-up radiographs should be used to confirm stability or detect resolution and thus rule out malignancy. In selected cases, percutaneous needle biopsy is necessary.

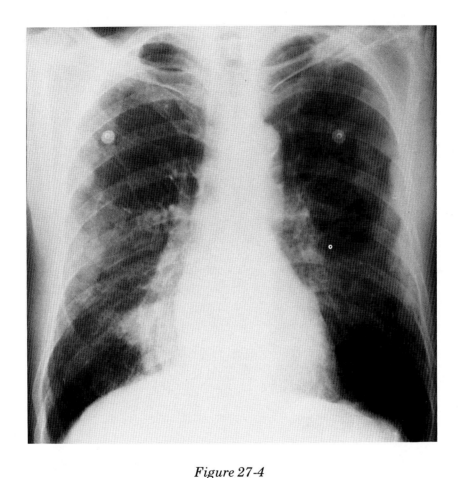

Figure 27-4
Figures 27-4 to 27-7. This 70-year-old patient with known previous asbestos exposure has a right lower lobe mass seen on posteroanterior (Figure 27-4) and lateral (Figure 27-5) chest radiographs, along with pleural plaques on both mid-lateral chest walls seen on the posteroanterior view. Two CT scans (Figures 27-6 and 27-7) show the mass but fail to display the comet tail of curving vessels essential for the diagnosis of rounded atelectasis (compare with Figure 27-3). Needle aspiration biopsy of the lung mass yielded adenocarcinoma.

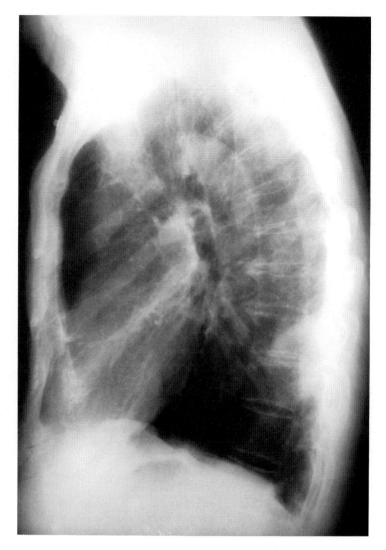

Figure 27-5

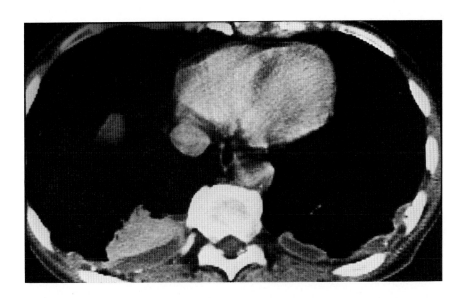

Figure 27-6

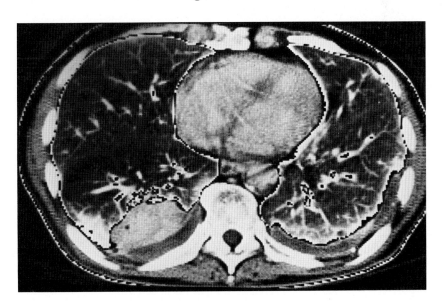

Figure 27-7

SUGGESTED READINGS

1. Bahadori M, Liebow A. Plasma cell granulomas of the lung. Cancer 1973; 31:191–208
2. Bone RC, Balk R. Staging of bronchogenic carcinoma. Chest 1982; 82:473–480
3. Chaudhuri MR. Primary pulmonary cavitating carcinomas. Thorax 1973; 28:354–366
4. Doyle TC, Lawler GA. CT features of rounded atelectasis of the lung. AJR 1984; 143:225–228
5. Fielding JE. Smoking: health effects and control. N Engl J Med 1985; 313:491–498
6. Hanke R, Kretzschmar R. Round atelectasis. Semin Roentgenol 1980; 15:174–182
7. Hill CA. "Tail" signs associated with pulmonary lesions: critical reappraisal. AJR 1982; 139:311–316
8. Loeb LA, Ernster VL, Warner KE, Abbotts J, Laszlo J. Smoking and lung cancer: an overview. Cancer Res 1984; 44(12 Pt 1):5940–5958
9. Siegelman SS, Zerhouni EA, Leo FP, Khouri NF, Stitik FP. CT of the solitary pulmonary nodule. AJR 1980; 135:1–13
10. Stark P. The plasma cell granuloma—an inflammatory pulmonary pseudotumor (author's transl). ROFO 1981; 134:265–268
11. Stark P. Round atelectasis: another pulmonary pseudotumor. Am Rev Respir Dis 1982; 125:248–250
12. Tylen U, Nilsson U. Computed tomography in pulmonary pseudotumors and their relation to asbestos exposure. J Comput Assist Tomogr 1982; 6:229–237
13. Webb WR. The pleural tail sign. Radiology 1978; 127:309–313
14. Woodring JH, Stelling CB. Adenocarcinoma of the lung: a tumor with a changing pleomorphic character. AJR 1983; 140:657–664

Notes

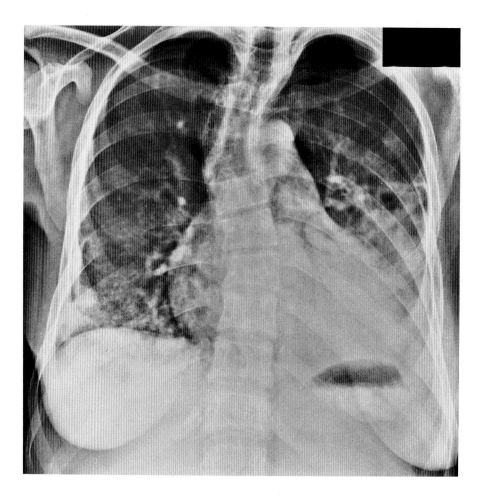

Figure 28-1

Figures 28-1 to 28-3. This 27-year-old woman presented with pneumonia. You are shown posteroanterior (Figure 28-1) and lateral (Figure 28-2) chest radiographs and a frontal view of the abdomen (Figure 28-3) taken at another time.

Case 28: Intrathoracic Manifestations of Sickle Cell Disease

Question 131

Which *one* of the following is the MOST likely diagnosis?

(A) Granulomatous infection
(B) Sickle cell disease
(C) Cystic fibrosis
(D) Leukemia
(E) Lupus erythematosus

The posteroanterior (Figure 28-1) and lateral (Figure 28-2) chest radiographs reveal bilateral lower lobe consolidations and pleural effusions, cardiomegaly, and end-plate deformity of midthoracic vertebral bodies (Figure 28-4, arrows). On the lateral view (Figure 28-4, arrowhead), an oval infradiaphragmatic calcification is visible posteriorly. The supine view of the abdomen confirms the presence of a calcified left upper quadrant structure, namely a shrunken calcified spleen (Figure 28-3). In essence, this patient exhibits radiographic hallmarks of sickle cell disease **(Option (B) is correct).**

Patients with granulomatous infections (Option (A)), including primary tuberculosis, would likely present with hilar and mediastinal lymph node enlargement. Postprimary tuberculosis has a bias for the upper regions of the lung, but basilar pneumonias might occur as a manifestation of bronchogenic spread. Splenic calcifications of a focal nature might be seen with granulomatous infections, unlike the dense diffuse calcification illustrated in Figure 28-3, so that granulomatous infection is not likely.

Cystic fibrosis (Option (C)) shows radiographic evidence for bronchiectasis and hyperexpansion of the lungs. Any parenchymal abnormality would usually show upper zonal and perihilar distribution, so that cystic fibrosis is also an unlikely diagnosis.

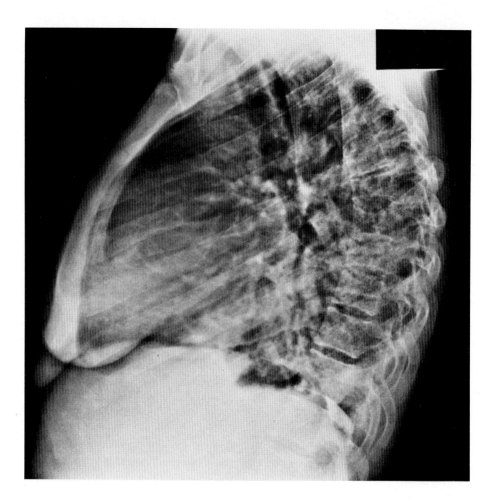

Figure 28-2

Patients with leukemia (Option (D)) do tend to develop bacterial or opportunistic pneumonias, and leukemic infiltration of the lung may occur as well, although the latter is infrequently visible on radiographs.[2] The type of splenic calcification illustrated in the test case is not a typical feature, and hence leukemia is unlikely.

In lupus erythematosus (Option (E)), pneumonia or pulmonary hemorrhage might produce parenchymal consolidation. Enlargement of the cardiac silhouette due to a pericardial effusion could also be a feature of the disease. However, the calcified shrunken spleen also militates against this diagnosis.

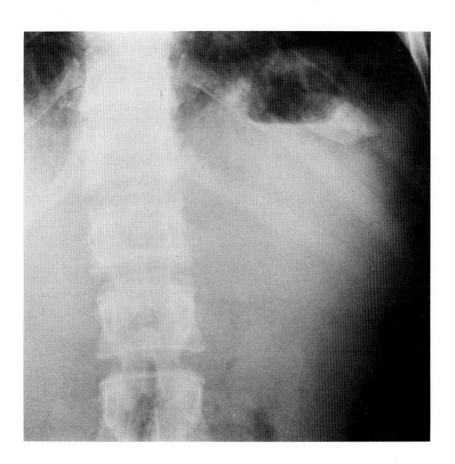

Figure 28-3

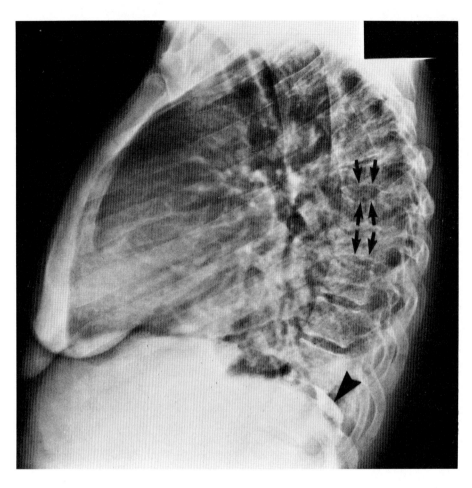

Figure 28-4 (Same as Figure 28-2).   Note end-plate deformity (arrows) and calcified spleen (arrowhead).

Question 132

Concerning patients with sickle cell disease,

(A) they have a higher incidence of pneumonia than do members of the general population
(B) they rarely develop pleural effusions
(C) the most common intrathoracic radiographic finding is cardiomegaly
(D) they have a high incidence of massive pulmonary embolism

In patients with sickle cell disease, pneumonia is a common complication and occurs 20 to 100 times more often than in the general population (**Option (A) is true**).[1] A high percentage of patients (approximately 50%) have pleural effusions (**Option (B) is false**). Cardiomegaly is the most common intrathoracic radiographic finding, occurring in up to 80% of patients older than 6 months (**Option (C) is true**).[9] Contrary to what one might expect, massive pulmonary embolism is infrequent (**Option (D) is false**) (see the Discussion section).

Question 133

Concerning cystic fibrosis,

(A) the pulmonary radiographic abnormalities occur predominantly in the lower lobes
(B) mucoid impaction is a rare radiographic feature
(C) pleural effusion is a common radiographic feature
(D) blood-streaked sputum is a common clinical sign

Cystic fibrosis is the most common inherited disease in people of Northern European descent, occurring in about 1 in 2,000 live births. About 5% of the aforementioned population carries the gene.[4] The estimated incidence of cystic fibrosis varies from 1 in 620 live births in Southwest Afrikaners of Dutch descent to 1 in 15,000 in Italians, 1 in 17,000 in blacks, and 1 in 90,000 in Orientals. In the United States, regional variations in incidence occur (in Minnesota, 1 in 1,000; in New England, 1 in 2,400; in Ohio, 1 in 3,700).[12]

Cystic fibrosis is characterized by a defective chloride transport mechanism at the level of the cell membrane with subsequent disturbance in the function of exocrine glands. Elevated levels of sodium and chloride can be found in the sweat of afflicted patients. Pancreatic insufficiency and chronic pulmonary disease predominate clinically. The diagnosis is made in 50% of patients within the first year of life and in 17% after age 15.

On pathologic examination, the lungs are normal at birth. Mucopurulent plugging of bronchi with bronchiectasis, destruction of bronchial epithelium, obliteration of small airways, and recurrent bronchopneumonia typically due to *Staphylococcus aureus* or *Pseudomonas aeruginosa* subsequently appear. Complications include spontaneous pneumothorax, cor pulmonale, abscess formation, allergic bronchopulmonary aspergillosis, and others (discussed below).

The radiographic distribution of abnormalities shows a preponderance of involvement of the upper lobes and perihilar areas **(Option (A) is false)**. Common radiographic findings include: bronchiectasis (90%), hyperinflated lungs (75%), hilar enlargement due to lymph nodes and pulmonary arteries (75%), atelectasis (50%), cystic air spaces (20%), and peripheral nodular and nonvascular linear opacities (Figure 28-5).[5]

Mucoid impaction is not a rare radiographic feature **(Option (B) is false)**, occurring approximately 30% of the time. Pleural effusions are not commonly seen, although a parapneumonic fluid collection may develop **(Option (C) is false)**. Blood-streaked sputum is a common clinical sign **(Option (D) is true)**, occurring in over 50% of patients reaching adulthood; massive hemoptysis (more than 500 mL in 24 hours) is found in approximately 8% of adults with cystic fibrosis.

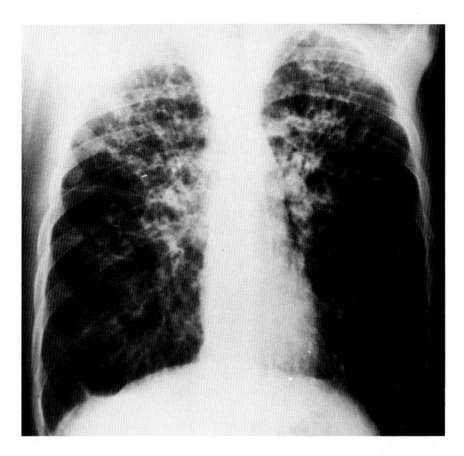

Figure 28-5. This posteroanterior radiograph of an adult patient with cystic fibrosis reveals hyperexpanded lungs, enlarged hila, bronchial wall thickening, and cystic areas suggesting bronchiectasis. Note the upper lobe preponderance.

Question 134

Concerning lupus erythematosus,

(A) it frequently produces a specific pneumonitis
(B) it leads to pulmonary hyperexpansion and a flat diaphragm
(C) hilar adenopathy is a common feature
(D) Libman-Sacks endocarditis frequently results in congestive heart failure

In lupus erythematosus, a nonspecific pneumonitis occurs in both acute and chronic forms **(Option (A) is false)**. The acute form is found in up to 12% of patients with active lupus. Pulmonary findings tend to be bilateral and are frequently accompanied by pleural effusions. The lung disease is characterized histologically by alveolar damage, interstitial edema, hyaline membrane formation, and perivascular lymphocytic and plasma cell infiltration.[7] The process may either clear completely or leave a residue. Cavitating pulmonary nodules (rare) have been described.[3,11] The chronic form of lupus pneumonitis is due to immune complex deposits in the alveolar walls and has the nonspecific feature of usual interstitial pneumonitis.[7] Radiographically, reticular opacities in the lower lung zones with an element of volume loss can be observed.

Patients with lupus tend to develop small lung volumes, and elevation of the hemidiaphragms is a well-recognized radiographic feature **(Option (B) is false)**.[7,10] The restrictive ventilatory defect may be caused by weakness of the diaphragmatic musculature, which is probably due to a localized myositis with intact phrenic nerve function. Diaphragmatic dysfunction is a reversible process.

Lymph node enlargement occurs in approximately 50% of all patients with lupus, although hilar adenopathy is distinctly uncommon **(Option (C) is false)**.[6]

Libman-Sacks endocarditis is the most characteristic cardiac lesion of lupus erythematosus. It is characterized by verrucous valvular lesions that are commonly found on the endocardial surfaces of the atrioventricular valves and less frequently found on the aortic valvular cusps. Despite the frequency and extent of these lesions, they do not often profoundly affect the function of the valves. Unlike rheumatic fever, Libman-Sacks endocarditis does not produce serious regurgitation during the acute phase of the disease. Thus, congestive heart failure due to Libman-Sacks endocarditis is unusual **(Option (D) is false)**.[9]

Discussion

Sickle cell disease affects 0.2% of the black population in the United States.[8] Its major clinical features result from chronic hemolysis, which is only moderately debilitating, and from acute vaso-occlusive crises, which account for most of the morbidity and mortality.

Patients with sickle cell disease frequently have an abnormal chest radiograph. Global cardiomegaly is the most common finding, occurring in up to 80% of patients older than 6 months (Figures 28-6 and 28-7). It may be the only detectable radiographic abnormality and is due to chronic anemia. High cardiac output, due to increased blood volume, and peripheral anoxia favor myocardial dilatation and hypertrophy.[8] The resting cardiac output doubles once the hemoglobin concentration falls below 7 mg/100 mL, resulting in hyperkinetic circulation and increased pulmonary vascularity. The circulatory system is stressed by sickled erythrocytes that occlude small blood vessels, including those of the pulmonary circulation. Pulmonary arterial hypertension and cor pulmonale may result. Occasionally, a striking similarity to the radiographic findings of mitral valvular disease or left-to-right shunts may be found.

Pulmonary parenchymal abnormalities are frequent. Subacute or chronic disease leads to reticular and small linear parenchymal opacities without definite consolidation. The opacities may result from interstitial pulmonary edema and obliterative changes in small blood vessels caused by stagnated, sickled erythrocytes. The findings are more marked in the lower lung zones, resulting in a reticular pattern.

Patients with sickle cell hemoglobinopathies have a well-known propensity to develop pneumonia. It occurs 20 to 100 times more often than in the general population and is a common reason for hospitalization.[1] The pneumonia often spreads rapidly and resolves slowly. There is a tendency for multilobar involvement and recurrence (Figure 28-8). An etiologic agent is recovered from bronchial secretions in less than 50% of patients with pneumonia. *Streptococcus pneumoniae* and *Haemophilus influenzae* are the responsible organisms in a relatively high percentage of cases.

Pulmonary vascular occlusion in sickle cell disease is usually due to in situ aggregation of erythrocytes, a phenomenon occurring preferentially in the unsaturated blood of the pulmonary arteries. Thrombosis ensues due to stasis. The differentiation of infarction from pneumonia may be difficult, and both may coexist. Infarcts occur commonly in the lower zones and tend to have a segmental configuration. Pneumonia may involve an entire lobe. Rarely, pulmonary vascular occlusion may

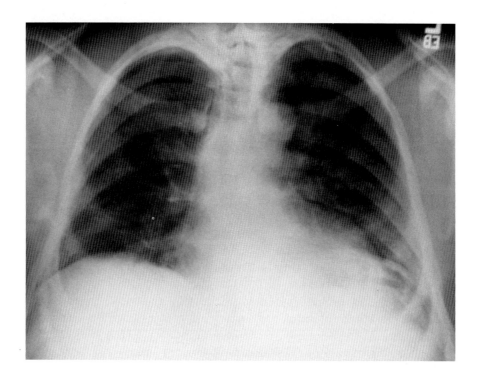

Figure 28-6
Figures 28-6 and 28-7. Cardiomegaly is noted on posteroanterior (Figure 28-6) and lateral (Figure 28-7) radiographs of a young adult patient with sickle cell disease, along with abnormal linear lung markings and "step-off" defects (arrow) of a thoracic vertebral body endplate (Reynold's sign).

progress rapidly and lead to complete opacification of a lobe or even of an entire lung. Radiographic resolution of an infarct is visible 7 to 10 days after the onset of symptoms. Major necrosis is rare, and linear scars are left behind.

A large number of patients with sickle cell disease (around 50%) will have pleural effusions related to either congestive heart failure or sickle cell crisis (Figure 28-9).[8]

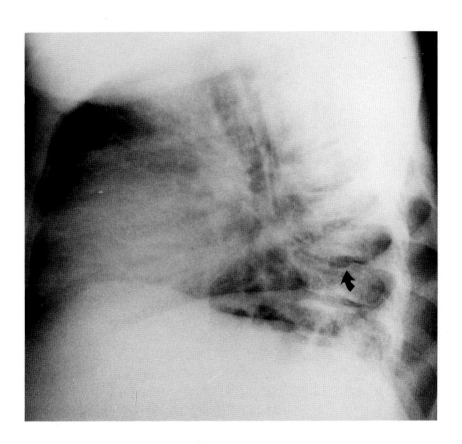

Figure 28-7

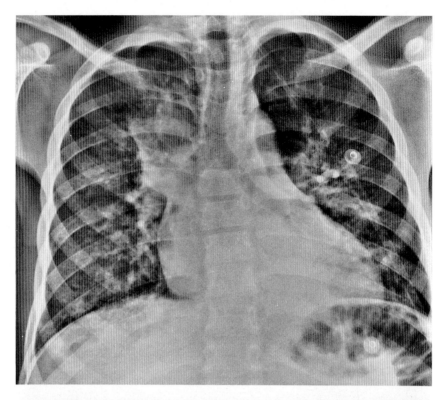

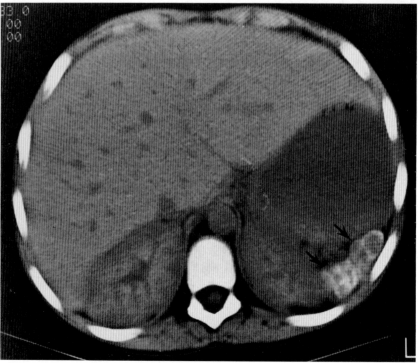

Figure 28-8. Sickle cell disease. (Top) Note cardiomegaly, linear parenchymal opacities, and right upper and left lower lobe pneumonia. (Bottom) CT scan of the upper abdomen in the same patient reveals a small calcified spleen (arrows).

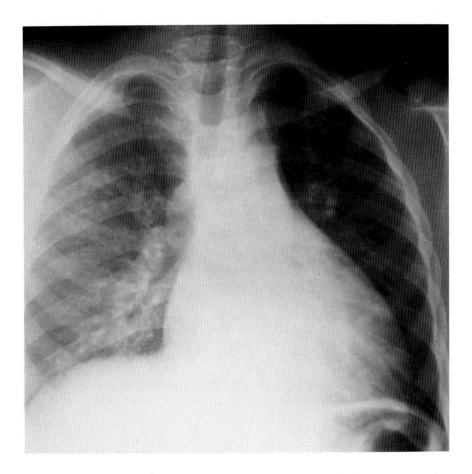

Figure 28-9. In this 5-year-old child with sickle cell disease, a supine chest radiograph reveals cardiomegaly and engorged pulmonary vessels. A right pleural effusion was also shown to be present, and this was the cause for the increased opacification of the right hemithorax on this supine examination.

SUGGESTED READINGS

1. Barrett-Connor E. Acute pulmonary disease and sickle cell anemia. Am Rev Respir Dis 1971; 104:159–165
2. Blank N, Castellino RA. The intrathoracic manifestations of the malignant lymphomas and the leukemias. Semin Roentgenol 1980; 15:227–245
3. Castaneda-Zuniga WR, Hogan MT. Cavitary pulmonary nodules in systemic lupus erythematosus. Radiology 1976; 118:45–48
4. Davis PB, di Sant'Agnese PA. Diagnosis and treatment of cystic fibrosis. An update. Chest 1984; 85:802–809
5. Friedman PJ, Harwood IR, Ellenbogen PH. Pulmonary cystic fibrosis in the adult: early and late radiologic findings with pathologic correlations. AJR 1981; 136:1131–1144
6. Kassan SS, Moss ML, Reddick RL. Progressive hilar and mediastinal lymphadenopathy in systemic lupus erythematosus on corticosteroid therapy. N Engl J Med 1976; 294:1382–1383
7. Pines A, Kaplinsky N, Olchovsky D, Rozenman J, Frankl O. Pleuro-pulmonary manifestations of systemic lupus erythematosus: clinical features of its subgroups. Prognostic and therapeutic implications. Chest 1985; 88:129–135
8. Stark P, Pfeiffer WR. Intrathoracic manifestations of sickle cell disease. Radiologe 1985; 25:33–35
9. Stollerman GH. Rheumatic and heritable connective tissue diseases of the cardiovascular system. In: Braunwald E (ed), Heart disease. A textbook of cardiovascular medicine, 3rd ed. Philadelphia: WB Saunders; 1988:1706–1733
10. Thompson PJ, Dhillon DP, Ledingham J, Turner-Warwick M. Shrinking lungs, diaphragmatic dysfunction, and systemic lupus erythematosus. Am Rev Respir Dis 1985; 132:926–928
11. Webb WR, Gamsu G. Cavitary pulmonary nodules with systemic lupus erythematosus. AJR 1981; 136:27–31
12. Wood RE, Boat TF, Doershuk CF. In: Murray JF (ed), Cystic fibrosis. American Lung Association lung disease—state of the art 1975–1976. 1976:275–320

Notes

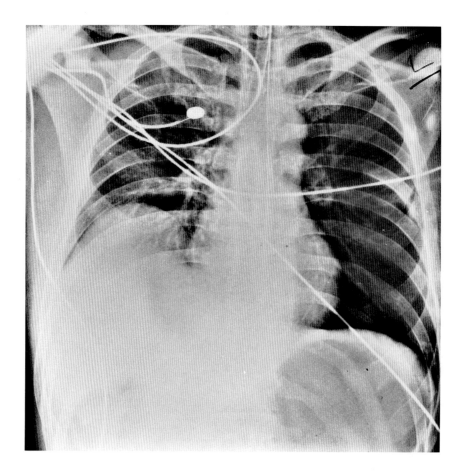

Figure 29-1. History withheld. You are shown an anteroposterior portable chest radiograph.

Case 29: Traumatic Rupture of the Diaphragm

Question 135

Based on the radiographic findings alone, diagnostic possibilities include:

(A) paralysis of the right hemidiaphragm
(B) eventration of the right hemidiaphragm
(C) right subpulmonic effusion
(D) right lower lobe collapse
(E) traumatic diaphragmatic rupture

The supine chest radiograph shows marked elevation of what appears to be the right hemidiaphragm (Figure 29-1). Paralysis, eventration due to replacement of muscle by collagenous connective tissue, and traumatic rupture may all produce a radiographic appearance similar to the one seen in this patient **(Options (A), (B), and (E) are true).**

A subpulmonic effusion should classically produce a lateral shift of the dome of the apparent elevated hemidiaphragm (actually a pseudohemidiaphragm produced by the interface between lung and fluid). Also, since the lung base in subpulmonic effusion would be displaced superiorly by the fluid beneath it, lower lobe pulmonary vascular branches should not be visible "through" the hemidiaphragm as we note in Figure 29-1 **(Option (C) is, therefore, false).**

Lower lobe collapse might produce elevation of the ipsilateral hemidiaphragm, but additional findings militate against that diagnosis; the wedge-shaped opacity of the collapsed lobe is missing,. and the lower lobe pulmonary artery branches are clearly visible **(Option (D) is also false).**

A delayed chest radiograph of the patient (a motor vehicle accident victim) shown in Figure 29-1 revealed nearly complete opacification of the right hemithorax, thus corroborating the diagnosis of ruptured right hemidiaphragm (Figure 29-2).

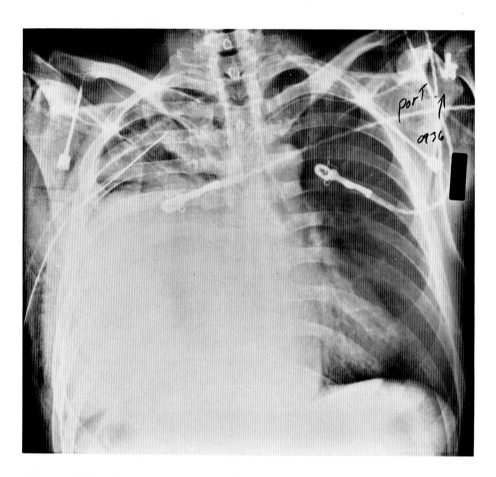

Figure 29-2. Same patient as in Figure 29-1, but 24 hours later. Note nearly complete opacification of the right hemithorax due to massive delayed herniation of the liver into the right hemithorax.

Question 136

Concerning diaphragmatic paralysis,

(A) the affected hemidiaphragm moves upward during sniffing
(B) at fluoroscopy, it is not easily differentiated from eventration
(C) it indicates unresectability in patients with bronchogenic carcinoma
(D) when bilateral it can be diagnosed easily by fluoroscopy
(E) the etiology is most often benign

With diaphragmatic paralysis, the affected hemidiaphragm moves paradoxically upward during sniffing (**Option (A) is true**). Sniffing usually elicits pure diaphragmatic breathing and a brisk downward motion of a normal hemidiaphragm. A paralyzed hemidiaphragm, on the other hand, moves upward with sniffing due to the vector force of the underlying abdominal organs, which are displaced upward by the downward movement of the normal contralateral hemidiaphragm.

At fluoroscopy, diaphragmatic paralysis is not easily differentiated from eventration (**Option (B) is true**). In both situations, decreased or paradoxical motion may occur. However, a fine point of differentiation is that an eventration will have an initial lag in downward motion or slight paradoxical motion, followed by an end-inspiratory downward motion as normal residual diaphragmatic muscle fibers contract.[10] A paralyzed hemidiaphragm is said to display only pure paradoxical motion.

Eventration is usually congenital and represents a diaphragmatic weakness due to intrauterine failure of migration of myoblasts with subsequent replacement of muscle fibers by collagenous connective tissue. Partial eventrations occur more commonly on the right, whereas complete eventrations are seen more frequently on the left. A paralyzed hemidiaphragm is more likely to be associated with atelectatic lung than is eventration, owing to the fact that an eventration still has a minimal residual net inspiratory downward motion.

Diaphragmatic paralysis does not necessarily indicate unresectability in patients with bronchogenic carcinoma (**Option (C) is false**). In contradistinction to recurrent laryngeal nerve involvement with vocal cord paralysis, which usually indicates mediastinal involvement, the phrenic nerve may be encased by the primary tumor to produce paralysis, and in the latter situation curative resection is still possible if the tumor is removed *in toto*.[4] Bilateral hemidiaphragmatic paralysis may cause problems in its diagnosis, since comparison of one side with another to detect paradoxical motion is then not possible at fluoroscopy (**Option (D) is false**). Careful observation of rib cage motion, however, may permit the diagnosis of paradoxical motion even in bilateral paralysis. Forceful expiration with abrupt relaxation of the anterior abdominal wall musculature may allow the paralyzed hemidiaphragms to passively move caudally at the beginning of inspiration. Fluoroscopy with the patient performing the sniffing maneuver helps avoid this pitfall.

Diaphragmatic paralysis may be due to malignant, inflammatory, and traumatic etiologies. The etiology is most often benign **(Option (E) is true)**. An idiopathic variety is known to occur, involving preferentially the right hemidiaphragm.[7]

In general, disease causing failure of normal diaphragmatic motion may occur at any of five levels.[3] Central disease leads to failure of respiratory centers (e.g., congenital hypoventilation syndrome; "Ondine's curse," in which the patient can breathe only through a conscious effort; tumors; trauma; multiple sclerosis; or intracerebral hemorrhage). Upper motor neuron damage may occur after high transection of the cord following trauma or may be due to transverse or ascending myelitis. Lower motor neuron (phrenic nerve) damage most commonly results from neoplastic, inflammatory, or traumatic etiologies. At the diaphragmatic level, there may be an abnormality of nerve conduction at the neuromuscular junction, degenerative change in the muscle itself (dystrophy, myositis), or total or partial congenital hypoplasia (eventration) of the diaphragm. At the paradiaphragmatic level, diminished diaphragmatic motion may result from pleural effusion, collapse of the lung, or a subphrenic abscess.

Paralysis of the right hemidiaphragm should be suspected when its dome is more than two posterior rib interspaces higher than that of the left hemidiaphragm. Paralysis of the left hemidiaphragm may be present when its dome is only one rib interspace higher than that of the right hemidiaphragm.

Diaphragmatic weakness and fatigue deserve mention at this juncture. Diaphragmatic weakness is the lack of muscular strength to perform adequate ventilation. It supervenes in patients who have been mechanically ventilated over extended periods of time. Diaphragmatic fatigue represents the inability to maintain the work necessary for adequate ventilation and occurs when the energy demand of the respiratory muscles exceeds the energy supply. Causes of fatigue are primarily increased respiratory work in asthma, chronic bronchitis, emphysema, pulmonary restrictive disease, high respiratory rate, or hyperinflation with chronic shortening of the diaphragmatic muscle. At fluoroscopy, the fatigued diaphragm is elevated. A decrease in or lack of motion is present, becoming more evident with rapid breathing. Whereas fatigue is bilateral, weakness is usually unilateral. Paradoxical motion with sniffing can occur in weakness, although a lag in motion is more likely when the weak hemidiaphragm is compared with the normal hemidiaphragm. Fluoroscopy should always be performed in the supine position to eliminate the effect of gravity, which may stress the diaphragm through the weight of the abdominal organs.

Question 137

Concerning subpulmonic effusions,

(A) they represent an uncommon distribution of pleural fluid
(B) the apparent hemidiaphragmatic dome is shifted medially
(C) they obscure vessels normally visible through the apparent hemidiaphragm on frontal radiographs
(D) they have a characteristic appearance on computed tomography (CT) when they invert the hemidiaphragm
(E) the majority are loculated

A subpulmonic distribution of pleural effusion occurs commonly **(Option (A) is false).** Nearly all pleural effusions accumulate in the subpulmonic space before they spill over into the costophrenic sulci.[6] Subpulmonic effusions are thus not atypical. On posteroanterior radiographs, the dome of the apparent hemidiaphragm (actually fluid against lung) is shifted laterally **(Option (B) is false).** This appearance is present in about 50% of cases, but it is accentuated on an expiratory view. The explanation for the appearance relates to the tethering of the medial part of the lower lobe by the inferior pulmonary ligament so that less fluid accumulates medially. The absence of lobar tethering laterally allows more fluid to accumulate there and explains the lateral shift of the dome of the apparent hemidiaphragm.[8] When a subpulmonic effusion is present, pulmonary vessels are not readily visible on frontal radiographs through the shadow of the presumed hemidiaphragmatic contour **(Option (C) is true).** This is explained by uplifting of the lung base by the fluid beneath it. Separation of the gastric air bubble from the lung base by subpulmonic effusion is another finding indicating its presence. On frontal views, the separation should be at least 2 cm. Lateral views are also helpful.

Subpulmonic effusions have a characteristic appearance on CT, especially when they invert the hemidiaphragm **(Option (D) is true).** As sequential cross-sections proceed from the thorax down to the upper abdomen, effusion is seen within the confines of the true hemidiaphragmatic musculature rather than the usual abdominal structures.[5] The majority of subpulmonic pleural effusions flow freely on decubitus views **(Option (E) is false)**. Encapsulation of pleural fluid in a subpulmonic location is the exception rather than the rule.

Question 138

Concerning diaphragmatic rupture secondary to blunt trauma,

(A) it is not diagnosed on initial radiographs in more than 50% of cases
(B) CT is the procedure of choice for confirming the diagnosis
(C) it occurs more commonly on the right side
(D) delayed herniation of abdominal contents is rare
(E) in most instances, it is an isolated injury

The diagnosis of traumatic diaphragmatic rupture is not made initially in 50 to 75% of cases **(Option (A) is true),** although it should be suspected. Coexistent injuries to the chest, abdomen, pelvis, and extremities detract from its recognition. Acute visceral herniation is diagnosed infrequently since it is initially misinterpreted or obscured by effusions or contusions. A CT scan may occasionally help by demonstrating abdominal viscera in the thorax and showing an interruption in the diaphragmatic muscle slips, but in most instances it is not necessary **(Option (B) is false)** (Figure 29-3). The rupture classically occurs on the left when due to blunt trauma **(Option (C) is false)**. Penetrating trauma obviously does not necessarily have such a left-sided predisposition. Delayed herniation of abdominal contents, as occurred in the test case, is a common event **(Option (D) is false).** The lag time may be several hours to several years. Once a ruptured hemidiaphragm is detected after blunt trauma, it is imperative to look for other injuries; associated major bone fractures, aortic rupture, or visceral abdominal injuries are often found **(Option (E) is false).**

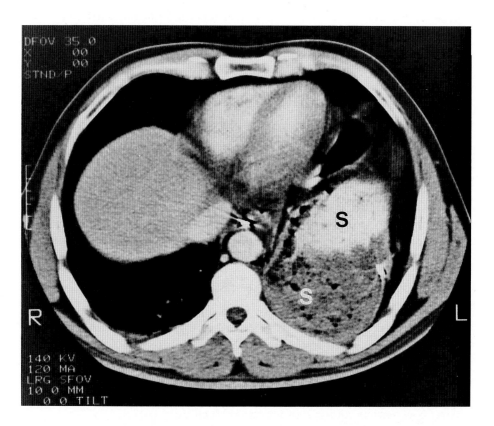

Figure 29-3. Patient with rupture of left hemidiaphragm. CT scan shows the stomach (S) in the left hemithorax abutting the posterior ribs and the left paraspinal region.

Discussion

Rupture of the diaphragm as a result of blunt or penetrating trauma is not always recognized promptly. An early diagnosis is impeded by a lack of specific clinical and radiographic findings. Other, more obvious injuries can divert attention from the possibility of an injury to the diaphragm. The main complication of a missed diaphragmatic tear is a hernia of abdominal viscera into the thoracic cavity, with subsequent incarceration. The mortality of such incarceration approaches 30%.[1] About 4.5% of all admissions for severe trauma will exhibit diaphragmatic rupture. Blunt injuries are usually the result of motor vehicle accidents. Penetrating injuries are usually the result of stab or gunshot wounds. With blunt trauma there is a predisposition for rupture of the left hemidiaphragm; rupture is 10 times more likely to occur on the left than on the right.[1,9] The liver, as might be expected, protects the right hemidiaphragm. Penetrating trauma due to missile injuries obviously does not favor one side over the other. However, stab wounds favor the left side since most assailants are right-handed.

The mechanism of injury in blunt trauma is an abrupt increase in intra-abdominal pressure with propagation of the pressure wave in all directions.[1] The weakest link, the central tendon, ruptures. Associated injuries of the spleen, liver, aorta, pelvis, ribs, and long bones are commonly found.

Herniation of abdominal viscera through the rupture may occur immediately after the accident or be delayed for days, months, or even years. Spontaneous healing of a diaphragmatic rupture is unlikely due to the pressure gradient from the peritoneal cavity to the pleural cavity, a gradient that keeps the tear open and favors herniation. The clinical picture is protean: abdominal pain with radiation to the shoulder region, bowel obstruction, and gastrointestinal bleeding.

In the vast majority of cases the chest radiograph is abnormal, although the initial findings can be subtle or nonspecific. Important signs include the following: elevation of the hemidiaphragm, opacification of the lower hemithorax, cystic lucencies above the presumed level of the hemidiaphragm, shift of the cardiomediastinal silhouette to the contralateral side, and subsegmental atelectasis on the ipsilateral side. Many of these aforementioned features usually indicate herniation of abdominal contents into the thorax. A ruptured hemidiaphragm without initial herniation of abdominal contents may be difficult to diagnose. At times, a small pleural effusion and an irregular hemidiaphragmatic contour may be the only radiographic findings (Figures 29-4 to 29-6). Differentia-

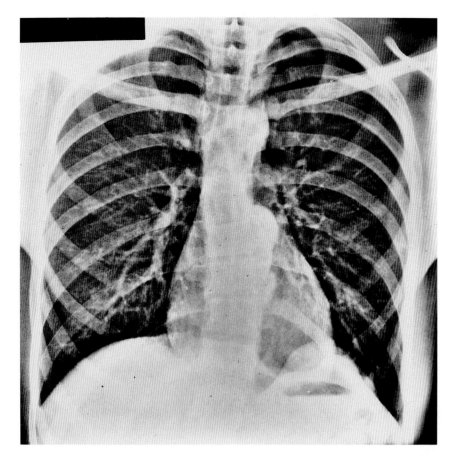

Figure 29-4. Asymptomatic patient with longstanding asymptomatic rupture of the left hemidiaphragm after a motor vehicle accident. Note the left paraspinal mass and the irregular contour of the left hemidiaphragm.

tion from scalloping of the hemidiaphragm, a normal variant, may be impossible (Figures 29-7 to 29-11). A pneumothorax that appears after a high abdominal stab wound should hint towards a concomitant injury to the hemidiaphragm.

In the radiographic work-up, an upper GI study or a barium enema will help clarify the structures that have entered the thorax. Diagnostic pneumoperitoneum was previously recommended, although it has a high rate of false-negative results. CT may elucidate the origin of abnormal opacities in the thorax and determine the relationship of abdominal viscera to the hemidiaphragm.[2]

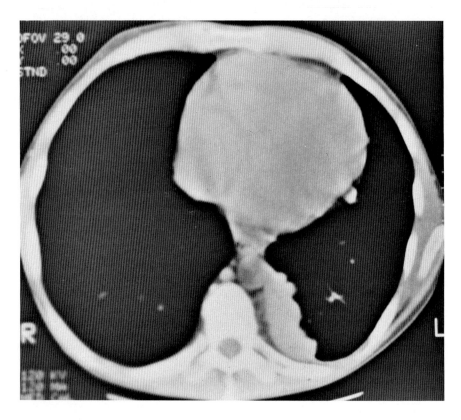

Figure 29-5. Same patient as in Figure 29-4. The CT scan reveals the left paraspinal mass with an irregular lateral margin.

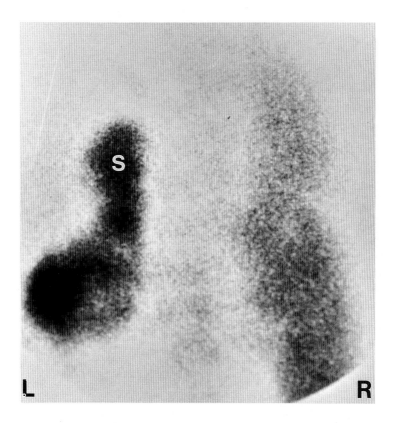

Figure 29-6. Same patient as in Figures 29-4 and 29-5. Posterior liver-spleen scintigram with Tc-99m sulfur colloid reveals splenic tissue (S) in the chest to explain the paraspinal mass seen in Figures 29-4 and 29-5. Implantation of splenic tissue in the thorax subsequent to a ruptured hemidiaphragm is termed splenosis.

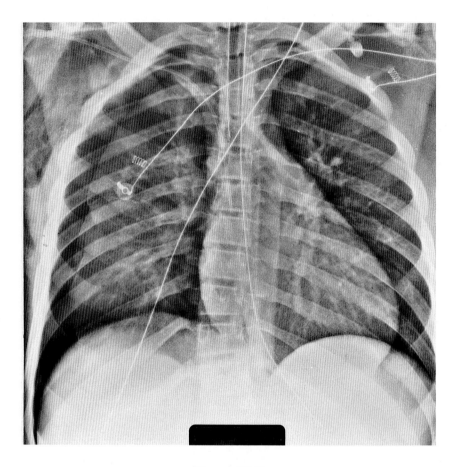

Figure 29-7

Figures 29-7 through 29-11. Traumatic rupture of the right hemidia-phragm. An anteroposterior supine radiograph (Figure 29-7) reveals a right-sided pneumothorax. One week later (Figure 29-8), the anteropos-terior supine radiograph shows scalloping of the right hemidiaphragm medially. Ten days after the first study (Figure 29-9), the anteroposterior supine radiograph reveals part of the liver above the level of the hemidiaphragm. Coronal (Figure 29-10) and sagittal (Figure 29-11) CT reconstruction images of the thorax confirm the presence of liver (L) entering the right hemithorax through the rupture of the right hemidiaphragm.

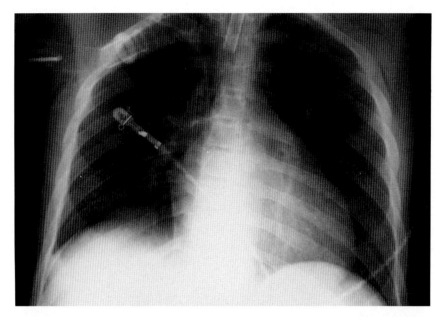

Figure 29-8

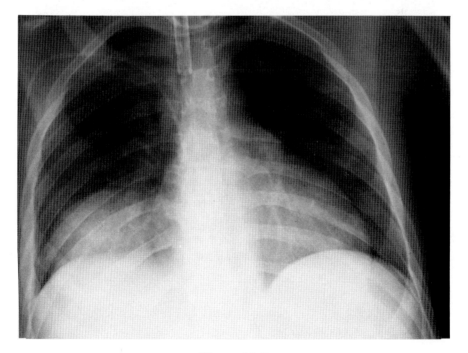

Figure 29-9

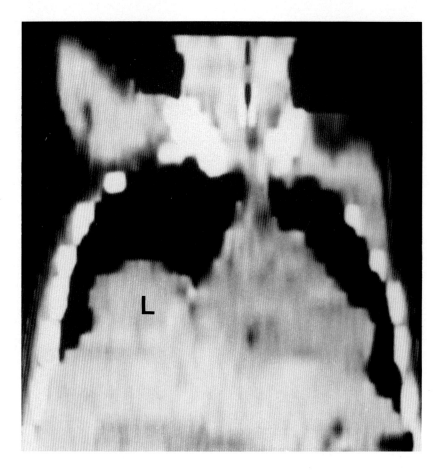

Figure 29-10

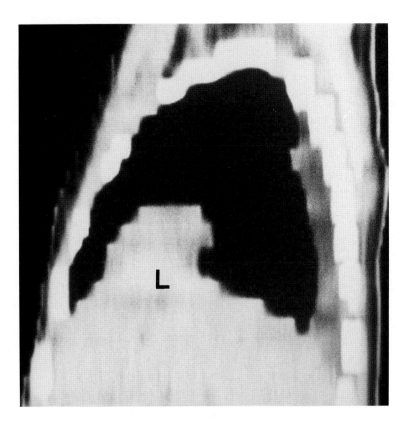

Figure 29-11

SUGGESTED READINGS

1. Fataar S, Schulman A. Diagnosis of diaphragmatic tears. Br J Radiol 1979; 52:375–381
2. Heiberg E, Wolverson MK, Hurd RN, Jagannadharao B, Sundaram M. CT recognition of traumatic rupture of the diaphragm. AJR 1980; 135:369–372
3. McCauley RG, Labib KB. Diaphragmatic paralysis evaluated by phrenic nerve stimulation during fluoroscopy or real-time ultrasound. Radiology 1984; 153:33–36
4. Mountain CF. A new international staging system for lung cancer. Chest (suppl) 1989; 89:225S–233S
5. Proto AV, Rost RC. CT of the thorax: pitfalls in interpretation. RadioGraphics 1985; 5:693–812
6. Raasch BN, Carsky EW, Lane EJ, O'Callaghan JP, Heitzman ER. Pleural effusion: explanation of some typical appearances. AJR 1982; 139:899–904
7. Riley EA. Idiopathic diaphragmatic paralysis. Am J Med 1962; 32:404–416
8. Rudikoff JC. The pulmonary ligament and subpulmonic effusion. Chest 1981; 80:505–507
9. Stark P. Traumatic rupture of the diaphragm—a problem of radiological diagnosis (author's transl). Radiologe 1982; 22:22–25
10. Tarver RD, Conces DJ, Cory DA, Vix VA. Imaging the diaphragm and its disorders. J Thorac Imaging 1989; 4:1–18

Notes

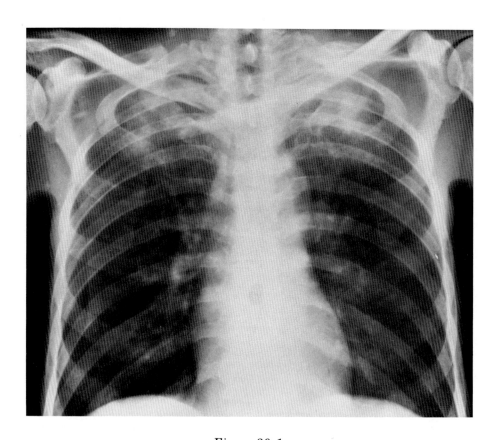

Figure 30-1
Figures 30-1 and 30-2. This 60-year-old man was evaluated for a 40-lb weight loss and anemia. You are shown a posteroanterior chest radiograph and an anterior bone scintigram. (Reprinted with permission. Armed Forces Institute of Pathology [AFIP] negs. 81-1085 and 81-1087, respectively.)

Case 30: Metastatic Calcification

Question 139

Which *one* of the following is the MOST likely diagnosis?

(A) Idiopathic pulmonary ossification
(B) Alveolar microlithiasis
(C) Metastatic calcification
(D) Tuberculosis
(E) Mucinous adenocarcinoma of the stomach

Figure 30-1 demonstrates poorly defined, bilateral apical opacities with some central coalescence. A close-up view of the left apex (Figure 30-3) shows the opacity to better advantage. The lungs are otherwise clear. A skin fold (not a pneumothorax) parallels the right lateral chest wall. On the bone scintigram, there is deposition of the radiopharmaceutical (Tc-99m diphosphonate) in the lungs, especially the pulmonary apices, and in the stomach (Figure 30-2). The lack of salivary gland or thyroid uptake suggests that the gastric activity is due to diphosphonate deposition rather than uptake of free Tc-99m pertechnetate. In addition, there are no bladder activity and only faint visualization of the right kidney, findings strongly suggestive of renal disease. Given these observations, the most likely diagnosis is metastatic calcification **(Option (C) is therefore correct).** The lung is one of the most common sites of such calcification, and a dominant upper lobe distribution has been well documented.[1,15] The deposition in the distal right tibia (Figure 30-2) was secondary to fibrous dysplasia.

Idiopathic pulmonary ossification (Option (A)) is unlikely. This uncommon condition is characterized by the presence of mature bone, often containing marrow, in the parenchyma of the lungs. The bone may be localized or diffuse and is visible on the chest radiograph (a trabecular pattern may be seen).[10] The radiographic opacity representing the bone does not resemble an alveolar infiltrate and is more common in the lung bases. While bone scintigraphy shows increased tracer accumulation in

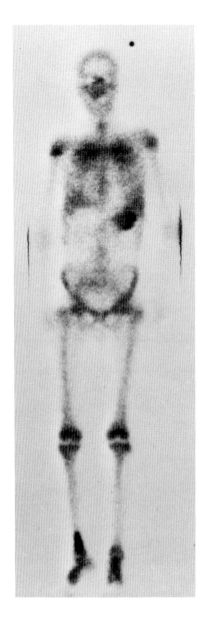

Figure 30-2

the lung, no other visceral or skeletal abnormalities are associated with this condition.

Alveolar microlithiasis (Option (B)) is another condition in which punctate pulmonary opacifications may be associated with increased tracer deposition in the lung on bone scintigraphy.[2] However, this diagnosis may be excluded on the basis of chest radiographic findings. Alveolar microlithiasis is a lower lobe disease. If the pulmonary apices are involved, there is usually extensive involvement of the remainder of the lungs. The disease is characterized by the presence of innumerable 1- to 3-mm calcific spherules in the alveolar spaces[24] that impart a granular texture to the involved lung (Figure 30-4). The infiltration is sometimes so intense that the pleura between the lung and the bony thorax is perceived as a lucency—the so-called "black pleura" sign.[11]

Tuberculosis (Option (D)) is also unlikely. Although the apices are a common site for post-primary tuberculosis, such infection would probably not be associated with pulmonary uptake on bone scintigraphy.

Mucinous adenocarcinoma of the stomach (Option (E)) is also not likely. Calcification has been described in primary mucinous carcinomas of the gastrointestinal tract and in their metastases,[18] but the radiographic appearance and the distribution to the lung apices in this patient would be extremely unusual for metastatic disease. Uptake of bone-seeking radiopharmaceuticals by pulmonary metastases from such mucinous adenocarcinomas is also a possibility.

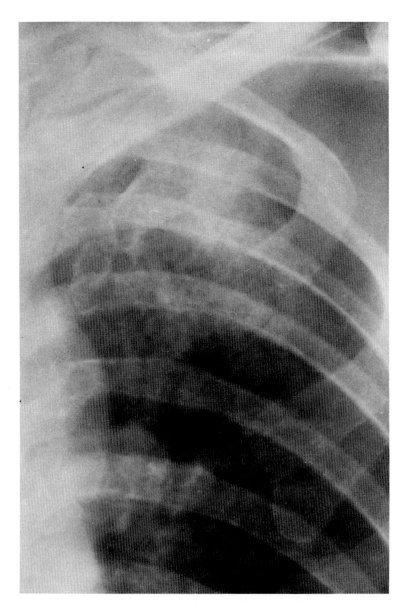

Figure 30-3. Photographic enlargement of the apex of the left lung shown in Figure 30-1 demonstrates a poorly defined opacity with central coalescence. (Reprinted with permission. AFIP neg. 81-1085.)

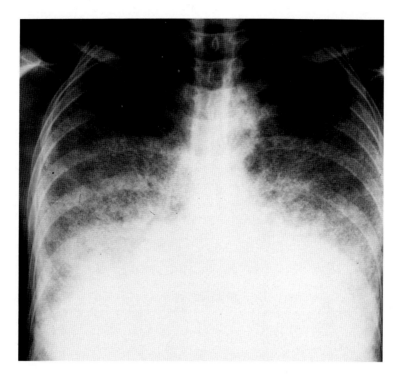

Figure 30-4A
Figure 30-4. Alveolar microlithiasis. Note the lower lobe distribution
in panel A and the granular texture of the lung on a close-up view (B)
from the same radiograph. The calcific spherules (arrowheads) are seen
in the air spaces in panel C (low-power view of gross specimen at ×10
magnification), and the widespread distribution of the spherules (black
structures) is noted on a low-power hematoxylin and eosin section of the
lung shown in panel D (×4 magnification). (Reprinted with permission.
AFIP negatives: 62-1856 (A and B), 62-2076 (C), and 62-2086 (D).)

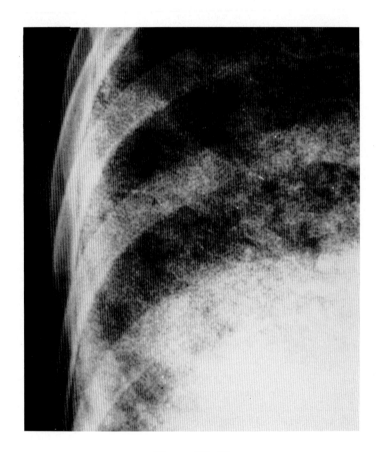

Figure 30-4B

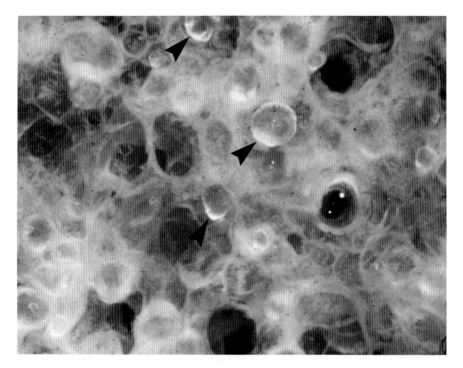

Figure 30-4C

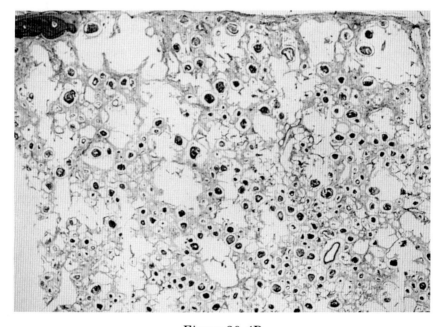

Figure 30-4D

Question 140

Concerning idiopathic pulmonary ossification,

(A) most patients have associated interstitial fibrosis
(B) its radiographic appearance is similar to that of the ossification associated with mitral stenosis
(C) the radiographic findings are most apparent in the lower lobes
(D) bone scintigraphy demonstrates pulmonary uptake
(E) serum calcium, phosphorus, and phosphatase levels are all normal

Most patients with idiopathic pulmonary ossification (IPO) do not have associated interstitial fibrosis **(Option (A) is false).** As the name implies, the etiology of this condition is unknown. Associations with amyloidosis, chronic venous stasis, and prior infections have been reported.[10]

The radiographic appearance of IPO is quite distinct from that of the pulmonary ossification associated with mitral stenosis **(Option (B) is false).** Bony deposits in the lungs of patients with mitral stenosis and other forms of rheumatic heart disease have been reported in as many as 13% of patients with long-standing disease. Small (2- to 8-mm) rounded nodules are visible in the lung bases and are usually few in number.[12] Cardiac abnormalities, including calcification of the mitral valve and left atrial enlargement, are invariably present and serve to further distinguish such patients from those with IPO.

There is a distinct predominance of lower lobe pulmonary involvement in patients with IPO **(Option (C) is true).**[22,25] This is true for both localized and diffuse forms of the disease.[10]

Bone scintigraphy may show pulmonary uptake in areas of involvement on the chest radiograph **(Option (D) is true).**[22,25] Since the lesions are composed of mature trabecular bone, this finding is not surprising.

Calcium metabolism is normal in patients with IPO. No consistent laboratory or clinical abnormalities are present **(Option (E) is true),** and no extrapulmonary sites of soft tissue ossification have been reported.[10]

Question 141

Concerning metastatic calcification,

   (A) the calcium is deposited in previously damaged tissues
   (B) the most commonly involved pulmonary structure is the alveolar basement membrane
   (C) the process is irreversible
   (D) it is commonly caused by renal failure

By definition, metastatic calcification occurs in morphologically normal tissues consequent to alterations in serum calcium and phosphorus levels **(Option (A) is false)**. The precipitation of calcium salts in normal soft tissues is facilitated by an alkaline environment and occurs most frequently in tissues involved with hydrogen ion secretion, i.e., the pulmonary capillaries, the gastric cardia, and the renal tubules. Dystrophic calcification, on the other hand, is the term applied to calcification occurring in previously damaged tissues.[27]

The deposition of calcium begins in the alveolar wall basement membrane between the epithelial and endothelial cells **(Option (B) is true)**.[7,27] As the process becomes more severe, vascular and bronchial walls become involved. The result of this process is a delicate encasement of the alveolar lumen by a lattice of soft tissue calcification (Figures 30-5, and 30-6).

Pulmonary metastatic calcification is in some instances reversible **(Option (C) is false)**.[9,19] Several cases document the regression of pulmonary calcification following parathyroidectomy and dialysis.[20]

Pulmonary metastatic calcification is a manifestation of a variety of disease states. Chronic renal failure is the most common **(Option (D) is true)**, but primary hyperparathyroidism and humoral hypercalcemia of malignancy have also been reported. Current evidence indicates that the latter is due to a recently identified protein hormone that is similar to parathyroid hormone, rather than to ectopic production of parathyroid hormone per se by a malignant tumor as was previously thought.[3] Other disease states associated with pulmonary metastatic calcification include vitamin D poisoning, sarcoidosis, intravenous calcium therapy, the milk-alkali syndrome, and massive bone destruction secondary to metastatic carcinoma, osteomyelitis, or multiple myeloma.[14]

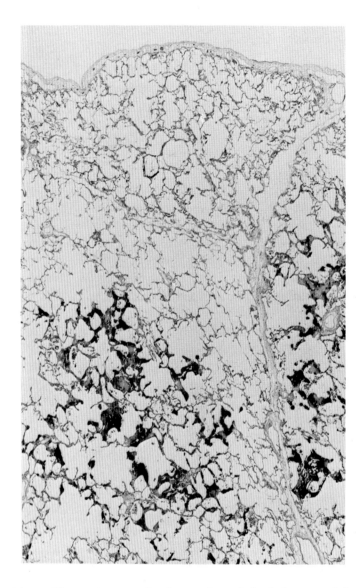

Figure 30-5. Photomicrograph of a section of the left upper lobe shows the visceral pleura at the top of the figure and an interlobular septum extending into the lung. On either side of the septum are dark-staining deposits of calcium in the alveolar walls. The air spaces are open, and adjacent noncalcified alveolar walls are also visible. (Reprinted with permission. AFIP neg. 82-2785.)

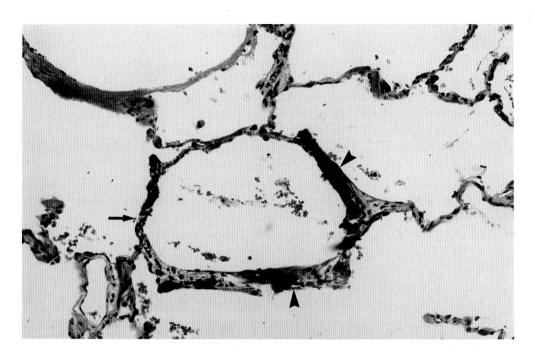

Figure 30-6. Same patient as in Figures 30-1 and 30-2. High-magnification photomicrograph better demonstrates the location of the dark-staining calcification. Early involvement of the alveolar basement membrane is visible on the left (arrow), while more extensive involvement is visible inferiorly and on the right (arrowheads). (Reprinted with permission. AFIP neg. 82-2789.)

Question 142

In the normal upright person,

    (A) the pO_2 is higher in the apex than in the base of the lung
    (B) the lung apices are better ventilated than the lung bases
    (C) the lung bases are better perfused than the lung apices
    (D) the tissue pH is higher in the lung apex than in the lung base

The pO_2 is higher in the lung apex than it is in the lung base **(Option (A) is true).** Under normal circumstances, the pO_2 in any region of the lung is dependent upon gas exchange across the alveolar wall, which, in turn, is determined by the ratio of ventilation to perfusion. The absolute values of ventilation and perfusion are not as important as the ratio of ventilation to perfusion in this regard. Both ventilation and perfusion decrease in actual amounts from the base of the lung to the apex, but blood flow decreases at a much higher rate than ventilation. This results in a gradient where the ratio of ventilation to perfusion is low (approximately 0.3) in the lung base and high (approximately 3.0) in the lung apex. Estimates of actual pO_2 have been in the range of 130 mm Hg for the apex of the lung and 90 mm Hg for the lung base.[28]

The lung apices are less well ventilated than the bases **(Option (B) is false)**. Ventilation is defined as the change in volume in a specific lung region per unit resting volume of that region per unit time. Since the resting volume of any lung unit is larger in the apex than in the base and since the amount of change in this resting volume is smaller in the apex for any given change in pressure, the resultant ventilation is less.[13]

The lung bases are better perfused than the apices **(Option (C) is true)**. This phenomenon is explained by the relative magnitudes of pulmonary arterial (P_a), venous (P_v), and alveolar (P_A) pressure at the top and bottom of the lung. The pulmonary alveolar pressure is constant throughout the lung; however, the pressure in the vascular system increases by approximately 1 cm of water for each centimeter of height of the lung. This produces a situation in the lung apices whereby the $P_A > P_a > P_v$ so that the pulmonary perfusion is markedly reduced. In the lung base, because of the hydrostatic pressure gradient in the vascular system of the upright patient, the $P_a > P_v > P_A$ to allow more blood flow to the lung bases as compared with that in the apices.[28]

The pH is higher in the lung apex than it is in the lung base **(Option (D) is true)**. The higher ventilation-to-perfusion ratio in the lung apex produces a lower pCO_2 in the upper portion of the lung. Since the pH is inversely related to the pCO_2, this decrease in pCO_2 produces an increase in the pH in the lung apex. The normal mean pH values are approximately 7.51 for the lung apex and 7.39 for the lung base.[28]

Discussion

The patient shown in Figures 30-1 through 30-3 presented with radiographic findings highly suggestive of metastatic pulmonary calcification. The matching of the areas of opacity on the chest radiograph with the areas of greatest tracer uptake on bone scintigraphy, coupled with the evidence of severe renal dysfunction on the latter, should lead to the correct diagnosis. The patient's serum calcium and phosphorus levels were both elevated (16.2 and 6.4 mg/dL, respectively). The patient died shortly after admission, and at autopsy small end-stage atherosclerotic

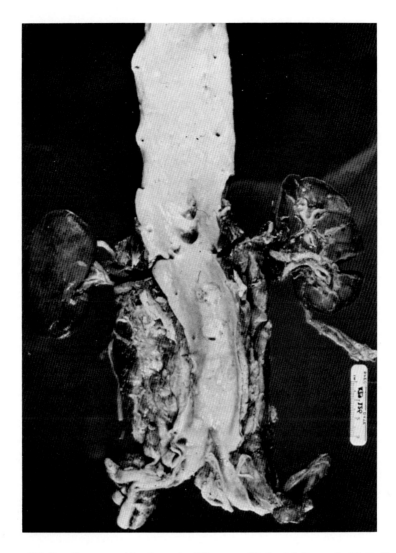

Figure 30-7. Same patient as in Figures 30-1, 30-2, and 30-6. Small end-stage, atherosclerotic kidneys on either side of the abdominal aorta. An unexpected finding was extensive enlargement of periaortic nodes (seen along lower aorta) by Hodgkin's lymphoma. (Reprinted with permission. AFIP neg. 84-2497.)

kidneys were found (Figure 30-7). In addition, extensive retroperitoneal nodal enlargement by Hodgkin's lymphoma was discovered. The apices of the lung were extensively calcified (Figure 30-8), as was the cardia of the stomach. A monostotic focus of fibrous dysplasia was found in the distal right tibia (Figure 30-2).

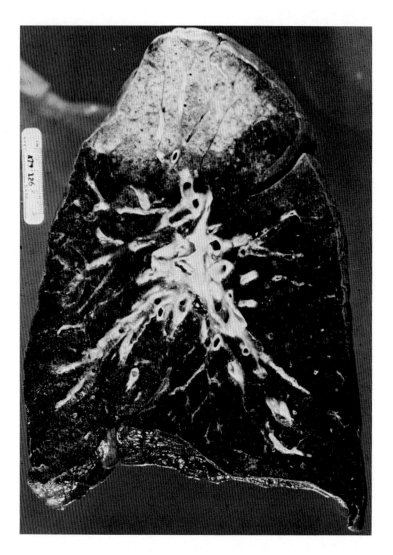

Figure 30-8. Gross lung specimen at autopsy reveals a whitish discoloration of the lung apex correlating with the radiographic and scintigraphic findings of metastatic calcification. The lung had a "gritty" texture when cut. (Reprinted with permission. AFIP neg. 81-2495.)

The lung is a common site of metastatic calcification in patients with chronic renal disease and hypercalcemia. In a prospective study of 31 patients undergoing chronic hemodialysis, autopsy was done on 15, of whom 9 showed parenchymal lung calcification.[7] In only one of the patients was the calcification evident on chest radiographs.

Clinical findings are often nonspecific. Difficult respiration and fever may suggest an infectious process. Pulmonary edema may be suggested by concomitant rales and peripheral edema. Most patients with metastatic pulmonary calcification suddenly deteriorate after the calcification decreases lung compliance and diffusing capacity.[5] When extensive, the pulmonary calcification may be a significant factor in the death of these patients.[8]

The cause of metastatic pulmonary calcification in patients with chronic renal failure and hypercalcemia is not fully understood. Precipitation of calcium salts in soft tissues occurs when the plasma calcium-phosphate product exceeds 70 mg/100 mL.[17] This precipitation takes place preferentially in healthy tissues with an alkaline environment (metastatic calcification) and in damaged tissues (dystrophic calcification). The lung, with its relatively high tissue pH and susceptibility to damage by pneumonia or edema, is particularly vulnerable to this process.[20]

Pulmonary calcification may be extremely difficult to detect since it generally cannot be seen on a routine chest radiograph.[7] Bone scintigrams have demonstrated pulmonary uptake in the absence of conventional radiographic abnormalities.[6,21] Although controversy exists concerning the sensitivity and specificity of bone scintigraphy, it may be the only method other than biopsy that can demonstrate these microscopic deposits of calcium.[6] However, the utility of dual-energy subtraction digital radiography and computed tomography in such detection has been reported.[13,23]

Metastatic calcification, when visible on the chest radiograph, presents in one of three patterns. The most common one is a diffuse alveolar pattern, which may mimic pulmonary edema or diffuse pneumonia.[16] This pattern develops slowly and is usually progressive. Occasionally, punctate calcifications are visible within the alveolar pattern and suggest the diagnosis. The possibility of metastatic pulmonary calcification should be considered for any patient with renal failure in whom persistent, relatively unchanging pulmonary opacities develop.

A second pattern of metastatic pulmonary calcification is that seen in our test case, i.e., bilateral areas of apical opacity. Even though this is less common than diffuse lung involvement, the presentation is well documented.[1,15] As stated above, the more alkaline environment of the pulmonary apices accounts for this preferential location of calcification.

The third pattern consists of large calcified nodules that appear within the lung.[4,26] This is the least common pattern of presentation, and only a few such cases have been reported. These localized mass-like lesions usually occur in areas of prior lung injury caused by either infection or chronic edema. They probably represent a combination of both metastatic and dystrophic calcification. Uptake of bone-seeking agents and high attenuation values on computed tomography should confirm the benign nature of these masses.

It is important to consider the possibility of pulmonary metastatic calcification in patients with severe renal disease. Progressive calcification may lead to severe cardiorespiratory compromise and death. There is evidence that parathyroidectomy and dialysis reverse the process and improve respiratory function if instituted early enough in the course of the disease.[20]

SUGGESTED READINGS

1. Bein ME, Lee DB, Mink JH, Dickmeyer J. Unusual case of metastatic pulmonary calcification. AJR 1979; 132:812–816
2. Brown ML, Swee RG, Olson RJ, Bender CE. Pulmonary uptake of ^{99m}Tc diphosphonate in alveolar microlithiasis. AJR 1978; 131:703–704
3. Burtis WJ, Wu TL, Insogna KL, Stewart AF. Humoral hypercalcemia of malignancy. Ann Intern Med 1988; 108:454–457
4. Chinn DH, Gamsu G, Webb WR, Godwin JD. Calcified pulmonary nodules in chronic renal failure. AJR 1981; 137:402–405
5. Cohen AM, Maxon HR, Goldsmith RE, et al. Metastatic pulmonary calcification in primary hyperparathyroidism. Arch Intern Med 1977; 137:520–522
6. Conger JD, Alfrey AC. Scanning for pulmonary calcification (comment). Ann Intern Med 1976; 84:224–225
7. Conger JD, Hammond WS, Alfrey AC, Contiguglia SR, Stanford RE, Huffer WE. Pulmonary calcification in chronic dialysis patients. Clinical and pathological studies. Ann Intern Med 1975; 83:330–336
8. Davidson RC, Pendras VP. Calcium-related cardio-respiratory death in chronic hemodialysis. Trans Am Soc Artif Intern Organs 1967; 13:36–40
9. Evans TW, Collins M, Adams JE, et al. Pulmonary calcification in renal transplant recipient. Br J Dis Chest 1983; 77:202–205
10. Felson B, Schwarz J, Lukin RR, Hawkins HH. Idiopathic pulmonary ossification. Radiology 1984; 153:303–310
11. Fraser RG, Paré JA. Diagnosis of diseases of the chest. Philadelphia: WB Saunders; 1979:1741–1744
12. Galloway RW, Epstein EJ, Coulshed N. Pulmonary ossific nodules in mitral valve disease. Br Heart J 1961; 23:297–307
13. Genereux GP. CT of acute and chronic distal airspace (alveolar) disease. Semin Roentgenol 1984; 19:211–221
14. Gilman M, Nissim J, Terry P, Whelton A. Metastatic pulmonary calcification in the renal transplant recipient. Am Rev Respir Dis 1980; 121:415–419

15. Jost RG, Sagel SS. Metastatic calcification in the lung apex. AJR 1979; 133:1188–1190
16. Karasick SR. Metastatic pulmonary calcification in a renal transplant recipient. Semin Roentgenol 1981; 16:5–6
17. Katz AI, Hampers CL, Merrill JP. Secondary hyperparathyroidism and renal osteodystrophy in chronic renal failure. Review of 195 patients with observations of the effects of dialysis, kidney transplantation and subtotal parathyroidectomy. Medicine 1969; 48:333–374
18. Libshitz HI, North LB. Pulmonary metastases. Radiol Clin North Am 1982; 20:437–451
19. McLachlan MS, Wallace M, Seneviratne C. Pulmonary calcification in renal failure. Report of three cases. Br J Radiol 1968; 41:99–106
20. Mootz JR, Sagel SS, Roberts TH. Roentgenographic manifestations of pulmonary calcifications. Radiology 1973; 107:55–60
21. Rosenthal DI, Chandler HL, Azizi F, Schneider PB. Uptake of bone imaging agents by diffuse pulmonary metastatic calcification. AJR 1977; 129:871–874
22. Saks DA, McClees EC, Fajman WA, Hollinger WM, Gilman MJ. Diffuse pulmonary ossification detected by bone scanning with Tc-99m hydroxymethylene diphosphate. Clin Nucl Med 1984; 9:594–595
23. Sanders CS, Frank MS, Rostand SG, Rutsky EA, Barnes GT, Fraser RG. Metastatic calcification of the heart and lungs in end-stage renal disease: detection and quantification by dual-energy digital chest radiography. AJR 1987; 149:881–887
24. Sears MR, Chang AR, Taylor AJ. Pulmonary alveolar microlithiasis. Thorax 1971; 26:704–711
25. Silberstein EB, Vasavada PJ, Hawkins H. Idiopathic pulmonary ossification with focal pulmonary uptake of technetium-99m HMDP bone scanning agent. Clin Nucl Med 1985; 10:436
26. Smith JC, Stanton LW, Kramer NC, Parrish AE. Nodular pulmonary calcification in renal failure. Report of a case. Am Rev Respir Dis 1969; 100:723–728
27. Spencer H. Pathology of the lung excluding pulmonary tuberculosis, 3rd ed. New York: Pergamon Press; 1977:685–688
28. West JB. Regional differences in the lung. Chest 1978; 74:426–437

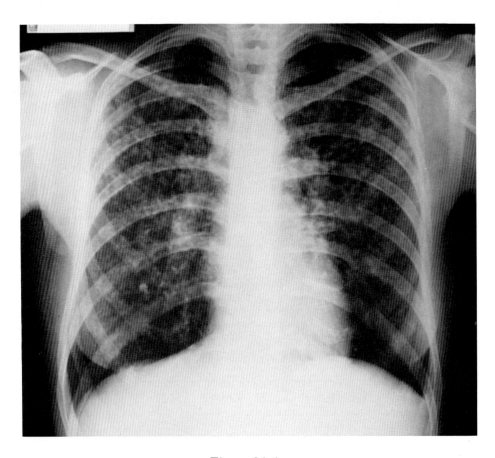

Figure 31-1
Figures 31-1 through 31-3. These three patients have the same disease. You are shown posteroanterior chest radiographs. (Reprinted with permission. Armed Forces Institute of Pathology [AFIP] negs. 64-6683, 60-4980, and 69-4018.)

Case 31: Eosinophilic Granuloma

Question 143

Which *one* of the following is the MOST likely diagnosis?

(A) Collagen vascular disease
(B) Asbestosis
(C) Eosinophilic granuloma
(D) Cystic fibrosis
(E) Acute farmer's lung

The three posteroanterior chest radiographs shown (Figures 31-1 through 31-3) have several features in common. All three patients have diffuse lung disease that primarily involves the middle and upper lung zones. The process appears nodular in the first patient, reticular in the second patient, and cystic and nodular in the third patient. None shows definite hilar adenopathy or pleural effusion. Evidence of decreased lung volume is seen only in the third patient. This spectrum of radiographic findings is characteristic of a granulomatous pneumonitis. Thus, eosinophilic granuloma is the most likely diagnosis **(Option (C) is correct).** The radiographic appearance of this disease depends to a large extent on the age of the lesion. Early in its development, poorly defined nodules ranging in size from 3 to 7 mm are diffusely scattered throughout the middle and upper lung zones (Figures 31-1 and 31-4).[2,11] Later in the course of the disease, the nodules fibrose and retract, giving rise to a reticular appearance (Figures 31-2 and 31-5). A small percentage of the cases progress to an end-stage honeycomb lung.[20,27] This finding virtually always occurs in the absence of hilar adenopathy or pleural effusion.[11,27]

Collagen vascular disease (Option (A)) would be an unlikely choice for two reasons. First, the five classic collagen vascular diseases (rheumatoid arthritis, scleroderma, systemic lupus erythematosus, polymyositis, and dermatomyositis) preferentially involve the lower lung zones when there is a zonal predominance.[13,21,26] For the three patients described here, the

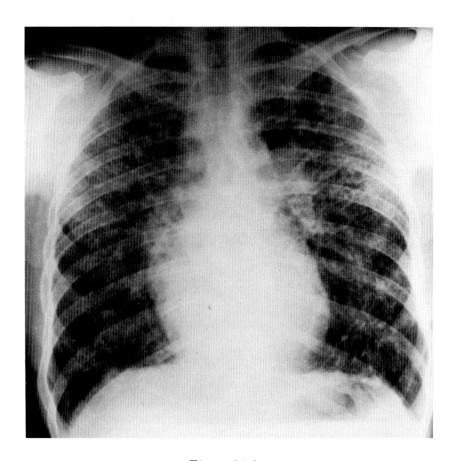

Figure 31-2

disease primarily involves the middle and upper lung zones. Second, the pleural manifestations commonly observed with some of the collagen vascular diseases listed above are not apparent in these three patients.

Asbestosis (Option (B)) is not likely since its zonal predominance is lower/middle rather than upper/middle. Moreover, the pulmonary opacities in asbestosis are less nodular and more linear and irregular than those shown in Figure 31-1.[5]

Cystic fibrosis (Option (D)) is not the most likely diagnosis, although it is more difficult to exclude on the basis of the radiographic findings. An increasing number of patients with cystic fibrosis present in early adult life with progressive pulmonary disease.[10,23,24] Friedman et al.[10] have reported the early radiographic features in a series of 50 patients 17 years of age or older, with cystic fibrosis. Upper lobe predilection and small nodular and linear opacities are findings in common with our three

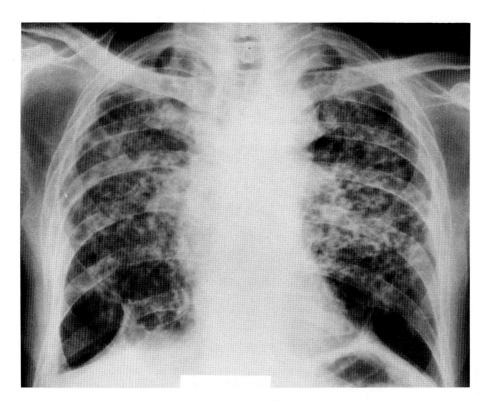

Figure 31-3

test cases. The granulomatous pneumonitis of eosinophilic granuloma and the lung involvement by cystic fibrosis may be distinguished by the more central distribution of the latter. Cystic fibrosis is primarily a disease of the airways, not of the pulmonary interstitium. Consequently, most of the nodular abnormalities of the lung in cystic fibrosis spare the outermost pulmonary periphery. Widespread bronchial wall thickening and frank bronchiectasis seen in cystic fibrosis should be distinguished from the cystic lucencies of eosinophilic granuloma. Other findings common in patients with pulmonary cystic fibrosis, but absent in our three test patients, include mucous plugs, atelectasis, and deformity of the thorax.[10]

Farmer's lung (Option (E)) is not the most likely diagnosis, although in its subacute or chronic form it may present with many of the radiographic features of our test cases. The lesions of the *acute* form resemble alveolar infiltrates and are the result of a hypersensitivity pneumonitis composed of chronic inflammatory cells. There is a tendency, however, in some cases to form sarcoid-like granulomas in the subacute

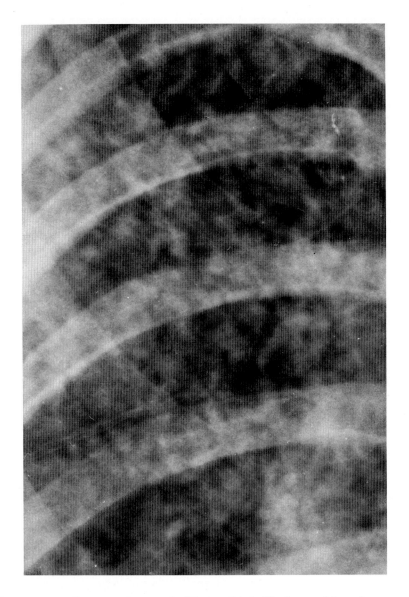

Figure 31-4. Same patient as in Figure 31-1. Photographic enlargement of the right upper lobe demonstrates the poorly defined nature of the small nodules. (Reprinted with permission. AFIP neg. 64-6683.)

form.[6,12,15,18,25] This gives the disease a nodular radiographic appearance. Moreover, the *acute* form of farmer's lung does not show the distinct upper zone predominance of the chronic form.[12]

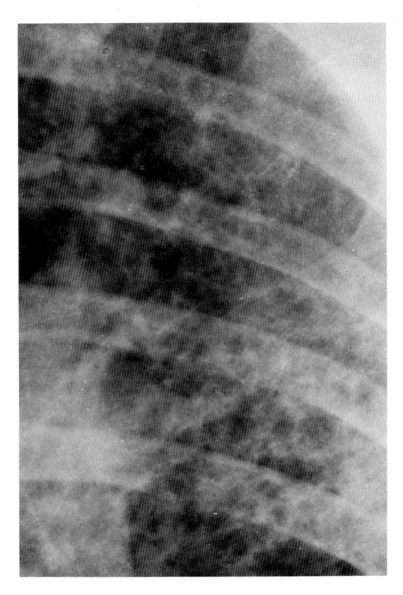

Figure 31-5. Same patient as in Figure 31-2. Photographic enlargement of the left upper lobe shows the reticular appearance (interlacing line shadows and delicate ring shadows) of this pattern to better advantage. (Reprinted with permission. AFIP neg. 60-4980.)

Question 144

Concerning pulmonary eosinophilic granuloma,

    (A) clinical symptoms correlate well with the severity of the radiographic abnormality

    (B) upper lobe disease is characteristic

    (C) reduction of lung volume occurs early in the course of the disease

    (D) acute chest pain is usually due to rib fracture from a concomitant rib lesion

    (E) peripheral blood eosinophilia is a reliable indicator of active disease

One of the hallmarks of pulmonary eosinophilic granuloma (PEG) is the lack of association between the mild clinical symptoms and the severity of radiographic abnormality **(Option (A) is false).** As many as one-third of patients present with no symptoms at all, the disease being discovered as the result of an abnormal chest radiograph.[2,11] A possible explanation for this observation is the focal nature of the lung involvement. Despite the widespread distribution of the individual lesions, intervening lung tissue is normal.

There is a definite upper lobe predilection in the distribution of the lesions of PEG **(Option (B) is true).** The disease may be diffuse and may then involve the lung bases, although there is usually sparing of the costophrenic angles.[2,11,16]

Reduction of lung volume is not an early feature of PEG **(Option (C) is false).** The maintenance of normal or slightly increased volume despite increasing fibrotic change in the lung is a recognized feature of the disease. In one report of 100 cases, pulmonary volumes were recorded as normal in 60 patients, increased in 31 patients, and decreased in only 9 patients.[11]

Acute chest pain in patients with PEG is most often due to pneumothorax (Figure 31-6) **(Option (D) is false).** The frequency of pneumothorax varies from 10 to 20% of reported cases,[11,17] and in one series a higher frequency of pneumothorax was reported in patients under 20 years of age. Bone lesions have been reported in 5 to 10% of patients.[11,16] Pathologic fracture of a rib lesion in association with parenchymal lung disease is a classic, but infrequent, presentation.

Peripheral blood eosinophilia is not an indicator of active disease **(Option (E) is false).** There are no consistent laboratory abnormalities reported for PEG.

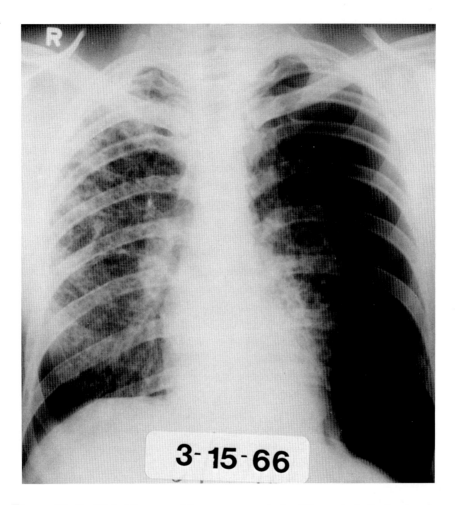

Figure 31-6. This 21-year-old man presented with acute left chest pain. The tension pneumothorax was secondary to underlying PEG. (Reprinted with permission. AFIP neg. 67-1136.)

Question 145

Concerning farmer's lung,

(A) peripheral eosinophilia is an important clinical finding
(B) the etiologic agents are spores of thermophilic fungi
(C) chronic exposure leads to hilar lymph node enlargement
(D) the primary injury occurs in the respiratory bronchiole
(E) end-stage pulmonary fibrosis is a result of chronic exposure

Peripheral eosinophilia is not a clinical feature of either the acute or the chronic form of farmer's lung **(Option (A) is false),** nor is wheezing. These features are common in type I immunologic reactions in the lung (for example, in allergic bronchopulmonary aspergillosis) but are not seen with type III or IV immunologic reactions responsible for the injury in farmer's lung.[19]

The etiologic agents of farmer's lung are the spores of the thermophilic fungi *Micropolyspora faeni* and *Thermoactinomyces vulgaris* **(Option (B) is true).** These organisms grow in moldy wet hay, producing vast numbers of spores that are released into the air when the hay is raked or unbailed. If the hay is gathered and stored with a moisture content of greater than 30%, conditions are favorable for fungal growth. The disease usually occurs in the winter when the hay is fed to livestock.[19]

Lymph node enlargement is not a feature of chronic farmer's lung disease **(Option (C) is false).**[25] As previously mentioned, chronic exposure may result in progressive pulmonary disease and lead eventually to an end-stage fibrotic lung; however, adenopathy is not a feature of the progression.

The primary site of injury in farmer's lung is the respiratory bronchiole **(Option (D) is true).** The hypersensitivity initiated in the bronchiole at the center of the pulmonary acinus extends to involve the adjacent interstitium.[15] The respiratory bronchiole is one of the more vulnerable regions of the tracheobronchial tree in inhalational diseases, because at the respiratory bronchiole small particles held in air suspension by laminar air flow tend to precipitate on the bronchial mucosa.

End-stage pulmonary fibrosis is a complication of chronic farmer's lung disease **(Option (E) is true).** The acute episode in this disease may be quite dramatic but is rarely fatal. Repeated symptomatic attacks have been correlated with increasing pulmonary function abnormalities and progressive worsening of the radiographic appearance.[6] A more subtle and insidious path to this progressive fibrosis is followed by the patient with numerous subacute exposures. In such cases, a variety of nonspecific pulmonary symptoms may be noted, none of which suggests a primary hypersensitivity reaction in the lung. This latter presentation is most common among patients exposed to small amounts of antigen on a regular basis over a long period of time. The frequency of progression to end-stage fibrosis in farmer's lung is difficult to determine, and avoidance of specific antigen exposure is the recommended treatment.

Discussion

Eosinophilic granuloma is a benign proliferative disorder of histiocytes. It is the least aggressive of the disorders collectively referred to as histiocytosis X. Lichtenstein introduced the term "histiocytosis X" in 1953 to encompass the following disorders: (1) localized eosinophilic granuloma of bone, (2) Hand-Schüller-Christian disease, and (3) Letterer-Siwe disease.[16] The lung is involved in all forms of the disease, either as the sole manifestation of the disorder (PEG) or as part of a multisystemic process.[7] Recent reports indicate that in most patients with pulmonary involvement, the disease is limited to the lung.[2,11]

The unit lesion of PEG is a focal, discrete stellate nodule usually centered on small airways and composed of a variable number of eosinophils, histiocytes, plasma cells, and lymphocytes (Figures 31-4 and 31-7). These cells are confined to the interstitium and tend to extend from a central nodular focus into adjacent lung by infiltrating and expanding adjacent alveolar septae (Figure 31-8). The Langerhans histiocyte is a histologic feature of PEG. This cell is a component of the interstitial process characteristic of this disease. The presence of eosinophils is variable and is not required for the diagnosis. Histologically, the histiocyte often has a large folded or indented nucleus (arrowheads, Figure 31-9) with eosinophilic cytoplasm. Electron microscopy demonstrates a pentalaminar inclusion in the cell's cytoplasm—the Langerhans granule or X-body (arrowheads, Figure 31-10). This racquet-shaped inclusion serves as a feature of eosinophilic granuloma, and recovery of the cell from bronchopulmonary lavage fluid may help to establish the diagnosis.[3,4] The presence of this cell also establishes a cytologic relationship between PEG and the other entities in the spectrum of histiocytosis X.

As the typical early lesion ages and begins to heal, the cellular infiltrate and the diagnostic cells are lost. In their place nonspecific scars develop (Figure 31-11). Diagnosis requires biopsy of the early cellular lesion. In a small number of patients progressive fibrosis ensues, with

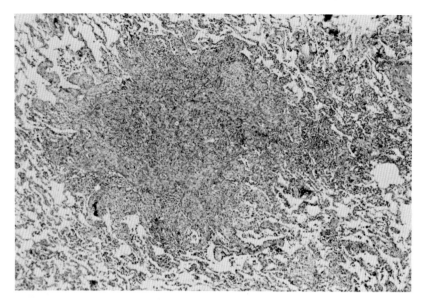

Figure 31-7. A low-power photomicrograph shows the early cellular nodule of PEG. (Reprinted with permission. AFIP neg. 79-12987.)

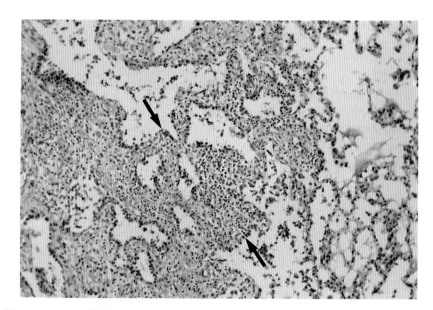

Figure 31-8. Higher-power view of the margin of the nodule shown in Figure 31-7 shows how the cellular infiltrate widens the interstitium (arrows) adjacent to the nodule and advances into the lung. These tentacles extending from the edge of the nodule help explain the indistinct margins visible radiographically. (Reprinted with permission. AFIP neg. 79-12987.)

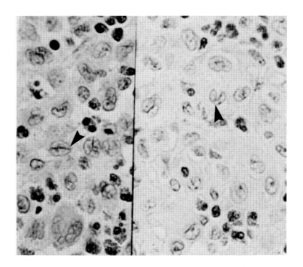

Figure 31-9. A composite high-power view of the cellular infiltrate demonstrated in Figure 31-8 shows the typical folded or cleft nucleus (arrowheads) of the Langerhans histiocyte, a feature of eosinophilic granuloma. The smaller darker-staining cells are eosinophils. (Reprinted with permission. AFIP neg. 79-12987.)

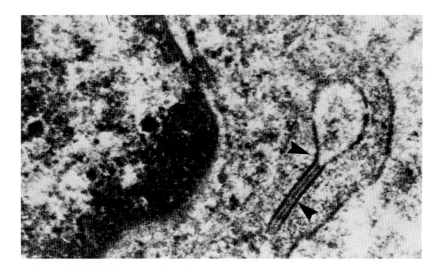

Figure 31-10. Electron micrograph of the cytoplasm of a Langerhans histiocyte shows the racquet-shaped X-body or Langerhans granule (arrowheads). (Reprinted with permission. AFIP neg. 79-12987.)

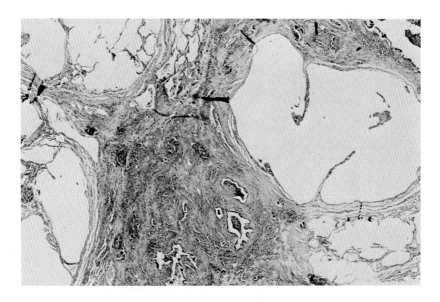

Figure 31-11. Low-power photomicrograph shows a stellate scar which has replaced an earlier cellular nodule. Once the lesions mature to this stage, the diagnosis may be extremely difficult to establish. (Reprinted with permission. AFIP neg. 80-463.)

coalescence of these isolated scars and resultant honeycomb lung. This progression was emphasized in a report of a patient followed for 25 years, whose autopsy findings were compared with his initial biopsy.[22]

Most of the initial cases of PEG were found by military physicians in a population of young soldiers,[1,9] so that the demographics were skewed to suggest that the disease was primarily one found in young white males. However, subsequent experience has shown a much wider age range and nearly equal sex distribution.[7] Presenting symptoms are often nonspecific or totally absent. Most patients complain of dyspnea, cough, sputum production, and, rarely, wheezing and hemoptysis. Only one-third of patients have systemic symptoms of weight loss, fever, or malaise. Acute chest pain due to pneumothorax is the presenting symptom in less than 3% of cases, although spontaneous pneumothorax has been reported in as many as 20% of patients at some point during their disease.[16] Diabetes insipidus has been reported in a few patients,[11] and bone lesions are found in approximately 5 to 10% of patients (Figure 31-12).[2,11,16]

The clinical outcome of the disease is difficult to predict and varies with the extent of organ involvement. If only patients with isolated lung disease are considered, the prognosis is good. Over 75% of such patients

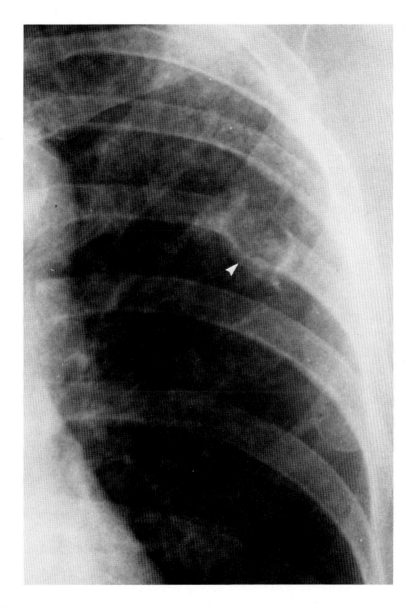

Figure 31-12. This 25-year-old man presented with acute left chest pain. The cause in this instance was a pathologic fracture of a rib (arrowhead) involved with eosinophilic granuloma. (Reprinted with permission. AFIP neg. 72-17554.)

show partial or complete resolution of their disease either spontaneously or following steroid therapy. About 20% have stable but definable pulmonary disease. Only 5 to 10% of patients have a progression that is eventually fatal—usually due to end-stage fibrosis. The prognosis is not as good for patients with multisystemic involvement.

Radiographic manifestations of PEG range from nodules to reticulation to frank fibrosis. It is tempting to equate these various radiographic patterns with stages of activity of the disease, but that is not entirely accurate. While it is true that biopsy of most nodules will yield the early cellular lesion diagnostic of PEG, it is not true that the reticular and cystic patterns represent quiescent, inactive, or burnt-out disease.[7] A peculiar feature of PEG is the poor correlation between the radiographic findings, clinical symptoms, and the pulmonary function studies. These parameters do not necessarily coincide with one another, so that resolution of the clinical symptoms is not necessarily associated with either radiographic clearing or marked improvement in pulmonary function. The active phase of the disease is extremely variable. One recent attempt to define activity in terms of a positive Ga-67 scintigram has been reported[14]; unfortunately, this has not proven to be a reliable marker for disease activity. Crystal et al. have reported that not all of their patients with biopsy-proven active disease have positive gallium studies.[8] It is not clear whether this is due to the minimal degree of inflammation that is present in some cases or whether the effector cells simply do not accumulate the radiopharmaceutical.

The well-defined, very delicate, thin-walled cystic spaces in the lungs of patients with PEG are usually attributed to fibrosis or "honeycombing." In certain instances this may be true. However, in many patients these cystic spaces actually resolve or show dramatic improvement over time. This suggests that at least some of these spaces are not the result of pulmonary fibrosis. Generally, they may represent dilated small airways instead (Figure 31-13). Radiographically visible cavitation is extremely rare, even though it is frequently seen histologically.

The association of PEG with spontaneous pneumothorax has been reported in as many as 20% of patients.[11,16] Recurrent pneumothorax is considered an unfavorable factor in prognosis.[2] It is more common in patients under 30 years of age and is more likely to occur in males than in females.[11] No correlation between pneumothorax and the pattern of parenchymal abnormality has been established. Pneumothorax occurs as frequently in patients with nodules as it does in those with cystic-appearing lungs.

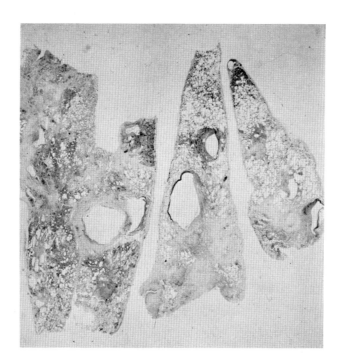

Figure 31-13. The cystic spaces in these low-power microsections are dilated airways with thickened walls. Smaller fibrosing lesions are present in each section as well. (Reprinted with permission. AFIP neg. 67-3397.)

Definite hilar adenopathy is rare. Enlargement of the central pulmonary arteries would be expected with extensive interstitial fibrosis. The absence of hilar adenopathy is a helpful distinction between PEG and sarcoidosis, but this distinction is probably more academic than useful since the treatments and prognoses for PEG and sarcoidosis are so similar.

SUGGESTED READINGS

1. Auld D. Pathology of eosinophilic granuloma of the lung. Arch Pathol 1957; 63:113–131
2. Basset F, Corrin B, Spencer H, et al. Pulmonary histiocytosis X. Am Rev Respir Dis 1978; 118:811–820
3. Basset F, Escaig J, Le Crom M. A cytoplasmic membranous complex in histiocytosis X. Cancer 1975; 29:1380–1386

4. Basset F, Soler P, Jaurand MC, Bignon J. Ultrastructural examination of broncho-alveolar lavage for diagnosis of pulmonary histiocytosis X: preliminary report on 4 cases. Thorax 1977; 32:303–306

5. Becklake MR. Asbestos-related diseases of the lung and other organs: their epidemiology and implications for clinical practice. Am Rev Respir Dis 1976; 114:187–227

6. Braun SR, doPico GA, Tsiatis A, Horvath E, Dickie HA, Rankin J. Farmer's lung disease: long-term clinical and physiologic outcome. Am Rev Respir Dis 1979; 119:185–191

7. Colby TV, Lombard C. Histiocytosis X in the lung. Hum Pathol 1983; 14:847–856

8. Crystal RG, Bitterman PB, Rennard ST, Hance AJ, Keogh BA. Interstitial lung disease of unknown cause. N Engl J Med 1984; 310:235–244

9. Farinacci CJ, Jeffrey HC, Lackey RW. Eosinophilic granuloma of the lung. US Armed Forces Med J 1951; 2:1085–1093

10. Friedman PJ, Harwood IR, Ellenbogen PH. Pulmonary cystic fibrosis in the adult: early and late radiologic findings with pathologic correlations. AJR 1981; 136:1131–1144

11. Friedman PJ, Liebow AA, Sokoloff J. Eosinophilic granuloma of lung. Clinical aspects of primary pulmonary histiocytosis in the adult. Medicine 1981; 60:385–396

12. Hapke EJ, Seal RM, Thomas GO, Hayes M, Meek JC. Farmer's lung. A clinical, radiographic, functional, and serological correlation of acute and chronic stages. Thorax 1968; 23:451–468

13. Hunninghake GW, Fauci AS. Pulmonary involvement in the collagen vascular diseases. Am Rev Respir Dis 1979; 119:471–503

14. Javaheri S, Levine BW, McKusick KA. Serial ^{67}Ga lung scanning in pulmonary eosinophilic granuloma. Thorax 1979; 34:822–823

15. Katzenstein AA, Askin FB. Surgical pathology of non-neoplastic lung disease. Philadelphia: WB Saunders; 1982:356–363

16. Lewis JG. Eosinophilic granuloma and its variants with special reference to lung involvement. A report of 12 patients. Q J Med 1964; 131:337–359

17. Lichtenstein L. Histiocytosis X. Arch Pathol 1953; 56:84–102

18. Metzger WJ, Fish J, Kelly JF, Rosenberg M, Patterson R. Hypersensitivity lung disease: early diagnosis. J Allergy Clin Immunol 1978; 61:67–72

19. Morgan WK, Seaton A. Occupational lung diseases, 2nd ed. Philadelphia: WB Saunders; 1984:564–590

20. Nadeau PJ, Ellis FH, Harrison EG, et al. Primary pulmonary histiocytosis X. Dis Chest 1960; 37:325–339

21. Olsen GN, Swenson EW. Polymyositis and interstitial lung disease. Am Rev Respir Dis 1972; 105:611–617

22. Powers MA, Askin FB, Cresson DH. Pulmonary eosinophilic granuloma. 25-year follow-up. Am Rev Respir Dis 1984; 129:503–507

23. Shwachman H, Kowalski M, Khaw KT. Cystic fibrosis: a new outlook. 70 patients above 25 years of age. Medicine 1977; 56:129–149

24. Tomashefski JF, Christoforidis AJ, Abdullah AK. Cystic fibrosis in young adults: an overlooked diagnosis, with emphasis on pulmonary function and radiological patterns. Chest 1970; 57:28–36

25. Unger GF, Scanlon GT, Fink JN, Unger J de B. A radiologic approach to hypersensitivity pneumonias. Radiol Clin North Am 1973; 11:339–356
26. Weaver AL, Divertie MB, Titus JL. Pulmonary scleroderma. Dis Chest 1968; 54:490–498
27. Weber WN, Margolin FR, Nielsen SL. Pulmonary histiocytosis X. A review of 18 patients with reports of 6 cases. AJR 1969; 107:280–289

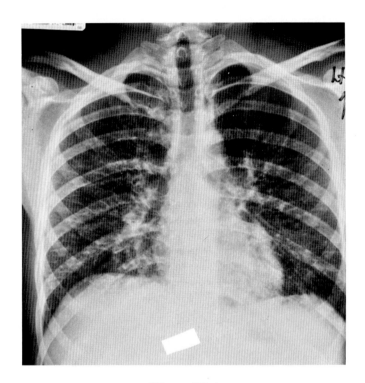

Figure 32-1
Figures 32-1 and 32-2. This 14-year-old boy presented with progressive dyspnea. You are shown a posteroanterior chest radiograph (Figure 32-1) and a close-up of the same radiograph (Figure 32-2). (Reprinted with permission. Armed Forces Institute of Pathology [AFIP] neg. 80-1169.)

Case 32: Pulmonary Veno-occlusive Disease

Question 146

Which *one* of the following is the LEAST likely diagnosis?

(A) Sclerosing mediastinitis
(B) Pulmonary veno-occlusive disease
(C) Left atrial myxoma
(D) Mitral insufficiency
(E) Cor triatriatum

The posteroanterior chest radiograph of this 14-year-old boy shows extensive interstitial pulmonary disease with Kerley B lines and peribronchial cuffing (Figures 32-1 and 32-2). There is no evidence of overall cardiomegaly, specific cardiac chamber enlargement, or upper lobe redistribution of vascular flow.

All of the diseases listed above may produce the interstitial pattern of edema shown in Figures 32-1 and 32-2. However, mitral insufficiency is least likely to present with a heart of normal size **(Option (D) is correct).** The incompetence of the mitral valve leads to enlargement of the left atrium in addition to, and usually before, pulmonary venous hypertension. If the degree of interstitial pulmonary edema seen in the test case were due to mitral insufficiency, one would expect the left atrium to be significantly larger.

Left atrial myxoma (Option (C)) may occasionally present with a similar pulmonary edema pattern and a heart of normal size.[11] Obstruction of pulmonary venous return with resultant radiographic findings similar to those in Figures 31-1 and 31-2 occurs with sclerosing mediastinitis (Option (A)), pulmonary veno-occlusive disease (Option (B)), and cor triatriatum (Option (E)). Although mediastinal widening is frequently seen with sclerosing mediastinitis, it is not invariably present,

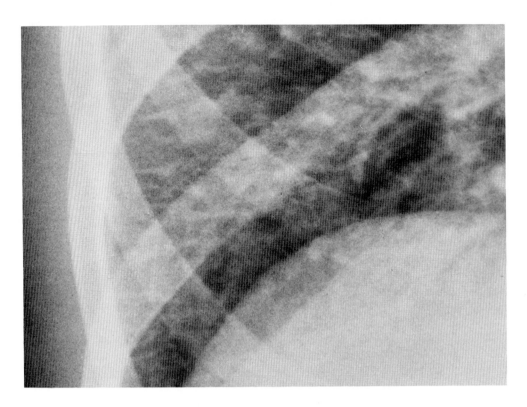

Figure 32-2

particularly if the sclerotic process originates from caseous subcarinal lymph nodes.[7]

Cor triatriatum is a rare congenital cardiac anomaly in which a fibromuscular membrane separates the pulmonary veins and the true left atrium. This membrane significantly impedes pulmonary venous return and causes severe pulmonary venous hypertension. Cardiac magnetic resonance imaging has been effective in imaging this anomaly.[1]

Question 147

Swan-Ganz catheterization of this patient demonstrated a normal pulmonary capillary wedge pressure. On the basis of this additional information, which *one* of the following is the MOST likely diagnosis?

(A) Sclerosing mediastinitis
(B) Pulmonary veno-occlusive disease
(C) Left atrial myxoma
(D) Mitral insufficiency
(E) Cor triatriatum

A normal pulmonary capillary wedge pressure of 10 mm Hg obtained in this patient with radiographic signs of interstitial edema was highly suggestive of pulmonary veno-occlusive disease **(Option (B) is correct)**.[13,18] Elevated pulmonary capillary wedge pressures are expected in patients with pulmonary venous obstruction at the level of the major pulmonary veins (Options (A) and (E)) or with mitral insufficiency (Option (D)) or left atrial myxoma (Option (C)). In pulmonary veno-occlusive disease, however, the venous obstruction occurs in scattered small pulmonary venules; thus, the capillary wedge pressure may be normal because drainage to the left atrium occurs through other patent venous channels.

Question 148

The anatomic components of a Kerley B line include:

(A) interlobular septum
(B) pulmonary venule
(C) pulmonary arteriole
(D) pulmonary lymphatics

The components of a Kerley B line are the structures found in the interlobular septum at the periphery of the secondary pulmonary lobule. These structures include the septum itself **(Option (A) is true)**, the pulmonary venule **(Option (B) is true)**, and the pulmonary lymphatics **(Option (D) is true)**. Pulmonary arterioles are central structures of the secondary lobule and are not a component of the Kerley B line **(Option (C) is false)**.[15]

Question 149

Concerning left atrial myxoma,

    (A) it is the most common primary tumor of the heart
    (B) it mimics mitral stenosis on the chest radiograph
    (C) computed tomography is preferable to echocardiography for establishing the diagnosis
    (D) the presence of calcification within the tumor allows distinction from left atrial thrombus
    (E) it most commonly arises from the left atrial appendage

Left atrial myxoma is the most common primary tumor of the heart **(Option (A) is true).** Although primary tumors of the heart are uncommon, the myxomas account for nearly one-fourth of such tumors. Two-thirds of cardiac myxomatous tumors are found in the left atrium.[9,14]

The radiographic findings of left atrial myxoma mimic those of mitral stenosis **(Option (B) is true).** As long as the tumors are small and do not obstruct blood flow, the chest radiograph is normal. When blood flow across the mitral valve is impeded, signs of pulmonary venous obstruction appear and are usually, but not necessarily, accompanied by left atrial enlargement.[8,20]

Echocardiography is the imaging method of choice when the diagnosis of cardiac myxoma is considered **(Option (C) is false).** Computed tomography has proven useful as a second method of noninvasive imaging and has provided information on location, mobility, and size of the myxoma.[10,17] Gated cardiac magnetic resonance imaging has shown promise as a useful method for demonstrating intracardiac neoplasms in selected patients. The ability to image the entire heart in any plane represents a distinct advantage over echocardiography; however, the requirement for a regular heart rhythm to gate data acquisition and the problem with magnetic life support apparatus in critically ill patients restrict the availability of this modality.[5,6]

The presence of calcification within an atrial myxoma does not allow distinction from an atrial thrombus, which may also show calcification **(Option (D) is false).** Radiographically visible calcification had been an unusual but not rare observation in atrial myxoma prior to the advent of computed tomography. Three of six atrial myxomas reported in one study showed calcification on the computed tomographic scan.[21] While calcification alone may not allow distinction of thrombus from myxoma, other features are more helpful. Atrial thrombi may be separate from the atrial septum, may have more homogeneous density (exclusive of the calcification), and frequently show a smooth or discrete angulated margin.[21]

Myxoma does not often arise from the atrial appendage **(Option (E) is false)**. It almost always develops in or near the fossa ovalis of the atrial septum.[16]

Discussion

The 14-year-old boy shown in the test case presented with dyspnea which progressed relentlessly over a 6-month period. The chest radiograph (Figure 32-1) was taken during his final hospital admission. Swan-Ganz catheterization revealed a pulmonary arterial pressure of 130/60 mm Hg, with a mean of 63 mm Hg and a mean pulmonary capillary wedge pressure of 10 mm Hg. Despite aggressive treatment for his pulmonary edema and pulmonary arterial hypertension, he died after experiencing cardiac arrhythmia and a sudden decrease in arterial oxygenation.

At autopsy, the heart showed marked right ventricular hypertrophy. The lungs were heavy and congested. Secondary hypertensive changes were found in the pulmonary arterioles. The most graphic finding, however, was a widespread fibrous narrowing or obliteration of the lumina of small pulmonary veins and venules (Figures 32-3 and 32-4). The final diagnosis was pulmonary veno-occlusive disease (PVOD).

Although PVOD is a rare condition, the number of reported cases has risen steadily over the past decade. While the diagnosis of PVOD is usually made histologically and frequently only at autopsy, this diagnosis may be suggested by characteristic radiographic and hemodynamic findings.

Well over 100 cases of PVOD have been described in the literature, and a characteristic clinical picture has emerged.[2-4,17-19,22,23] Generally, PVOD affects children and young adults; the average age of such patients is less than 20 years. Unlike primary pulmonary artery hypertension, there is no sexual predilection; males and females are equally affected. Shortness of breath, particularly on exertion, is invariably the presenting symptom. This dyspnea is progressive and may be accompanied by syncope, dizziness, hemoptysis, and cyanosis. The duration of the disease varies considerably, and since no adequate therapy is yet available, death occurs within a few years of the onset of symptoms.

The pathologic findings in PVOD are limited to the thoracic organs, and the lesion common to all cases is a fibrous narrowing or obliteration

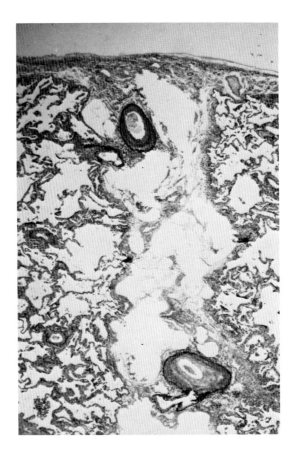

Figure 32-3. Same patient as in Figures 32-1 and 32-2. Low-power photomicrograph of a peripheral lung section taken at autopsy shows the pleural surface at the top. A grossly dilated, markedly edematous interlobular septum extends downward vertically from the pleura and contains two abnormal small pulmonary veins (thickened walls). The normally delicate thin-walled veins are here narrowed by intimal fibrosis. The alveoli adjacent to the interlobular septum contain hemosiderin-laden macrophages, and the alveolar walls are congested. (Reprinted with permission. AFIP neg. 80-2087.)

of the lumina of many small veins and venules. In many vessels, the lumina are completely occluded. In others, there are a concentric thickening of the intima and hypertrophy of the media of the wall to the point that the vein resembles a pulmonary arteriole, a process called venous arterialization. The pulmonary arterioles show secondary hypertensive changes. Dilated lymphatic channels are present. Alterations common to other causes of postcapillary hypertension are present as well

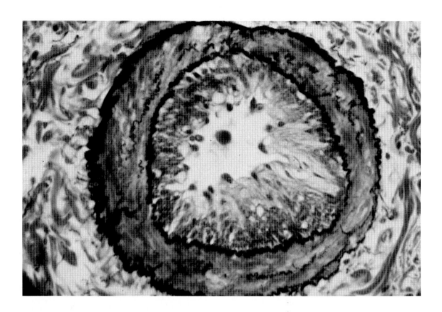

Figure 32-4. Same patient as in Figures 32-1 to 32-3. High-power photomicrograph of a pulmonary venule shows "venous arterialization." Elastin stains outline prominent elastic lamina with medial hypertrophy. Bizarre endothelial proliferation and fibrosis narrow the venous lumen. (Reprinted with permission. AFIP neg. 80-2089.)

(focal hemorrhage and hemosiderosis). The major pulmonary veins are usually normal.

The chest radiograph reflects many of the secondary effects of PVOD (Figure 32-1). Kerley B lines are invariably present, resulting from interstitial edema. The heart is normal in size until late in the course of the disease, when right ventricular decompensation and cor pulmonale result. The left atrium and left ventricle are normal. The major pulmonary arteries are enlarged due to the secondary pulmonary arterial hypertension. Important observations are the lack of upper lobe vascular redistribution and the presence of major pulmonary veins of normal size. Pleural effusion is common, and pulmonary opacities due to hemorrhage or infarction are not unusual. Pulmonary angiograms show a prolonged circulation time, and pulmonary perfusion scintigraphy is normal.[12,19]

PVOD is suggested by the triad of severe pulmonary arterial hypertension, pulmonary edema with Kerley B lines on the chest radiograph, and a normal pulmonary capillary wedge pressure.[18] Once the clinical problem of pulmonary arterial hypertension is recognized, the chest radiograph plays a key role in placing the level of pulmonary vascular disease in the postcapillary venous circulation. Kerley B lines and generalized pulmonary edema are not features of primary pulmonary arterial hypertension and would not be expected with recurrent pulmonary emboli unless left ventricular failure were associated. The absence of left-sided heart enlargement and the absence of upper lobe vascular redistribution of flow exclude intrinsic heart disease as the cause of the interstitial edema. The normal pulmonary capillary wedge pressure is not seen in the extrapulmonary obstruction of venous return encountered with mediastinal fibrosis, anomalous pulmonary venous return, cor triatriatum, or pulmonary vein stenosis.

Reasons for the normal to slightly increased pulmonary capillary wedge pressure in patients with PVOD are not fully understood. Carrington and Liebow explain this observation by the fact that, once arterial inflow into a capillary bed has been interrupted by the wedged catheter, the capillary pressure will gradually fall if drainage is through a partially obstructed venule or collateral bronchial vein.[3] They further indicate that, in contrast, when obstruction to venous return is in a major pulmonary vein or at the mitral valve, the wedged catheter measures pressure reflected from veins still receiving inflow from other nearby arteries.[3]

The etiology of PVOD is unknown. There is fairly wide acceptance that the condition is acquired and not the result of a congenital malformation of pulmonary veins. A wide range of insults, from environmental factors and toxic substances to immune complexes and infection, have been implicated as causative agents in the obstruction of the postcapillary venules. Wagenvoort has suggested that several different and distinct agents may be responsible for the initial injury to the pulmonary circulation and that PVOD might well be a syndrome rather than a discrete disease.[22]

SUGGESTED READINGS

1. Bisset GS, Kirks DR, Strife JL, Schwartz DC. Cor triatriatum: diagnosis by MR imaging. AJR 1987; 149:576–586
2. Brown CH, Harrison CV. Pulmonary veno-occlusive disease. Lancet 1966; 2:61–65
3. Carrington CB, Liebow AA. Pulmonary veno-occlusive disease. Hum Pathol 1970; 1:322–324
4. Crissman JD, Koss M, Carson RP. Pulmonary veno-occlusive disease secondary to granulomatous venulitis. Am J Surg Pathol 1980; 4:93–99

5. Freedberg RS, Kronzonm I, Rumancik WM, Leibeskind D. The contribution of magnetic resonance imaging to the evaluation of intracardiac tumors diagnosed by echocardiography. Circulation 1988; 77:96–103

6. Go RT, O'Donnell JK, Underwood DA, et al. Comparison of gated cardiac MRI and 2D echocardiography of intracardiac neoplasms. AJR 1985; 145:21–25

7. Goodwin RA, Nickell JA, DesPres RM. Mediastinal fibrosis complicating healed primary histoplasmosis and tuberculosis. Medicine 1972; 51:227–246

8. Greenwood WF. Profile of atrial myxoma. Am J Cardiol 1968; 21:367–375

9. Heath D. Pathology of cardiac tumors. Am J Cardiol 1968; 21:315–327

10. Huggins TJ, Huggins MJ, Schnapf DJ, Brott WH, Sinnott RC, Shawl FA. Left atrial myxoma: computed tomography as a diagnostic modality. J Comput Assist Tomogr 1980; 4:253–255

11. Hurst JW, Logue RB. The heart, 5th ed. New York: McGraw-Hill; 1982:1403–1413

12. Koerner SK. Pulmonary hypertension: etiology and clinical evaluation. J Thorac Imaging 1988; 3:25–31

13. Liebow AA, Moser KM, Soothgate MT. Rapidly progressive dyspnea in a teenage boy. JAMA 1973; 223:1243–1253

14. McAllister HA, Fenoglio JJ. Tumors of the cardiovascular system. Atlas of tumor pathology, 2nd series, fasc 15. Washington, DC: Armed Forces Institute of Pathology; 1978:1–3

15. Murray JF. The normal lung. The basis for diagnosis and treatment of pulmonary disease, 2nd ed. Philadelphia: WB Saunders; 1986:43–46

16. Nasser WK, Davis RH, Dillon JC, et al. Atrial myxoma. I: clinical and pathologic features in nine cases. Am Heart J 1972; 83:694–704

17. Norlindh T, Lilja B, Nyman U, Hellekant C. Left atrial myxoma demonstrated with CT. AJR 1981; 137:153–154

18. Rambihar VS, Fallen EL, Cairns JA. Pulmonary veno-occlusive disease: antemortem diagnosis from roentgenographic and hemodynamic findings. Can Med Assoc J 1979; 120:1519–1522

19. Scheibel RL, Dedeker KL, Gleason DF, Pliego M, Kieffer SA. Radiographic and angiographic characteristics of pulmonary veno-occlusive disease. Radiology 1972; 103:47–51

20. Steiner RE. Radiologic aspects of cardiac tumors. Am J Cardiol 1968; 21:344–356

21. Tsuchiya F, Kohno A, Saitoh R, Shigeta A. CT findings of atrial myxoma. Radiology 1984; 151:139–143

22. Wagenvoort CA. Pulmonary veno-occlusive disease. Entity or syndrome? Chest 1976; 69:82–86

23. Wagenvoort CA, Wagenvoort N. The pathology of pulmonary veno-occlusive disease. Virchows Arch (Pathol Anat) 1974; 364:69–79

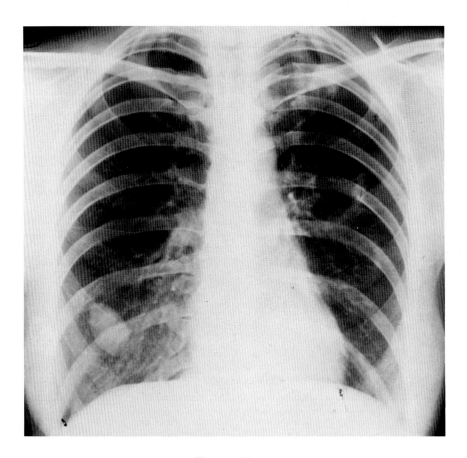

Figure 33-1
Figures 33-1 and 33-2. This 50-year-old woman was asymptomatic. You are shown two posteroanterior chest radiographs taken 1 month apart. (Reprinted with permission. Armed Forces Institute of Pathology [AFIP] negs. 56-571 and 56-573, respectively.)

Case 33: Localized Fibrous Mesothelioma

Question 150

Which *one* of the following is the MOST likely diagnosis?

   (A) Inflammatory pseudotumor
   (B) Pleural pseudotumor (fluid)
   (C) Lipoma
   (D) Localized fibrous mesothelioma
   (E) Rounded atelectasis

The two posteroanterior chest radiographs of this 50-year-old asymptomatic woman demonstrate a well-defined oval mass that has changed position during the 1-month interval of observation. Note that the patient's positioning and degree of inspiration are similar for both radiographs. No other significant positive findings are present. Important negative findings are the absence of any evidence of atelectasis or free pleural fluid.

Inflammatory pseudotumor (Option (A)) is not likely. Although this entity frequently presents as a circumscribed mass, it is located within the lung parenchyma and does not change position unless some volume alteration occurs within the lung.[12,16]

Pleural pseudotumor (fluid) (Option (B)), although more likely than inflammatory pseudotumor, is still not very likely. Fluid may become loculated in the pleural space and present as a mass. It may shrink or even disappear, but it does not usually shift to another location. The absence of any radiographic or clinical evidence of congestive heart failure, trauma, infection, or other cause of pleural effusion further reduces the likelihood of this diagnosis.

A thoracic lipoma (Option (C)) is also unlikely. It may arise from the extrapleural tissues of the chest wall, the bronchial wall, or rarely, the

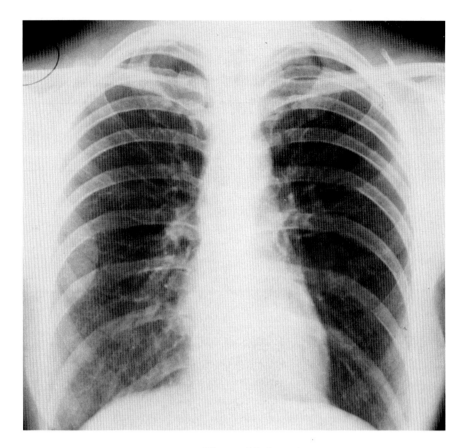

Figure 33-2

lung parenchyma, but none of these locations would allow the remarkable mobility of the mass demonstrated in Figures 33-1 and 33-2.

The pleura-based mass of rounded atelectasis (Option (E)) would not change its position on serial radiographs as in Figures 33-1 and 33-2. Rounded atelectasis is thus unlikely.

Localized fibrous mesothelioma is the most likely diagnosis **(Option (D) is correct).** This predominantly benign tumor of the pleura pedunculates into the pleural space in 30 to 50% of reported cases.[2] If the fibrovascular pedicle is long enough, the tumor may move around within the pleural space and present, as in this case, in a different position at different times (Figures 33-1 through 33-3).

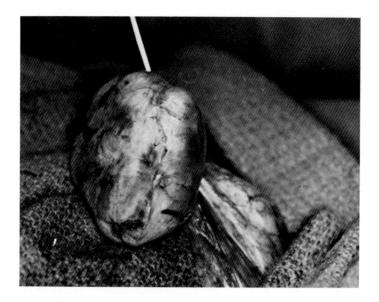

Figure 33-3. The operative specimen from the patient in Figures 33-1 and 33-2 shows a well-circumscribed tumor attached to the visceral pleura. (Reprinted with permission. AFIP neg. 85-10488.)

Question 151

Concerning pleural pseudotumor (fluid),

    (A) the most common location is in the minor fissure
    (B) it resorbs spontaneously
    (C) elliptical or biconvex margins are characteristic
    (D) the most common etiology is closed chest trauma

While loculated fluid may be found between any two layers of visceral pleura, it has a predilection for the minor fissure **(Option (A) is true).** In one series of 41 pleural pseudotumors, 32 were located in the minor fissure.[9] Pleural pseudotumor resorbs spontaneously **(Option (B) is true).** The spontaneous resorption of the loculated fluid collections has given rise to the names "pseudotumor" and "vanishing tumor."[7] Elliptical or biconvex margins are characteristic of pleural pseudotumor **(Option (C) is true).** Such margins are due to the bulging of adjacent pleural surfaces by the trapped fluid. Finally, the most common cause of pleural pseudotumors (fluid) is congestive heart failure **(Option (D) is false).**[21]

Question 152

Concerning intrathoracic lipoma,

(A) it is more common in female patients
(B) parenchymal lesions change shape with phases of respiration
(C) its fat density is rarely recognized on routine radiographs
(D) hypertrophic pulmonary osteoarthropathy occurs in 10% of patients

Intrathoracic lipomas are benign neoplasms and show a male predilection of almost 5 to 1 **(Option (A) is false).**[18] Since parenchymal lesions are compact and encapsulated, they do not change shape with phases of respiration **(Option (B) is false).**[17] Lipomas arising within the lung are usually associated with the major bronchi and present as rounded solitary nodules or with manifestations of bronchial obstruction. Extrapleural lipomas arising from the connective tissue beneath the parietal pleura do change shape during respiration, becoming smaller and flatter during inspiration.[8]

The true fat density of intrathoracic lipomas is often difficult to see on routine radiographs **(Option (C) is true).** These tumors usually appear on chest radiographs as water-density lesions. The explanation for this phenomenon may be related to the adjacent pulmonary air density or, less frequently, to a peculiar type of fat with a high phospholipid content (so-called brown fat of hibernomas).[6,14] Computed tomography invariably demonstrates the fat density of these lesions.[13] Hypertrophic pulmonary osteoarthropathy has not been associated with intrathoracic lipomas **(Option (D) is false).**

Question 153

Concerning localized fibrous mesothelioma,

(A) it is associated with asbestos exposure
(B) there is potential for malignancy
(C) it arises predominantly from the parietal pleura
(D) it is associated with hypertrophic pulmonary osteoarthropathy
(E) an apical location is characteristic

Localized fibrous mesothelioma (LFM) has no known association with asbestos exposure **(Option (A) is false).** The malignant mesothelioma, on the other hand, is definitely associated with asbestos exposure.[5,19] The malignant potential of LFM is small and is more often expressed by local invasion and recurrence than by distant metastasis **(Option (B) is true)**.[11,20] Approximately 80% of the time, LFM arises from the visceral pleura **(Option (C) is false)**.[3]

Hypertrophic pulmonary osteoarthropathy has been associated with LFM in as many as 50% of patients in some series **(Option (D) is true)**.[3] Although the frequency of this finding has decreased in more recent reviews, it remains one of the significant clinical manifestations of LFM.

The most common location for LFM is the dependent portions of the pleural space **(Option (E) is false)**.[5,10] The reason appears to be twofold: (1) there is a greater surface area of the larger lower lung covered by visceral pleura from which the lesion may arise, and (2) pedunculated tumors arising from the middle and upper pleura tend to "drop" to the lower pleural space.

Discussion

Primary tumors of the pleura present in either a diffuse or a localized form. Diffuse mesothelioma is noted for its highly malignant nature, its dramatic radiographic appearance, and its association with asbestos exposure. Localized mesothelioma, on the other hand, is a much less aggressive tumor and may present with a variety of interesting clinical and radiographic manifestations.

Localized fibrous mesothelioma (LFM) is but one of many names given to this particular tumor. Other names include benign mesothelioma, fibrous mesothelioma, localized mesothelioma, subpleural fibroma, and localized fibrous tumor of the pleura.[3] These various names reflect the basic nature of this tumor. Consisting primarily of benign fibrous tissue (Figure 33-4), it remains localized to its point of origin in the majority of cases. The tumor arises from the visceral pleura in more than 80% of reported cases.[3] As many as 30 to 50% of these tumors are attached to the pleura by a fibrovascular pedicle, which allows the tumor to change its location (Figures 33-1 and 33-2).

Clinically, pulmonary manifestations of these tumors are often absent or nonspecific. Many tumors are found as incidental abnormalities on chest radiographs of asymptomatic patients, as in our test case. Extrapulmonary symptoms, on the other hand, are not uncommon. Thirty-five to 50% of patients have associated hypertrophic osteoarthropathy (Figures 33-5 and 33-6), while 4% have hypoglycemia.[1,15] The latter two manifestations are particularly common with lesions

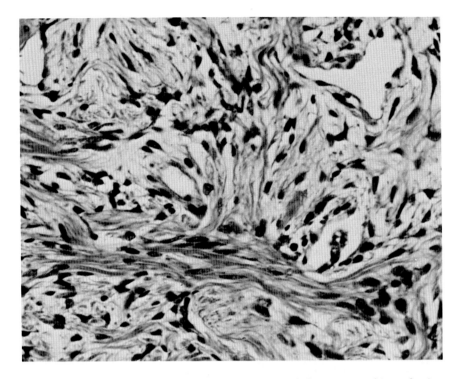

Figure 33-4. This microsection shows the typical pattern of interlacing bundles of spindle cells that characterizes the localized fibrous mesothelioma. (Reprinted with permission. AFIP neg. 85-10493.)

greater than 10 cm in diameter and are relieved after removal of the mass.[1] An association with asbestos exposure or some other causative agent has not been established.

The most common chest radiographic finding in patients with LFM is an isolated pleura-based mass. This mass may vary in size from a small nodule to a large tumor occupying the entire hemithorax with mediastinal shift. They are most commonly found in the lower thorax but may be seen along any portion of the pleural surface.[4,5] The tumor margins are sharp and present a convex border indenting the lung when seen in profile. Pleural effusion, tumor calcification, and rib erosion are rare. Computed tomography may demonstrate low-density areas of necrosis within larger tumors. Commonly, the tumor is suspended by a vascular pedicle, which allows a change in its position on sequential radiographs or with a change in the position of the patient. The remarkable mobility of these pedunculated pleural masses is an important clue to their diagnosis. Figures 33-7 through 33-17 illustrate further examples of radiographic findings in LFM.

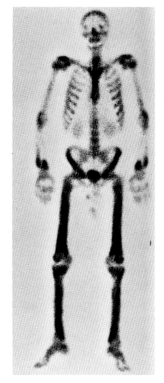 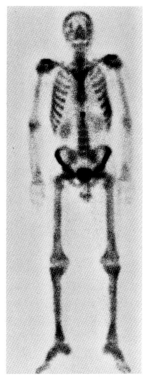

Figure 33-5   *Figure 33-6*

Figures 33-5 and 33-6. Preoperative (Figure 33-5) and 6-week postoperative (Figure 33-6) anterior-view bone scintigrams in a patient with LFM show dramatic improvement in the hypertrophic pulmonary osteoarthropathy following removal of the lesion. This is indicated by diminished uptake of the radionuclide in the upper and lower extremities. (Reprinted with permission. AFIP neg. 80-2190.)

The prognosis for patients with LFM is generally good; it can be cured by surgical resection in most cases. Recurrence of tumor following resection occurs in less than 10% of cases[7,21] and is almost invariably associated with the nodular rather than the pedunculated pattern of growth.

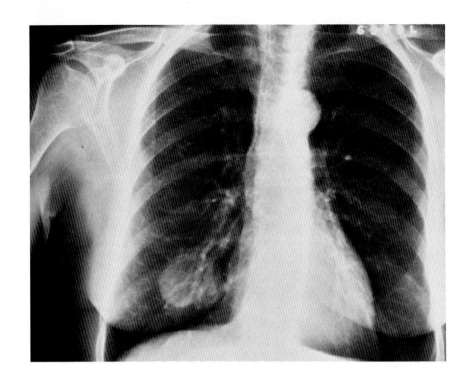

Figure 33-7

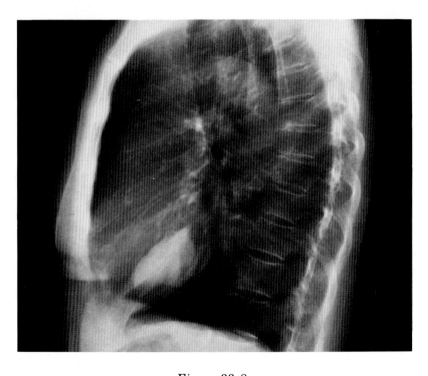

Figure 33-8
Figures 33-7 and 33-8. LFM arising in the major fissure shows, on the lateral view, a small "beak" superiorly where the two layers of visceral pleura converge above the mass. (Reprinted with permission. AFIP neg. 80-1163.)

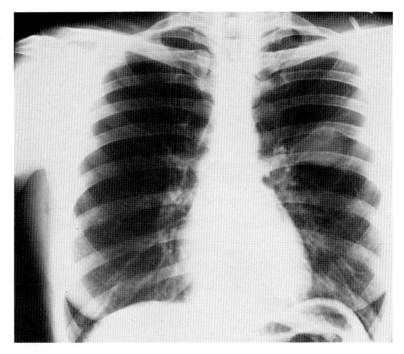

Figure 33-9

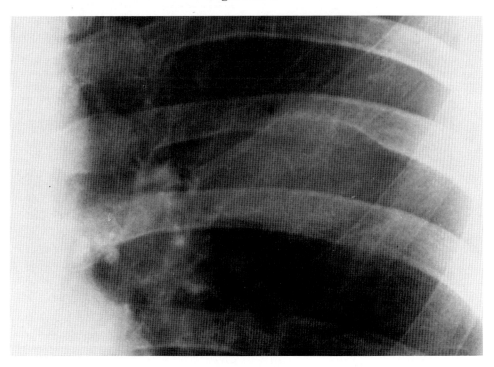

Figure 33-10
Figures 33-9 and 33-10. The posteroanterior view and a close-up of the same view show left rib erosion, which is rarely found with LFM (Reprinted with permission. AFIP neg. 62-15048.)

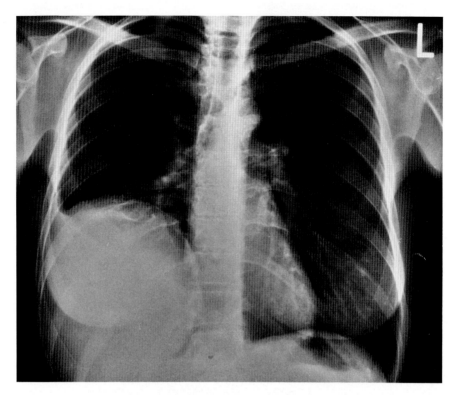

Figure 33-11

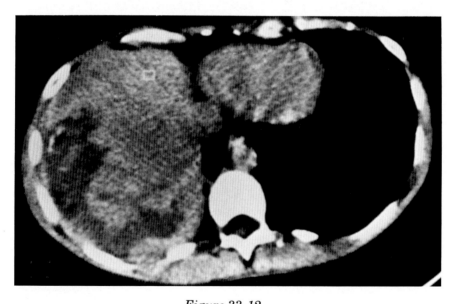

Figure 33-12
Figures 33-11 and 33-12. A large LFM is visible in the lower right hemithorax (Figure 33-11). A computed tomographic scan of the same area (Figure 33-12) shows focal areas of decreased attenuation within the tumor, correlating with areas of tumor necrosis. (Reprinted with permission. AFIP neg. 79-5069.)

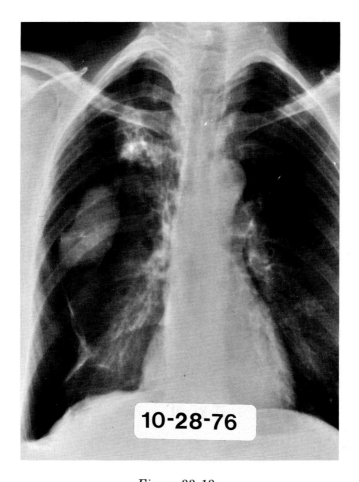

Figure 33-13
Figures 33-13 to 33-17. This series of posteroanterior radiographs illustrates the 1979 and 1981 recurrences of an LFM on the right, following two attempts at surgical excision. The initial study, in 1976, was taken after percutaneous biopsy and resultant pneumothorax. (Reprinted with permission. AFIP neg. 85-403.)

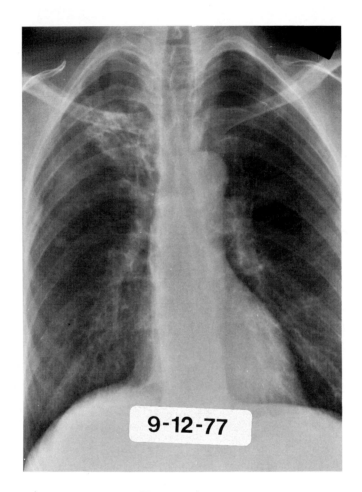

Figure 33-14

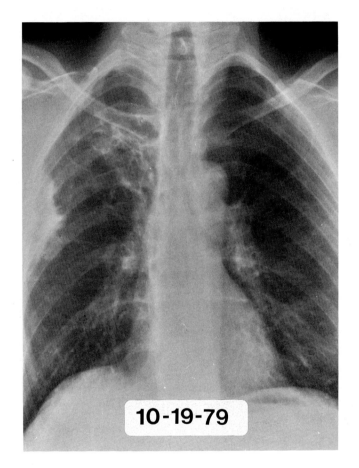

Figure 33-15

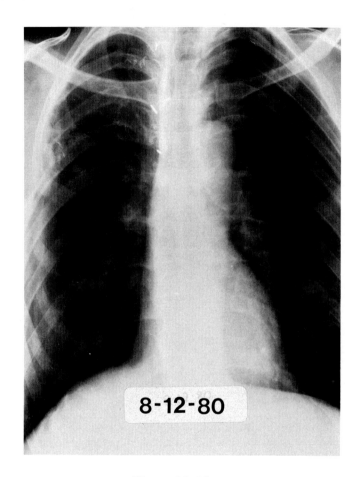

Figure 33-16

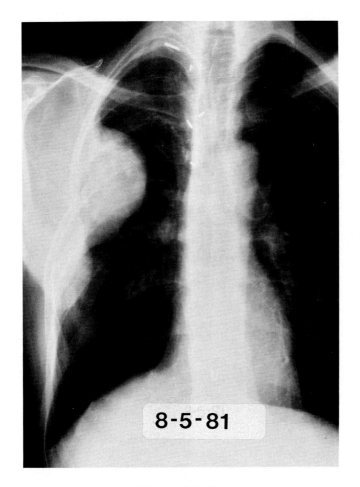

Figure 33-17

SUGGESTED READINGS

1. Antman KH, Corson JM. Benign and malignant pleural mesothelioma. Clin Chest Med 1985; 6:127–140
2. Berne AS, Heitzman ER. The roentgenologic signs of pedunculated pleural tumors. AJR 1962; 87:892–895
3. Briselli M, Mark EJ, Dickersin GR. Solitary fibrous tumors of the pleura: eight new cases and review of 360 cases in the literature. Cancer 1981; 47:2678–2689
4. Dalton WT, Zolliker AS, McCaughey WT, Jacques J, Kannerstein M. Localized primary tumors of the pleura: an analysis of 40 cases. Cancer 1979; 44:1465–1475
5. Ellis K, Wolff M. Mesotheliomas and secondary tumors of the pleura. Semin Roentgenol 1977; 12:303–311
6. Felson B. Chest roentgenology. Philadelphia: WB Saunders; 1973:55
7. Fraser RG, Paré JAP, Paré D, Fraser RS, Genereux GP. Diagnosis of diseases of the chest, 3rd ed. Philadelphia: WB Saunders; 1988:677–682
8. Gramiak R, Koerner HJ. A roentgen diagnostic observation in subpleural lipoma. AJR 1966; 98:465–467
9. Higgins JA, Juergens JL, Bruwer AJ, Parkin TW. Loculated interlobar pleural effusion due to congestive heart failure. Arch Intern Med 1955; 96:180–187
10. Hutchinson WB, Friedenberg MJ. Intrathoracic mesothelioma. Radiology 1963; 80:937–945
11. Kerr WF, Nohl HC. Recurrence of "benign" intrathoracic fibromas. Thorax 1961; 16:180–189
12. Madewell JE, Feigin DS. Benign tumors of the lung. Semin Roentgenol 1977; 12:175–186
13. Mendelsohn SL, Fagelman D, Zwanger-Mendelsohn S. Endobronchial lipoma demonstrated by CT. Radiology 1983; 148:790
14. Morgan AD, Jepson EM, Billimoria JD. Intrathoracic hibernoma. Thorax 1966; 21:186–192
15. Nelson R, Burman SO, Kiani R, Chertow BS, Shah J, Cantave I. Hypoglycemic coma associated with benign pleural mesothelioma. J Thorac Cardiovasc Surg 1975; 69:306–314
16. Pearl M. Postinflammatory pseudotumor of the lung in children. Radiology 1972; 105:391–395
17. Peleg H, Pauzner Y. Benign tumors of the lung. Dis Chest 1965; 47:179–186
18. Plachta A, Hershey H. Lipoma of the lung. Review of the literature and report of a case. Am Rev Respir Dis 1962; 86:912–916
19. Shabanah FH, Sayegh SF. Solitary (localized) pleural mesothelioma. Report of two cases and review of the literature. Chest 1971; 60:558–563
20. Utley JR, Parker JC Jr, Hahn RS, Bryant LR, Mobin-Uddin K. Recurrent benign fibrous mesothelioma of the pleura. J Thorac Cardiovasc Surg 1973; 65:830–834
21. Weiss W, Boucet KR, Gefter WI. Localized interlobar effusion in congestive heart failure. Ann Intern Med 1953; 38:1177–1186

Notes

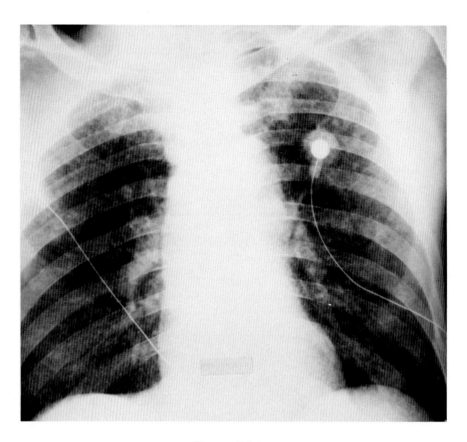

Figure 34-1
Figures 34-1 and 34-2. This 41-year-old foundry worker was admitted
to the emergency room after a cerebrovascular accident. You are shown
a portable chest radiograph (Figure 34-1) and a close-up of the same
radiograph (Figure 34-2). (Reprinted with permission. Armed Forces
Institute of Pathology [AFIP] neg. 76-6820.)

Case 34: Siderosis

Question 154

Which *one* of the occupational diseases listed below is the LEAST likely diagnosis?

(A) Silicosis
(B) Asbestosis
(C) Coal worker's pneumoconiosis
(D) Siderosis
(E) Stannosis

The portable chest radiograph taken in the emergency room (Figure 34-1) demonstrates diffuse small nodular opacities evenly distributed throughout the lung. On the photographic enlargement of the right mid lung (Figure 34-2), these rounded opacities are fairly discrete. There is no evidence of calcification or hilar adenopathy. The patient had no pulmonary symptoms and was brought to the emergency room with a ruptured intracranial aneurysm. You are asked which one of five pneumoconioses would be least compatible with the radiographic findings. Of the choices listed, silicosis (Option (A)), coal worker's pneumoconiosis (Option (C)), siderosis (Option (D)), and stannosis (Option (E)) present initially with small rounded opacities on the chest radiograph. Asbestosis does not; it is characterized by small irregular opacities with a predominant lower lobe distribution (Figures 34-3 to 34-6). Asbestosis is thus the least likely diagnosis **(Option (B) is correct).**

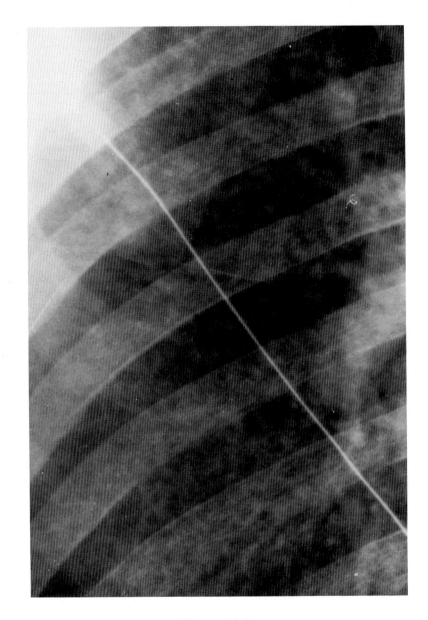

Figure 34-2

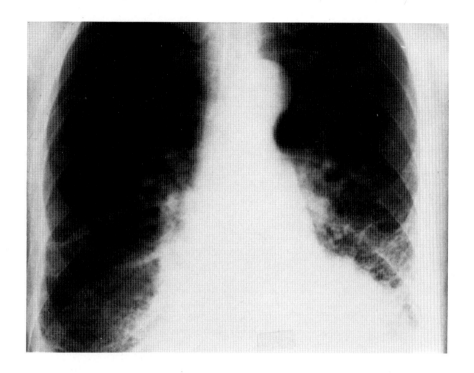

Figure 34-3
Figures 34-3 through 34-6. Asbestosis. Note the typical basilar distribution of small irregular opacities on the posteroanterior radiograph (Figure 34-3) and on a close-up view of the left base (Figure 34-4). A low-power photomicrograph (Figure 34-5) of lung tissue from a patient with asbestosis shows nonspecific fibrosis. A high-power photomicrograph (Figure 34-6) of similar tissue shows the interstitial fibrosis. (Reprinted with permission. AFIP negs. 69-1083, 75-4296, and 75-4290, respectively.)

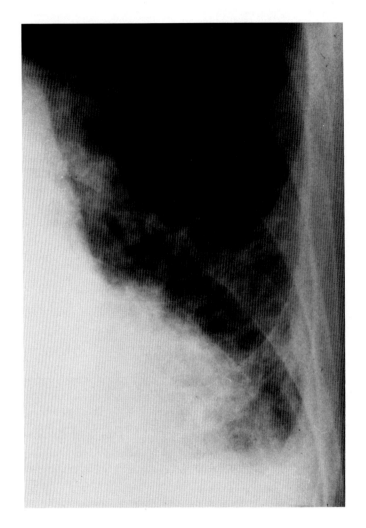

Figure 34-4

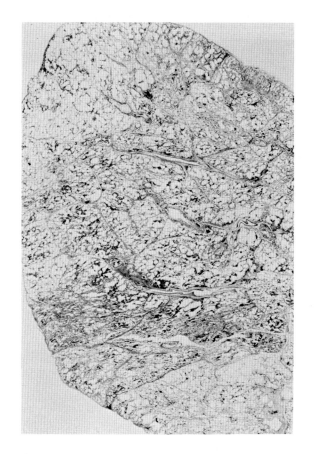

Figure 34-5

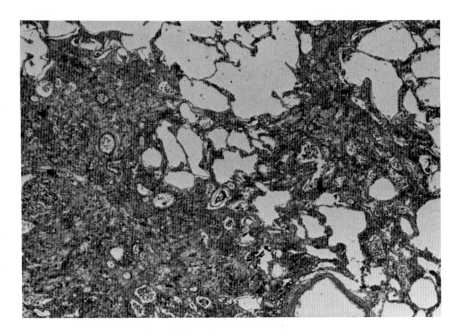

Figure 34-6

Question 155

In comparing silicosis and siderosis,

    (A) pulmonary fibrosis caused by silicosis is less severe than that caused by siderosis

    (B) there are fewer clinical symptoms in siderosis

    (C) the exposure time required to produce radiographic abnormality is greater for silicosis

    (D) conglomerate masses (large opacities) are seen in both

Silicosis and siderosis are two distinct pathologic entities that share many clinical and radiographic features, at least in their early stages. Silicosis results from inhalation of silica dust and is by far the more common and clinically significant problem. Siderosis results from inhalation of metallic iron or iron oxide and is much less frequently seen.

The most significant difference between silicosis and siderosis is the marked pulmonary fibrosis found in silicosis **(Option (A) is false)**.[1,5,6,8,9] Histologically, the silicotic nodule is rich in collagen. No collagenous fibrosis is produced in siderosis, since the inhaled iron or iron oxide is inert. The radiographic nodule in siderosis is produced by focal deposits of the heavy metal itself within the lung.

There are fewer clinical symptoms in siderosis than in silicosis (**Option (B) is true**). Both diseases are essentially asymptomatic during the early phases. However, the progression to large opacities and pulmonary disability that may be seen with silicosis is not seen with siderosis.[1]

The exposure time required to produce a radiographic abnormality is not greater for silicosis than for siderosis (**Option (C) is false**). The length of exposure, the concentration of dust particles in the exposure environment, and the composition of the dust may all influence the appearance and progression of radiographic abnormality. In general, however, previously healthy patients exposed to low levels of relatively pure dusts require 10 to 15 years of exposure before the appearance of radiographic abnormality.[1,8] Acute silicosis may result from massive inhalation.

Conglomerate masses (large opacities) are seen in patients with silicosis but not in patients with siderosis (**Option (D) is false**). Such masses are reported to occur in up to 15 to 20% of patients.[8]

Question 156

Concerning coal worker's pneumoconiosis,

- (A) the unit pathologic lesion is similar to that of silicosis
- (B) lower lung zones are more frequently involved than upper zones
- (C) calcification of pulmonary nodular opacities occurs frequently
- (D) the "simple" form progresses even in the absence of further exposure
- (E) the distinction between "simple" and "complicated" forms of the disease is based on the radiographic findings

The unit pathologic lesion in coal worker's pneumoconiosis (CWP) is distinctly different from the collagenous nodule characteristic of silicosis (**Option (A) is false**). The coal macule is the primary lesion of CWP (Figures 34-7 to 34-9). Histologically, it is a stellate accumulation of dust-laden macrophages and irregular fibrosis situated in or near the terminal bronchiole. Silicotic nodules contain concentric, laminated bands of hyalinized collagen (Figures 34-10 to 34-13). Particles of silica are inconspicuous in the lesion but may be demonstrated under polarized light as birefringent specks scattered throughout the nodule. Radiogra-

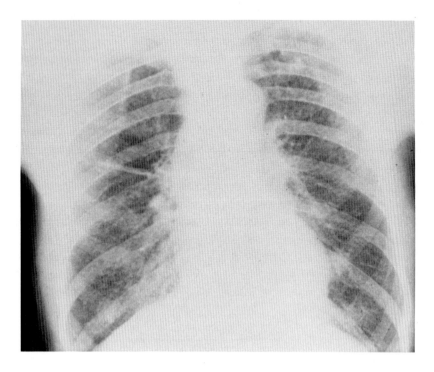

Figure 34-7

Figures 34-7 through 34-9. Coal worker's pneumoconiosis. Small rounded opacities, which may have an upper zone distributional predominance, are visible on the posteroanterior (Figure 34-7) and close-up (Figure 34-8) views of the left lung. A low-power photomicrograph (Figure 34-9) shows the unit lesion of CWP—the coal macule. Black pigment (single arrows) is trapped in radiating spokes of fibrosis, producing a stellate scar. The lesion has obliterated a small bronchiole adjacent to a pulmonary arteriole (double arrows). (Figure 34-9 is reprinted with permission. AFIP neg. 71-926.)

phically, both silicosis and CWP may present with small rounded opacities showing a tendency for middle and upper zonal pulmonary distribution.

The early nodular opacities in CWP frequently show a middle and upper zonal distribution similar to that seen in early silicosis **(Option (B) is false).** The reasons for this selective distribution are unclear but may be related to better clearance of the dust from the lower lobes.[8]

If a patient with CWP develops calcification within the small rounded opacities visible on the chest radiograph, one must consider a mixed dust

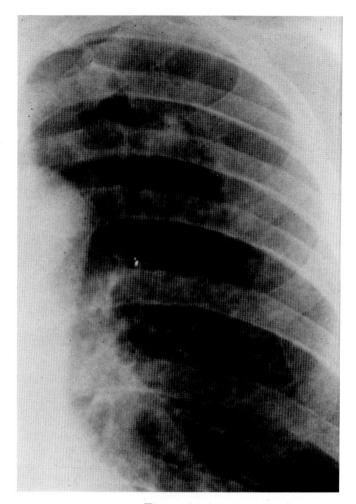

Figure 34-8

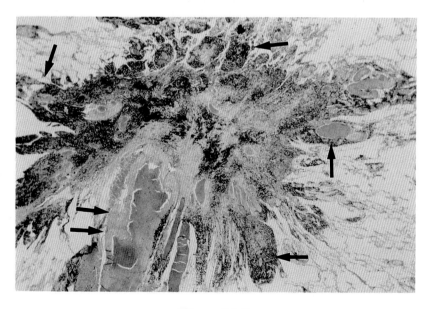

Figure 34-9

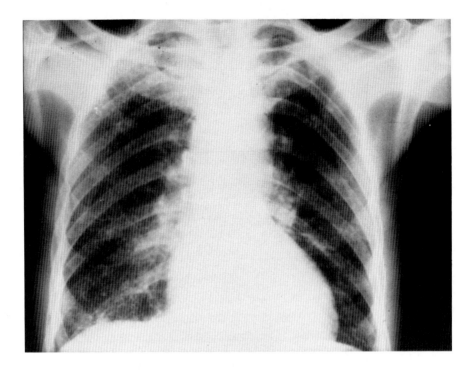

Figure 34-10

Figures 34-10 through 34-13. Silicosis. The chest radiographic appearance of silicosis (posteroanterior view [Figure 34-10] and close-up of right lung [Figure 34-11]) is indistinguishable from that of siderosis and CWP (all may show small rounded opacities). A low-power photomicrograph of a silicotic nodule (Figure 34-12) shows swirls of hyalinized collagen in the nodule. Nonpolarized (left) and polarized (right) views of a silicotic nodule (Figure 34-13) reveal birefringent specks in the matrix of dense fibrosis on the polarized view. (Figures 34-10 through 34-12 reprinted with permission. AFIP negs. 68-427 and 69-126, respectively.)

exposure that includes a significant component of silica **(Option (C) is false).**

"Simple" CWP rarely progresses in the absence of continued exposure **(Option (D) is false).**[8] The severity of simple CWP is clearly related to the amount and duration of dust exposure, but there is no convincing evidence of progression in the absence of further exposure.[6]

The distinction between "simple" and "complicated" forms of CWP is made on the basis of radiographic findings **(Option (E) is true).**[4] Simple pneumoconiosis is present if the rounded opacities on the chest radiograph measure less than 1 cm in diameter. Complicated pneumoconiosis refers to the presence of conglomerate masses (large opacities) and

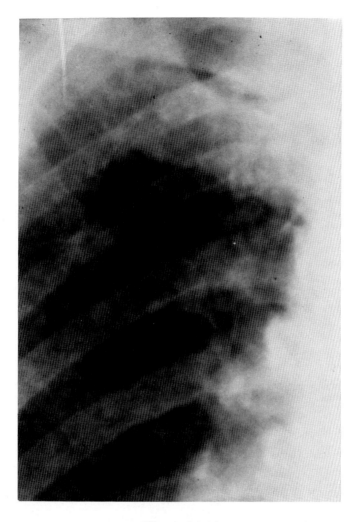

Figure 34-11

is diagnosed when one or more opacities larger than 1 cm in diameter are present. This definition excludes opacities resulting from other causes, such as cancer of the lung, granulomatous disease, etc.

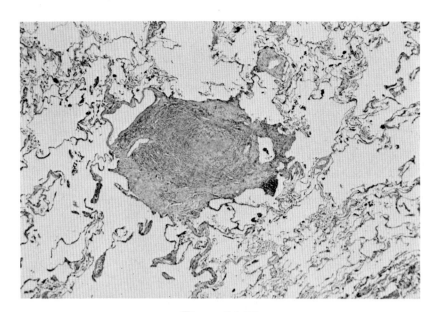

Figure 34-12

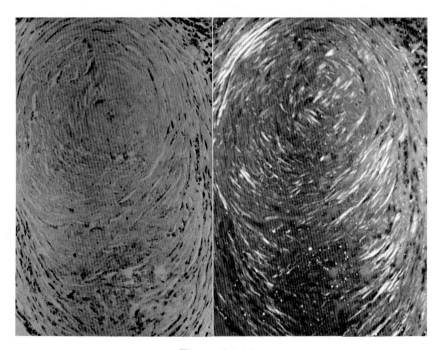

Figure 34-13

Question 157

Which *one* of the following pulmonary structures is MOST susceptible to deposition and accumulation of inhaled dust?

(A) Subpleural lymphatics
(B) Interlobular septum
(C) Alveolar wall
(D) Terminal bronchiole
(E) Alveolar sac

The pulmonary structure most susceptible to deposition and accumulation of inhaled dust is the terminal bronchiole **(Option (D) is correct).** The subpleural lymphatics (Option (A)), interlobular septum (Option (B)), alveolar wall (Option (C)), and alveolar sac (Option (E)) are all less susceptible. The terminal bronchiole is the last purely conductive portion of the airway.[9] Proximal to this structure are progressively larger bronchioles and bronchi. The respiratory bronchioles, alveolar ducts, atria, alveolar sacs, and alveoli are found distal to the terminal bronchiole.

The terminal bronchiole is vulnerable to dust deposition and accumulation for two reasons. First, at the junction of the terminal and respiratory bronchioles, mass air flow ceases to be the primary mechanism for gas delivery to the alveolus (Figures 34-14 and 34-15). Beyond this point, gas molecules proceed more as a result of diffusion. The terminal bronchiole is like the needle valve of a carburetor in that there is a rapid increase in volume just distal to its tiny lumen. Any particulate foreign matter that had escaped more proximal clearance mechanisms and that was held in suspension by mass air flow would tend to fall out of suspension in this region of the airway. Second, the mucociliary escalator and the central lymphatic channels usually begin at the terminal bronchiole. Alveolar macrophages, which patrol the alveolar surface and remove debris, are cleared from the alveolus by migrating more centrally toward the terminal bronchiole to be transported by either the mucociliary escalator or the central lymphatics.

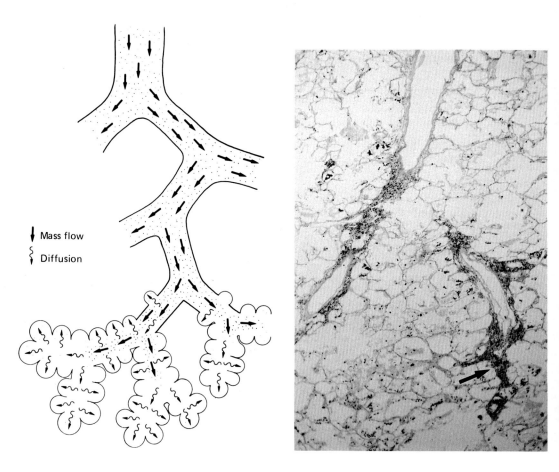

Figure 34-14   *Figure 34-15*

Figures 34-14 and 34-15. A diagram of the terminal bronchiole/
respiratory bronchiole junction (Figure 34-14) shows that mass air flow
ceases just distal to the terminal bronchiole. Thereafter, diffusion
becomes the mechanism of gas delivery to the alveolus. A low-power
photomicrograph (Figure 34-15) demonstrates the peribronchiolar accumulation (arrow) of pigmented particles in a patient with early siderosis.
Note that very few particles appear in the alveoli or more proximal
bronchiole (top of figure). (Reprinted with permission from AFIP.)

Discussion

Siderosis is an inhalational disease of the lung in which metallic iron and/or iron oxide is deposited in the lower respiratory tract. It is classified as a benign or inert pneumoconiosis since the retained dust is not toxic, allergenic, or pathogenic to the lung.[5,10,11] Siderosis produces no clinical symptoms and causes no impairment of pulmonary function.[1,10] The diagnosis is suggested on the basis of an abnormal chest radiograph and a history of exposure to iron dust or fumes. Since the radiographic findings are nonspecific and evoke a broad differential diagnosis, this condition may be overlooked if an adequate history is not obtained.

Obvious sources of exposure include occupations involved with mining, transporting, and processing iron ores or with milling and refining metals from that ore. The patient in our test case was employed in one such high-risk occupation; he was a foreman in an iron foundry. Two less obvious occupations with significant risk of exposure are welders and silver polishers. The high temperatures of electric arc or oxyacetylene torches produce large amounts of ferric oxide fumes, which can reach critical concentrations if the welding is performed in poorly ventilated areas such as tanks, boilers, or a ship's hold. "Jeweler's rouge" or "crocus" is a fine-powder abrasive made from ferric oxide. This powder is used with mechanical buffers to polish silver, glass, and cutlery.

Radiographic findings in siderosis are caused by focal deposits of the heavy metal in pulmonary tissues. Small, nodular opacities are the typical finding.[2,3,7,10] These opacities are diffusely distributed throughout the lung and may become strikingly dense over time despite their small size. This density is due to the high absorptive capacity of iron (atomic number 26). Occasionally, these nodular capacities are associated with faint linear opacities and Kerley B lines caused by deposition of iron in the pulmonary interstitium. The hilar lymph nodes may appear unusually dense due to their iron content, but they are rarely enlarged.[10] Lengthy exposures are required for these classic appearances to occur; however, there have been reports of radiographic abnormalities developing within 3 years when high concentrations of dust were involved. One interesting feature of this form of pneumoconiosis is the tendency for partial or complete resolution of radiographic abnormality after the patient leaves the source of exposure.[10]

Pathologically, peribronchial/perivascular aggregations of dark-pigmented iron oxide particles are found. Alveolar macrophages with intracellular particles may be found within the alveolar lumen. Typically, no fibrosis is present and very little distortion of the normal lung architecture occurs.[5]

The patient in our test case offers an excellent opportunity to correlate the radiologic and pathologic findings in siderosis. At autopsy, the lungs were fixed in an inflated state, sectioned, and radiographed (Figure 34-16). Prominent radiodense cuffs were noted about the small bronchioles. The normal architecture was disturbed very little, and only in the posterior segment of the upper lobe was there any evidence of fibrosis. This fibrosis was due to concomitant, mild silicosis. The peribronchiolar location of the abnormal density in the specimen radiograph is consistent with the histologic distribution observed in other cases of siderosis (Figures 34-17 to 34-19). Other heavy metals, such as tin (Figures 34-20 and 34-21), antimony, barium, and aluminum, may also be deposited in the lung.

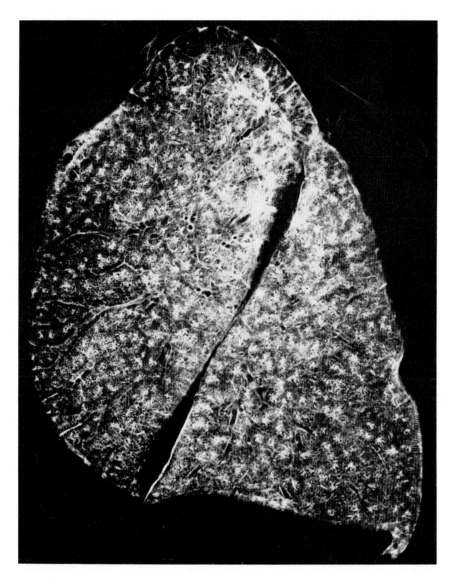

Figure 34-16. A radiograph of a section of the fixed inflated lung from the patient with siderosis shows very little architectural distortion. Note radiodense cuffs around bronchioles visible in the middle of the figure. See the text for further discussion. (Reprinted with permission. AFIP neg. 78-69032.)

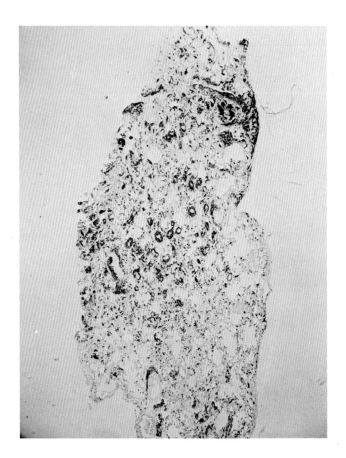

Figure 34-17. On a low-power photomicrograph of a siderotic lung, the absence of fibrosis or tissue distortion may be noted. (Reprinted with permission. AFIP neg. 76-7509.)

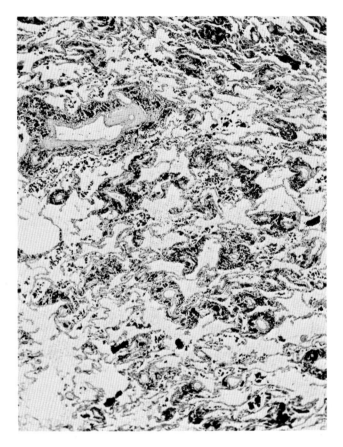

Figure 34-18. A higher-power photomicrograph of the siderotic lung shown in Figure 34-17 demonstrates the peribronchiolar/perivascular distribution of the black iron pigment in siderosis. (Reprinted with permission. AFIP neg. 76-7509.)

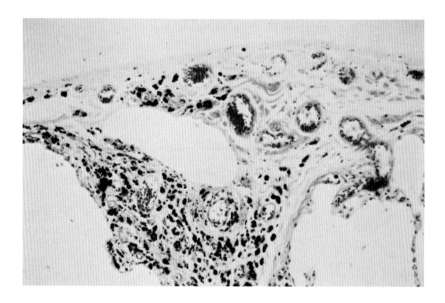

Figure 34-19. A peripheral section of the lung at the junction of an interlobular septum with the visceral pleura (top of figure) shows black iron deposited in the interlobular septum. (Reprinted with permission. AFIP neg. 78-1076.)

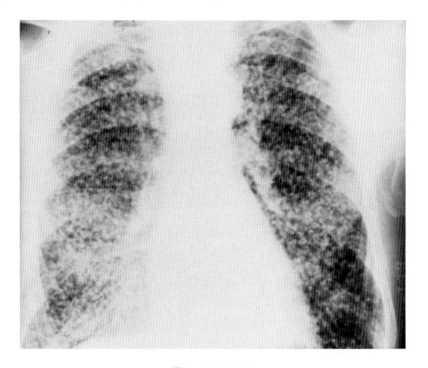

Figure 34-20
Figures 34-20 and 34-21. Stannosis. Tin is another heavy metal that
may produce a "benign" or "inert" pneumoconiosis. Note the radiographic
appearance on the posteroanterior view (Figure 34-20) and on a close-up
of the left lung from the same view (Figure 34-21). Again, these nodules
have a peribronchiolar distribution. (Reprinted with permission. AFIP
neg. 75-620.)

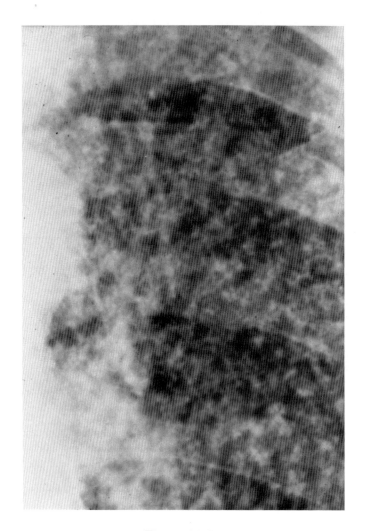

Figure 34-21

SUGGESTED READINGS

1. Brooks SM. Lung disorders resulting from the inhalation of metals. Clin Chest Med 1981; 2:235–254
2. Charr R. Pulmonary changes in welders, a report of three cases. Ann Intern Med 1956; 44:806–812
3. Doig AT, McLaughlin AIG. X-ray appearance of lung of electric arc welders. Lancet 1936; 1:771–775
4. Guidelines for the use of the ILO international classification of radiographs of pneumoconioses, no. 22, rev ed. Occupational Safety and Health Series. Geneva: International Labor Organisation; 1980:1–48
5. Katzenstein A, Askin FB. Surgical pathology of non-neoplastic lung disease. Philadelphia: WB Saunders; 1982:73–107
6. Lapp NL. Lung disease secondary to inhalation of nonfibrous minerals. Clin Chest Med 1981; 2:219–233
7. McLaughlin AI, Grout JL, Barre HJ, Harding HE. Iron oxide dust and the lungs of silver finishers. Lancet 1945; 1:337–341
8. Morgan WK, Seaton A. Occupational lung diseases, 2nd ed. Philadelphia: WB Saunders; 1984:250–294
9. Murray JF. The normal lung. The basis for the diagnosis and treatment of pulmonary disease, 2nd ed. Philadelphia: WB Saunders; 1986:43–50
10. Parkes WR. Occupational lung disorders. London: Butterworths; 1982:113–116
11. Spencer H. Pathology of the lung. Oxford: Pergamon Press; 1977:371–462

Index

Where there are multiple page references, **boldface** indicates the main discussion of a topic.

Adenopathy *(continued)*
  nontuberculous mycobacterial infection, 461
  Pneumocystis carinii pneumonia, 459
  primary tuberculosis, 269–70, 277
  sarcoidosis, 423–24
  siderosis, 623
  thoracic amyloidosis, 106
 inflammatory, granulomatous, 38
 intrathoracic
  AIDS-related complex (ARC), 459, 462
  non-Hodgkin lymphoma, 462
 ipsilateral, in granulomatous infections, 277
 lupus erythematosus, 518
 mesenteric, in lymphoma, 215
 methotrexate-induced, 109
 paratracheal, in sarcoidosis, 37, 423–24
 pneumocystis pneumonia and, 260
 retroperitoneal
  invasive thymoma, 216
  lymphoma, 215, 557
 subcarinal, 3, **5–6**
  differential diagnosis
   bronchogenic cyst, 3, **15–19**
   in pulmonary arterial hypertension, 417
   in sarcoidosis, 423–24
 see also Lymph node(s)
Adenovirus, Swyer-James syndrome, 166
Adriamycin (Doxorubicin) toxicity
 cardiotoxicity, 251, **254–55**
 radiation pneumonitis reactivation by, 202
AIDS. *See* Acquired immunodeficiency syndrome
AIDS-related complex (ARC), 459
Air
 extra-alveolar, in pneumocystis pneumonia, 260
 pulmonary artery (*see* Pulmonary artery air)
Air bronchogram
 alveolar disease, 73
 alveolar sarcoidosis, 72
 bilateral pneumothorax, 154
 interstitial emphysema, simulated by, 291
 Pneumocystis carinii pneumonia, 455
 Streptococcus pneumoniae, 263
Air collection, subphrenic, and postoperative pleural effusion, 379

Air cyst. *See* Cyst(s), air
Air embolism
 arterial, 297
 venous, 286, **287–309**
Air trapping
 carcinoid bronchial adenoma, 395
 hypogammaglobulinemia, 23
 laryngotracheal papillomatosis, 343
Air-space disease
 acute, 75–77
 in Legionnaires' disease, 259, 265
 pneumocystis pneumonia, 260
 pneumonia, 277
 see also Alveolar disease
Alcoholism
 hepatic hydrothorax cause, 404
 pneumococcal pneumonia and, 261
Alpha-1-antiprotease inhibitor, emphysema and, 173
Alpha-1-antitrypsin deficiency, 151, **157**, 166, 167, **173–74**, 313, **316**
 differential diagnosis
  cysts, giant bullous, 151, **154–55**, **157–63**, 166
  emphysema with pulmonary edema, **313–14**, 328, **331–33**
Aluminum inhalation, siderosis due to, 624
Alveolar cell carcinoma. *See* Carcinoma, bronchioloalveolar cell
Alveolar disease
 acute, hemorrhage in, 75–77
 interstitial lung disease simulating, 67, **72–73**
 see also Air-space disease
Alveolar formation, postpneumonectomy, 138, **141–42**
Alveolar hemorrhage syndromes, 75–77
Alveolar microlithiasis. *See under* Microlithiasis
Alveolar proteinosis. *See* Proteinosis, pulmonary alveolar
Alveolar silicolipoproteinosis, 62
Alveolitis
 drug-induced, 108, 109
 Pneumocystis carinii pneumonia and, 460
Aminorex fumarate, primary pulmonary arterial hypertension due to, 422
Amiodarone toxicity, 235, **236–40**
 differential diagnosis
  aspiration pneumonia, 235, **236**
  congestive heart failure, 235, 236, 238
  digitalis toxicity, 235–36

Arthritis *(continued)*
  rheumatoid
    and rheumatoid lung, 235, **241–42**
    vs. eosinophilic granuloma, 563
  systemic lupus erythematosus, 244
Asbestos exposure
  malignant mesothelioma due to, 402, 594, 595
  rounded atelectasis due to, 502, 503, 504
Asbestosis, 61, 563, **564**, 609
  differential diagnosis
    eosinophilic granuloma, 563, **568, 571–77**
    siderosis, 609, **614–15, 623–24**
Ascites
  in Meigs' syndrome, 403
  pleural effusion due to, 378
  with cirrhosis, in hepatic hydrothorax, 403–4
Aspergilloma, 63
Aspergillosis
  AIDS secondary infection, 459
  allergic bronchopulmonary, 60, **62**, 63
    complication of cystic fibrosis, 516
    peripheral eosinophilia/wheezing in, 570
  alveolar proteinosis secondary infection, 78
  disseminated, 63
  invasive primary/secondary, 62
  saprophytic, noninvasive, 60, **62**, 63
  semi-invasive, 57, 60, **62–63**
    differential diagnosis
      collagen vascular disease, 57, 64
Aspergillus fumigatus mycetoma (fungus ball), 60
Aspergillus sp.
  alveolar proteinosis secondary infection, 466
  ankylosing spondylitis secondary infection, 64
  empyema, 145
  infectious pneumonia, 101
Aspiration
  blood, pulmonary hemorrhage due to, 75
  lung abscess due to, 489
  massive, and amniotic fluid embolization, 300
  of food particles, parenchymal disease due to, 126
  of foreign body, and wheezing, 332
  of gastric contents, basilar pneumonitis due to, 356

Aspiration *(continued)*
  of nasal regurgitation, in polymyositis, 247
  pneumonia *(see under* Pneumonia)
  pulmonary hemorrhage due to, 244
Asthma
  and allergic bronchopulmonary aspergillosis, 62
  and pneumothorax, 290–91
  atypical, and endobronchial lesion, 42–43
  clinical definition, 332
  diaphragmatic fatigue due to, 530
  eosinophilic pneumonia, chronic, and, 455
  misdiagnosis
    of malignant tracheal tumor, 480
    of postintubation tracheal lesion, 353
Astrocytoma, and central neurofibromatosis, 88
Atelectasis
  associated with
    adult respiratory distress syndrome, 323
    alveolar proteinosis, 78
    carcinoid bronchial adenoma, 395
    cystic fibrosis, 516, 565
    immotile cilia syndrome, 26
    pulmonary sling, 475
    subphrenic abscess, 378, **379**
    systemic lupus erythematosus, 244
    tracheal tumor, 481
    venous air embolism, 287
  basilar, in systemic lupus erythematosus, 244
  bilateral lower lobe, 151, **154**
    differential diagnosis
      giant bullous cysts, 151, **154–55, 157–63**, 166
  cicatrization, in atypical mycobacterial disease, 457–58
  lobar, in thoracic amyloidosis, 106
  lower lobe, following coronary artery surgery, 375, **378**
  paralyzed hemidiaphragm and, 529
  right lung, 401, 402
    differential diagnosis
      hepatic hydrothorax, 401, **403–4**
  rounded, 497, **502, 503–4**, 591, 592
    differential diagnosis
      bronchogenic carcinoma, 497, **500–501**
      cryptococcal granuloma, 497

Atelectasis *(continued)*
  fibrous mesothelioma, localized, 591, 592, **594–97**
  organized pulmonary infarct, 497
  plasma cell granuloma, 497, **502–3**
  subsegmental, and diaphragmatic rupture, 534
Atopy, and chronic eosinophilic pneumonia, 455
Atrial septal defect, 429, **430–32**, **433**
  differential diagnosis
    pulmonary thromboembolism, 429, **434–36**
  double aortic arch and, 477
Atrioventricular conduction disturbance, in digitalis toxicity, 236
Atrioventricularis communis, of ostium primum defect, 430–31
Azotemia, due to Wegener's granulomatosis, 491
Azygos vein, dilated, and tricuspid insufficiency, 407, 408, **414**

Bacterial pneumonia, acute, 261, **277–83**
Bactrim. *See* Trimethoprim/sulfamethoxazole
Balloon embolotherapy, of pulmonary arteriovenous malformation, 397, **398**
Barium (metal) inhalation, siderosis due to, 624
Barotrauma, ventilator-induced, 288, **290–93**
Behcet's disease, sulfonamide-induced, 253
Black pleura sign, in metastatic pulmonary calcification, 547
Blastomyces dermatitidis
  blastomycosis, 216–18, 261
  empyema, 145
Blastomycosis, 215, **216–18**, 259, **260–61**
  differential diagnosis
    Legionnaires' disease, 259, **261–64**, **265–66**
Bleb rupture, pneumothorax due to, 290
Bleeding
  amniotic fluid embolization and, 299
  gastrointestinal, diaphragmatic rupture and, 534
Blood
  aspiration, pulmonary hemorrhage due to, 75
  extravascular collection, stages of evolution, 379–82

Blood *(continued)*
  transfusion, and AIDS, 458
Bone
  abnormalities, rhinoscleroma, 355
  bowing of, with pseudoarthroses, in peripheral neurofibromatosis, 90
  destruction, due to metastatic carcinoma, 553
  long/pelvic, fractures, fat embolism syndrome cause, 300
  see also specific type or location
Bowel
  involvement, in lymphoma, 215
  obstruction, due to diaphragmatic rupture, 534
Bradycardia, in Legionnaires' disease, 262
Brain abscess. *See* Abscess, brain; Dementia; Encephalopathy
Breast carcinoma. *See under* Carcinoma
Bronchial adenoma, 42, 480
Bronchial tumor, 480, 481
Bronchial wall thickening, in
  cystic fibrosis, 565
  hypogammaglobulinemia, 23
  immotile cilia syndrome, 26
Bronchiectasis
  cystic fibrosis, 565
  hypogammaglobulinemia, 23
  immotile cilia syndrome, 26
  Kartagener syndrome, 23
  Mounier-Kuhn syndrome and, 354
  proximal, in allergic bronchopulmonary aspergillosis, 62
  sickle cell disease and, 511, 516
  tracheobronchomegaly and, 21, **31**
  upper lobe, hemoptysis secondary to, 60
Bronchiolectasis, secondary to tracheobronchomegaly, 31
Bronchiolitis, obliterative, in Swyer-James syndrome, 154, 166, 333
Bronchioloalveolar cell carcinoma. *See under* Carcinoma
Bronchitis
  bullous disease and, 160
  chronic
    acquired diverticula in, 32
    centriacinar emphysema and, 331
    clinical definition, 331, 332
    diaphragmatic fatigue and, 530
    tracheobronchomegaly and, 31
  in alpha-1-antitrypsin deficiency, 316
  Mounier-Kuhn syndrome and, 354
  recurrent, in hypogammoglobulinemia, 23

Bronchitis *(continued)*
vs. alveolar edema, 313
Bronchoesophageal fistula. *See under* Fistula
Bronchogenic carcinoma. *See under* Carcinoma
Bronchogenic cyst. *See under* Cyst(s)
Bronchopleural fistula. *See under* Fistula
Bronchopneumonia
and bacterial pneumonia, 277
and influenza, 279
recurrent, cystic fibrosis causing, 516
Bronchopulmonary foregut malformation, 6–7
Bronchopulmonary sequestration, 6–7
Bulla(e)
formation, in atypical mycobacterial infection, 465
in ankylosing spondylitis, 64
infected, 485, **492–93**
differential diagnosis
anaerobic lung abscess, 485, **489–91, 493**
empyema, 485, **489–91, 493**
tuberculosis, 485
Wegener's granulomatosis, 485, **491–92**
paramediastinal, 287, **288**
differential diagnosis
pulmonary artery air, 287–88
peripheral
as form of paraseptal emphysema, 332
rupture, pneumothorax due to, 290
Bullous cyst, giant. *See under* Cyst(s)
Busulfan (Myleran)
lung toxicity, in leukemia, **108–9**, 110–12
potentiates effects of radiotherapy, 202

Calcification
anterior mediastinal masses, 18
aortic wall, atherosclerotic, 17–18
atrial myxoma, 584
atrial thrombus, 584–85
bronchogenic carcinoma, 500
coal worker's pneumoconiosis, 616–18
dystrophic
bronchogenic carcinoma, 500
pulmonary, 553, 559, 560
eggshell, of sarcoidosis/silicosis, 423, **424**
localized fibrous mesothelioma, 596
lymph node, 15, **16**, **17–18**, 37, 38, 106
malignant bronchial adenoma, 394, **395**

Calcification *(continued)*
metastatic, pulmonary, 545, **553–60**
bilateral apical opacity pattern, 545, **553–60**
calcified nodules pattern, 559–60
differential diagnosis
alveolar microlithiasis, 545, **546–47**
idiopathic pulmonary ossification, 545–46, **552**
mucinous adenocarcinoma of stomach, 545, **547**
tuberculosis, 545, **547**
diffuse alveolar pattern, 559
neuroblastoma, 93
neurogenic tumors, 15, 91–92, 93
plasma cell granuloma, 502
primary carcinoma, at hilum, 46
pulmonary nodule, 16
rounded atelectasis, 502
spleen, in sickle cell disease, 511, 512
thoracic amyloidosis, 106
thymoma, 449
tracheal stenosis, 351
tracheopathia osteochondroplastica, 29
Calcium therapy, intravenous, and metastatic pulmonary calcification, 553
Candida sp.
candidiasis, 216
costochondral junction infection, 211
infectious pneumonia, 101, 211
sternal osteomyelitis infection, 211
Candidiasis, 207, **211**, **215–16**
alveolar proteinosis secondary infection, 78
differential diagnosis
lymphoma, 207, **211–12**, 215
esophageal, acquired bronchoesophageal fistula cause, 143
Capillary block, alveolar, in alveolar proteinosis, 77
Capillary permeability increase
adult respiratory distress syndrome due to, 316, 319, **323**, 324
edema formation and, 324
endothelial cell injury causing, 323, 324
fat embolism syndrome causing, 300
oil embolism causing, 304
venous air embolization causing, 297
Capillary wall injury, and systemic vasculitis, 77
Capillary wedge pressure. *See* Pulmonary capillary wedge pressure

Cardiomyopathy *(continued)*
  adriamycin-induced, 255
  congestive, and AIDS, 464
Cardiopulmonary disease, pneumococcal
    pneumonia and, 264
Cardiopulmonary insufficiency, amniotic
    fluid embolization causing, 300
Cardiopulmonary surgery, complications
    following, 375–78, 382–84
Cardiotoxicity, adriamycin-induced, 254–
    55
Cardiovascular defects, congenital, and
    Hughes-Stovin syndrome, 419
Cardiovascular effects, of monitoring/
    support device use, 306–9
Cardiovascular rhythm disturbance, digi-
    talis-induced, 236
Carotid artery stenosis, radiotherapy-
    induced, 201
Catecholamine production, in thoracic
    pheochromocytoma, 84, 94
Catheter positioning, complications of,
    306–9
Catheterization
  extrapulmonary air after, 287–88
  venous air embolism after, 287–88, 297
Cavity/cavitation
  adenocarcinoma, 500
  alveolar proteinosis, 78
  amyloid pulmonary nodules, 106
  atypical mycobacterial disease, 457
  blastomycosis, 261
  bronchogenic carcinoma, 500
  cavity wall thickness, differentiates be-
    nign/malignant disease, 486
  eosinophilic granuloma, 576
  intracavitary mycetoma and, 60, 62–63
  large-scale carcinoma, 500
  laryngotracheal papillomatosis, 343
  Legionnaires' disease, 265
  lung abscess, 485, 489
  Mycobacterium avium-intracellulare in-
    fection, in AIDS, 462
  Pittsburgh pneumonia, 266
  plasma cell granuloma, 502
  pneumocystis pneumonia, 260
  rheumatoid arthritis, 242
  semi-invasive aspergillosis and, 62–63
  silicosis, 61
  squamous cell carcinoma, 500
  systemic lupus erythematosus, 244
  tuberculosis, 61, 270, 485
  Wegener's granulomatosis, 485, 491
Cells, capillary endothelial, injury

Cells *(continued)*
  from leukemic drug therapy, 108
  in adult respiratory distress syndrome,
    323
Cellular immunity defect, in leukemia
    patient, 101
Central venous pressure (CVP) catheter
  technique, 306
  venous air embolism due to, 287–88
Chemotherapy
  antileukemic, 97–98, **108–15**
  concomitant, potentiates effects of ra-
    diotherapy, 109, 202
  mediastinal carcinoma, complicated by
    tracheoesophageal fistula, 356
  toxicity, **254–55**, 396
Chest drainage tube, placement/technique,
    363–68, 375
Chest pain
  acute, due to pneumothorax, in eosino-
    philic granuloma, 568, 574
  pleuritic
    in radiation pneumonitis, 201
    infected bullae and, 492
    Wegener's granulomatosis and, 491
  Pneumocystis carinii pneumonia, 259
  pneumonitis, drug-induced, 251
  venous air embolization causing, 297
Chest wall involvement
  lymphoma, 211–12
  malignant mesothelioma, 209, 218, **221**
  open wound, pneumothorax due to, 290
  thymoma, 211
Chickenpox, and adenopathy, 277
Childbirth
  amniotic fluid embolization and, 299–
    300
  pleural effusion after, 378
  venous air embolism due to, 297
Chill(s)
  acute pneumonitis, drug-induced, 251
  amiodarone toxicity causing, 235
  infected bullae and, 493
  oil embolism causing, 304
  recurrent, in Legionnaires' disease, 262
  single shaking, in pneumococcal pneu-
    monia, 262
Chlorambucil-induced lung disease, 108
Chlorpromazine, antinuclear antibodies
    due to, 246
Chlorpropamide-induced toxicity, 253
Chondrosarcoma, vs. malignant tracheal
    tumor, 481

Crocidolite asbestos, and malignant meso-
thelioma, 402
Cromolyn sulfate-induced toxicity, 253
Cryptococcosis
    AIDS secondary infection, 459
    alveolar proteinosis secondary infection,
        78
Cryptococcus, alveolar proteinosis sec-
    ondary infection, 466
Cryptococcus neoformans empyema, 145
Cushing's syndrome, carcinoid thymus
    gland associated with, 450
Cutis laxa, tracheal widening in, 32, 343
Cyanosis
    amniotic fluid embolization causing,
        299
    and dyspnea, of pulmonary veno-
        occlusive disease, 585
    and trilogy of Fallot, 421
Cyclophosphamide
    lung toxicity due to, 108
    potentiates radiotherapy effects, 202
Cylindroma. (*See* Adenoid cystic carci-
    noma)
Cystic air spaces, in cystic fibrosis, 516
Cystic disease, fibrobullous, upper lobe, 60
Cystic fibrosis, 511, **515–16**, 563, **564–65**
    differential diagnosis
        eosinophilic granuloma, 563, **568,**
            571–77
        sickle cell disease, 511, **515**, **519–20**
Cyst(s)
    air, round or oval
        interstitial emphysema and, 291
        /postinfectious pneumatocele differen-
            tiation, 291
        subpulmonic pneumothorax mimic,
            291
    bronchogenic, 3, **5–19**, 471
        and bronchogenic carcinoma, 5
        differential diagnosis
            achalasia, esophageal, 3, **4–5**
            adenopathy, subcarinal, 3, **5–6**
            aneurysm, aortic, 3–4, **17–18**
            childhood respiratory illness,
                acute/chronic, 17
            teratoma, 3
            tracheal neoplasm, 471, **476**, **480–
                82**
        /esophageal cyst, distinguished, 10–
            13
        hilar, 10
        lung, 6
        mediastinal, 6, **7–10**, 11, **12–13**

Cyst(s) *(continued)*
    paraesophageal, 10
    paratracheal, 10
    parenchymal, **7–10**, 11
    duplication, as non-neurogenic mass, 94
    enteric, 13
    esophageal, 6
        /bronchogenic cyst, distinguished, 10–
            13
    foregut (*see* Cyst(s), bronchogenic)
    gastroenteric, 6
    giant bullous, 151, **154–55**, **157–63**, 166
        differential diagnosis
            alpha-1-antitrypsin deficiency,
                151, **157**, 166, 167, **173–74**
            atelectasis, bilateral lower lobe,
                151, **154**
            pneumothorax, bilateral, **151–54**,
                155, **160–61**
            Swyer-James syndrome, 151, **154,**
                166
    in ankylosing spondylitis, 64
    intradural, spinal cord, 84
    mediastinal, 6, **7–10**, 11, **12–13**
    neurenteric, 83–84
        bronchogenic cyst and, 12
        differential diagnosis
            lateral meningocele, 83, **92–93**
            neurofibroma, 83, 86, 87, 88, 90,
                91–92
    residual, and intracavitary mycetoma,
        60
Cytomegalovirus pneumonia, 459, 461
Cytosine-arabinoside-induced lung dis-
    ease, 108

Da Nang lung, 319
Dactinomycin, potentiates radiotherapy
    effects, 202
Daunorubicin cardiotoxicity, 108, **109–11**
Dehiscence, sternal, postoperative, 375,
    377–78
Dementia, AIDS, 459
Dermatomyositis
    /polymyositis, 241, **246–49**
    vs. eosinophilic granuloma, 563
Dermatomyositis/polymositis, 241, **246–49**
Diabetes insipidus, and eosinophilic
    granuloma, 574
Diabetes mellitus, and semi-invasive pul-
    monary aspergillosis, 63
Dialysis
    peritoneal, hepatic hydrothorax cause,
        404

Erythrocyte *(continued)*
    in nitrofurantoin-induced interstitial fibrosis, 252
    in postpericardiotomy syndrome, 384
Escherichia coli
    aerobic gram-negative pneumonia, 279
Esophagopleural fistula. *See under* Fistula
Esophagus
    achalasia, 3, **4–5**
        differential diagnosis
            bronchogenic cyst, 3, **15–19**
            /esophageal carcinoma, distinguished, 5
    carcinoma (*see under* Carcinoma)
    cyst (*see* Cyst(s), esophagus)
    dilatation, bronchoesophageal fistula due to, 143
    dilated
        bronchoesophageal fistula due to, 143
        in scleroderma, 246
    diverticula, 6–7
    leiomyoma of, 471
        differential diagnosis
            tracheal neoplasm, 471, **476**, **480–82**
    rupture
        complication of Sengstaken-Blakemore tubes, 356–58
        pulmonary ligament air due to, 288
    tumor, primary, and tracheal invasion, 481
Eventration, of hemidiaphragm. *See under* Hemidiaphragm

Fallot trilogy
    /Fallot tetralogy, distinguished, 420, **421**
    /pulmonic valvular stenosis, distinguished, 420, **421**
Farmer's lung
    acute, 563, **565–66**, **570–71**
        differential diagnosis
            eosinophilic granuloma, 563, **568**, **571–77**
Fat, brown, of hibernoma, 594
Fat embolism syndrome, 297, **300**
    vs. *Pneumocystis carinii* pneumonia, 455
Fetal death, intrauterine, amniotic fluid embolization due to, 299
Fever
    acute pneumonitis, 251
    AIDS, 459
    alveolar proteinosis secondary infection, 78

Fever *(continued)*
    amiodarone toxicity, 236
    antineoplastic drug toxicity, 108, 109
    bronchopleural fistula, 121
    chronic eosinophilic pneumonia, 455
    eosinophilic granuloma, 574
    high
        in Legionnaires' disease, 262
        in pneumococcal pneumonia, 262
    infected bullae, 493
    low-grade, in blastomycosis, 261
    lupus erythematosus, 76
    methysergide-induced, 253
    oil embolism causing, 304
    Pneumocystis carinii pneumonia, 259
    postpericardiotomy syndrome, 384
    pulmonary hemorrhage, in leukemic patient, 99
    radiation pneumonitis, 201
Fibroma
    benign ovarian, in Meigs' syndrome, 403
    subpleural (benign mesothelioma), 595
Fibrosis
    basilar interstitial
        scleroderma and, 246
        systemic lupus erythematosus and, 244
    cystic (*see* Cystic fibrosis)
    interalveolar, and ankylosing spondylitis, 64
    interstitial
        idiopathic pulmonary ossification and, 552
        in alveolar proteinosis, 78
        in rheumatoid lung, 235
        in scleroderma, 241, **246**
        nitrofurantoin-induced, 251–53
        pulmonary hemorrhage, 75, 76
    pulmonary
        antineoplastic drugs causing, 98, 101, **108–15**, 238
        bronchioloalveolar cell carcinoma and, 246
        end-stage
            in eosinophilic granuloma, 576
            in farmer's lung, 570–71
        Hamman-Rich, 246
        hypogammaglobulinemia and, 23
        in silicosis, 61, 614–15, 624
        miliary tuberculosis mimicked by, 242
        Mounier-Kuhn syndrome and, 354
        nitrofurantoin-induced, 251
        rheumatoid arthritis and, 242

Fibrosis *(continued)*
    tracheobronchomegaly and, 31
    radiation, **185–90**, 202
        /recurrent neoplasm, distinguished, 190–94
        semi-invasive pulmonary aspergillosis and, 63
    secondary to impaired respiratory mechanism of ankylosing spondylitis, 64
    terminal bronchiole, in Swyer-James syndrome, 166
Fibrothorax, tuberculosis and, 272, 274
Fistula
    bronchoesophageal, postpneumonectomy, 119, **125–26**, 135
    acquired, 143–44
    differential diagnosis
        empyema, 119, 121, **125–26, 128–29, 135–36, 145**
        recurrent carcinoma, 119, 121, 126, **130, 143–44**
    /lung abscess, distinguished, 369–70
    bronchopleural
        rheumatoid arthritis and, 242
        tuberculous, 272
    bronchopleural, postpneumonectomy, 119, 120, **121–25**, 126, **128–29**, 135
    differential diagnosis
        empyema, 119, 121, **125–26, 128–29, 135–36, 145**
        recurrent carcinoma, 119, 121, 126, **130, 135–36, 143–44**
    esophagopleural, postpneumonectomy, **125**, 135
    associated with
        bronchoesophageal fistula, 125–28
        empyema, 125–26, 128–29
        recurrent carcinoma, 126
    formation, venous air embolism due to, 297
    hemoptysis surgery complicated by, 64
    patent, spinal cord, and neurenteric cyst, 84
    tracheoesophageal, 143, 337, 343, **356–59**
    differential diagnosis
        postintubation tracheal stenosis, 337–40, 351–53
Fixed splitting of second heart sound, in atrial septal defect, 430, **431**
Fluid collection
    loculated

Fluid collection *(continued)*
    post-thoracotomy, 363, 365, 366, 369
    resorption of, 593
    parapneumonic, due to cystic fibrosis, 516
    post-thoracotomy
        extrapleural, 363, 365
        in anterior mediastinum, 362, **363–84**
        in major fissure, 363–68
Focal dust emphysema, 167
Folded lung. *See* Atelectasis, rounded
Foramen, enlarged
    intervertebral, and intraspinal lesion extension, 92, 93
    neural, and intraspinal lesion extension, 92
Forced expiratory volume (FEV)
    and tracheal function, 351, **352–53**
    postpneumonectomy, 138, **142–43**
Foregut cyst. *See* Cyst(s), bronchogenic
Fracture, long/pelvic bone, fat embolism syndrome due to, 300
Fungus ball. *See* Mycetoma
Fungus infection
    alveolar proteinosis secondary infection, 78
    chronic, alveolar pattern in, 67
    granulomatous infection due to, 60
    infectious pneumonia due to, 101
    pulmonary hemorrhage due to, 75
Furadantin. *See* Nitrofurantoin

Ganglioneuroblastoma, 91, 94
Ganglioneuroma, 86, 87, 91, **93**
Ganglionic tumor, 91–94
Gastric diverticula, 6–7
Gastroenteric cyst, 6
Gastrointestinal perforation, and pneumoperitoneum, 293
Ghon lesion, in primary tuberculosis, 269
Gingivitis, chronic mercurialism causing, 300
Glomerulitis, in Goodpasture syndrome, 76
Glomerulonephritis
    Goodpasture syndrome and, 76, 77
    lupus erythematosus and, 77
Goodpasture syndrome (anti-basement membrane antibody disease), 75–76
Gram-negative bacillus
    aerobic/anaerobic, empyema cause, 128, 145
    alveolar proteinosis, 78
    pneumonia, 98, 101, 459

Gram-positive bacillus
  aerobic/anaerobic, empyema cause, 128, 145
  pneumonia, 101
Granuloma
  caseating/noncaseating, 423
  cryptococcal, 497
    differential diagnosis
      rounded atelectasis, 497, **502, 503–4**
  eosinophilic, 563, **568, 571–77**
    differential diagnosis
      acute farmer's lung, 563, **565–66, 570–71**
      asbestosis, 563, **564**
      collagen vascular disease, 563–64
      cystic fibrosis, 563, **564–65**
  mediastinal, bronchoesophageal fistula cause, 143
  methotrexate toxicity in leukemia causing, 109
  plasma cell, 497, **502–3**
    differential diagnosis
      rounded atelectasis, 497, **502, 503–4**
    see also Pseudotumor, inflammatory
Granulomatosis
  lymphomatoid, and malignant lymphoma, 492
  Wegener's, 143, 485, **491–92**
    differential diagnosis
      infected bulla, 485, **492–93**
Granulomatous infection, 277, 511
  and tracheal mass/stenosis, 481
  differential diagnosis
    adenopathy and parenchymal disease, 277
    sickle cell disease, 511, **515, 519–20**
  hilar adenopathy due to, 38
  pulmonary hemorrhage due to, 75
  systemic, sarcoidosis as, 423–25
  upper-lobe fibrobullous cystic changes due to, 60
Gravitational shift test, for lung water detection, 324, **326–29**
Gynecomastia, in digitalis toxicity, 236

Haemophilus influenzae pneumonia, 519
Hair-spray pneumonia, 67
Hamman-Rich pulmonary fibrosis, and scleroderma, 246
Hand-Schüller-Christian disease, 571
Headache
  AIDS, 459
  intrathoracic pheochromocytoma, 84

Headache *(continued)*
  prodromal, in methotrexate toxicity, 109
Head/neck surgery, aspiration pneumonia due to, 236
Heart disease, congestive, pneumococcal pneumonia and, 261
Heart failure, congestive, 235, 236, 238, 332, 333, 384
  adriamycin-induced, 255
  AIDS and, 464
  atrial septal defect causing, 431
  azygos vein dilatation and, 414
  basilar interstitial infiltration mimicking, 106
  cardiomegaly mimicking, 106
  chronic, **429–30**, 431, 432, 433
    differential diagnosis
      pulmonary thromboembolism, 429, **434–36**
  complication in daunorubicin cardiotoxicity, 109–11
  differential diagnosis
    amiodarone toxicity, 235, **236–40**
    postpericardiotomy syndrome, 384
  intra-aortic counter-pulsation balloon support, 307
  Libman-Sacks endocarditis of lupus erythematosus and, 518
  lung infiltrates, in leukemia patients, due to, 98
  pleural effusion due to, and rounded atelectasis, 503
  pneumothorax causing, 325–26
  postoperative effusion due to, 379
  pulmonary edema due to, 244, 73
  pulmonary hemorrhage due to, 75, 244
  right, complication in idiopathic pulmonary hemorrhage, 76
  sickle cell disease and, 520
  ventricular septal defect causing, 432
  with pulmonary edema complicating emphysema, **313–14**, 328, **331–33**
Hematogenous dissemination, empyema due to, 128–29
Hematologic malignancy
  alveolar proteinosis and, 78, 466
  and lymphoma, alveolar proteinosis associated with, 466
  Pneumocystis carinii lung infection and, 145
Hematoma, mediastinal
  postoperative effusion and, 381
  radiotherapy-induced, 200

Hilar enlargement *(continued)*
  associated diseases, 417
  see also Adenopathy
Hilum
  55° oblique tomography of, 34, **35–54**
  mass in malignant mesothelioma, 218,
    219
Histiocytoma. *See* Granuloma, plasma cell
Histiocytosis X, 571
Histoplasma capsulatum empyema, 145
Histoplasmosis
  acquired bronchoesophageal fistula
    cause, 143
  AIDS and, 459
  fibrosing mediastinitis and, 277
  hilar/mediastinal adenopathy of, 277
HLA-B27 histocompatibility antigen, in
    ankylosing spondylitis, 64
Hoarseness, due to malignant tracheal
    tumor, 480
Hodgkin/non-Hodgkin lymphoma. *See un-
    der* Lymphoma
Honeycomb lung. *See under* Lung
Hughes-Stovin syndrome, 417, **419**
  differential diagnosis
    pulmonary arterial hypertension,
      417–18, **421–22**
Human immunodeficiency virus (HIV),
    and AIDS, 458–59
Humoral hypercalcemia of malignancy,
    and metastatic pulmonary calcifi-
    cation, 553
Humoral immunity defect, in leukemia
    patient, 101
Hyaline-membrane formation, alveolar
    space, associated with
  adult respiratory distress syndrome, 323
  antileukemic chemotherapy, 108
  lupus erythematosus, 518
  radiotherapy injury, 187
Hydralazine, antinuclear antibodies due
    to, 246
Hydrostatic pressure, capillary, and edema
    formation, 324–28
Hydrothorax
  hepatic, 401, **403–4**
    differential diagnosis
      atelectasis of right lung, 401, 402
      Klebsiella pneumonia, 401
      malignant mesothelioma, 401, **402**
      Meigs' syndrome, 401, **403**
  unilateral pulmonary edema and, 324
Hypercalcemia, and metastatic pulmonary
    calcification, 553, 558, 559

Hyperinflation
  diaphragmatic fatigue due to, 530
  in alveolar proteinosis, 78
  in cystic fibrosis, 511, 516
  in immotile cilia syndrome, 26
  obstructive, in thoracic amyloidosis, 106
  postpneumonectomy, 138
Hypernephroma, metastatic/vascular
    structures, distinguished, 17
Hyperparathyroidism, and metastatic pul-
    monary calcification, 553
Hyperplasia
  thymic, 441, 447
    differential diagnosis
      anterior mediastinal thymoma,
        441, 447–48, **449–50**
Hypersalivation, chronic mercurialism
    causing, 300
Hypertension
  in intrathoracic pheochromocytoma, 84
  pulmonary
    idiopathic, and rheumatoid arthritis,
      242
    secondary to alpha-1-antitrypsin
      edema, 174
    vasculitis causing, 244
    venous air embolization causing, 297
  pulmonary arterial, 398, 417–18, **421–
    22**
    amniotic fluid embolization causing,
      299
    arteriovenous malformation, re-
      secting or embolizing, and, 398
    complication of sickle cell disease, 519
    differential diagnosis
      Hughes-Stovin syndrome, 417, **419**
      lymphoma, 417, 418
      pulmonic valvular stenosis, 417,
        418–19, **420–21**
      sarcoidosis, 417, 418, **423–25**
    in centriacinar emphysema, 331–32
    in polymyositis, 247–49
    in vasculitis, 246
    primary, **421–22**, 585
    pulmonary thromboembolism with,
      429, **434–35**
    pulmonary veno-occlusive disease
      and, 585, 587–88
  pulmonary venous, cor triatriatum and,
    582
Hyperventilation
  at rest, in alveolar proteinosis, 77
  in adult respiratory distress syndrome,
    319

Hypocarbia, in adult respiratory distress syndrome, 319
Hypogammaglobulinemia, 21, **23**
    acquired, associated with thymoma, 450
    differential diagnosis
        Mounier-Kuhn syndrome, 21, **31–33**
Hypoglycemia, and localized fibrous mesothelioma, 595–96
Hypoproteinemia, secondary to
    cardiopulmonary bypass, 376
    lupus nephrosis, 242
Hypotension
    after coronary artery surgery, 375
    venous air embolization causing, 297
Hypothermia, topical cardiac, diaphragm paresis due to, 375, **378**
Hypoventilation syndrome, congenital, paralyzed diaphragm and, 530
Hypovolemia. *See* Oligemia
Hypoxemia
    arterial, venous air embolization and, 299, 299
    pulmonary hemorrhage, in leukemia patients, due to, 99
Hypoxia
    adult respiratory distress syndrome, 319, 320, 322, 323
    chronic, and primary pulmonary arterial hypertension, 422
    fat embolism syndrome causing, 300

Idiopathic and immune disorders, 75–77
Idiopathic pulmonary hemorrhage, 75, **76**
Idiopathic pulmonary ossification. *See* Ossification, idiopathic pulmonary
Immotile cilia syndrome, 24–26
Immune defect, in leukemia patient
    cellular defect, 101
    humoral defect, 101
Immunocompromised host, associated diseases
        AIDS, 454, **455–65**
        hypogammaglobulinemia, 23
        invasive aspergillosis, 62
        Legionnaires' disease, 265
        leukemia, 101
            chemotherapy, 101, 108
        mediastinitis, 211
        semi-invasive aspergillosis, 63
        systemic lupus erythematosus, 244
Immunodeficiency-state infections
    Candida, 211, 216

Immunodeficiency *(continued)*
    Mycobacterium avium-intracellulare (MAI), 459, 462, 465
    Mycobacterium kansasii, 465
    Nocardia, 244
    Pneumocystis carinii, 145, 259, 455, **458–64**
    Pseudomonas aeruginosa, 279–80
    Toxoplasma gondii, 455
Infarct
    in sickle cell disease, 520
    organized pulmonary, 497
        differential diagnosis
            rounded atelectasis, 497, **502**, **503–4**
Infarction
    angina, and intra-aortic counterpulsation support, 307
    myocardial, 384
        acute, 429
            differential diagnosis
                pulmonary thromboembolism, 384, 429, **434–36**
    pulmonary
        lupus erythematosus with cavitary lesions due to, 244
        pleural effusion and rounded atelectasis due to, 503
        /pneumonia, in sickle cell disease, compared, 519–20
    pulmonary artery, due to wedging, 306–7
    syndrome, postmyocardial, pleural effusion due to
        and postpericardiotomy syndrome, 384
        and rounded atelectasis, 503
Infection(s)
    acute pulmonary hemorrhage due to, 244
    alveolar proteinosis complicated by, 78
    chronic recurrent, in hypogammaglobulinemia, 23
    lupus erythematosus, with cavitary lesions, due to, 244
    peripheral, pneumothorax due to, 290
    postoperative, vs. postpericardiotomy syndrome, 384
    prior, and idiopathic pulmonary ossification, 552
    tracheoesophageal fistula and, 343, 356
    tuberculosis, silicosis cavitation due to, 61
Infiltrates, pulmonary
    basilar, interstitial, congestive heart failure mimic, 106

Infiltrates *(continued)*
    complicating leukemia, 96, **97–115**
    cytotoxic, drug-induced, 115
    in alveolar proteinosis, 78
    in Goodpasture syndrome, 76
    reticular, in thoracic amyloidosis, 106
Inflammatory disease, postpneumonectomy empyema and, 128
Influenza
    adenopathy and, 277
    staphyloccocal infection following, 279
    virus, bronchiolitis/Swyer-James syndrome due to, 166
Injury
    alveolar, in leukemia, 99
    capillary wall, and systemic vasculitis with alveolar hemorrhage, 77
    pneumocyte, from antileukemic chemotherapy, 108
    pulmonary radiation, 180, **181–204**
    tracheal postintubation, 336, **337–40, 351–53**
    tracheoesophageal fistula due to, 356
    see also Trauma
Intercostal vein
    left superior, dilated, 407–8
        differential diagnosis
            aortic diverticulum, 407, 409, **410–11**
            ductus arteriosus, 407, 409
            lymph node, 407
            persistent left superior vena cava, 407–9
Interstitial fibrosis. *See under* Fibrosis
Interstitial infiltration, basilar, congestive heart failure mimic, 106
Interstitial lung disease
    diffuse bilateral, in pneumocystis pneumonia, 260
    diffuse, in amiodarone toxicity, 236
    in pneumococcal pneumonia, 263
    in polymyositis, 247
    in rheumatoid arthritis, 242
    in sytemic lupus erythematosus, 244
    simulating air-space disease, 67, **72–73**
    see also Fibrosis, pulmonary
Interstitial pneumonitis. *See under* Pneumonitis
Intra-aortic counter-pulsation balloon, technique, 307–9
Intradural cyst. *See under* Cyst(s)
Intubation
    endotracheal, acquired bronchoesophageal fistula cause, 143

Intubation *(continued)*
    postintubation tracheal stenosis *(see under* Stenosis, tracheal)
    prolonged, fistulas due to, 356
Iritis, in ankylosing spondylitis, 63
Iron oxide/metallic iron inhalation, siderosis due to, 614, 623–24
Irradiation, for carcinoma, bronchoesophageal fistula cause, 143
Ischemia
    intra-aortic counter pulsation balloon use causing, 308–9
    postpneumonectomy esophagopleural fistula related to, 126
    silicosis cavitation and, 61
Isoniazid, antinuclear antibodies due to, 246

Juxtaphrenic peak sign, and lower lobe atelectasis, 168, **170–72**

Kaposi's sarcoma, **458**, 459, **462**
Kartagener syndrome, 21, **23–26**
    differential diagnosis
        Mounier-Kuhn syndrome, 21, **32–33**
Kerley lines
    asymmetric pulmonary edema, 328
    interstitial edema, 73
    pulmonary veno-occlusive disease, 581, 583, 587–588
    siderosis, 623
Kidney
    atherosclerotic, small end-stage, and metastatic pulmonary calcification, 556–57
    involvement, in lymphoma, 215
    see also terms beginning with Renal
Klebsiella pneumonia, 401
    differential diagnosis
        hepatic hydrothorax, 401, **403–4**
Klebsiella rhinoscleromatis rhinoscleroma, 355
Kultschitzky cell neural crest, carcinoid tumor origin, 394–95
Kyphosis, in neurofibromatosis, 88

Labor (childbirth) amniotic fluid embolization cause, 299
Laceration, lung, pulmonary hemorrhage due to, 75
Langerhans histiocyte, of eosinophilic granuloma, 571
Laparotomy, pleural effusion after, 378
Large-cell carcinoma. *See under* Carcinoma

Lupus *(continued)*
    drug-induced, 236, 241, **242–46**
      table of drugs, 246, **247**
    non-drug-induced, 244
    vs. eosinophilic granuloma, 563
Lymph node(s), 407
  calcification (*see under* Calcification)
  differential diagnosis
    intercostal vein, left superior, dilated, 407–8
  enlarged
    AIDS-related complex, 459
    atypical mycobacterial infection and AIDS, 458
    human immunodeficiency virus infection, 459
    Kaposi's sarcoma, 462
    lupus erythematosus, 518
    non-Hodgkin lymphoma, 462
    Pneumocystis carinii pneumonia, 459
    /vascular structures, distinguished, **35–41**, 51–53
  granulomatous/neoplastic, distinguished, 16
  see also Adenopathy
Lymphadenopathy
  hilar enlargement due to, and arterial hypertension, 417
  sarcoidosis, 423–24
  see also Adenopathy
Lymphangiographic contrast medium, embolization of, 304
Lymphocytic interstitial pneumonia (LIP), and AIDS, 463
Lymphographic contrast material, causing alveolar hemorrhage syndrome, 77
Lymphoma, 207, **211–12**, **215**, 277, 417, 418
  adriamycin therapy, cardiotoxicity due to, 254–55
  and enlarged lymph nodes, as mediastinal mass, 17
  and hematologic malignancy, associated with alveolar proteinosis, 466
  and tracheal tumor, malignant, 481
  and Wegener's granulomatosis, 491, **492**
  bronchoesophageal fistula, acquired, due to, 143
  differential diagnosis
    adenopathy and parenchymal disease, 277
    candidiasis, 207, **211**, **215–16**

Lymphoma *(continued)*
    invasive thymoma, 207, **211**, 212, 215, **216**
    malignant mesothelioma, 207, **209–11**, **215**, **218–23**
    pulmonary arterial hypertension, 417–18, **421–22**
    thoracic actinomycosis, 207–9, **229–30**
  hilar adenopathy due to, 38
  Hodgkin, 211, 212, **215**, 387, 388, **396–97**
    differential diagnosis
      arteriovenous malformation, 387, **397–98**
      metastatic pulmonary calcification and, 557
  noncaseating granulomas in, 423
  non-Hodgkin, 211, **215**, 396, 462
  primary pulmonary, 67, **69**, **72–73**
    differential diagnosis
      alveolar proteinosis, 67, **74**, **77–78**
  radiotherapy, pulmonary injury due to, 181, **182**, 184, 199
  tracheobronchial/tracheopathia osteochondroplastica, distinguished, 29

Macule, coal, in coal worker's pneumoconiosis, 615
Malaise, associated with
  AIDS, 459
  eosinophilic granuloma, 574
  methotrexate toxicity, 109
Malformation
  bronchopulmonary foregut, 6–7
  orbital, in peripheral neurofibromatosis, 90
  pulmonary arteriovenous, 387, 389, **397–98**
    differential diagnosis
      carcinoid tumor, 387, 388–89, **394–95**
      Hodgkin lymphoma, 387, 388, **396–97**
      metastatic carcinoma, 387, 388
      primary tuberculosis, 387, 388
  systemic arteriovenous, 397
Measles, and adenopathy, 277
Mediastinal adenopathy. *See* Adenopathy, hilar/mediastinal
Mediastinal air, 287, **288**, 290, **291–93**
  differential diagnosis
    pulmonary artery air, 287–88
Mediastinal carcinoma, 356

Microlithiasis (continued)
    metastatic pulmonary calcifica-
      tion, 545, **553–60**
  chronic, 595
    alveolar pattern in, 67, **72**
Micropolyspora faeni farmer's lung, 570
Miliary disease, with atypical myco-
    bacterial infection, in AIDS pa-
    tient, 458
Milk-alkali syndrome, and metastatic pul-
    monary calcification, 553
Mineral oil pneumonia, 67
Mitral insufficiency, 581, 583
  differential diagnosis
    pulmonary veno-occlusive disease,
    581, **583**, **585–88**
Mitral stenosis. *See under* Stenosis
Mitral valve disease
  complication of atrial septal defect, 432
  sickle cell disease and, 519
Mononucleosis, and adenopathy, 277
Mononucleosis-like infection, with AIDS,
    459
Mounier-Kuhn syndrome (tracheobron-
    chomegaly), 21, **31–33**, 337, 343,
    354
  differential diagnosis
    hypogammaglobulinemia, 21, **23**
    Kartagener syndrome, 21, **23–26**
    polychondritis, chronic relapsing, **21–
    23**, 29
    postintubation tracheal stenosis,
      337–40, 351–53
    tracheopathia osteochondroplastica,
      21, **29**
Mucinous adenocarcinoma, of stomach. *See*
    Stomach, mucinous adenocar-
    cinoma of
Mucoepidermoid carcinoma, 395
Mucoid impaction
  in allergic bronchopulmonary aspergil-
    losis, 62, 63
  in cystic fibrosis, 515, 516
Mucor, alveolar proteinosis secondary in-
    fection, 466
Mucous
  plug
    allergic bronchopulmonary aspergil-
      losis, 62
    centriacinar emphysema, 331
    cystic fibrosis, 565
    radiation pneumonitis, 202
  thickening, in rhinoscleroma, 355

Multiparity, amniotic fluid embolization
    due to, 299
Multiple sclerosis, and paralyzed dia-
    phragm, 530
Murmur
  "mill wheel," venous air embolization
    causing, 297
  systolic
    atrial septal defect, 431
    ventricular septal defect, 432
Muscle weakness, generalized, and res-
    piratory failure, in polymyositis,
    247
Muscular prowess increase attempt, by
    intravenous metallic mercury,
    300
Myalgia, with AIDS, 459
Myasthenia gravis, 441, **447–48**
Mycetoma (fungus ball), 60
  ankylosing spondylitis, 57, 64
  aspergillosis, 62
  collagen vascular disease, 57, 64
  semi-invasive aspergillosis, 62–63
Mycobacteria, granulomatous infection
    cause, 60
Mycobacterial infection, atypical, 57, **60**,
    455, **457–58**, **465**
  differential diagnosis
    alveolar proteinosis, pulmonary, 455,
      458, **466**
    collagen vascular disease, 57, 64
    edema, pulmonary, due to heroin
      abuse, 455, **458**
    Pneumocystis carinii pneumonia,
      with AIDS, 455, **458–64**
Mycobacterium avium-intracellulare in-
    fection, and AIDS, 459, 462, 465
Mycobacterium kansasii
  infection, immunocompromised host,
    465
Mycobacterium tuberculosis empyema, 145
Mycoplasma pneumonia, 277
Mycotic infections, noncaseating granulo-
    mas in, 423
Myelitis, transverse or ascending, and
    paralyzed diaphragm, 530
Myeloma, multiple
  bone destruction effects, and metastatic
    pulmonary calcification, 553
  plasma cell granuloma and, 502
Myocardial depression, amiodarone tox-
    icity causing, 236
Myocardial dilatation/hypertrophy, in
    sickle cell disease, 519

Oligemia *(continued)*
    pulmonary periphery, in primary pulrmonary arterial hypertension, 422
    pulmonary thromboembolism and, 429
"Ondine's curse," and paralyzed diaphragm, 530
Opacities/opacification
    adult respiratory distress syndrome, 319, 321
    alveolar microlithiasis, 546
    alveolar proteinosis, 74, 78, 466
    amiodarone-induced, 235–38
    asbestosis, 61, 564
    bacterial pneumonia, 278
    candidiasis, 211
    coal worker's pneumoconiosis, 616, 618–19
    cystic fibrosis, 516
    fat embolism syndrome, 300
    lower lobe atelectasis, 168, 170–71
    lupus pneumonitis, 244, 518
    mediastinal, pulmonary sling and, 475
    metastatic pulmonary calcification, 545, 559
    methadone-induced, 253–54
    nitrofurantoin-induced pneumonitis, 251
    of hemithorax
        diaphragmatic rupture and, 534
        hepatic hydrothorax and, 401
        malignant mesothelioma, 222
        postpneumonectomy and, 119, 121
    Pneumocystis carinii pneumonia, 455
    polymyositis, 247
    pulmonary edema due to heroin abuse, 458
    pulmonary veno-occlusive disease, 587
    radiotherapy-induced, **181–94**, 199, **201–1**
    reticular/reticulonodular/patchy, with lymphocytic interstitial pneumonia, and AIDS, 463–64
    reticulonodular perihilar, with *Pneumocystis carinii* pneumonia, and AIDS, 455, 459
    sickle cell disease, 519, 520
    siderosis, 609, 615, 623
    silicosis, 61, 615, 616
    sinus opacification, in rhinoscleroma, 355
    sulfonamide-induced, 253
    Wegener's granulomatosis, 491

Orbital malformation, in peripheral neurofibromatosis, 90
Ornithosis, and adenopathy, 277
Orthopedic procedures, fat embolism syndrome cause, 300
Ossification, idiopathic pulmonary, 545–46, **552**
    differential diagnosis
        metastatic pulmonary calcification, 545, **553–60**
Osteoarthropathy, hypertrophic, associated with
    arteriovenous malformation, 397
    benign mesothelioma, 402
    localized fibrous mesothelioma, 594, **595–96**
Osteochondroplastica, tracheopathia. *See* Tracheopathia osteochondroplastica
Osteomyelitis
    bone destruction effects, and metastatic pulmonary calcification, 553
    in blastomycosis, 261
    sternal, 211
        after median sternotomy, 376–77
Osteoradionecrosis, radiotherapy-induced, 201
Ostium primum, atrial septal defect, 430
Ostium secundum, atrial septal defect, 430
Otitis media, recurrent, in immotile cilia syndrome, 26
Ovarian fibroma, in Meigs' syndrome, 403

Palpitations, in intrathoracic pheochromocytoma, 84
Pancreatic insufficiency, and cystic fibrosis, 515–16
Pancreatic pseudocyst, as non-neurogenic mass, 94
Pancreatitis, postoperative effusion due to, 379
Papillomatosis
    laryngotracheal, 337, **342–43**
        childhood vs. adult form, 354–55
        differential diagnosis
            postintubation tracheal stenosis, 337–40, 351–53
        tracheobronchial, and tracheopathia osteochondroplastica, distinguished, 29
Paradoxical embolism, 300
Paraganglioma, 91, 92, 94
Paralysis, of hemidiaphragm. *See under* Hemidiaphragm

Pneumonomediastinum. *See* Mediastinal air

Pneumoperitoneum, following ventilator-induced barotrauma, 293

Pneumoretroperitoneum, result of ventilator-induced barotrauma, 293

Pneumothorax
and ventilator-induced barotrauma, 290–91
bilateral, **151–54**, 155, **160–61**
differential diagnosis
giant bullous cysts, 151, **154–55**, **157–63**, 166
complication of cystic fibrosis, 516
diaphragmatic paralysis due to, 530
following pneumomediastinum, 293
in ankylosing spondylitis, 64
in bronchopleural fistula, 124
in bullous disease, 160
in pulmonary eosinophilic granuloma, 568, 574, 576
interstitial edema progressing to, 290–91
pneumatocele simulation, in pneumonia, 278
pulmonary edema after, 325–26
radiotherapy-induced, 200
re-expansion of lung after, 324
subpulmonic, air cyst mimicking, 291
trauma, blunt or penetrating, causing, 290

Polychondritis, chronic relapsing, **21–23**, 29, 343
differential diagnosis
Mounier-Kuhn syndrome, 21, **31–33**

Polymyositis
/dermatomyositis, 241, **246–49**
vs. eosinophilic granuloma, 563

Polyposis, nasal, in immotile cilia syndrome, 26

Positive end-expiratory pressure (PEEP), 307
in adult respiratory distress syndrome, 322–23

Positive pressure therapy, pneumothorax and, 290–91

Postmyocardial infarction (Dressler's) syndrome, pleural effusion due to, 384

Postpartum pleural effusion, 378

Postpericardiotomy syndrome, 378, **382–84**
differential diagnoses, 384

Prednisone, treatment for methotrexate toxicity, 108, **109**

Pregnancy, azygos vein dilatation and, 414

Procainamide, antinuclear antibodies due to, 246

Prominent venous confluence, 35, **40–41**, **43**

Protease/antiprotease imbalance, in emphysema, 173

Proteinosis, pulmonary alveolar, 67, **74**, **77–78**, 455, 458, **466**
differential diagnosis
atypical mycobacterial infection, 455, **457–58**, **464**
bronchioloalveolar cell carcinoma, 67–68
chronic eosinophilic pneumonia, 455–57
edema, pulmonary, due to heroin abuse, 455, **458**
hydrostatic pulmonary edema, 67, **69**, 73, 75
Pneumocystis carinii pneumonia, with AIDS, 455, **458–64**
primary pulmonary lymphoma, 67, **69**, **72–73**
pulmonary hemorrhage, 67, **69**, **71**, **75–77**
silicosis and, 62

Pseudoaneurysm formation, and mediastinitis, 4

Pseudocyst, pancreatic, 94

Pseudomonas aeruginosa
aerobic gram-negative pneumonia, 277, **279**, **280–83**
bronchopneumonia, 516
cystic fibrosis, 516

Pseudotumor
atelectatic (*see* Atelectasis, rounded)
inflammatory
differential diagnosis
fibrous mesothelioma, localized, 591, 592, **594–97**
see also Granuloma, plasma cell
pleural asbestotic (*see* Atelectasis, rounded)
pleural (fluid), 591, **593**
differential diagnosis
fibrous mesothelioma, localized, 591, 592, **594–97**

Pulmonary artery
anomalous left (*see* Pulmonary sling)
atrophy, radiotherapy-induced, 200–1

Renal failure *(continued)*
  peritoneal dialysis for, and hepatic hydrothorax, 404
  pulmonary edema, in lupus erythematosus, due to, 244
Renal transplant patient, Legionnaires' disease in, 265
Rendu-Osler-Weber syndrome, and arteriovenous malformation, 397
Respiratory disease, in alveolar proteinosis, 77
Respiratory distress. *See* Dyspnea
Respiratory distress syndrome, adult, 313, 316, **319–24**
  differential diagnosis
    emphysema with pulmonary edema, 312, **313–14**, **328**, **331–33**
    fat embolism syndrome causing, 297, **300**
  table of associated diseases, 319, **320**
  table of synonyms, 319, **320**
  v. *Pneumocystis carinii* pneumonia, 455
  see also Dyspnea
Respiratory equipment, aerosol pneumonia spread, 279–80
Respiratory failure, due to
  diaphragmatic weakness, in polymyositis, 247
  radiation fibrosis, 202
  tracheal tumor, malignant, 480
  Wegener's granulomatosis, 492
Respiratory infection, recurrent
  bronchogenic mediastinal cyst and, 8
  in immotile cilia syndrome, 24, 26
Respiratory insufficiency, chronic, pneumonectomy and, 142–43
Respiratory mechanism, impaired, in ankylosing spondylitis, 63–64
Respiratory syncytial virus, Swyer-James syndrome, 166
Restrictive disease, pulmonary, diaphragmatic fatigue due to, 530
Retrovirus (HTLV-III), and AIDS, **458–59**, 463
Rheumatoid arthritis vs. eosinophilic granuloma, 563
Rheumatoid lung, 235, **241–42**
  differential diagnosis
    amiodarone toxicity, 235, **236–40**
Rhinoscleroma, 354, **355**
Rib abnormalities/involvement
  eosinophilic granuloma, 568, 574
  lateral meningocele, 93
  leukemia, 102

Rib *(continued)*
  localized fibrous mesothelioma, 596
  malignant mesothelioma, 221
  neuroblastoma, 93
  parenchymal lung disease, 568
  peripheral neurofibromatosis, 90
Ring-sling complex, 475

Sacroiliac joint, arthropathy, in ankylosing spondylitis, 63
Salivary gland
  and adenoid cystic carcinoma, 476, 480
  and tracheal neoplasm, 480
Salivation. *See* Hypersalivation
Sansert. *See* Methysergide
Sarcoidosis, 57, 277, 417, 418, **423–25**
  alveolar, 67, **72–73**
  chronic pulmonary, and fibrobullous/cystic disease, 60
  differential diagnosis
    adenopathy/parenchymal disease, 277
    collagen vascular disease, 57, 64
    pulmonary arterial hypertension, 417–18, **421–22**
  hilar adenopathy of, 35, **37**
  /Hodgkin lymphoma, differentiated, 396
  metastatic pulmonary calcification and, 553
  noncavitary, and semi-invasive pulmonary aspergillosis, 63
  /pulmonary eosinophilic granuloma, distinguished, 577
  radiographic staging, 424–25
Schistosomiasis, pulmonary arterial hypertension due to, 422
Schwannoma (neurilemmoma)
  and central neurofibromatosis, 88
  benign, 86, **87**, **91–92**, 93
    /neurofibroma, distinguished, 91
  malignant, 91
  /meningocele differentiation, 15
Scleroderma
  pulmonary fibrosis in, 241, **246**
  vs. eosinophilic granuloma, 563
Sclerosing mediastinitis. *See under* Mediastinitis
Sclerosis, multiple. *See* Multiple sclerosis
Scoliosis
  in lateral meningocele, 93
  in neurofibromatosis, 88
  in peripheral neurofibromatosis, 90
  neurenteric cyst and, 84

Spinal canal (continued)
posterior mediastinal neurofibroma and, 83
Spinal cord, anomaly, and neurenteric cyst, 84
Spinal ligament ossification, in ankylosing spondylitis, 63
Spine
destruction
in neuroblastoma, 93
thoracic, anomalies
in ankylosing spondylitis, 57, 63
Spleen
calcification, in sickle cell disease, 511, 512
dense, in rheumatoid arthritis, 240
Splenosis, due to ruptured hemidiaphragm, 537
Split-pleura sign, in empyema, 369
Spondylitis, ankylosing, 57, 60, **63–64**
Sputum
blood-streaked
blastomycosis, 261
cystic fibrosis, 515, **516**
production
alpha-1-antitrypsin deficiency, 316
eosinophilic granuloma, 574
purulent
Legionnaires' disease, 262
or increasing, due to infected bullae, 492–93
pneumococcal pneumonia, 262
Squamous cell carcinoma. See under Carcinoma
Stannosis, 609
differential diagnosis
siderosis, 609, **614–15, 623–24**
Staphylococci alveolar proteinosis, 78
Staphylococcus aureus
bronchopneumonia, 278–79, 516
cystic fibrosis, 516
empyema, 145
postpneumonectomy, 128
pneumonia, and leukemia, 101
Stenosis
aortic valvular, and double aortic arch, 477
carotid/subclavian artery, radiotherapy-induced, 201
esophageal
radiotherapy-induced, 201
infundibular pulmonic/valvular stenosis, distinguished, 420

Stenosis (continued)
mitral
/idiopathic pulmonary ossification, distinguished, 552
mimicked by left atrial myxoma, 584
pulmonic valvular, 417, 418–19, **420–21**
differential diagnosis
pulmonary arterial hypertension, 417–18, **421–22**
secondary to chronic pulmonary emboli, 436
transglottic, in rhinoscleroma, 355
Stenosis, tracheal
adenoid cystic carcinoma causing, 481
postintubation, 337–40, 351–53
differential diagnosis
laryngotracheal papillomatosis, 337, **342–43, 354–55**
Mounier-Kuhn syndrome, 337, 343, **354**
saber-sheath trachea, 337, 342, 354, **355**
tracheoesophageal fistula, 337, 343, **356–59**
pulmonary sling and, 475
thoracic amyloidosis and, 106
Sterility, male, in immotile cilia syndrome, 26
Sternotomy, median, complications following, 375–78
Sternum
dehiscence, postoperative, 375, **377–78**
osteomyelitis of, 211, 376–77
Steroid therapy, and semi-invasive pulmonary aspergillosis, 63
Stevens-Johnson syndrome, sulfonamide-induced, 253
Stomach, mucinous adenocarcinoma of, 545, **547**
differential diagnosis
metastatic pulmonary calcification, 545, **553–60**
Streptococcus pneumoniae
bronchopneumonia, 263
empyema, 145
pneumococcal pneumonia, 262, 263, 519
Stridor, associated with
double aortic arch, 477
malignant tracheal tumor, 480
Stroke, due to pulmonary arteriovenous malformation embolization, 397
Subcarinal adenopathy. See under Adenopathy

Subclavian artery
    right or left aberrant, and aortic diverticulum, 410
    stenosis, radiation-induced, 201
Suicide gesture
    ingestion of mercury, 301
    injection of mercury, 300
Sulfamethoxazole. *See* Trimethoprim/sulfamethoxazole
Sulfonamide-induced diseases, 251, **253**
Superior vena cava. *See* Vena cava, superior
Swallowing disorder. *See* Dysphagia
Swan-Ganz catheter, technique, 306–7
Sweats, associated with
    AIDS, 459
    eosinophilic pneumonia, chronic, 455
Swyer-James syndrome, 151, **154**, **166**, 313, **315–16**, 328, 331, **333**
    differential diagnosis
        cysts, giant bullous, 151, **154–55**, **157–63**, 166
        emphysema with pulmonary edema, 312, **313–14**, **328**, **331–33**
Syncope, and dyspnea, in pulmonary veno-occlusive disease, 585
Synovial joint of spine, in ankylosing spondylitis, 63
Syphilis, bronchoesophageal fistula cause, 143
Systemic lupus erythematosus. *See* Lupus erythematosus, systemic

Tachycardia
    in Legionnaires' disease, 262
    in pneumococcal pneumonia, 262
    venous air embolization causing, 297
Tachypnea
    in adult respiratory distress syndrome, 319
    in methotrexate toxicity, 109
    venous air embolization causing, 297
Tamponade, cardiac, associated with
    coronary bypass surgery, 375
    CVP catheter positioning, 306
    pericardial effusion, in postpericardiotomy syndrome, 384
Taste, metallic, chronic mercurialism causing, 301
Telangiectasia, hereditary hermorrhagic, and arteriovenous malformation, 397
Teratoma, 3
    differential diagnosis
        bronchogenic cyst, 3, **5–19**

Teratoma *(continued)*
    mediastinal, calcification in, 18
Tethering, spinal cord, and neurenteric cyst, 84
Tetralogy of Fallot. *See* Fallot trilogy
Thalassemia, extramedullary hematopoiesis and, 83
Therapy
    immunosuppressive, and invasive secondary pulmonary aspergillosis, 62, 63
    steroid, and semi-invasive pulmonary aspergillosis, 63
Thermoactinomyces vulgaris farmer's lung, 570
Thoracic disease processes, abdominal involvement in, 215–18
Thoracotomy, fluid collection following, 362, **363–84**
Thorax
    deformity, in cystic fibrosis, 565
    see also Hemithorax
Thromboembolism
    pulmonary, 429, **434–36**
        differential diagnosis
            acute myocardial infarction, 429
            atrial septal defect, 429, **430–32**, **433**
            chronic congestive heart failure, 429–30
            ventricular septal defect, 429, **432–33**
        in Hughes-Stovin syndrome, 419
        pulmonary arterial hypertension due to, 421
    venous
        amniotic fluid embolization and, 300
        fat embolism syndrome and, 297
    see also Embolism
Thrombosis
    peripheral veins/dural sinuses, in Hughes-Stovin syndrome, 419
    pulmonary artery
        due to wedging, 306–7
        vascular occlusion, in sickle cell disease, and, 519
Thrombus/myxoma, distinguished, 584–85
Thymolipoma, 441, **448–49**
    differential diagnosis
        anterior mediastinal thymoma, 441, 447–48, **449–50**

Veno-occlusive disease *(continued)*
    mitral insufficiency, 581, 583
    sclerosing mediastinitis, 581, 583
Venous air embolism, 286, **287–88**, **297–300**
Venous arterialization, in pulmonary veno-occlusive disease, 586
Venous stasis, chronic, and idiopathic pulmonary ossification, 552
Ventilator-induced barotrauma, 287–88, **290–93**
Ventricular arrhythmia
    amiodarone treatment for, 236
    CVP catheter positioning causing, 306
    in digitalis toxicity, 236
Ventricular dysfunction, radiotherapy-induced, 199
Ventricular failure, complication of
    alveolar proteinosis, 78
    atrial septal defect, 432
Ventricular filling pressure, elevated left, and pulmonary arterial hypertension, 421–22
Ventricular premature beats, in digitalis toxicity, 236
Ventricular septal defect, 429, **432–33**
    differential diagnosis
        pulmonary thromboembolism, 429, **434–36**
Vertebral anomaly
    ankylosing spondylitis and, 63
    neurenteric cyst and, 12, 83, **84**
Vertebral body, mid-thorax, end-plate deformity of, in sickle cell disease, 511
Vincristine
    neural toxicity, in leukemia, 108, **111**
    potentiates radiotherapy effects, 202

Viral infection
    in alveolar proteinosis, 78
    see also name of virus
Visual disturbances, in digitalis toxicity, 236
Vitamin D poisoning, and metastatic pulmonary calcification, 553
Vocal cord
    papillomas, in laryngotracheal papillomatosis, 342
    paralysis, in tracheal stenosis, 352
Vomiting, in digitalis toxicity, 236

Web, associated with chronic pulmonary emboli, 434, **436**
Wedging/wedge pressure, Swan-Ganz catheter and, 306–7
Wegener's granulomatosis. *See under* Granulomatosis
Weight loss, associated with
    chronic eosinophilic pneumonia, 455
    eosinophilic granuloma, 574
Wheezing, associated with
    allergic bronchopulmonary aspergillosis, 570
    asthma, 332
    bronchogenic cyst, 8
    chronic bronchitis, 332
    congestive heart failure, 332
    eosinophilic granuloma, 574
    foreign body aspiration, 332
    postintubation tracheal stenosis, 353
    pulmonary embolism, 332
    venous air embolization, 297
Whooping cough, and adenopathy, 277
Wound infection
    deep, and sternal dehiscence after median sternotomy, 377–78
    local, intra-aortic counter-pulsation balloon causing, 308–9